CHILDES/BIB

An annotated bibliography of child language and language disorders

1994 Supplement

Roy Higginson
Center for Research in Language
University of California
San Diego

Brian MacWhinney
Carnegie Mellon University

LAWRENCE ERLBAUM ASSOCIATES, PUBLISHERS
1994 Hillsdale, New Jersey Hove and London

Lawrence Erlbaum Associates, Inc., Publishers
365 Broadway
Hillsdale, New Jersey 07642

Library of Congress Cataloging-in-Publication Data

Higginson, Roy.
CHILDES/BIB : an annotated bibliography of child language and language disorders : 1994 supplement / [compiled by] Roy Higginson, Brian MacWhinney.
p. cm.
"The supplement covers North American research since late 1990 and international research published outside North America since 1970. It also includes a few North American items published prior to 1990 that were omitted from the earlier work"--Pref.
ISBN 0-8058-1478-7
1. Children--Language--Bibliography. 2. Language acquisition--Bibliography. 3. Language disorders--Bibliography.
I. MacWhinney, Brian. II. Title.
Z5814.C5H54 1991 Suppl.
[LB1139.L3]
016.1554'136--dc20 93-34993
CIP

Books published by Lawrence Erlbaum Associates are printed on acid-free paper, and their bindings are chosen for strength and durability.

Printed in the United States of America

10 9 8 7 6 5 4 3 2 1

Dedicated to Allen Gilbert

ACKNOWLEDGMENTS

The compilers wish to acknowledge their gratitude to Ragnhild Soederbergh and Barbara Gelbart for their permission to include the references from the 1990 *Stockholm bibliography of child language* in the present book, and their contributions to the 1991 book. Thanks are also due to Dan Slobin and Adele Abrahamsen for their generous contributions to the 1991 book, which helped to make *CHILDES/BIB* so comprehensive. We would also like to repeat our previous acknowledgment of Werner Leopold's bibliographic work.

For the present volume, we are not only indebted to the above people, but also to those colleagues from all around the world who responded to the 1990 call for the submission of bibliographies. Their response was so great that regrettably we will not be able to acknowledge each of them individually, and hope that as a group they will accept our gratitude. Many of these individuals were kind enough to send us abstracts of their publications; their kindness in providing this extra information is acknowledged by appending their initials to their abstracts.

Since the publication of the first volume of *CHILDES/BIB* in 1991, the electronic underpinning of the database has been changed twice. The first change was based upon a program specially created for *CHILDES/BIB* by Leonid Spektor of Carnegie Mellon University, to whom we are also grateful for advice and help with the various computer problems that struck during the last two years. The second change was the adoption of *Endnote* as the database program, and we are grateful to Niles and Associates for extending to us a licensed version of their program for distribution with the electronic version.

Thanks are also due to Bev Arthur who spent many long hours entering the international bibliographies into the database, and to Smokey McKinley and Erik Johansen who did an excellent job of checking the incoming bibliographies against the existing database to avoid unnecessary duplications. *Endnote* was used in conjunction with *WordPerfect* to produce the text version of *CHILDES/BIB*, and we would like to thank Martin Arthur of Atelier 88 for help and advice regarding *WordPerfect*.

Funding for the research assistants and the hardware and software needs of the project was provided by *CHILDES* at Carnegie Mellon University. The Regents of the University of California extended professional support, and e-mail access to the project.

Finally, the compilers wish to once again acknowledge the Society for Research in Child Development for its permission to include materials from *Child Development Abstracts* in the database, and the Linguistic Society of America for its permission to include materials previously published in *Language*.

PREFACE

In 1990, after the Budapest Congress, a request was sent out to members of the International Association for the Study of Child Language asking them to submit their personal bibliographies for inclusion in the *CHILDES/BIB* database. The request was sent to all "non-North-American" members and the response was great. During the past two years the bibliographies we received have been assembled into the database together with current journal articles and books. The result is this supplement, which adds 3,000 new references to the original work, and brings the total number of references in *CHILDES/BIB* to 10,400. Approximately 33% of the new references are drawn from the bibliographies of "non-North-American" scholars, 6% are drawn from *Child Development Abstracts**, and *Language†*, and 1% from the *Stockholm bibliography of child language,‡* (1990). All of the abstracts include keyword annotations, and 38% have additional abstracts.

In the organization of this supplement we have tried to give regard to the comments of the reviewers of our earlier work. The supplement includes in the printed version, the keywords used in the electronic version, and indicates the language the text is written in if the text language is not English. The keywords appear at the end of each citation, prior to the abstract (if one is available). The text language appears after the ":" symbol in the keywords listing. The absence of any notation for English texts is neither meant to bestow any special status upon English, nor to convey any lack of respect for other languages; it merely reflects the fact that this is an English language publication. As in the earlier work, the references are arranged alphabetically by the name of the first author, and an extensive index provides access to them through the keywords used in the electronic version.

The supplement covers North American research since late 1990 and international research published outside North America since 1970. It also includes a few North American items published prior to 1990 that were omitted from the earlier work. At the time of publication, *CHILDES/BIB* betokens the state of child language and language disorders research worldwide, and we believe it to be the most comprehensive access to the literature currently available to researchers in acquisition related fields.

* *Child Development Abstracts*, published three times a year by the University of Chicago Press for the Society for Research in Child Development.

† *Language* published four times a year by the Linguistic Society of America

‡ Gelbart, Barbara and Soederbergh, Ragnhild (Eds). *Bibliography of child language.* Published annually by the Child Language Institute, Stockholm University.

CONTENTS

A

Abbeduto, Leonard, Nuccio, J. B., Almabuk, R., & Rotto, P., et al. (1992). Interpreting and responding to spoken language: children's recognition and use of a speaker's goal. *Journal of Child Language*, 19, 677-693. COMPREHENSION COMMUNICATIVE COMPETENCE:

Abkarian, G. G., Jones, A., & West, G. (1992). Young children's idiom comprehension: trying to get the picture. *Journal of Speech and Hearing Research*, 35, 580-587. FIGURATIVE LANGUAGE:

Abunuwara, E. (1993). The structure of the trilingual lexicon. In A. M. B. de Groot, & C. Barry (Eds), *The multilingual community*. Hillsdale, NJ: Lawrence Erlbaum Associates. BILINGUALISM-LEXICAL DEVELOPMENT BILINGUALISM-SEMANTIC DEVELOPMENT:

Ackerman, Brian P., & Glickman, Ilene. (1989). Place and action in children's representations of stories. *Journal of Experimental Psychology*, 48, 246-269. NARRATIVES TEXT/STORY GRAMMARS EVENTS/SCRIPTS:

Place inconsistency is more important than action inconsistency in children's judgements of story adequacy, except when the action involves the story theme. Developmental differences in story judgements generally were larger for inconsistent actions than for inconsistent places.

Ackerman, Brian P., & Jackson, Megan. (1991). When is a guess a guess: Children's sensitivity to inference constraint in assessing understanding of story information. *Journal of Experimental Child Psychology*, 52, 117-146. NARRATIVES IMPLICATURE CAUSALITY:

Four experiments determined if second and fourth grade children and college students are sensitive to inference constraint both in making causal inferences and in assessing understanding of a story. The results were that both inference likelihood and understanding ratings varied with constraint for all grades. Findings included the competence of second graders in assessing understanding, marked differences with grade in dealing with uncertainty, and contrasting patterns of performance for the children in evaluating understanding and story adequacy. From Child Development Abstracts.

Ackerman, Brian P., & McGraw, Megan. (1991). Constraints on the causal inferences of children and adults in comprehending stories. *Journal of Experimental Child Psychology*, 51, 364-394. NARRATIVES CAUSALITY IMPLICATURE:

Second, fifth, and college grade students listened to stories with an early stated goal, and an end result inconsistent with the goal statement. The results showed consistent encoding x retrieval interactions, with inferences reflecting weak encoding constraint varying with retrieval support, and the effect decreases with grade. From Child Development Abstracts.

Acredolo, Linda, & Goodwyn, Susan W. (1991). Sign language in babies: the significance of symbolic gesturing for understanding language development. In R. Vasta (Ed.), *Annals of Child Development*. Greenwich, CT: JAB Press. SIGNING:

Adamik-Jaszó, Anna. (1976). Megjegyzések a kiejtés tanitásához. (Remarks on teaching enunciation.). *Magyar Nyelvör*, 100, 316-319. ARTICULATION: HUNGARIAN

Adamik-Jaszó, Anna. (1979). Tanitóképzös hallgatók kiejtésének vizsgálata. (An analysis of the pronounciation of college students.). *A Budapesti Tanitóképzö Föiskola Kiadványai*, 4, 80-85. ARTICULATION: HUNGARIAN

Adamik-Jaszó, Anna. (1982). Föiskolai hallgatók kiejtésének vizsgálata. (An analysis of the pronounciation of high-school students.). *Magyar Nyelvör*, 106, 73-97. ARTICULATION: HUNGARIAN

Adamik-Jaszó, Anna. (1982). Irányzatok a XIX. század végi olvastanításban. (Trends in teaching reading at the end of the

19th century.). *Pedagógiai Szemle*, 32, 20-32,119-130. LITERACY: HUNGARIAN

Adamik-Jaszó, Anna. (1983). Beszéd- és értelemgyakorlatok az óvodában a XIX. század végén. (Exercises for developing speech and understanding in the preschool at the end of the 19th century.). *Pedagógiai Szemle*, 38(7-8), 668-674. OVERVIEW-GENERAL LANGUAGE AND EDUCATION: HUNGARIAN

Adamik-Jaszó, Anna. (1990). Az anyanyelvi tárgyak tanítása a magyar népiskolában 1868-tól 1905-ig. (Teaching language arts in the Hungarian elementary schools between 1865-1905.). *A Budapesti Tanítóképzö Föiskola Tudományos Közleményei.*, 8, 345. LANGUAGE AND EDUCATION: HUNGARIAN

Adamik-Jaszó, Anna. (1990). Speech and thought developing exercises (STD) in Hungarian education. *Education Today*, 40(2), 32-36. LANGUAGE AND EDUCATION:

Adamson, Hugh D. (1989). *Variation theory and second language acquisition*. Washington, DC: Georgetown University Press. L2 VARIATION:

Reviewed by Coppieters in Language 66(1).

Adamson, L. B. (1992). Variations in the early use of language. In L. T. Winegar, & J. Valsiner (Eds), *Children's development within social context, (Vol. 1)*. Hillsdale, NJ: Lawrence Erlbaum Associates. INDIVIDUAL VARIATION:

Adrien, J. L., Barthelemy, C., Perrot, A., & Roux, S., et al. (1992). Validity and reliability of the Infant Behavioral Summarized Evaluation (IBSE)-a rating scale for the assessment of young children with autism and developmental disorders. *Journal of Autism and Developmental Disorders*, 22, 375-394. CLASSIFICATION OF DISORDERS AUTISM DEVELOPMENTAL DISORDERS INFANT BEHAVIOR SUMMARIZED EVALUATION:

Adrien, J. L., Faure, M., Perrot, A., Hameury, L., Garreau, B., Barthelemy, C., & Sauvage, D. (1991). Autism and family home movies: Preliminary findings. *Journal of Autism and Developmental Disorders*, 21, 43-49. AUTISM:

Analyses of home movies taken by parents before the recognition of autistic disorders of their own child confirm the major value of this method for describing early signs: anomolies of eye contact, deficient variability of emotional expression, defect of attention, initiation of communication, motor abnormalities etc.

Akamatsu, C. T., & Fischer, Susan D. (1991). Using immediate recall to assess language proficiency in deaf students. *American Annals of the Deaf*, 136, 428-434. LANGUAGE AND MEMORY DEAF CHILDREN:

Akhtar, Nameera, Dunham, Frances, & Dunham, Philip J. (1991). Directive interactions and early vocabulary development: the role of joint attentional focus. *Journal of Child Language*, 18, 41-49. SOCIAL INTERACTION ATTENTION JOINT REFERENCE ADULT-CHILD INTERACTION:

Mothers were videotaped interacting with their children and 100 maternal utterances were coded for pragmatic intent. Prescriptives were coded as either changing (leading) or following the child's focus of attention. Only the frequency of mothers' follow-prescriptives correlated significantly with a productive vocabulary measure.

Akiyama, M. Michael. (1992). Cross-linguistic contrasts of verification and answering among children. *Journal of Psycholinguistic Research*, 21, 67-85. CROSSLINGUISTIC STUDY-DISCOURSE CHILDREN'S DISCOURSE:

Alahuhta, Eila. (1976). Afaattisen lapsen terapian suunnittelusta primaarioreita kartioittavan tutkimuksen perusteella. (Planning the therapy of an aphasic child on the basis of investigation recording the primary symptoms.). *Publications of the Department of Phonetics (University of Helsinki)*, 29, FINNISH APHASIAS INTERVENTION PROGRAMS: FINNISH

Alahuhta, Eila. (1976). CP-lapsen kielellisten hairioiden taustaoireista ja niiden kuntoutuksesta. (On the underlying symptoms of the linguistic defects of CP children and their rehabilitation.). *CP-lehti*, 2, FINNISH CEREBRAL PALSY: FINNISH

Alahuhta, Eila. (1976). Esikouluikaisten kuntoutusta ja valmennusta Ranskassa. (Rehabilitation and training of pre-school age children in France.). *CP-lehti*, 4, INTERVENTION PROGRAMS FRENCH: FINNISH

Alahuhta, Eila. (1976). On the defects of perception, reasoning and spatial orientation ability in linguistically handicapped children (abstract in Swedish). *Membership Periodical of the Association of Clinic Education*, 3, FINNISH LANGUAGE AND COGNITIVE DEVELOPMENT:

Alahuhta, Eila. (1976). Onko piileva lukemis- ja kirjoittamishairioisyys koulujen tyorauhaongelmien yksi syy. (Are the undetected defects of reading and writing one of the causes behind the problem of disturbances in the classroom.). *Opettaja*, 23, FINNISH READING DISORDERS LANGUAGE AND EDUCATION: FINNISH

Alahuhta, Eila. (1976). Puhumisen, lukenisen ja kirjoittamisen hairioiden yhteidet primaarit oireet tri R. Hussonin kuvaaman aivotoiminnallisen mekanismin valossa. (Primary symptoms common to defects of speech, reading and writing, in the light of the cerebral function model described by Dr. R. Husson.) *Publications of the Department of Phonetics, University of Helsinki*. LANGUAGE DISORDERS FINNISH READING DISORDERS LITERACY: FINNISH

Alahuhta, Eila. (1976). Sur les déficienses dans la perception, le raisonnement et l'orientation spatiale chez les enfants linguistiquement handicapes. (On the defects of perception, reasoning and spatial orientation ability in linguistically handicapped children.). *Rééducation Orthophonique*, 14 (90), LANGUAGE AND COGNITIVE DEVELOPMENT: FRENCH

Alahuhta, Eila. (1977). Gemensamma primarysympton for storingar i tal-, las- och skrivfunktionerna i belysning ac R- Hussons beskrivning av den cerebrala mekanismen. (Primary symptoms common to defects of speech, reading and writing in the light of the cerebral function model described by Dr. R. Husson.). *Faculty of Education, Abo Akademi*, 4, READING DISORDERS FINNISH LITERACY LANGUAGE DISORDERS NEUROLINGUISTICS: SWEDISH

Alahuhta, Eila. (1977). Kielellisten hairioiden yhteisista taustatekijoista ja kantouttamismahdollisuuksista. (On the underlying causes common to linguistic defects and their prospects of rehabilitation.). *Sellista*, 4, FINNISH LANGUAGE AND COGNITIVE DEVELOPMENT INTERVENTION PROGRAMS LANGUAGE PRECURSORS: FINNISH

Alahuhta, Eila. (1978). BM-testi, Suzanne Borel-Maisonnyn nonverbaalinen testi alyllisen kehitystason ja kielellisen kehityksen edellytyksena olevan perusvalmiuden kartoittamiseksi. (The BM test, a non-verbal test by Suzanne Borel-Maisonny to determine intellectual development level and the basic capacities required for proper linguistic development.). *Publications of the Institute for Educational Research*, 291, FINNISH LANGUAGE AND COGNITIVE DEVELOPMENT ASSESSMENT PROCEDURES: FINNISH

Alahuhta, Eila. (1978). BMA-testi. Testi puhe-, lukemis- ja kirjoittamishairioiden primaarioireiden kartoittamiseksi. Eila Aluhuhdan mouokkaama ja vaakaama osoipatteristo Suzanne Borel-Maisonnyn testeista. (The BMA test: a test for determining the primary symptoms of defects in speech, reading and writing. A battery of test sections adapted and adjusted by by Eila Alahuhta, on the basis of the tests of Suzanne Borel-Maisonny.). *Publications of the Institute for Educational Research*, 292, FINNISH LANGUAGE AND COGNITIVE DEVELOPMENT ASSESSMENT PROCEDURES: FINNISH

Alahuhta, Eila. (1978). Motorisen suuntautumiskyvyn harjoittamisesta valmentautumisena optimaaliseen puhumiseen, lukemiseen ja kirjoittamisen hallintaan. (On improving the ability of motor orientation as a means of preparing for an optimal command of speech, reading and writing.). *Lastentarha*, 10 (11), LANGUAGE AND MOTOR DEVELOPMENT FINNISH: FINNISH

Alahuhta, Eila. (1978). Sur les facteurs primaires affectant les facultés du langage chez les enfants d'âge prescholaire. (On the primary factors effecting the language faculties of preschool children.). *Rééducation Orthophonique*, 16 (101), LANGUAGE PRECURSORS LANGUAGE AND COGNITIVE DEVELOPMENT: FRENCH

Alahuhta, Eila. (1978). Sur les facteurs primaires affectant les facultés du langage chez les enfants d'âge prescolaire. (On the primary factors effecting the language faculties of preschool children.).

Bulletin d'Audiophonologie, 2, LANGUAGE PRECURSORS LANGUAGE AND COGNITIVE DEVELOPMENT: FRENCH

Alahuhta, Eila. (1978). Voiko luki-hairioita ehkaista? (Can defects of reading and writing be prevented?). *Lastentarha*, 3, LITERACY LANGUAGE AND EDUCATION READING DISORDERS FINNISH: FINNISH

Alahuhta, Eila. (1979). Tidig diagnostisering som urgangspunkt for optimal rehabilitering. (Early diagnostics as the foundation for optimal rehabilition.). *Nordisk Tidsskrift for Specialpaedagogik*, 4, ASSESSMENT PROCEDURES INTERVENTION PROGRAMS FINNISH: NORWEGIAN

Alahuhta, Eila. (1979). Tutkimusprojekti esikouluikaisten paivakotilasten mahdollisten lukivaikeuksien ennakoimiseksi ja lieventamiseksi. (Research project on predicting and mitigating the possible reading problems of pre-school age kindergarten children.). *Lastentarha*, 7, FINNISH READING DISORDERS: FINNISH

Alahuhta, Eila. (1981). Esikoululaisten kielellista kykya ennustavista primaaritekijoista. (On the primary factors predicting the linguistic abilities of preschool chlidren.). In *EASE 80: The Conference for Special Education 4*. ASSESSMENT PROCEDURES FINNISH: FINNISH

Alahuhta, Eila. (1981). Om de primara faktorer som forutsager spraklig formaga i forskolealdern. (On the primary factors affecting linguistic abilities at pre-school age.). *Nordisk Tidsskrift for Specialpaedagogik*, 2, LANGUAGE PRECURSORS LANGUAGE AND COGNITIVE DEVELOPMENT: NORWEGIAN

Alahuhta, Eila. (1982). Kirjoittamisen eri ulottuvuuksista. (On the different dimensions of writing.). *Kirjoituksia kirjoittamisesta*, XXLX, 32-43. WRITTEN LANGUAGE: FINNISH

Alahuhta, Eila. (1982). Las- och skrivsvarigheter-komplexa svarigheter-beteende-storningar. (Defects of reading abd writing-complex defects-disturbances in behavior.). *Lasning: Membership Periodical of SCIRA*, 1, READING DISORDERS AGRAPHIA: SWEDISH

Alahuhta, Eila. (1982). On the primary factors predicting linguistic abilities of pre-school children. In *Communication and Handicap Report of EASE 80, Congress for Special Education 4*. Finland: ASSESSMENT PROCEDURES FINNISH:

Alahuhta, Eila. (1983). Spastinen dysarthria-eras hoitokertomus. (Spastic dysarthria-a case study.). In *Erityispedagogiikka-logopedia, Opetusmonisteita & selosteita, 2*. Jyvaskyla, Finland: DYSARTHRIA: FINNISH

Alahuhta, Eila. (1983). Vieraan kielen omaksumisen hairioista-erityispedagoginen ja logopedinen nakokulma. (On disabilities in the filed of acquiring a foreign language: considerations from the viewpoints of special education and logopedics.). In *Seminar report: Seminar on experimenting with the starting time of foreign-language teaching*. Finland: National Board of General Education, Bureau of Experimenting and Research. L2 EDUCATION: FINNISH

Alahuhta, Eila. (1984). Logopediassa on monta tiedetta. Puheen ja lielen hairioiden pedagogista kuntoutusta. (Logopedics involves several disciplines: on the pedagogicla treatment of speech and language disorders.). *Aamulehti*, 17, LANGUAGE AND EDUCATION INTERVENTION PROGRAMS: FINNISH

Alahuhta, Eila. (1989). Die Symptome einer leichten neurologischen Fehlleistung und ihre Korrelation im Schulerfolg. (The symptoms of a mild neurological performance error and their correlation in the classroom.). *Jyvaskyla Studies in Education Psychology and Social Research*, 71, FINNISH LANGUAGE AND EDUCATION CEREBRAL DISORDERS NEUROLINGUISTICS: GERMAN

Alahuhta, Eila. (1989). Fields of applied research at the Institute of Logopedics and Phonetics (ILP), University of Oulu. *Publications of the Finnish Association of Logopedics and Phoniatrics*, 23, FINNISH:

Alahuhta, Eila. (1989). Forskning i barnets sprak vid institutionen for logopedi och fonetik vid Uleaborgs universitet. (Research in child language at the department of logopedics and phonetics.). In R. Soederbergh (Ed.), *The Second Scandinavian Child Language*

Symposium. Lund, Sweden: Lund University, Department of Linguistics. FINNISH: SWEDISH

Alahuhta, Eila. (1989). Occurence of functional voice disorders in the population of northern Finland. In *Publications of the 21st Congress of the International Association of Logopedics and Phoniatrics*. Prague: FINNISH LANGUAGE DISORDERS ARTICULATION DISORDERS:

Alahuhta, Eila. (1989). Vuorovaikutus ja sen ongelmat dysfasialapsen perheessa. (Interaction and its problems in the family of an aphasic child.). *Afasia*, 2, 16. INTERVENTION PROGRAMS APHASIAS DEVELOPMENTAL DISORDERS: FINNISH

Alatis, James E. (1990). *Language teaching, testing, and technology: Lessons from the past with a view toward the future*. Washington, DC: Georgetown University Press. LANGUAGE AND EDUCATION L2 READING PROFICIENCY L2 ACQUISITION THEORIES L2 ASSESSMENT PROCEDURES L2 SEMANTICS C.A.L.L. MACHINE TRANSLATION:

Alatis, James E. (1990). *Linguistics, language teaching and language acquisition : the interdependence of theory, practice and research*. Washington, D.C.: Georgetown University Press. LANGUAGE AND EDUCATION L2 EDUCATION:

A volume in the Georgetown University Round Table on Languages and Linguistics series.

Alberts, Jeffrey R., & Decsy, G. J. (1990). Terms of endearment. *Developmental Psychobiology*, 23(7), NATIVISM:

Aldridge, Michelle. (1990). *The acquisition of INFL*. Bloomington, IN: Indiana University Linguistics Publications. PARAMETER SETTING SYNTACTIC DEVELOPMENT:

This study analyses, within Chomsky's Barriers framework, the development of the I-system in the speech of children between 18 and 36 months acquiring English as their native language. It is argued that early child clauses (in children roughly under two years of age) lack an I-system, and in consequence show no evidence of mastery of infinitival to, Modals, Tense/ Agreement inflections, Nominative case-marking, and the syntax of pro. It is claimed that the I-system begins to be acquired from around two years of age, and various transitional phases in its acquisition are examined.

Allen, Gary L., Kirasic, Kathleen C., & Beard, Rebecca L. (1989). Children's expression of spatial knowledge. *Journal of Experimental Child Psychology*, 48, 114-130. SPATIAL TERMS DEIXIS-SPATIAL:

First-, fourth-, and sixth-grade children performed model construction, verbal description, and route reversal tasks. Age-related improvement was found in the rate of learning the maze and in the accuracy of verbal descriptions. All children performed well in sequencing intersections in the model but performed poorly in choosing path options in the model.

Allen, M. H., Lincoln, A. J., & Kaufman, A. S. (1991). Sequential and simultaneous processing abilities of high-functioning autistic and language-impaired children. *Journal of Autism and Developmental Disorders*, 21, 483-502. AUTISM LANGUAGE AND COGNITIVE DEVELOPMENT:

Allen, R. (1991). Integration of communicational cues by very young children. *Journal of Psycholinguistic Research*, 20, 389-402. CUES-PRAGMATIC:

Altmann, Gerry T. (1990). *Cognitive models of speech processing*. Cambridge, MA: MIT/Batsford. LANGUAGE PROCESSING COMPUTER SIMULATIONS WORD RECOGNITION LEXICAL ACCESS SPEECH PERCEPTION:

A review of current theory in psycholinguistics and computational models of speech perception and natural language processing. Provides new information on computer simulations and experimental research from topics such as: lexical access, word recognition, syntactic processing, and prosodic cues.

Altmann, Gerry T. (1992). *Parsing and interpretation*. Hillsdale, NJ: Lawrence Erlbaum Associates. LANGUAGE PROCESSING CONNECTIONISM SYNTACTIC STRUCTURES AMBIGUITY SEMANTIC RELATIONS ANAPHORA:

A special issue of Language and Cognitive Processes dealing with various aspects of sentence interpretation. The book has a section on connectionist views of thematic relations, and includes and a discussion of architectures for modeling language functions. Other topics covered include: empty categories, anaphora, subcategorization, ambiguiyt, and local and on-line processing.

Ambert, Alba N. (1991). *Bilingual education and English as a second language : a research handbook, 1988-1990*. New York, NY : Garland. REFERENCE MANUAL BILINGUALISM-EDUCATION L2 EDUCATION:

Ambrus, M., Farkas, Zsolt, Hirschberg, Jenö, Nagy, E., & Simon-Nagy, E. (1989). Experiences with the G-O-H hearing screening method. *Hungarian Papers in Phonetics*, 21, 160-163. AUDIOLOGY LANGUAGE TESTING G-O-H SYSTEM HUNGARIAN:

Anden, G., & Brodin, Jane. (1984). *Min kropp-mina ord, kommunikation for forstandshandikappade. (My body-my words: Communication for the mentally reatrded.)*. Stockholm: The Swedish Handicap Institute. RETARDED CHILDREN INTERVENTION PROGRAMS BLISS SYMBOLS SIGNING: SWEDISH

A presentation of various systems of alternative ways to communicate. Includes: Bliss, Pictogram, Picture communication, Amerind, Sign language for deaf and hearing impaired, Adapted sign language for mentally retarded, Music, Signs in hand for deaf-blind, Body language, etc. The aim is to give an overall view of different ways to communicate for people with mental retardation. Also available in an English translation.

Andersen, Elaine S. (1990). *Speaking with style : the sociolinguistic skills of children*. London, UK : Routledge. SOCIOLINGISTIC FACTORS COMMUNICATIVE COMPETENCE:

Anderson, A. B., & Stromqvist, Sven. (1990). Adult L2 acquisition of gender: A crosslinguistic and crosslearner types perspective (Project Report No. 4). *Gothenburg Papers in Theoretical Linguistics.* GENDER CROSSLINGUISTIC STUDY-MORPHOSYNTAX:

Anderson, Anne H., Clark, A., & Mullin, J. (1991). Introducing information in dialogues-forms of introduction chosen by young speakers and the responses elicited from young listeners. *Journal of Child Language*, 18, 663-687. TOPIC INITIATION CHILDREN'S DIALOGUES SOCIAL SPEECH:

Anderson, Anne H., Garrod, S. C., Clark, A., & Boyle, E., et al. (1992). The Human-Communication-Research-Centre dialogue database. *Journal of Child Language*, 19, 711-716. CHILD LANGUAGE CORPORA:

Aparicio, Maria T. (1989). Modelling and early language acquisition in Down's syndrome. *Early Child Development and Care*, 44, 51-59. DOWN SYNDROME INTERVENTION PROGRAMS MODELING:

From Stockholm Bibliographies.

Appel, Gabriela., & Dechert, Hans W. (1991). *A case for psycholinguistic cases.* Amsterdam, The Netherlands: John Benjamins. CASE MORPHOSYNTACTIC DEVELOPMENT:

Papers from the Second International Congress of the International Society for Applied Psycholinguistics held from July 27-31, 1987 at the University of Kassel.

Appleyard, J. A. (1990). *Becoming a reader: the experience of fiction from childhood to adulthood.* New York, NY: Cambridge University Press. LITERACY:

In the first study of the psychological development of readers of fictional stories across the whole lifespan, J.A. Appleyard argues that regardless of personality and background, readers go through a sequence of stages as they mature from childhood to adulthood which affects how they experience and respond to stories. Each subsequent stage requires an advance to a way of thinking about a story which is qualitatively different from the previous one. Appleyard's evidence for these claims is drawn from numerous studies of reading and from interviews with readers of all ages. The developmental perspective provides a useful framework for assessing the implications of competing theories of reading, for charting the evolution of young readers as they mature, and for locating and understanding the varied responses of adult readers.

Aram, Dorothy M., Gillespie, L. L., & Yamashita, T. S. (1990). Reading among children with left and right brain lesions. *Developmental Neuropsychology*, 6, 301-317. TRAUMATIC DISORDERS READING DISORDERS:

Arena, Louis A. (1990). *Language proficiency: Defining, teaching, and testing*. New York, NY: Plenum. L2 INPUT FACTORS L2 ASSESSMENT PROCEDURES L2 EDUCATION INTERLANGUAGE-PHONOLOGY INTERLANGUAGE-MORPHOLOGY L2 READING PROFICIENCY BILINGUALISM-MOTIVATION:

A collection of papers examining second language proficiency and the factors which impact upon L2 speakers' ability to gain proficiency in L2. Topics covered include: attitudinal factors, pedagogical methods, and means of assessing L2 proficiency..

Argyle, M., & Ingham, R. (1972). Gaze, mutual gaze, and proximity. *Semiotica*, 4(1), 32-49. GAZE JOINT REFERENCE:

Arlinger, Stig. (1989). *Manual of practical audiometry*, vol 1. San Diego, CA: Singular Publishing Group. AUDIOMETRY:

General prerequisites for audiometry. Psychoacoustic test methods using pure tone stimulation. Psychoacoustic test methods using speech stimulation. Audiometry with children. Impedance audiometry. Electrophysiological Tests-Electric Response Audiometry (ERA). The audiogram format and symbols. Explanations of terms and abbreviations. Index.

Arlinger, Stig. (1991). *Manual of practical audiometry*, vol. 2. San Diego, CA: Singular Publishing Group. AUDIOMETRY:

Expertly details auditory anatomy, physiology and pathophysiology, acoustics, and psychology for the tests described in volume I.

Armstrong, S. L., Gleitman, Lila R., & Gleitman, Henry. (1982). What some concepts might not be. *Cognition*, 13, 263-308. CONCEPT DEVELOPMENT LEXICAL DEVELOPMENT SEMANTIC DEVELOPMENT:

Aronson, Karin, & Rundstrom, Bengt. (1989). Cats, dogs, and sweets in the clinical negotiation of reality: on politeness and coherence in pediatric discourse. *Language in Society*, 18(4), 483-504. CHILDREN'S DISCOURSE COMMUNICATIVE COMPETENCE:

From Stockholm Bibliographies.

Ashmead, D. H., Davis, D. L., Whalen, T., & Odom, R. D. (1991). Sound localization and sensitivity to interaural time differences in human infants. *Child Development*, 62, 1211-1226. INFANT PERCEPTION:

Astington, Janet W. (1991). Intention in the child's theory of mind. In D. Frye, & C. Moore (Eds), *Children's theories of mind.* Hillsdale, NJ: Lawrence Erlbaum Associates. THEORY OF MIND INTENTIONALITY:

Astington, Janet W. (1991). Narrative and the child's theory of mind. In B. Britton, & A. Pellegrini (Eds), *Narrative thought and narrative language.* Hillsdale, NJ : Lawrence Erlbaum Associates. NARRATIVES THEORY OF MIND:

Astington, Janet W., & Gopnik, Alison. (1991). Theoretical explanations of children's understanding of the mind. *British Journal of Developmental Psychology*, 9, 7-31. THEORY OF MIND:

Astington, Janet W., Harris, Paul L., & Olson, David R. (Eds) (1988). *Developing theories of mind.* New York, NY: Cambridge University Press. THEORY OF MIND LANGUAGE AND COGNITION LANGUAGE AND COGNITIVE DEVELOPMENT:

A collection of empirical reports and conceptual analyses written by leading reseachers in an exciting new area of the cognitive sciences. It provides numerous answers to the question of when and how children develop theories of mind: theories that enable them to give commonsense predictions and explanations of behavior by ascribing mental states to themselves and to other people. The authors examine children's increasing awareness and understanding of these mental states, such as beliefs, desires, intentions, and emotions. They consider how this understanding is expressed in talk and action, and the consequence of this awareness for other aspects of children's cognition and behavior.

Atkins, B., & Levin, B. (1991). Admitting impediments. In U. Zernik (Ed.), *Lexical acquisition: Exploiting on-line resources to build a lexicon*. Hillsdale, NJ : Lawrence Erlbaum Associates. LEXICAL DEVELOPMENT LEXICAL ACCESS:

Atkinson, Martin. (1992). *Children's syntax : An introduction to principles and parameters theory*. Oxford, UK: Basil Blackwell. PARAMETER SETTING SYNTACTIC DEVELOPMENT QUESTIONS:

Atkinson begins by illustrating the differences between a parameter based acquisition system and a rule-based acquisition system and then takes a closer look at the development of questions.

Au, Terry Kit-Fong. (1990). Children's use of information in word learning. *Journal of Child Language*, 17, 393-416. LEXICAL DEVELOPMENT MUTUAL EXCLUSIVITY CONTRAST-SEMANTIC:

This work examined if and how children's beliefs about word meanings may affect their use of contrastive linguistic information in the input in word meaning. In the study 1, 3- and 4-year-olds were introduced to a novel material or shape name and heard it contrasted with familiar words. Others merely heard the novel word used for referring to an object. In study 2, another group of 3- and 4-year- olds were asked to name the materials and shapes used for introducing these novel terms. Children made use of linguistic contrast only in some situations. They benefitted more when the novel term did not overlap much in denotation with any terms commonly known by 3- and 4-year-olds. These results suggest that children can use information in the input very efficiently in learning a term for an as-yet-unnamed catagory, but not in learning a term similar in denotation to a word they already know.

Au, Terry Kit-Fong, & Glusman, Mariana. (1990). The principle of mutual exclusivity in word learning: To honor or not to honor. *Child Development*, 61, 1474-1490. MUTUAL EXCLUSIVITY SEMANTIC MAPPING LEXICAL DEVELOPMENT CONCEPT DEVELOPMENT:

Six studies examined whether knowledge about hierarchical organization of catagories and about cross-language equivalents for ogject labels can help children limit their use of mutual exclusivity assumption appropriately. Adults as well as children resisted assigning 2 novel names to the same object in some situations. By 4, children accepted 2 names for an object if the names picked out categories from different levels of a hierarchy but not if they picked out categories from the same level. Two names from different languages were accepted.

Au, Terry Kit-fong, & Laframboise, Denise E. (1990). Acquiring color names via linguistic contrast: The influence of contrasting terms. *Child Development*, 61, 1808-1823. MUTUAL EXCLUSIVITY CONTRAST-SEMANTIC COLOR NAMES LEXICAL DEVELOPMENT:

Contrasting a new color term with childrens' own label helped 5-year-olds learn but contrasting the new term with randomly chosen familiar color terms did not last. For 4-year-olds neither contrast helped. When the contrastive information was presented more than once, 3- and 4-year-olds performed much like the 5-year-olds.

B

Babai, László. (1978). Az emlékezeti hangoztatások (beszéltetések) jelentösége, szerkezeti és kivitelezési formai a dadogás terápiájában. (The importance of structural and exceptional forms of memorized speech in stuttering therapy.). *Magyar Fonetikai Füzetek*, 1, 120-125. STUTTERING LANGUAGE AND MEMORY HUNGARIAN: HUNGARIAN

Babic, Nada. (1983). *Djecja pitanja. (Children's questions.).* Zagreb: Skolska knjiga. QUESTIONS SERBOCROATIAN: SERBOCROATIAN

> The results of an investigation of the development of questions by pre-school children, 4-7 years of age.

Babic, Nada. (1984). Razvitie voprosov u doskoljnikov. (Development of questions in preschool children.). *Voprosy psihologii*, 30 (2), 67-74. SERBOCROATIAN QUESTIONS: SERBOCROATIAN

> The aim of the study was to reveal basic trends in appearance of questions in children and to establish corresponding factors.

Babic, Nada. (1988). Funkcije govora (jezika) odgajatelja u komunikaciji s predskolskom djecom. (Speech functions of the preschool teacher in communication with preschool children.). *Zivot i skola*, 37 (4), 337-355. METHODOLOGY ADULT-CHILD INTERACTION PARENTAL SPEECH SERBOCROATIAN: SERBOCROATIAN

> The author presents methodological advantages of a three-set functional model for studying forms of adult language behavior in communication with pre-school children.

Babic, Nada. (1989). *Govor odgajatelja i djecje aktivnosti. (Preschool teacher's speech (language) and children's activities.).* Zagreb: Skolske novine. LANGUAGE AND EDUCATION SERBOCROATIAN ADULT-CHILD INTERACTION: SERBOCROATIAN

An investigation of the influence of teacher's language on non-verbal and verbal behavior of children in pre-schools.

Babic, Nada. (1989). Razvoj govora predskolske djece u komunikaciji s odraslima. (The development of preschool children's speech (language) in communication with adults.). In *Predsolski otrok med druzinsko in drusbeno organizirano vzgojo.*. Maribor: Pedkagoska fakulteta, Univerza u Mariboru. SERBOCROATIAN PARENTAL SPEECH: SERBOCROATIAN

The author offers methodological solutions, whose essential message is: it is necessary to offer a wide language framework in order to acquire and develop linguistic and communicative competence.

Bacri, N., & de Boysson-Bardies, Bénédicte. (1977). Portée de la négation et référenciation. (The scope of negation and referencing.). *L'Année Psychologique*, 77 (1), 117-136. NEGATION REFERENCE: FRENCH

Badaf, G. (1984). Niños confrontados a enunciados en lengua desconocida formulados en un contexto pragmatico. (Children confronted with utterances in an unknown language formulated in a pragmatic context.). In M. Siguan (Ed.), *Adquisición precoz de una segunda lengua. (Precocious acquisition of a second language.).* Barcelona, Spain: Ediciónes de la Universidad. BILINGUALISM: SPANISH

Badaf, G. (1986). Étude sur le rôle des connaissances contextuelles dans la formation du sens. (Study of the role of contextual knowledge in the formations of meaning.). *Communication et Cognition*, 19, 85-97. CONTEXT SEMANTIC DEVELOPMENT LEXICAL DEVELOPMENT CONCEPT DEVELOPMENT: FRENCH

Badaf, G. (1987). Problemas de lenguaje y modelos evolutivos. (Problems of language and developmental models.). In *Actes du XIV Congreso Nacional de Logopedia, Foniatria y Audiologia.* Burgos, Spain. LANGUAGE AND COGNITIVE DEVELOPMENT: SPANISH

Badaf, G. (1987). Quelques éléments pour une discussion autour et à propos de 'mais'. (Some elements for a discussion around and about 'but'.). *Communication et Cognition*, 20, 311-318. CONNECTIVES-CONDITIONAL FRENCH: FRENCH

Badaf, G. (1988). L'examen du langage d'un enfant est un art difficile. (The investigation of child language is a difficult art.). *Parole d'Or*, 1, 11-13. METHODOLOGY: FRENCH

Badaf, G. (1988). Quelques réflexions à propos du retard de langage chez l'enfant. (Some reflections on language delay in children.). *Journal de l'Association Romande des Logopédistes Diplomes*, 8, 11-12. LANGUAGE DISORDERS LANGUAGE DELAY: FRENCH

Badaf, G. (1989). Le rôle des répétitions dans la description des conduites inférentielles à partir de phrases avec 'mais'. (The role of repetitions in the description of inferential paths for phrases with "but".). *Klagenfurter Beitrage zur Sprachwissenschaft.* CONNECTIVES-CONDITIONAL: FRENCH

Badaf, G. (1989). Mise en perspectif psycholinguistique de 'mais'. (Putting 'but' in a psycholinguistic perspective.). *Bulletin CILA*, 50, 42-47. CONNECTIVES-CONDITIONAL: FRENCH

Badaf, G. (1989). Psycholinguistique de 'mais'. (The psycholingistics of "mais".). *Cahiers de l'Institut de Linguistique de Louvain*, 14, 27-37. CONNECTIVES-CONDITIONAL: FRENCH

Badalamenti, A. F. (1992). Ontogenesis of object discrimination. *Journal of Psycholinguistic Research*, 21, 219-247. CONCEPT DEVELOPMENT CATEGORIZATION:

Badzinksi, Diane M., Cantor, Joanne, & Hoffner, Cynthia. (1989). Children's understanding of quantifiers. *Child Study Journal*, 19, 241-258. RELATIONAL TERMS QUANTIFIERS:

Children from grade 4 understood the count quantifiers: 'no, not any, a few, not many, a lot, ' and 'many.' For the relational quantifiers: 'none, some, most' and 'all' mastery followed the expected pattern of none < some < most < all and was age related.

Bailey, Ch-J. N., & Harris, R. (1985). *Developmental mechanisms of language*. New York, NY: Pergamon. PHONOLOGICAL DEVELOPMENT NATIVISM SEMANTIC DEVELOPMENT BIOLOGICAL FOUNDATIONS LANGUAGE AND COGNITIVE DEVELOPMENT PRAGMATIC DEVELOPMENT:

A collection of articles which view language as a mode of human development at the individual and social level. Includes chapters on phonetological development, nativism, semantic developoment, biological bases of language, pragmatic development, and language and cognitive development.

Baillargeon, Renee, & Devos, J. (1991). Object permanence in young infants-further evidence . *Child Development*, 62, 1227-1246. OBJECT PERMANENCE:

Bain, Ann M., Bailet, Laura Lyons, & Moats, Louisa Cook. (1991). *Written language disorders: Theory into practice.* San Diego, CA: Singular Group. WRITTEN LANGUAGE LITERACY LANGUAGE DISORDERS AGRAPHIA LANGUAGE AND EDUCATION COMPUTER ASSISTED THERAPY LANGUAGE TESTING:

Contents include: spelling disorders, handwriting disorders, expression disorders, process and product in writing, computer assisted therapy and instruction, and reviews of language tests.

Baken, Ronald J. (1987). *Clinical measurement of speech and voice.* San Diego, CA: Singular Group. ACOUSTIC PHONETICS ARTICULATION SPEECH PRODUCTION ASSESSMENT PROCEDURES:

The use of general purpose tools and sound spectrography to measure: speech movements, airflow, volume, intensity, and other aspects of speech production and acoustic phonetics.

Baken, Ronald J. (1991). *Readings in clinical spectrography of speech.* San Diego, CA: Singular Group. ACOUSTIC PHONETICS SPEECH PRODUCTION:

Baker, C. L., & McCarthy, J. J. (Eds). (1981). *The logical problem of language acquisition.* Cambridge, MA: MIT Press. ACQUISITION AND LINGUISTIC THEORY LEARNABILITY:

Balázs, Boglárka. (1990). Utmutató a gyermekkori diszfonia javításához. (Guide to the correction of childhood phonological disorders.). Budapest, Hungary. HUNGARIAN PHONOLOGICAL DISORDERS: HUNGARIAN

Baldwin, Dare A. (1989). Priorities in children's expectations about object label reference: Form over color. *Child Development*, 60, 1291-1306. CATEGORIZATION LABELING:

Toddlers sorted 10 sets of 3 pictures that contrasted form with color. Half were shown a target and asked to 'find another one' while the others heard a novel label for the target and were asked to extend the label. Three year olds sorted on the basis of form while 2 year olds frequently chose the color match when labels were absent, but form when asked to extend a novel label. - From Child Development Abstracts.

Baldwin, Dare A. (1991). Infant's contribution to the achievement of joint reference. *Child Development*, 62, 875-890. JOINT REFERENCE:

Baldwin, Dare A., & Markman, Ellen M. (1989). Establishing word-object relations: a first step. *Child Development*, 60(2), 381-398. SEMANTIC MAPPING MUTUAL EXCLUSIVITY:

From Stockholm Bibliographies.

Ball, Martin J. (1982). Asesu iaith. (Assessing language.). *Y Gwyddonydd*, 20, 126-130. ASSESSMENT PROCEDURES WELSH: WELSH

Ball, Martin J. (1984). Phonological development and assessment. In N. Miller (Ed.), *Bilingualism and language disability*. London: Croom Helm. PHONOLOGICAL DEVELOPMENT PHONOLOGICAL DISORDERS BILINGUALISM-LANGUAGE DISORDERS BILINGUALISM-PROBLEMS/EFFECTS:

Ball, Martin J. (1984). X-ray techniques. In C. Code & M. Ball (Eds), *Experimental clinical phonetics*. London: Croom Helm. ASSESSMENT PROCEDURES LANGUAGE DISORDERS:

Ball, Martin J. (1987). Clinical linguistics. *Revue de l'AILA/AILA Review*, 4, 69-87. LANGUAGE DISORDERS:

Ball, Martin J. (1987). Linguo-labials revisited: the PRDS solution. *Journal of the International Phonetic Association*, 17, 115-117. PHONETIC FEATURES:

Ball, Martin J. (1988). Clinical linguistics encounters. *Clinical Linguistics and Phonetics*, 2, 143-151. LANGUAGE DISORDERS:

Ball, Martin J. (1988). The contribution of speech pathology to the development of phonetic description. In M. Ball (Ed.), *Theoretical linguistics and disordered language*. London: Croom Helm. PHONOLOGICAL DEVELOPMENT PHONOLOGICAL DISORDERS METHODOLOGY-TRANSCRIPTION:

Ball, Martin J. (1988). A diacritic range for phonation types. *Journal of the International Phonetic Association*, 18, 39-40. METHODOLOGY-TRANSCRIPTION:

Ball, Martin J. (1988). Investigating performance and competence in variation studies: adapting tecniques from speech pathology. In A. Thomas (Ed.), *Methods in dialectology*. Clevedon: Multilingual Matters. METHODOLOGY-ANALYSIS SOCIOLINGUISTIC FACTORS NONSTANDARD DIALECTS:

Ball, Martin J. (1988). LARSP to LLARSP. Designing a Welsh grammatical profile. *Clinical Linguistics and Phonetics*, 2, 55-73. WELSH LARSP ASSESSMENT PROCEDURES:

Ball, Martin J. (1988). *Theoretical linguistics and disordered language*. San Diego, CA: College Hill. LANGUAGE DISORDERS:

Ball, Martin J. (1988). The transcription of phonation types. *Clinical Linguistics and Phonetics*, 2, 253-256.
METHODOLOGY-TRANSCRIPTION PHONOLOGICAL DISORDERS:

Ball, Martin J. (1989). *Phonetics for speech pathology*. San Diego, CA: Singular Group. ARTICULATION AUDITORY PHONETICS ACOUSTIC PHONETICS METHODOLOGY-TRANSCRIPTION PHONETIC VARIATION:

Includes: auditory, acoustic and articulatory phonetics, and notes on transcription. Also available from Taylor & Francis (London).

Ball, Martin J. (1991). *The clinician's guide to linguistic profiling of language impairment*. Kibworth: Far Communications.
ASSESSMENT PROCEDURES CLASSSIFICATION OF DISORDERS:

Ball, Martin J. (1991). Recent developments in the transcription of non-normal speech. *Journal of Communication Disorders*, 25.
METHODOLOGY-TRANSCRIPTION ATYPICAL DEVELOPMENT:

Ball, Martin J., Davies, E., Duckworth, M., & Middlehurst, R. (1991). Assessing the assessments: a comparison of two clinical pragmatic profiles. *Aphasiology*, 5. ASSESSMENT PROCEDURES:

Ball, Martin J., Duckworth, M., & Munro, S. M. (1984). Transcription of disordered phonology in Welsh. *Cardiff Working Papers in Welsh Linguistics*, 3, 21-30. METHODOLOGY-TRANSCRIPTION WELSH:

Ball, Martin J., & Munro, S. M. (1981). Language assessment procedures for linguistic minorities: an example. *Journal of Multilingual and Multicultural Development*, 2, 231-241.
ASSESSMENT PROCEDURES SOCIOLINGUISTIC FACTORS:

Ball, Martin J., & Tench, P. (1992). *Phonetic transcription: theory and application*. Amsterdam, The Netherlands: John Benjamins.
METHODOLOGY-TRANSCRIPTION:

Ballo, Larissza. (1983). *Hungarian verbal associations*. Szeged: Hungary. SEMANTIC ORGANIZATION HUNGARIAN:

Balota, David A., Ferraro, R., & Connor, L. T. (1991). On the early influence of meaning in word recognition: a review of the literature. In P. Schwanenflugel (Ed.), *The psychology of word meanings*. Hillsdale, NJ: Lawrence Erlbaum Associates. LEXICAL DEVELOPMENT VOCABULARY DEVELOPMENT SEMANTIC DEVELOPMENT:

Balota, David A., Flores d'Arcais, G. B., & Rayner, Keith. (1991). *Comprehension processes in reading*. Hillsdale, NJ: Lawrence Erlbaum Associates. LITERACY DYSLEXIA DISCOURSE COMPREHENSION READING DISORDERS LANGUAGE AND MEMORY:

> This book addresses the interrelationship among several areas relevant to understanding how people comprehend text. The contributors focus on the on-line processes associated with text understanding rather than simply with the product of that comprehension-what people remember from reading. Presenting the latest theories and research findings from a distinguished group of contributors, Comprehension Processes in Reading is divided into four major sections. Each section, concluding with a commentary chapter, discusses a different aspect of reader understanding or dysfunction such as individual word comprehension, sentence parsing, text comprehension and comprehension failures and dyslexia.

Baltaxe, Christine A. M., & d'Angiola, N. (1992). Cohesion in the discourse interaction of autistic, specifically language-impaired, and normal children. *Journal of Autism and Developmental Disorders*, 22, 1-21. AUTISM DISCOURSE COHERENCE SPECIFIC LANGUAGE IMPAIRMENT:

Bamberg, Michael, & Damrad-Frye, R. (1991). On the ability to provide evaluative comments: further explorations of children's narrative competencies. *Journal of Child Language*, 18, 689-710. NARRATIVES:

Bamberg, Michael, & Marchman, Virginia A. (1991). Binding and unfolding-towards the linguistic construction of narrative discourse. *Discourse Processes*, 14, 277-305. NARRATIVES:

Bamford, John, & Saunders, Elaine. (1991). *Hearing impairment, auditory perception, and language disability*. San Diego, CA: Singular Group. DEAF CHILDREN AUDIOLOGY SPEECH PERCEPTION READING DISORDERS:

Includes chapters on: the normal development of auditory and speech perception, language development, deaf children, reading disabilities and hearing problems, and neuropsychological aspects of deafness.

Banks, James, Gray, Colin, & Fyfe, Ronald. (1990). The written recall of printed stories by severely deaf children. *British Journal of Educational Psychology*, 60, 192-206. SEQUENCING DEAF CHILDREN LITERACY LANGUAGE AND MEMORY:

The recall of written stories by severely deaf children was compared with that of hearing slow-readers. Although the results showed a similarity between the two groups, the recall of the deaf children showed a greater problem with temporal sequencing.

Barbieri, Maria S. (1977). *Gli inizi del linguaggio: aspetti cognitivi e comunicativi (The emergence of language: Cognitive and communicative aspects.)*. Firenze, Italy: La Nuova. LANGUAGE AND COGNITIVE DEVELOPMENT COMMUNICATIVE DEVELOPMENT INTERSUBJECTIVITY: ITALIAN

Barbieri, Maria S. (1978). Interpretare e sovrainterpretare: un problema nello studio primo linguaggio infantile (Interpreting and overinterpreting: A problem in studying early language development.). *Giornale Italiano di Psicologia.*, 5, 174-189. CONTEXT SEMANTIC DEVELOPMENT LEXICAL DEVELOPMENT SINGLE-WORD STAGE: ITALIAN

Using the Antinucci and Parisi model for semantic development, the author studied the evolution of language in two children. They were 14 and 18 months old respectively at the beginning of the research and 20 and 27 months old at the end of it. As for the time and modalities of appearance of the optional semantic configurations, the results are thoroughly consistent with the model adopted. Some problems arose since the data were mainly collected during the single word stage. It seems that the model might be unsuitable to interpret the early word utterances as it overestimates the child's linguistic competence, attributing to it what could be supported by the verbal interaction with the adult. In this way it is difficult to notice the development taking place during the single-word stage. It is proposed that this stage be not considered a homogeneous one, but a set of subsequent stages, and that the Antinucci and Parisi model could only be correctly applied to the last of these stages. The author further suggests as interpretation of the child's first words greatly emphasizing contextual factors, but not combining them with the linguistic description of the child's competence.

Barbieri, Maria S. (1979). Le prime conversazioni non verbali. (The first non-verbal conversations.). *Giornale Italiano di Psicolgia*, 6, 67-89. INTERSUBJECTIVITY ADULT-CHILD INTERACTION PRELINGUISTICS: ITALIAN

In this research 56 episodes of interaction between one adult and one child are analyzed. The data were collected following the observational method in a group of six preverbal or the single-word stage children ages 14 to 18 months. The author wants to apply some models used in describing adult conversation to the analysis of early non-verbal interactions in order to point out their rich and complex organization. Through a qualitiative analysis such interactions are demonstrated to have a different structure depending on their different goal (interactions for the sake of interaction versus interactions having a defined goal) and to follow the conversational rules according to Goffman's Model.

Barbieri, Maria S. (1981). Uno studio sull'interpretazione materna del pianto infantile. (A study of maternal interpretation of child crying.). *Eta Evolutiva.*, 8, 28-37. CRYING: ITALIAN

Taking a pragmatic appraoch, maternal interpretation seems to be very important in establish a smooth and effective communication.Mother gives significance to her child's behaviour by interpreting it, and, as a result, she behaves as if he were a real partner in the interaction and in thisway the child learns the effect of his own behavior on the enviroment: therefore maternal interpretation is a focal point in the development af any further communicative competence. The aim of this research is to analyze the maternal representation of child's mind as this emerges from her interpretation of child'scrying. A mother-child pair has been studied from child's birth to his sixth month. The author analyzed mother's comments on child's crying in one hour's recording once a week. The comments have been classified in three catagories: descriptions, intstructions for behavior, interpretations. It has been possibleto isolate three different kinds of interpretations: physiological, intermediate and psychological. They occur one after the other in the course of four months. mother's representation of the child seems to change from a simple organism soon after the birth to a person. There is as well a change in the subjective certainty of interpretations, ranging from the greatest uncertainty in the first month to the possibilty of anticipating child's behavior in the third.

Barbieri, Maria S. (1982). Esperienze e ruolo dell'adulto nello sviluppo infantile, 1,2. (Experience and role of the adult in child development, 1 and 2.). *Scuola e Citta*, 33, 256-267(328-335).
ADULT-CHILD INTERACTION INTERVENTION PROGRAMS LANGUAGE AND SOCIAL CLASS PARENTAL SPEECH INPUT FACTORS ENVIRONMENTAL FACTORS SOCIOLINGUISTIC FACTORS: ITALIAN

The two papers together constitute a review chapter dealing with the issue of the nature of experience that fosters cognitive and linguistic development in infancy and early childhood. Particular attention is paid to social class differences and to their related outcomes. Within this framework, typologies and results of early intervention are examined. The author concludes that continuity of experience seems to be the main feature accounting for different outcomes in development and that, therefore, particular attention has to be paid to maternal styles and strategies of interaction deriving from different and often implicit 'theories' of the child held by different social and cultural groups.

Barbieri, Maria S. (1989). Introduction: Explanations as social acts. In M. S. Barbieri (Ed.), *La speigazione nell'interazione sociale* . Torino, Italy: Loescher. CHILDREN'S EXPLANATIONS CONNECTIVES-CAUSAL CONNECTIVES-CONDITIONAL ADULT-CHILD INTERACTION: ITALIAN

A presentation of the book including a review of different approaches to the concept of explanation in philosophy and in psychology, from Hempel's formal definition to a more interactional and contextual-bound perspective.

Barbieri, Maria S. (1989). *La speigazione nell'interazione sociale. (Ordinary explanations in social interaction.).* Torino, Italy: Loescher. CHILDREN'S EXPLANATIONS CONNECTIVES-CAUSAL CONNECTIVES-CONDITIONAL ADULT-CHILD INTERACTION SPEECH ACTS COMMUNICATIVE COMPETENCE: ITALIAN

A collection of papers dealing with adult-child interaction, the connective "because", causality, speech acts, communicative competence, and children's explanations.

Barbieri, Maria S. (1990). Cosa vuol dire imparare a spiegare? (What does it mean elanring to explain?). In A. Doria, & W. Zudini (Eds), *Festschrift in onore di G. Francescato.* CHILDREN'S EXPLANATIONS PIAGETIAN THEORY VYGOTSKYAN THEORY CAUSALITY: ITALIAN

The Piagetian and the Vygotskian approaches to the development of the explaining capacity in children are reviewed. The first uses mainly an experimental methodology and comes to the conclusion that children are unable to master causality and explanations until 7 or 8 years. These results are nevertheless challanged on linguistic grounds by studies relying on spontaneous production and on cognitive grounds by somerecent results. The author argues in favor of a Vygotskian perspective which seems to be more suitable than the other to encompass into a unitary perspective the results presently available in the literature.

Barbieri, Maria S. (1990). Determinati sociali e familiari dello sviluppo linguistico. (Social and family determinants of linguistic development.). In M. Battacchi (Ed.), *Trattato enciclopedico di psicologia dell'eta evolutiva, vol 2, tomo 1.* Padova: Piccin. LANGUAGE AND SOCIAL CLASS SIBLING EFFECTS: ITALIAN

This paper deals with the issue of social and family determinants of language development. The Italian literature in the field is reviewed.

Barbieri, Maria S., Colavita, F., & Scheuer, N. (1989). Some pragmatic aspects of the explaining competence in early childhood. *Papers in Pragmatics*, 3 (1), 129-154. CHILDREN'S EXPLANATIONS:

Explaining is a frequently occurring communicative act in every-day interaction. We focus on the social dimension of the act of giving an explanation. The authors assume that explaining is more than finding and relating causes and expressing them linguistically. Our work has both theoretical and empirical purposes. On a theoretical level, they identify the features that enable an explanation to be recognized as such in social interaction: i.e. the conditions that need to be met when giving an explanation. On an empirical level, they explore how three-year old children honour these conditions in spontaneous interaction. Following Searle's work on promises, they distinguish between preparatory conditions which lay the appropriate grounds for the speech act, essential conditions which indicate the speaker's concern for his partner's logic, sincerity conditions which refer to the speaker's honesty in relation to a speech act, and affilative conditions which refer to the symmetrical-asymmetrical axis of the speaker-partner relationship.

Barbieri, Maria S., & Devescovi, A. (1982). Different ways of explanation in two social classes: story telling to children from 18 to 36 months. In C. Johnson, & C. Thew (Eds), *Proceeding of the 2nd International Congress for the Study of Child Language*. Lanham: University Press of America. LANGUAGE AND SOCIAL CLASS PARENTAL INPUT LANGUAGE AND SOCIAL TRANSMISSION:

The paper analyzes the differences in mothers' talk according to the age of the child (18 to 36 months) and the socio-cultural level of the mother (high or low). Mother-child pairs (16) were videotaped while the mother was reading a short picture-story. Eight mothers had University degrees and eight the minimum level of schooling (8 years). Children were divided into four age groups (18,24,30, and 36 months). Each group was balanced by sex. Mothers' language was analyzed using two main measures: interactive speech acts and story speech acts. The story speech acts were further subdivided into several categories such as explanations linking events and explanations clarifying word meanings. Results show that in both social classes the quantity of language increases according to the age of the child, but that in the low social class the proportion of interactive speech acts is greater. Moreover, the overall number of explanations and the distribution of their types is different in the two socio-cultural groups, showing a greater sensitivity to the cognitive possibilities of the child in the higher socio-cultural group. MSB.

Barbieri, Maria S., & Devescovi, A. (1983). Lo sforzo di comprendere: inferenze e spiegazioni nel racconot di una ai bambini ai 18 ai 36 mesi. (Efforts to be understood: inferences and explanations in story telling to children from 18 to 36 months.). *Giornale Italiano di Psicologia*, 10, 61-78. PARENTAL SPEECH-STYLE: ITALIAN

This research compares mother's speech to children between 18 and 36 months, with the speech addressed to an adult interlocutor, in telling a short picture story. In order to point out the cognitive adaptation to different interlocutors, the authors analyzed the explanations which were given to the interlocutors and the inferences that were explicated. The results show that the qualitative and quantitative changes occur according both to the type of interlocutor (adult or child) and to the different ages of the children..

Barbieri, Maria S., & Devescovi, A. (1989). Reading a story together: adult's explanations to children. In M. S. Barbieri (Ed.), *La speigazione nell'interazione sociale*. Torino, Italy: Loescher. ADULT-CHILD INTERACTION PARENTAL SPEECH-STYLE:

An analysis of explanations that adults give to children from 18 to 36 months, in the context of book-reading, showing different types and levels of adaption to the knowledge and understanding capabilities of the partner.

Barbieri, Maria S., Devescovi, A., & Bonardi, P. (1984). L'interazione verbale tra bambini ed educatrice durante il racconto di una storia. (Verbal interaction between children and educator during story telling.). In S. Mantovani, & T. Musatti (Eds), *Tra adulto e bambini: educare e communicare*. Bergamo: Juvenilia. SOCIAL INTERACTION ADULT-CHILD INTERACTION LANGUAGE AND EDUCATION: ITALIAN

In this paper mother's story telling strategies are compared to those of teachers dealing with small groups (3 to 5) of children aged 18 to 36 months. The qualitative analysis points out two main strategies: a 'monologic' strategy where the speaker first tells the story and then assesses the child's comprehension of it, and a more 'dialogic' strategy where the adult tries to make the child reconstruct the story and the assessment of the child's comprehension is carried out at the same time. The latter seems to be more typical of day-care teachers, possibly as a consequence of the necessity of keeping alive the attention and involvment of several children.

Barbieri, Maria S., et al. (1989). A pragmatic basis for children's explaining competence at three years. In M. S. Barbieri (Ed.), *La speigazione nell'interazione sociale*. Torino, Italy: Loescher. CHILDREN'S EXPLANATIONS COMMUNICATIVE COMPETENCE:

A qualitative analysis of three-year-olds use of explanations during free play interaction, with the aim of pointing out the possible cues which might indicate whether the pragmatic rules governing the act of explaining are honoured or not.

Barbieri, Maria S., & Scheuer, N. (1988). The emergence of the explaining capacity. *IPRA Bulletin*, 5, 3-4. CHILDREN'S EXPLANATIONS:

This is a shorter version of the paper 'Some pragmatic aspects of the explaining competence in early childhood.'.

Bardovi-Harlig, K. (1992). The relationship of form and meaning-a cross-sectional study of tense and aspect in the interlanguage of learners of English as a second language. *Applied Psycholinguistics*, 13, 253-278. TENSE ASPECT L2 MORPHOSYNTAX:

Barkmeier, Julie, Jordan, Linda S., Robin, Donald A., & Schum, Robert L. (1991). Inexperienced listener ratings of dysarthric speaker intelligibility and physical appearance. In C. A. Moore, K. M. Yorkston, & D. R. Beukleman (Eds), *Dysarthia and apraxia of speech*. Baltimore, MD: Paul H. Brookes Publishing Co. DYSARTHRIA INTELLIGIBILITY:

Baron, Naomi S. (1990). *Pigeon-birds and rhyming words : the role of parents in language learning*. Englewood Cliffs, NJ: Prentice-Hall. PARENTAL INPUT PARENTAL SPEECH ADULT-CHILD INTERACTION BIBLIOGRAPHY:

Baron, Naomi S. (1992). *Growing up with language : how children learn to talk*. Reading, MS : Addison-Wesley. OVERVIEW-GENERAL:

Baron-Cohen, S. (1991). The theory of mind deficit in autism-how specific is it. *British Journal of Developmental Psychology*, 9, 301-314. AUTISM THEORY OF MIND:

Baroni, Maria R., & Axia, Giovanna. (1989). Children's metapragmatic abilities and the identification of polite and impolite requests. *First Language*, 9, 285-297. METALINGUISTICS COMMUNICATIVE COMPETENCE REQUESTS:

Two aspects of 5-and 7-year-old children's metapragmatic knowledge are examined. The first is the ability to attribute polite and impolite requests according to degrees of perceived familiarity among participants in a verbal exchange. The second is the representational explicitness of the pragmatic rule involved in the task. Results showed a developmental difference both in the attribution task and in metapragmatic awareness, confirming an age-related increase in the ability to establish representational links among pragmatic procedures. - From Child Development Abstracts.

Barratt, L., & Kassai, Ilona. (1989). Early second language contact: Acquisition or learning?. In *Proceedings of the International Speech Research Conference 1989*. Budapest: L2 ACQUISITION HUNGARIAN:

Barrenechea, Ilse L., & Schmitt, John F. (1989). Selected pragmatic features in Spanish-speaking preschool children. *Journal of Psycholinguistic Research*, 18, 353-367. SPANISH PRAGMATIC DEVELOPMENT LANGUAGE FUNCTIONS COMMUNICATIVE COMPETENCE:

Spontaneous speech from eighteen Spanish preschoolers (3:0-4:0) was examined for the development of seven language functions and three discourse features. All of the features and functions we represent in the sampled speech.

Barrett, Martyn D. (1979). Semantic development during the single-word stage of language acquisition. SINGLE-WORD SPEECH SEMANTIC DEVELOPMENT LEXICAL DEVELOPMENT:

Unpublished doc. diss., University of Sussex, England.

Barrett, Martyn D. (1982). A data-sensitive method for the functional analysis of early child language. *Working Papers of the London Psycholinguistics Research Group*, 4, 11-19. METHODOLOGY-ANALYSIS LANGUAGE FUNCTIONS:

Proposes a data-sensitive method for the functional analysis of early child language. This method is illustrated by means of a detailed analysis of two children's early linguistic productions with a particular focus upon the children's use of language to transfer objects and to request actions. The advantages and limitations of this method of analysis are discussed. MDB.

Barrett, Martyn D. (1983). The course of early lexical development: a review and an interpretation. *Early Child Development and Care*, 11, 19-32. LEXICAL DEVELOPMENT EVENTS/SCRIPTS NOUNS LABELING:

Provides a review of recent findings concerning the early acquisition of word meaning. It is argued that these findings can best be explained by postulating that the young child uses scripts to mentally represent events, and initially maps words directly onto these scripts. The development of word meaning subsequently occurs through the partitioning of these scripts into their constituent elements, with the prototypes that are disembedded from these scripts providing the ontogenetic source of the meanings of object names. MDB.

Barrett, Martyn D. (1983). Scripts, prototypes, and the early acquisition of word meaning. *Working Papers of the London Psycholinguistics Research Group*, 5, 17-26. LEXICAL DEVELOPMENT SEMANTIC DEVELOPMENT EVENTS/SCRIPTS:

Some phenomena that characterize the early acquisition of word meaning which have not previously received much theoretical attention are discussed. It is argued that script theory can provide a useful framework for interpreting these phenomena.

Barrett, Martyn D. (1986). Early semantic representations and early word-usage. In S. A. Kucsaj, II & M. D. Barrett (Eds), *The development of word meaning*. New York, NY: Springer-Verlag. REPRESENTATIONS-SEMANTIC REPRESENTATIONS-LEXICAL LEXICAL DEVELOPMENT DECONTEXTUALIZATION SEMANTIC DEVELOPMENT:

Provides a detailed review of the principal phenomena which characterize early word-usage. These phenomena are illustrated with some new data from a diary-based single-case study, as well as with data from other existing studies. A new theoretical framework is proposed in order to account for these phenomena. This framework which incorporates notions drawn from script theory, prototype theory and lexical contrast theory postulates that there are two main routes in early lexical development, one for context-bound words, the other for decontextualized nominal and non-nominal words. These two routes together can account for at least eight different patterns of change that have been observed to occur in the use of individual words. MDB.

Barrett, Martyn D. (1989). Early language development. In G. Bremner, & A. Slater (Eds), *Infant development.* London, UK: Lawrence Erlbaum Associates. FIRST WORDS SINGLE-WORD SPEECH OVERGENERALIZATION UNDERGENERALIZATION LANGUAGE FUNCTIONS CONVERSATIONAL SKILLS TRANSITIONAL PHASES INDIVIDUAL VARIATION EARLY SYNTACTIC DEVELOPMENT DECONTEXTUALIZATION:

Provides a detailed review of recent research into early language development. The following topics are discussed: the first words of the infant covering context-bound words, affect expressions and referential words: lexical development in the single-word period covering the acquisition of nominal and non-nominal words, and the phenomena of decontextualization, underextension, overextension, and the rescission of overextensions, pragmatic development in the single-word period covering the communicative functions of the first words, the emergence of new communicative functions, and the development of conversation, and the transition to two-word speech covering the acquisition of combinatorial rules, the analytic and synthetic routes into multi-word speech, the use of dummy forms, and individual differences in the transition to two-word speech. MDB.

Barrett, Martyn D., & Diniz, F. (1989). Lexical development in mentally handicapped children. In M. Beveridge, G. Conti-Ramsden, & I. Leudar (Eds), *Language and communication in mentally handicapped people.* London, UK: Chapman & Hall. RETARDED CHILDREN LEXICAL DEVELOPMENT LANGUAGE AND COGNITION LANGUAGE AND COGNITIVE DEVELOPMENT CATEGORIZATION CONNECTIVES ADJECTIVES PREPOSITIONS DEMONSTRATIVES:

A comparison of the overall patterns of lexical development in mentally handicapped children and in non-handicapped children, possible syndromic differences in the lexical development of mentally handicapped children, the acquisition and mental representation of the meanings of words by mentally handicapped children covering object names, action names, personal-social words, formulaic phrases, adjectives, prepositions, proforms, demonstratives, and connectives, and mentally handicapped children's knowledge of superordinate and subordinate lexical relations. MDB.

Barrett, Martyn D., & Harris, Margaret. (1986). Language and cognition in early social interaction. *British Journal of Developmental Psychology*, 4(3), SOCIOLINGUISTIC FACTORS SOCIAL INTERACTION LANGUAGE AND COGNITIVE DEVELOPMENT INPUT FACTORS:

A special issue of the British Journal of Developmental Psychology. Contains the reports of original empirical studies investigating the nature of the social-linguistic environment of the language-learning child and the effects of that environment upon the child's linguistic and cognitive development. Contributing authors are: Barrett & Harris, Halliday & Leslie, Zukow, Woollett, Beeghly Bretherton & Mervis, Harris Jones Brookes & Grant, Durkin, Shire, Riem, Crowther & Rutter, and Kuczaj. MDB.

Barrett, Martyn D., Harris, Margaret, & Chasin, Joan. (1991). Early lexical development and maternal speech: A comparison of children's initial and subsequent use of words. *Journal of Child Language*, 18, 21-40. LEXICAL DEVELOPMENT PARENTAL SPEECH-VOCABULARY CONTRASTIVE HYPOTHESIS:

The results of an analysis of 40 words are reported. This analysis reveals that seven qualitatively different patterns of change occurred between the children's initial and subsequent use of these words. The particuklar patterns of change which occurred support Barrett's (1986) model of early lexical development and there was a strong relationship between maternal speech and the children's initial word uses. The relationship between maternal speech and the children's subsequent word uses was very much weaker.

Barrett, Martyn D., Harris, Margaret, Jones, David, & Brookes, Susan. (1986). Linguistic input and early context-bound word use. In *Proceedings of the Child Language Seminar, 1986*. LEXICAL DEVELOPMENT FIRST WORDS INPUT FACTORS:

A longitudinal, observational study of two mother-child dyads, in which it was found that the majority of the children's first words were context-bound, although a minority of words were used referentially right from the outset. It was also found that there was a strong relationship between the children's initial uses of words and the most frequently occurring uses of these words by the mothers. The theoretical implications of these findings are discussed. MDB.

Barthelemy, C., Adrien, J. L., Tanguay, P., Garreau, B., Fermanian, J., Roux, S., Sauvage, D., & Lelord, G. (1990). The Behavioral Summarized Evaluation: Validity and reliability of a scale for the assessment of autistic behaviors. *Journal of Autism and Developmental Disorders*, 20, 189-204. ASSESSMENT PROCEDURES BEHAVIORAL SUMMARIZED EVALUATION AUTISM:

The BSE is a 20 item paper/pencil rating scale designed for the measurement of behavioral parameters which could be related to biological data in autistic children involved in educational programs, neurophysiological studies, and therapeutic trials. The results suggest that BSE is an acceptable tool for the assessment of autistic behaviors.-From Child Development Abstracts.

Bartlett, Elsa J. (1978). The acquisition of the meaning of color terms: A study of lexical development. In R. N. Campbell, & P. T. Smith (Eds), *Recent advances in the psychology of language*. New York, NY: Plenum. COLOR NAMES LEXICAL DEVELOPMENT:

Barton, David. (1992). The emergence of sounds: parallels between learning to read and learning to speak. In C. A. Ferguson, L. Menn, & C. Stoel-Gammon (Eds), *Phonological development: Models, research, implications*. Monkton, MD: York Press. LITERACY:

Bassano, Dominique, & Champaud, Christian. (1989). The argumentative connective 'meme' in French: an experimental study in eight- to ten-year-old children. *Journal of Child Language*, 16(3), 643-664. FRENCH CONNECTIVES RELATIONAL TERMS:

From Stockholm Bibliographies.

Bassano, Dominique, Hickmann, Maya, & Champaud, Christian. (1992). Epistemic modality in French children's discourse-to be sure or not to be sure. *Journal of Child Language*, 19, 389-413. FRENCH CHILDREN'S DISCOURSE:

Batchelor, Ervin S., Jnr, Kixmiller, Jeffrey S. , & Dean, Raymond S. (1990). Neuropsychological aspects of reading and spelling performance in children with learning disabilities. *Developmental Neuropsychology*, 6, 183-192. READING DISORDERS DYSLEXIA WRITTEN LANGUAGE:

Scores on the Halstead-Reitan Neuropsychological Battery and Wechsler Intelligence Scale for Children-Revised were regressed on both reading and spelling subtests of the Wide Range Achievement Test. The results showed 39% of reading and 33% of spelling variability was accounted for by neuropsychological functioning.

Bates, Elizabeth. (1990). Crosslinguistic study of aphasia. *Brain and Language*. APHASIAS CROSSLINGUISTIC STUDY-DISORDERS:

A special issue of Brain and Language.

Bates, Elizabeth, Camaioni, Luigia, & Volterra, Virginia. (1977). The Acquisition of performatives prior to speech. In M. S. Barbieri (Ed.), *Gli inizi del linguaggio: aspetti cognitivi e comunicativi (The emergence of language: cognitive and communicative aspects).*. La Nuova, Italy: Firenze. PERFORMATIVES PRELINGUISTICS ITALIAN:

Bates, Elizabeth, & MacWhinney, Brian. (1989). Functionalism and the competition model. In B. MacWhinney and E. Bates (Eds), *The crosslinguistic study of sentence processing*. New York: Cambridge University Press. COMPETITION MODEL:

Bates, Elizabeth, McDonald, Janet L., MacWhinney, Brian, & Appelbaum, M. (1991). A maximum likelihood procedure for the analysis of group and individual data in aphasia research. *Brain and Language*, 40, 231-265. METHODOLOGY-ANALYSIS APHASIAS:

Bates, Elizabeth, Thal, Donna, Fenson, Larry, Whitesell, Kimberly, & Oakes, Lisa M. (1989). Integrating language and gesture in infancy. *Developmental Psychology*, 25, 1004-1019. GESTURE FIRST WORDS:

Parental reports for 1-year-olds suggested that word comprehension and production are dissociated and that comprehension and production map onto districts aspects of gesture. Thirteen 15-month-olds were tested so the modeled gesture was accompanied by supportive, contradictory, or neutral narratives. Infants can use adult speech as an aid in reproduction of modeled gestures (comprehension mediation). Additional variance exists in gestural production that correlates with expressive vocabulary. -From Child Development Abstracts.

Bates, Elizabeth, Thal, Donna, & MacWhinney, Brian. (1991). A functionalist approach to language and its implications for assessment and intervention. In T. M. Gallagher, & N. Rees (Eds), *Pragmatics of language: Clinical practice issues*. San Diego, CA: Singular Group. COMPETITION MODEL ACQUISITION THEORIES PRAGMATIC DISORDERS:

A contrastive review of the competition model and other functionalist views. A discussion of the application of the competition model to language disorders.

Bates, Elizabeth, Thal, Donna, & Marchman, Virginia A. (1991). Symbols and syntax: a Darwinian approach to language development. In N. A. Krasnegor, et al. (Eds), *Biological and behavioral determinants of language development*. Hillsdale, NJ: Lawrence Erlbaum Associates. GESTURE SYMBOL DEVELOPMENT SYNTACTIC DEVELOPMENT LANGUAGE PRECURSORS PRELINGUISTCIS:

Bateson, M. C. (1975). Mother-infant exchanges: The epigenesis of conversational interaction. In D. Aaronson, & R. W. Rieben (Eds), *Annals of the New York Academy of Sciences, #263*. New York, NY: New York Academy of Sciences. ADULT-CHILD INTERACTION PRELINGUISTICS SOCIAL INTERACTION HYPOTHESIS INTERSUBJECTIVITY:

Bauer, Patricia J., & Mandler, Jean M. (1989). Taxonomies and triads: conceptual organization in one-to two-year-olds. *Cognitive Psychology*, 21(2), 156-184. CATEGORIZATION CONCEPT DEVELOPMENT SEMANTIC ORGANIZATION:

Baum, S. R., & Waldstein, R. S. (1991). Perseveratory coarticulation in the speech of profoundly hearing-impaired and normally hearing children. *Journal of Speech and Hearing Research*, 34, 1286-1292. COARTICULATION ARTICULATION DEAF CHILDREN:

Bavin, Edith L. (1985). Issues in first language acquisition research. *Australian Review of Applied Linguistics*, 8(2), 13-26. METHODOLOGY ACQUISITION THEORY:

Bavin, Edith L. (1987). Anaphora in children's Warlpiri. *Australian Review of Applied Linguistics*, 10(2), 1-11. WARLPIRI ANAPHORA:

Bavin, Edith L. (1988). Teaching Warlpiri as a community language. In E. L. Bavin & L. Wales (Eds), *Languages programs in primary schools: Some Australian experiences*. Geelong, Australia: Deakin University Press. WARLPIRI L2 EDUCATION BILINGUALISM-EDUCATION WARLPIRI-ENGLISH ENGLISH-WARLPIRI LANGUAGE AND EDUCATION:

Bavin, Edith L. (1989). Some lexical and morphological changes in Warlpiri. In N. Dorian (Ed.), *Studies in language death and contraction*. Cambridge, MA: Cambridge University Press. WARLPIRI LANGUAGE CHANGE:

Bavin, Edith L. (1990). Locative terms and Warlpiri acquisition. *Journal of Child Language*, 17, 43-66. WARLPIRI LOCATIVES RELATIONAL TERMS ORIENTATIONAL TERMS:

A series of tests examining children's use of the equivalent expressions in Warlpiri for the English terms: 'in, on, under, in front of, behind' and 'between.' The results indicate that locative case forms are first used without the more specific locative nominal. 'Between' is understood before 'front' and 'behind', and children aged 4:0-5:0 do not understand that 'front- behind' is unidimensional. The use of features on a referent for orientational purposes does not develop before about 6:0, but the orientation of the referent itself in addition to its features) may affect interpretation.

Bavin, Edith L. (1992). The acquisition of Warlpiri. In D. I. Slobin (Ed.), *The crosslinguistic study of language acquisition* . Hillsdale, NJ: Lawrence Erlbaum Associates. WARLPIRI:

Bavin, Edith L., & Shopen, Timothy A. (1985). Warlpiri and English: Languages in contact. In M. Clyne (Ed.), *Australia; Meeting place of languages*. Canberra: Pacific Linguistics. WARLPIRI-ENGLISH ENGLISH-WARLPIRI BILINGUALISM-LANGUAGE CONTACT:

Bavin, Edith L., & Shopen, Timothy A. (1985). Warlpiri children's development of narrative: The social context of language acquistion in an aboriginal community. *Language in Aboriginal Australia.*, 11, 1-13. WARLPIRI NARRATIVES ABORIGINES CROSSLINGUISTIC STUDY:

Bavin, Edith L., & Shopen, Timothy A. (1987). Innovations and neutralizations in the Warlpiri pronominal system. *Journal of Linguistics*, 23, 149-175. WARLPIRI PRONOUNS LANGUAGE CHANGE:

Bavin, Edith L., & Shopen, Timothy A. (1989). Warlpiri children's processing of transitive sentences. In E. Bates, & B. MacWhinney (Eds), *Crosslinguistic studies of sentence processing*. Cambridge, MA: Cambridge University Press. WARLPIRI LANGUAGE PROCESSING BILINGUALISM-LANGUAGE PROCESSING COMPLEX SENTENCES VERBS-TRANSITIVE:

Bavin, Edith L., & Shopen, Timothy A. (1990). Warlpiri in the 80's: An overview of research into language variation and child language. In S. Romaine (Ed.), *Language of Australia*. Cambridge, MA: Cambridge University Press. WARLPIRI VARIATION SOCIOLINGUISTIC FACTORS:

Beal, Carole R. (1990). Development of knowledge about the role of inference in text comprehension. *Child Development*, 61, 1011-1023. IMPLICATURE:

First, second, and third-grade children were presented with stories in which the physical cause of a target event was described explicitly, implied, or not mentioned. Sometimes children judged whether they had inferred the cause or if it had been explicitly mentioned. For stories with implicit causes, first and second-grade children tended to report that the cause had been explicitly mentioned, while third-graders correctly reported that the causes were inferred.

Beal, Carole R. (1990). The development of text evaluation and revision skills. *Child Development*, 61, 247-258. LITERACY WRITTEN LANGUAGE TEXT/STORY GRAMMARS DISCOURSE DEVELOPMENT:

Fourth-grade and sixth-grade students were asked to evaluate 3 types of problematic texts and suggest changes. Others were asked whether 4 types of revisions improved the comprehensibility of problematic stories. Older children detected more of the text problems. When younger children spontaneously detected a text problem they were as likely as older children to revise the text adequately. Younger children were less able to revise text problems that they had originally overlooked. Younger children overestimated the informativeness of several types of revisions. - From Child Development Abstracts.

Beal, Carole R., & Belgrad, Susan L. (1990). The development of message evaluation skills in young children. *Child Development*, 61, 705-712. COMMUNICATIVE COMPETENCE AMBIGUITY:

Children (4:0-8:0) evaluated the communicative quality of informative, ambiguous, and ineffective picture messages in a communication game. Younger children tended to overestimate the informativeness of ambiguous and ineffective messages. Older children were more successful at evaluating the message quality. Younger children recognized the ambiguity more when they were not aware of the target reference.

Bebko, James M., & McKinnon, Elaine E. (1990). The language experience of deaf children: Its relation to spontaneous rehearsal in a memory task. *Child Development*, 61, 1744-1752. DEAF CHILDREN LANGUAGE AND MEMORY:

A lag of several years was noted in the emergence of spontaneous rehearsal for the deaf in an empirical study.

Language history was a nearly perfect mediator of the relation between the age and rehearsal use.

Bebout, L., & Arthur, B. (1992). Cross-cultural attitudes toward speech disorders. *Journal of Speech and Hearing Research*, 35, 45-52. CROSSCULTURAL STUDY LANGUAGE DISORDERS CULTURAL FACTORS:

Bechtel, William. (1993). Knowing how to use language: Developing a rapprochement between two theoretical traditions. In L. M. Herman, H. L. Roitblat, & P. E. Nachtigall (Eds), *Language and communication: Comparative perspectives*. Hillsdale, NJ: Lawrence Erlbaum Associates. ACQUISITION THEORIES ACQUISITION AND LINGUISTIC THEORY:

Bechtel, William, & Abrahamsen, Adele A. (1991). *Connectionism and the mind: An introduction to parallel processing in networks*. Cambridge, MA: Basil Blackwell. CONNECTIONISM:

An introductory text which examines the application of connectionist models (parallel distributed processing models and neural networks) to both philosophical and psychological theories of the mind.

Becker, Joseph. (1989). Preschoolers' use of number words to denote one-on- one correspondence. *Child Development*, 60, 1147-1157. NUMERALS LANGUAGE AND COGNITIVE DEVELOPMENT:

Children matched 2 sets to determine whether they could be put in one-to-one correspondence and then judged whether the same number word should be used for both. Then children counted 2 sets and used the final number words of the count to determine whether the sets could be put in one-to-one correspondence. Most 4-year-olds and some 3:6-year-olds use number words to denote one-to-one correspondence in each task.-From Child Development Abstracts.

Beckwith, Richard T. (1991). The language of emotions, the emotions, and nominalist bootstrapping. In D. Frye, & C. Moore (Eds), *Children's theories of mind*. Hillsdale, NJ: Lawrence Erlbaum Associates. THEORY OF MIND LANGUAGE AND AFFECT BOOTSTRAPPING:

Beckwith, Richard T., Fellbaum, C., Gross, D., & Miller, George A. (1991). WordNet: a lexical database organized on psycholinguistic principles. In U. Zernik (Ed.), *Lexical acquisition: Exploiting on-line resources to build a lexicon*. Hillsdale, NJ: Lawrence Erlbaum Associates. LEXICAL DEVELOPMENT CONNECTIONISM COMPUTER SIMULATIONS:

Beech, John. (1985). *Learning to read: a cognitive approach to reading and poor reading*. San Diego, CA: Singular Publishing Group. LITERACY READING DISORDERS DYSLEXIA:

Introduction. Dyslexia and the incidence of reading problems. Teaching children to learn to read. Cognitive factors behind poor reading. Developmental and biological factors behind poor reading. Evironmental factors behind poor reading. The theory anmd practice of learning to read. References. Author index. Subject index. Appendix.

Beertema, A., Koetsenruyter, P., Postama, P., & de Saint Aulaire, R. (1980). Deafness and speech motor aspects (in Dutch). *Logopedie en Foniatrie*, 52, 146-160. DEAF CHILDREN LANGUAGE AND MOTOR DEVELOPMENT ARTICULATION: DUTCH

Analysis of rate of diadochokinesis in two groups of deaf children with emphasis on regularity of the movement.

Behrend, Douglas A. (1990). The development of verb concepts: Children's use of verbs to label familiar and novel events. *Child Development*, 61, 705-712. VERBS:

Three year olds used action verbs more frequently than older children and adults and showed a preference for them over result verbs. Reflecting the use of older children and adults, the instrument verb was most often used as a first response.

Beilin, Harry, & Pufall, Peter B. (1992). *Piaget's theory: prospects and possibilities*. Hillsdale, NJ: Lawrence Erlbaum Associates. PIAGETIAN THEORY NEOPIAGETIAN THEORY:

The twentieth anniversary volume of the Jean Piaget Society sets out how the theory has developed and its implications for current research.

Beitchman, Joseph H., Hood, Jane, & Inglis, Alison. (1990). Psychiatric risk in children with speech and language disorders. *Journal of Abnormal Child Psychology*, 18, 282-296. AT-RISK CHILDREN LANGUAGE DISORDERS PSYCHOPATHOLOGICAL CHILDREN:

Language disordered children appear to be at some risk of developing psychiatric disorders, and females are at greater risk than males.

Bell, M. A., & Fox, N. A. (1992). The relations between frontal brain electrical activity and cognitive development during infancy. *Child Development*, 63, 1142-1163. NEUROLINGUISTICS LANGUAGE AND COGNITIVE DEVELOPMENT:

Bellugi, Ursula. (1991). Brain organization underlying dissociations of language and cognition. In M. Gunner, & C. Nelson (Eds), *Developmental behavioral neuroscience*. Hillsdale, NJ: Lawrence Erlbaum Associates. NEUROLINGUISTICS CEREBRAL DISORDERS CENTRAL LANGUAGE DISORDERS:

Bellugi, Ursula, Bihrle, A., & Corina, D. (1991). Linguistic and spatial development: dissociations between cognitive domains. In N. A. Krasnegor, et al. (Eds), *Biological and behavioral determinants of language development*. Hillsdale, NJ: Lawrence Erlbaum Associates. SIGNING:

Bellugi, Ursula, Blumstein, Sheila E., Fodor, J., Mann, V., & Samuel, A. (1990). The modularity of speech and language. In I. G. Mattingly, & M. Studdert-Kennedy (Eds), *Modularity and the motor theory of speech perception*. Hillsdale, NJ: Lawrence Erlbaum Associates. MODULARITY:

Bendell-Estroff, Debra, Greenfield, Daryl B., Hogan, Anne E., & Claussen, Angelika H. (1989). Early assessment of sensorimotor and cognitive development in high-risk infants. *Journal of Pediatric Psychology*, 14, 549-557. ASSESSMENT PROCEDURES BAYLEY SCALES:

Eighty eight infants at risk for mental retardation on the Bayley Scales of Infant Development and a measure of visual recognition memory at three months corrected age were assessed. At three months of age the Bayley scales and the measure of visual recognition memory were not significantly correlated. Both measures, however, showed significant correlation to the Bayley scales administered at 1 year of age.-From Child Development Abstracts.

Benelli, Beatrice, D'Odorico, Laura, Levorato, Maria C., & Simion, Francesca. (1977). Formation and extension of a concept in a prelinguistic child. *Giornale Italiano di Psicologia*, 4, 429-448.
CONCEPT DEVELOPMENT PRELINGUISTICS: ITALIAN

A case study of concept formation in a prelinguistic child.

Benelli, Beatrice, D'Odorico, Laura, Levorato, Maria C., & Simion, Francesca. (1980). *Formedi conoscenza prelinguistica e linguistica. (Linguistic and prelinguistic knowledge.).* Florence, Italy: Giunti.
PRELINGUISTICS LABELING VOCALIZATIONS: ITALIAN

Experimental studies of: concept formation, the communicative functions of prelinguistic vocalizations, and labelling.

Benton, Shlomo, Deutsch, Avital, & Liberman, Isabelle Y. (1990). Syntactic competence and reading ability in children. *Journal of Experimental Child Psychology*, 49, 147-172. READING DISORDERS SYNTACTIC DEFICIT HYPOTHESIS:

The effect of syntactic context on auditory word identification and on the ability to detect and correct syntactic errors in speech was examined in severely reading disabled children and in good and poor readers selected from the normal distribution of fourth graders. The results suggest that the severely disabled readers were inferior to both good and poor readers in syntactic awareness and inability to use syntactic rules, while poor readers were equal to good readers in syntactic awareness but were relatively impaired in using syntactic knowledge productively. - From Child Development Abstracts.

Berczyné, Somogyi V., & Gerebenné, Várbíró K. (1989). A Marianne Frostig féle vizuális percepciótvizsgálóteszt müködésére vonatkozó tapasztalatok 5 éves gyermekeknél. (Experiences with the Frostig test for 5-year-old children). In V. K. Gerebenné & T. Vidakovich (Eds), *A differenciált beiskolázás nehány méröeszköze.* Budapest: Akadémiai. ASSESSMENT PROCEDURES FROSTIG TEST HUNGARIAN: HUNGARIAN

Berg, T. (1992). Phonological harmony as a processing problem. *Journal of Child Language*, 19 , 225-257. HARMONY LANGUAGE PROCESSING PHONOLOGICAL DEVELOPMENT:

Berghout Austin, Ann M., & Braeger, T. J. (1990). Gendered differences in parents' encouragement of sibling interaction: Implications for the construction of a personal premise system. *First Language*, 10, 181-197. PARENTAL SPEECH-SEX DIFFERENCES SEX DIFFERENCES LANGUAGE AND SOCIAL TRANSMISSION SIBLING EFFECTS:

Fathers' and mothers' encouragement of sibling interaction was examined in two-child families. Fathers' and mothers' own linguistic behavior as well as their encouragement of their children's behavior reflected gender- specific patterns with fathers demonstrating as well as encouraging more accomodative or agentic patterns and mothers demonstrating as well as encouraging more assimilative or communion-enhancing patterns.

Berk, Laura E., & Potts, Michael K. (1991). Developmental and functional significance of private speech among Attention-Deficit Hyperactive Disordered and normal boys. *Journal of Abnormal Child Psychology*, 19, 357-377. REGULATIVE FUNCTION OF SPEECH PRIVATE SPEECH INNER SPEECH VYGOTSKYAN THEORY:

Comparison of the development of private speech in normal and disordered populations showed that ADHD children were delayed in private speech development. They engaged in more externalized, self-guiding speech than inner, private speech. Subjects on medication showed a substantially increased maturity in their use of private speech. From Child Development Abstracts.

Berkell, Diane E. (Ed.). (1992). *Autism: Identification, education, and treatment, vol.*. Hillsdale, NJ: Lawrence Erlbaum Associates. AUTISM INTERVENTION PROGRAMS ASSESSMENT PROCEDURES LANGUAGE AND EDUCATION:

A collection of papers from 12 experts on autism which aims to provide the reader with information on the extent of the syndrome, the diagnosis of autism, treatment programs, and the education of autistic children.

Berko-Gleason, Jean, Perlmann, R., Ely, R., & Evans, D. (1993). The baby-talk register: Parents' use of diminutives. In J. L. Sokolov, & C. E. Snow (Eds), *Handbook of research in language development using CHILDES*. Hillsdale, NJ: Lawrence Erlbaum Associates. PARENTAL SPEECH-STYLE METHODOLOGY-ANALYSIS METHODOLOGY-COMPUTERS CHILDES:

Berkson, Gershon. (1993). *Children with handicaps: A review of behavioral research*. Hillsdale, NJ: Lawrence Erlbaum Associates. HANDICAPPED CHILDREN LANGUAGE AND PLAY DEVELOPMENTAL DISORDERS INTERVENTION PROGRAMS:

Berlin, Charles I. (1984). *Hearing science: Recent advances*. San Diego, CA: Singular Publishing Group. AUDIOLOGY:

Comparative psychoacoustics: new directions. Developmental mechanisms of mammalian inner ear formation. Recent advances toward understanding auditory system development. Neurotransmitters of the cochlea and lateral line organ. Anatomical measures of physiological parameters in the cochlea. Inner ear function based on the mechanical tuning of the hair cells. Functional roles of the inner-and-outer-hair-cell subsystems in the cochlea and brainstem. Speech encoding in the auditory nerve. Cochlear implants. Neurotransmitters of the auditory nerve and central auditory system. The structual basis for stimulus coding in the cochlear nucleus of the cat. Response characteristics of neurons of the cochlear nuclei. Asymmetries in evoked potentials. Author index. Subject index.

Berman, Ruth A. (1990). On acquiring an (S)VO language - subjectless sentences in children's Hebrew. *Linguistics*, 28(6), 1135-1166. NULL SUBJECTS HEBREW SYNTACTIC STRUCTURES:

Berman, Ruth A., & Clark, Eve V. (1989). Learning to use compounds for contrast. *First Language*, 9, 247-270. CONTRAST-SEMANTIC HEBREW COMPOUNDS PREPOSITIONS RELATIVIZATION:

> This study investigated children's ability to produce compounds by asking them to label contrasting subcategories as distinct from generic categories. 60 Hebrew speakers (2:0 to 7:4), and 12 adults, answered questions about a series of picture sets. Adults and older children produced compound nouns as labels for subcategories, and favored one-word labels for generic categories. Two and three year olds produced mostly inappropriate, one-word labels for both levels of categories. But children's subcategory labels, whether compound or nouns with relative clause or prepositional phrase adjuncts, consistently included a dimension contrast, while their generic category labels mentioned the absence of such a dimension.-From Child Development Abstracts.

Bernstein-Ratner, Nan. (1992). Measurable outcomes of instructions to modify normal parent-child verbal interactions: Implications for indirect stuttering therapy. *Journal of Speech and Hearing Research*, 35, 14-20. INTERVENTION PROGRAMS FOR PARENTS STUTTERING:

Bernstein-Ratner, Nan. (1993). Phonological analysis of children's speech. In J. L. Sokolov, & C. E. Snow (Eds), *Handbook of research in language development using CHILDES*. Hillsdale, NJ: Lawrence Erlbaum Associates. PHONOLOGICAL DEVELOPMENT METHODOLOGY-ANALYSIS METHODOLOGY-COMPUTERS CHILDES:

Bernthal, John E., Beukelman, David R., Healy, E. Charles, Kenyon, Karen K., & Stuart, Sheela L. (1991). Dysarthria followings Reye's syndrome: A case report. In C. A. Moore, K. M. Yorkston, & D. R. Beukleman (Eds), *Dysarthria and apraxia of speech*. Baltimore, MD: Paul H. Brookes. DYSARTHRIA REYE'S SYNDROME:

Berry, V. (1992). Communication priorities and strategies for the mainstreamed child with hearing loss. *Volta Review*, 94, 29-36. DEAF CHILDREN LANGUAGE AND EDUCATION:

Bertelson, P., & de Gelder, B. (1991). The emergence of phonological awareness: Comparative approaches. In I. G. Mattingly, & M. Studdert-Kennedy (Eds), *Modularity and the motor theory of speech perception*. Hillsdale, NJ: Lawrence Erlbaum Associates. PHONOLOGICAL DEVELOPMENT ACQUISITION THEORIES-PHONOLOGICAL METALINGUISTICS:

Berthoud-Papandropoulou, Ioanna. (1979). L'élaboration du concept de mot chez l'enfant. (The elaboration of the concept of the word by the child.). *Éducateur*, 13, 362-365. LEXICAL DEVELOPMENT CONCEPT DEVELOPMENT: FRENCH

Berthoud-Papandropoulou, Ioanna. (1987). L'élaboration du concept de traducteur chez les enfants de 4 à 9 ans. (The elaboration of the concept of translation by children aged 4-9 years.). *Cahiers du Departement des Langues et des Sciences du Langage Université de Lausanne*, 5, 19-29. BILINGUALISM-EDUCATION: FRENCH

Berthoud-Papandropoulou, Ioanna. (1990). Comment les enfants entre quatre et dix ans s'y prennent pour produire des énonces qu'ils considérent comme déviants? (How do children between four and ten produce utterances that they consider ungrammatical?). *Bulletin CILA*, 51, 83-91. GRAMMATICALITY: FRENCH

Berthoud-Papandropoulou, Ioanna, & Kilcher, H. (1985). The concept of operation: A comparison between the Piagetian perspective and the UNITYP linguistic approach. In H. Seiler, & G. Brettschneider (Eds), *Language invariants and mental operations*. Tubingen, Germany: Gunter Narr. PIAGETIAN THEORY:

Berthoud-Papandropoulou, Ioanna, & Kilcher, H. (1987). Que faire quand on me did de dire? L'enfant messager des paroles d'autrui dans une situation de communication: recherche exploratoire. (What do you do when someone tells you to talk? The child as a carrier of other people's utterances in a communicative situation.). *Archives de Psychologie*, 55, 219-239. COMMUNICATIVE COMPETENCE CHILDREN'S SUMMARIES: FRENCH

Berthoud-Papandropoulou, Ioanna, Kilcher, H., & Veneziano, Edy. (1989). What can children do with utterances? Linguistic and metalinguistic activities: Theory, methods and results. *Cahiers de la Fondation Archives Jean Piaget*, 10, METALINGUISTICS:

Berthoud-Papandropoulou, Ioanna, & Mello, D. (1985). Was macht ein Übersetzer? Ideen des Kindes über die Tätigkeit des Übersetzens. (What makes a translator? Children's ideas about the activity of translations.). In T. B. Seiler, & W. Wannenmacher (Eds), *Begriffs-und Wortbedeutungsentwicklung.*. Berlin: Springer Verlag. LEXICAL DEVELOPMENT SEMANTIC DEVELOPMENT CONCEPT DEVELOPMENT BILINGUALISM: GERMAN

Berthoud-Papandropoulou, Ioanna, & Othenin-Girard, C. (1978). Quelques aspects du raisonnement chez des adolescents récemment immigrés à Geneve et mal scolarisés. (Some aspects of reasoning in children recently immigrated to Geneva with low scholastic performance.). *Bulletin CILA*, 27, 10-22. LANGUAGE AND EDUCATION ACCULTURATION: FRENCH

Berthoud-Papandropoulou, Ioanna, & Othenin-Girard, C. (1983). L'étude génétique des subordonnées: Propositions méthodologiques. (Genetic study of subordination: Methodological proposals.). In J. P. Bronckart, E. M. Kail, & J. Noizet (Eds), *Psycholinguistique de l'enfant: Recherches sur l'acquisition du langage.* Neuchatel, France: Delachaux & Niestle. SUBORDINATION METHODOLOGY CATEGORIZATION: FRENCH

Berthoud-Papandropoulou, Ioanna, & Sinclair, Hermina. (1974). What is a word? Experimental study of children's ideas on grammar. *Human Development*, 17, 214-258. LEXICAL DEVELOPMENT PIAGETIAN THEORY METALINGUISTICS:

Berthoud-Papandropoulou, Ioanna, & Sinclair, Hermina. (1978). L'expression d'éventualités et de conditions chez l'enfant. (Children's expression of eventualities and conditions.). *Archives de Psychologie*, 46, 205-233. CONDITIONALS CONTINGENCY: FRENCH

Berthoud-Papandropoulou, Ioanna, & Veneziano, Edy. (1989). La signification énonciatif dans les débuts du langage. (Vocalization at the onset of language.). *Archives de Psychologie*, 57, 271-281. INTENTIONALITY PRELINGUISTICS VOCALIZATIONS: FRENCH

Besner, Derek, & Humphreys, Glyn. (1991). *Basic processes in reading-Visual word recognition*. Hillsdale, NJ: Lawrence Erlbaum Associates. LITERACY CONNECTIONISM:

The chapters in this book span the range of reading processes from early visual analysis to semantic influences on word identification, thus providing a state-of-the-art summary of current work and offering important contributions to prospective reading research. The book examines both future plans and past accomplishments in the world of word identification research. Three chapters provide a futuristic view taking a parallel distributed processing approach to semantic priming, phonology, and the identification of old words and the learning of new words. Reviews on eye movements in reading and semantic priming on word identification provide a retrospective summary of work on these issues as well as solid pointers for future investigations. Other chapters provide new demonstrations of the importance of phonological contributions to word identification, of interactive processes in the identification of handwritten words, and a re-evaluation of the processes involved in the neuropsychological syndrome described as 'letter-by-letter' reading. This is a key reference for courses in visual information processing in general, and reading in particular.

Bettinghaus, E. P., & Selnow, G. W. (1982). Television exposure and language development. *Journal of Broadcasting*, 26, 469-479. TELEVISION AND LANGUAGE DEVELOPMENT:

Beukelman, David R., & Yorkston, Kathryn M. (1991). *Communication disorders following traumatic brain injury: Management of cognitive, language and motor impairments*. San Diego, CA: Singular Group. TRAUMATIC DISORDERS MOTOR DISORDERS INTERVENTION PROGRAMS ASSESSMENT PROCEDURES LANGUAGE AND MEMORY:

Bever, Thomas G. (1992). The logical and extrinsic sources of modularity. In M. R. Gunnar, & M. Maratsos (Eds), *Modularity and constraints in language and cognition*. Hillsdale, NJ: Lawrence Erlbaum Associates. MODULARITY CONSTRAINTS:

Beveridge, Michael, & Conti-Ramsden, Gina. (1987). *Children with language disabilities*. Milton Keynes: Open University Press. LANGUAGE DISORDERS: PORTUGUESE SPANISH FRENCH GERMAN

Reprinted in 1990 in several languages including English, French, German and Portuguese.

Beveridge, Michael, & Conti-Ramsden, Gina. (1987). Social cognition and problem-solving in persons with mental retardation. *Australian and New Zealand Journal of Developmental Disabilities*, 13, 99-106. RETARDED CHILDREN LANGUAGE AND COGNITIVE DEVELOPMENT:

Beveridge, Michael, Conti-Ramsden, Gina, & Leudar, I. (1989). *Language and communication in mentally handicapped people*. London, UK: Routledge, Chapman and Hall. RETARDED CHILDREN ATYPICAL DEVELOPMENT:

Beveridge, Michael, & Marsh, Lesley. (1991). The influence of linguistic context on young children's understanding of homophonic words. *Journal of Child Language*, 18, 459-467. POLYSEMY AMBIGUITY CONTEXT:

An examination of children's comprehension of homophones in two contexts showed that children provided with an expanded version with full linguistic details and explanations of the words it contained were more readily able to identify the meaning of the homophone than children provided with less contextual and linguistic information. Age and type of story impacted on the results. - From Child Development Abstracts.

Bialystok, Ellen. (1990). *Communication strategies in second language acquisition*. Oxford, England: Blackwell. L2/L1 ACQUISITION L2 ACQUISITION STRATEGIES L2 COMMUNICATION STRATEGIES L2 EDUCATION:

How do learners manage when their command of language is limited? The tecniques and approximations they use are known as communication strategies. Understanding these strategies adds to our knowledge of linguistic structure and psychological processing. It also adds significantly to the practical business of language teaching. In this book Bialystok addresses central issues in the study of communication strategies. How can we determine when language use is strategic? How are strategies best conceptualized and classified? Can communication strategies be taught? Is there any advantage in doing so? In answering such theoretical and practical questions, Bialystok places her subject firmly within the broader framework of language processing, adding to our understanding of both first and second language acquisition.

Bialystok, Ellen. (1991). *Language processing in bilingual children*. New York, NY: Cambridge University Press. LANGUAGE PROCESSING BILINGUALISM-LANGUAGE PROCESSING BILINGUALISM-EDUCATION BILINGUALISM-LANGUAGE POLICY:

This book is a collection of papers that explore the ways in which bilingual children cope with two language systems. The papers address issues in linguistics, psychology, and education that bear on the abilities that bilingual children use to understand language, to perform highly specialized operations with language, and to function in school settings. All the papers provide detailed analysis about how specific problems are solved, how bilingualism influences those solutions, and how social conflict affects the process. Finally, the implications of those findings for policy setting and the development of bilingual education programs are explored.

Bialystok, Ellen. (1991). Letters, sounds, and symbols: Changes in children's understanding of written language. *Applied Psycholinguistics*, 12, 75-89. WRITTEN LANGUAGE:

Children between 3-5 years who knew the alphabet but could not read were given three tasks. Although all the children had explicit knowledge of letters and sounds, they lacked symbolic knowledge of how letters represent sounds.

Bialystok, Ellen, & Niccols, Alison. (1989). Children's control over attention to phonological and semantic properties of words. *Journal of Psycholinguistic Research*, 18, 369-387. SEMANTICS AND PHONOLOGY SEMANTIC MAPPING LEXICAL DEVELOPMENT REPRESENTATIONS-PHONOLOGICAL REPRESENTATIONS-SEMANTIC PHONOLOGICAL PATTERNS WORD RECOGNITION:

Children aged 5:0 to 9:0 were asked to match words either against their meaning or against their sounds. Although all of the children were capable of paying attention to both aspects of the word, younger children were unable to select the focus of their attention when they were distracted. Under the same conditions, older children showed a bias for the phonological form when distracted and only the oldest children could attend to both meaning and sound when distracted.

Bideau, Jacqueline, Meljac, Claire, & Fischer, Jean-Paul. (1992). *Pathways to number: Children's developing numerical abilities*. Hillsdale, NJ: Lawrence Erlbaum Associates. NUMERALS:

Bigler, Erin D. (1990). *Traumatic brain injury*. San Diego, CA: Singular Publishing Group. TRAUMATIC DISORDERS:

Neuropathology of traumatic brain injury. Epidemiology of traumatic brain injury. Incidence, clinical characteristics, and risk factors. Epidemiology of traumatic brain injury in adults. Neuropsychological assessment of traumatic brain injury in adults. Cognitive dysfunction and psychoeducational assessment in traumatic brain injury. Disorders of communication in traumatic brain injury. Neuropsychiatric evaluation and treatment of traumatic brain injury. Behavioral change strategies for children and adolescents with traumatic brain injury. Management of academic and educational problems in traumatic brain injury. Recovery and cognitive retraining after traumatic brain injury. Effective traumatic brain injury rehabilitation: team/patient interaction. Psychotherapy and neurospychological assessment after brain injury. Disorders of attention and their treatment in traumatic injury rehabilitation. Acquisition and domain-specific knowledge in patients with organic memory disorders. Chronic emotional, social, and physical changes after traumatic brain injury. Family issues in traumatic brain injury. Legal challanges in traumatic brain injury. Author index. Subject index.

Bijou, Sidney W. (1989). Psychological linguistics: Implications for a theory of individual development and a method for research. In H. W. Reese (Ed.), *Advances in child development and behavior*. New York, NY: Academic Press. METHODOLOGY:

Birdsong, D. (1992). Ultimate attainment in second language acquisition. *Language*, 68, 706-755. L2 ACQUISITION L2 VARIATION L2 COMMUNICATIVE COMPETENCE:

Bishop, Dorothy V. M. (1990). *Handedness and developmental disorders*. New York, NY: Camridge/MacKeith. AUTISM LATERALIZATION DEVELOPMENTAL DISORDERS LANGUAGE AND HANDEDNESS CEREBRAL DISORDERS:

Comprehensive account of the development of handedness and its relationship to lateralization which also reviews the connections between handedness and developmental disorders such as epilepsy, autism, retardation, and speech/language disorders.

Bishop, Dorothy V. M., & Adams, C. (1990). A prospective study of the relationship between specific language impairment, phonological disorders and reading retardation. *Journal of Child Psychology and Psychiatry*, 31, 1027-1050. READING DISORDERS PHONOLOGICAL DISORDERS SPECIFIC LANGUAGE IMPAIRMENT:

Language and literacy skills were assessed in 8 1/2-year-olds whose language development had been impaired at 4 years of age. Provided that language problems had vbeen resolved by age 5 1/2 years, literacy development was normal, but many of the children who still had verbal deficits at 5 1/2 years of age did have reading difficulties and persisting oral language impairments later on.

Bishop, Dorothy V. M., & Adams, C. (1991). What do referential communication tasks measure-a study of children with specific language impairment. *Applied Psycholinguistics*, 12, 199-215. SPECIFIC LANGUAGE IMPAIRMENT REFERENTIAL COMMUNICATION ASSESSMENT PROCEDURES:

Bishop, Dorothy V. M., & Adams, C. (1992). Comprehension problems in children with specific language impairment-literal and inferential meaning. *Journal of Speech and Hearing Research*, 35, 119-129. COMPREHENSION DISORDERS IMPLICATURE SPECIFIC LANGUAGE IMPAIRMENT:

Bishop, Julie, Knights, Robert M., & Stoddart, Clare. (1990). Rey Auditory-Verbal learning Test: Performance of English and French children aged 5 to 16. *Clinical Neuropsychologist*, 4, 133-140. ASSESSMENT PROCEDURES REY AUDITORY-VERBAL LEARNING TEST CROSSLINGUISTIC STUDY FRENCH:

> Rey Auditory-Verbal learning Test performance by 252 patients between the ages of 5:0 and 16:0 showed a high positive correlation between the test result and age, and a moderate one with IQ.

Bisping, Rudolph, Steingrueber, Hans J., Oltmann, Martine, & Wenk, Christine. (1990). Adults' tolerance of cries: An experimental investigation of acoustic features. *Child Development*, 61, 1218-1229. CRYING:

> Experimental manipulation of 3 acoustic features of the cry (fundamental frequency, intonation, spectral complexity) and of the information given to subjects about the infants' health status were varied. Medical were allowed to control the sound pressure level. For the original cry version, the accepted sound level pressure decreased as fundamental frequency increased. Listener's reaction to certain physical cry characteristics can be altered substantially by inducing different cognitive sets.

Bittera, Tiborné. (1986). Az akadályozott beszéd fejlödésü gyermekek terápiájának sokrétüsége (Multiple therapy in speech retardation.). *Gyógypedagógiai Szemle*, 4, 10-12. INTERVENTION PROGRAMS LANGUAGE DELAY HUNGARIAN: HUNGARIAN

Bivens, Jennifer A., & Berk, Laura E. (1990). A longitudinal study of the development of elementary school children's private speech. *Merrill-Palmer Quarterly*, 36, 443-463. INNER SPEECH PRIVATE SPEECH VYGOTSKYAN THEORY REGULATIVE FUNCTION OF SPEECH:

A three year study of the development of inner speech with regard to mathematical problems in the first three grades. Results conform to Vygotskyan expectations. From Child Development Abstracts.

Bjorck-Akesson, E., & Brodin, Jane. (1990). *Forskning om alternativ kommunikation i Holland och Kanada. (Research in alternative communication in Holland and Canada.).* Umea University. INTERVENTION PROGRAMS BLISS SYMBOLS SIGNING RETARDED CHILDREN: SWEDISH

This report is a compilation from a round table discussion and workshop on alternative and augmentative communication with participants from Canada, Holland, Norway, and Sweden. The workshop took place in Hoensbroek, Holland, in October 1989. The aim was to exchange experiences within this area and to discuss how researchers from different countries can meet and cooperate.JB

Bjorklund, David F. (1990). *Children's strategies: Contemporary views of cognitive development.* Hillsdale, NJ: Lawrence Erlbaum Associates. COGNITIVE DEVELOPMENT:

Blake, J., & de Boysson-Bardies, Bénédicte. (1992). Patterns in babbling-a cross-linguistic study. *Journal of Child Language*, 19, 51-74. BABBLING CROSSLINGUISTIC STUDY-PHONOLOGY:

Blanken, G., Dittman, J., Grimm, Hannelore, Marshall, John C., & Wallesch, C. (1993). *Linguistic disorders and pathologies: An international handbook.* Berlin: De Gruyter. LANGUAGE DISORDERS CLASSIFICATION OF DISORDERS DEVELOPMENTAL DISORDERS APHASIAS:

Bleile, Kenneth M. (1991). *Child phonology: A book of exercises for students.* San Diego, CA: Singular Group. METHODOLOGY-ANALYSIS METHODOLOGY-TRANSCRIPTION PHONOLOGICAL DEVELOPMENT:

A workbook to accompany introductory courses in phonological development and speech pathology.

Bleile, Kenneth M., & Tomblin, J. Bruce. (1991). Regressions in the phonological development of 2 children. *Journal of Psycholinguistic Research*, 20, 483-499. PHONOLOGICAL DEVELOPMENT UNLEARNING:

Blewitt, Pamela, & Toppino, Thomas C. (1991). The development of taxonomic structure in lexical memory. *Journal Of Experimental Child Psychiatry*, 51, 296-319. LANGUAGE AND MEMORY CATEGORIZATION LEXICAL DEVELOPMENT:

Subjects in five different cue conditions were presented with same to-be-remembered (TBR) items. In different conditions, cues were related to the TBR items either schematically (zoo-elephant) or taxonomically. Schematic and superordinate cues were most effective in aiding recall, and coordinate cues were least effective. The relative strength of different relationships, as reflected in cued recall performance, does not appear to change with age.

Bloodstein, O. (1990). On pluttering, skivering, and floggering-a commentary. *Journal of Speech and Hearing Disorders*, 55, 392-393. STUTTERING:

Bloom, Lois. (1991). *Language development from two to three.* New York, NY: Cambridge University Press. EARLY SYNTACTIC DEVELOPMENT COMPLEX SENTENCES DISCOURSE DEVELOPMENT CONTEXT VERBS SEMANTICS AND SYNTAX BOOTSTRAPPING SEMANTIC HYPOTHESIS INDIVIDUAL VARIATION LANGUAGE AND COGNITIVE DEVELOPMENT:

The time between two to three years of age is a time of great achievement in language development in children as they acquire a basic knowledge of semantics, syntax, and discourse. The chapters in this volume were originally published between 1970 and 1989 as separate research reports from a longitudinal study of a group of four children. As a collection, the reports present a developmental story of the children's language acquisition. The early chapters show the children learning to form simple sentences: later chapters show them beginning to acquire the structures of complex sentences. Two chapters in particular describe the children's development in contingent discourse from their first simple sentences through the age of three. Several conceptual themes in current language acquisition research and theory were first articulated in the studies reproduced here: the centrality of verbs for learning syntax, the role of meaning in acquisition, the importance of context: the relationshis of language learning to other aspects of cognitive development and individual differences among children learning the same language. These themes are discussed in an introductory chapter that unifies the studies and places the reports in the context of the current research and theory in child language.

Bloom, Lois. (1991). On the acquisition of negation in Tamil and English . *Journal of Child Language*, 18, 715-716. CROSSLINGUISTIC STUDY-SYNTAX NEGATION TAMIL:

Bloom, Lois. (1991). Representation and expression. In N. A. Krasnegor, et al. (Eds), *Biological and behavioral determinants of language development*. Hillsdale, NJ: Lawrence Erlbaum Associates. REPRESENTATIONS:

Bloom, Lois. (1993). Language acquisition and the power of expression. In H. L. Roitblat, L. M. Herman, & P. E. Nachtigall (Eds), *Language and communication: Comparative perspectives*. Hillsdale, NJ: Lawrence Erlbaum Associates. LANGUAGE AND OTHER PRIMATES ANIMAL COMMUNICATIONS LANGUAGE AND AFFECT:

Bloom, Paul. (1990). Syntactic distinctions in child language. *Journal of Child Language*, 17, 343-355. TWO-WORD SPEECH SYNTACTIC STRUCTURES WORD ORDER:

In two analyses, the spontaneous speech of 14 one- and two-year-old children was studied. These analyses show that even in children's very first word combinations, they almost never say things like big Fred or big he. A theory is proposed as to how children could use semantic information to draw the noun/NP distinction and to acquire this restriction on English word order.

Boada, H., Triado, C., & Vila, Ignasi. (1986). El acceso a las primeras palabras. (The step of the first words.). *Cahiers de l'Institut de Louvain*, 12(3-4), 77-102. FIRST WORDS: SPANISH

Bock, K. (1991). A sketchbook of production problems. *Journal of Psycholinguistic Research*, 20, 141-160. PRODUCTION/PERCEPTION ARTICULATION DISORDERS PHONOLOGICAL DISORDERS SYNTACTIC DISORDERS LANGUAGE DISORDERS:

Boden, Margaret A. (1988). *Computer models of the mind.* New York, NY: Cambridge University Press. COMPUTER SIMULATIONS CONNECTIONISM:

This book shows how computer models are used to study many aspects of the mind including language, and learning. It outlines the differences between traditional computer models and parallel-distributed processing models.

Bodin, L., & Snow, Catherine E. (1993). Lexical analyses of superordinates. In J. L. Sokolov, & C. E. Snow (Eds), *Handbook of research in language development in CHILDES*. Hillsdale, NJ: Lawrence Erlbaum Associates. CATEGORIZATION SEMANTIC ORGANIZATION LEXICAL ACCESS LEXICAL DEVELOPMENT METHODOLOGY-DESIGN CHILDES METHODOLOGY-COMPUTERS:

Boer, Frits, & Dunn, Judy. (1992). *Children's sibling relationships: Developmental and clinical issues*. Hillsdale, NJ: Lawrence Erlbaum Associates. SIBLING EFFECTS RETARDED CHILDREN:

This collection contains the proceedings from the First International Symposium on Siblings held in Leyden. The topics cover the range of sibling effects on development.

Boeschoten, Hendrik. (1990). *Acquisition of Turkish by immigrant children : a multiple case study of Turkish children in the Netherlands aged 4 to 6*. Wiesbaden, Germany: O. Harrassowitz. TURKISH METHODOLOGY-DIARY/CASE STUDY L2/L1 ACQUISITION:

Bohannon, Neil, MacWhinney, Brian, & Snow, Catherine E. (1990). No negative evidence revisited: Beyond learnability or who has to prove what to whom. *Developmental Psychology*, 26, 221-226. CHILDES RECASTS NEGATIVE EVIDENCE LEARNABILITY:

Bolander, Maria. (1990). On the acquisition of word order rules in Swedish as a second language. In M. A. K. Halliday, J. Gibbons, & H. Nicholas (Eds), *Learning, keeping and using language* . Amsterdam, The Netherlands: John Benjamins. SWEDISH L2 EDUCATION L2 WORD ORDER:

Selected paper from the proceedings of the Eighth World Congress of Applied Linguistics, Sydney, 1987.

Bolger, F., & Karmiloff-Smith, Annette. (1990). The development of communicative competence: are notational systems like language? *Archives de Psychologie*, 58, 257-273. LANGUAGE AND COGNITIVE DEVELOPMENT:

Bonvillian, John D., & Folven, R. J. (1992). Early sign language development. In M. Marschark, & M. D. Clark (Eds), *Psychological perspectives on deafness*. Hillsdale, NJ: Lawrence Erlbaum Associates. DEAF CHILDREN SIGNING:

Borel-Maisonny, Suzanne. (1985). Symposium of logopedics in Oulu: a summation (Logopedian symposium Oulussa, jalkitarkastelua). *Korkeakoulutieto*, 2, 23-25. LANGUAGE AND EDUCATION: FINNISH

Borel-Maisonny, Suzanne. (1986). Les problèmes des écoliers qui ne savent par écouter. (The problems of school children who cannot hear). *Bulletin D'Audiophonologie*, 2, 615-622. DEAF CHILDREN LANGUAGE AND EDUCATION: FRENCH

Borel-Maisonny, Suzanne. (1987). Die Symptome einer leichten neurologischen Fehlleistung und ihre Korretation zum Schulerfolg. (The symptoms of a mild neurological fault and their correction...). In *Pädagogisch-psychologische Prophylaxe bei 4-8 jahrigen Kinder: International Kolloquium in Finland*. Joensuu, Finland: Publications in Education, University of Joensuu. LANGUAGE AND EDUCATION LANGUAGE DISORDERS: GERMAN

Borel-Maisonny, Suzanne. (1988). Logopedinen tutkimus Oulun yliopistossa. (Logopedic research at Oulo University.). *Logopedic and Phoniatric Research and Therapy*, 21, FINNISH: FINNISH

Borel-Maisonny, Suzanne. (1988). Logopedisen tutkimuksen sykytilanne Oulun yliopiston logopedian ja fonetiikan laitoksella. (The present state of logopedic research in the department of logopedics and phonetics, Oulu University.). *Sellista*, 2, 8-9. LANGUAGE AND EDUCATION: FINNISH

Borland, Helen. (1990). A crossover effect in interlanguage: Learners' use of English predicate complement constructions. In M. A. K. Halliday, J. Gibbons, & H. Nicholas (Eds), *Learning, keeping and using language* . Amsterdam, The Netherlands: John Benjamins. INTERLANGUAGE-SYNTAX:

Selected paper from the proceedings of the Eighth World Congress of Applied Linguistics, Sydney, 1987.

Bornstein, Marc H. (1989). Information processing (habituation) in infancy and stability in cognitive development. *Human Development*, 32, 129-136. INDIVIDUAL VARIATION:

Recent longitudinal study indicates that this type of information processing in infancy also predicts mental status later in child development. In this paper, data and theory on individual differences and stability in mental development are evaluated with respect to predictive validity of information-processing measures made near the beginning of life to normative indices of mental development and performance in childhood. - From Child Development Abstracts.

Bornstein, Marc H., & Lamb, Michael E. (1992). *Developmental psychology: An advanced textbook*, 3rd Ed. Hillsdale, NJ: Lawrence Erlbaum Associates. ADULT-CHILD INTERACTION PARENTAL INPUT COGNITIVE DEVELOPMENT SOCIAL INTERACTION METHODOLOGY CROSSCULTURAL STUDY:

The third edition has been extensively revised and includes chapters on: methodology, adult-child interaction, parental input, and a chapter newly written for this edition on cross-cultural aspects of development.

Bornstein, Marc H., & Tamis-LeMonda, Catherine S. (1990). Activities and interactions of mothers and their first born infants in the first six months of life: Covariation, stability, continuity, correspondance, and prediction. *Child Development*, 61, 1206-1217. ADULT-CHILD INTERACTION SOCIAL INTERACTION:

Mothers' activities did not positively covary at either age, nor did those of infants. Infants' activities were unstable, but most increased over time. Over time, mothers and infants influenced one another in specific ways. In the first half-year, infants appear to be flexible and plastic and are influenced by their mothers. Mothers are somewhat consistent, but they also adapt to their infants.

Bornstein, Marc H., Tamis-LeMonda, Catherine S., Tal, J., & Ludemann, P., et al. (1992). Maternal responsiveness to infants in 3 societies-the United-States, France, and Japan. *Child Development*, 63, 808-821. ADULT-CHILD INTERACTION CROSSLINGUISTIC STUDY CROSSCULTURAL STUDY PARENTAL INPUT:

Boscolo, Pietro. (1990). The construction of expository text. *First Language*, 10, 217-230. WRITTEN LANGUAGE DISCOURSE STRUCTURE:

This study analyzed the ways in which elementary school children construct an expository text. Eighty subjects from grade 2 to 8 were requested to write a text about the wind. Data showed a developmental trend in expository writing, which concerns strategies of content generation, the changes from dictation to text production, and the organization of the final text.

Botuck, Shelly, & Turkewitz, Gerald. (1990). Intersensory functioning: Auditory-visual pattern equivalence in younger and older children. *Developmental Psychology*, 26, 115-120. MODALITY:

Increased accuracy was associated with increased age on both intra- and intersensory matching whether or not transposition was required. For the 7-year-old children, intrasensory matching was easier when transposition was not required, intersensory matching was easier when transposition was required. The requirement of transposition facilitated the performance of 13-year-old children on intersensory tasks, there was no effect of transposition on the oldest subjects' performance.-From Child Development Abstracts.

Boucher, Jill, Lewis, Vicky, & Collis, Glyn. (1990). Hand dominance of parents and other relatives of autistic children. *Developmental Medicine and Child Neurology*, 32, 304-313. LANGUAGE AND HANDEDNESS ANNETT HANDEDNESS QUESTIONNAIRE ASSESSMENT PROCEDURES AUTISM LANGUAGE DISORDERS:

A study of approximately 400 parents of autistic children used the Annett Handedness Questionnaire to determine whether or not handedness and language disorders were associated. No significant correlation was found between handedness and language problems.

Boueke, Dietrich. (1990). Wie lernen Kinder, eine Geschichte zu erzählen? (How do children learn to tell a story?). In W. Dinkelacker, et al. (Eds), *Ja muz ich sunder ruhe sin. Festschrift für Karl Stackmann*. Gottingen: TEXT/STORY GRAMMARS NARRATIVES METHODOLOGY-DESIGN METHODOLOGY-ANALYSIS: GERMAN

An introduction to the work carried out in the Bielefeld University study, "Understanding the development of narrative capabilities in children" which describes the methodology for the collection and analysis of the data and discusses the theoretical issues involved in the development of children's narrative capability.

Boueke, Dietrich, & Klein, Wolfgang. (1980). Kindersprachforschung 1977/78. (Child language research 77-78.). In H. Muller-Michaels (Ed.), *Jahrbuch der Deutschdidaktik 1979*. Germany: Konigstein/Ts. GERMAN OVERVIEW-THEORY: GERMAN

Overview of research in child language.

Boueke, Dietrich, & Klein, Wolfgang. (1981). Alltagsgesprache von Kindern als 'Interaktionsspiele.' (Children's everyday language as social interaction play.). In *Pragmatik: Theorie und Praxis*. Amsterdam, The Netherlands: Amsterdamer Beitrage zur Neuren Germanistik. METHODOLOGY-ANALYSIS DISCOURSE ANALYSIS: GERMAN

> This paper uses the 'play' metaphor to develop a method for examining children's discourse.

Boueke, Dietrich, & Klein, Wolfgang (Eds). (1983). *Untersuchungen zur Dialogfahigkeit von Kindern. (Investigation of children's dialogue capabilities.), vol.*. Tubingen, Germany: CHILDREN'S DISCOURSE CONVERSATIONAL SKILLS NARRATIVES GERMAN TURN TAKING: GERMAN

> This volume contains 13 articles on the development of children's dialogue capabilities. Its themes include the acquisition of narrative strategies and the conduct of children in disputes.

Boueke, Dietrich, & Schulein, Frieder. (1988). 'Story grammars.' Zur Diskussion um ein erzählstrukturelles Konzept und seine Konsequenzen fur die Erzähldidaktik. (Story Grammars: A discussion of the story grammar concept and its consequences for narrative instruction.). *Wirkendes Wort*, 38, 125-143. TEXT/STORY GRAMMARS LANGUAGE AND EDUCATION: GERMAN

> An introduction to Rumelhart et al's concept of the story grammar and a look at its impact on teachers, learners, and the school curriculum.

Boueke, Dietrich, & Schulein, Frieder. (1988). Von der Lehr- und Lernbarkeit des Erzählens. (On the teachability and learnability of narratives.). *Diskussion Deutsch 19*, 102, 386-403. NARRATIVES LANGUAGE AND EDUCATION: GERMAN

Boueke, Dietrich, & Schulein, Frieder. (1991). Beobachtungen zum Verlauf der Entwicklung kindlicher Erzählfähigkeit. (Observations on the course of children's narrative knowledge development.). In E. Neuland, & H. Bleckwenn (Eds), *Stil-Stilistik-Stilisierung*. Tübingen, Germany: NARRATIVES: GERMAN

Proposes four stages of narrative knowledge development in children: 1. Representation of isolated events, 2. Linearly connected events, 3. Development of logically structured events, 4. Narrative setting of events.

Boueke, Dietrich, & Schulein, Freider. (1991). Kindliches erzählen als Realisierung eines narrativen Schemas (Children's narratives and the realization of narrative schemata.). In B. Dolle-Weinkauff, & H. Ewers (Eds), *Erzählen und Erzählliteratur von Kindern*. Weinheim: NARRATIVES TEXT/STORY GRAMMARS EVENTS/SCRIPTS: GERMAN

A discussion of schema theory and the development and construction of narrative schemata for children's stories.

Bountress, Nicholas G., Sever, Joseph C., & Williams, Joyce T. (1989). Relationship between two nontraditional procedures for assessing speech-sound discrimination. *Perceptual and Motor Skills*, 69, 499-503. ASSESSMENT PROCEDURES AUDITORY DISCRIMINATION:

The reliability and validity of established speech-sound discrimination tests has been questioned during the last 10 years. The authors, therefore, propose two new techniques for the assessment of school-age children, and examine them to see if they elicit responses in a similar fashion.

Bouton, Charles P. (1991). *Neurolinguistics: Historical and theoretical perspectives*. New York, NY: Plenum. NEUROLINGUISTICS CORTICAL STRUCTURES CEREBRAL DISORDERS LANGUAGE AND COGNITION:

Text covers the history and origins of neurolinguistics, language and perception, neural substrates of language, and neurally motivated language disorders.

Bowerman, Melissa F. (1988). The 'No Negative Evidence' Problem: How Do Children Avoid Constructing an Overly General Grammar? In J. A. Hawkins (Ed.), *Explaining Language Universals.*. Oxford: Blackwell. NEGATIVE EVIDENCE ACQUISITION THEORIES:

Bowerman, Melissa F. (1989). Learning a Semantic System: What Role Do Cognitive Predispositions Play? In M. L. Rice, & R. L. Schiefelbusch (Eds), *The Teachability of Language..* Baltimore: Brookes. SEMANTIC DEVELOPMENT LANGUAGE PRECURSORS LANGUAGE AND COGNITIVE DEVELOPMENT LANGUAGE AND COGNITION SEMANTIC MAPPING:

Bowerman, Melissa F. (1990). Mapping Thematic Roles Onto Syntactic Functions. Are Children Helped By Innate Linking Rules? *Linguistics*, 28(6), 1253-1289. LEXICAL DEVELOPMENT SEMANTIC MAPPING NATIVISM CONCEPT DEVELOPMENT:

Bowerman, Melissa F., & Perdue, Clive. (1990). The structure of the simple clause in language acquisition. *Linguistics*, 28(6). SYNTACTIC STRUCTURES:

Bowey, J. A., Cain, M. T., & Ryan, S. M. (1992). A reading-level design study of phonological skills underlying 4th-grade children's word reading difficulties. *Child Development* , 63, 999-1011. READING DISORDERS LITERACY:

Bowey, J. A., & Francis, J. (1991). Phonological analysis as a function of age and exposure to reading instruction. *Applied Psycholinguistics*, 12, 91-121. LITERACY:

Bracken, Bruce A. (Ed.). (1991). *The psychoeducational assessment of preschool children, vol..* Boston, MA: Allyn & Bacon. ASSESSMENT PROCEDURES BILINGUALISM-ASSESSMENT PROCEDURES L2 ASSESSMENT PROCEDURES:

This book provides tips on establishing rapport with preschoolers and discusses how to overcome the limits imposed on preschool assessment by the testing environment. Many popular tests are reviewed and their use with preschoolers is discussed. There are chapters on: adaptive behavior, language, motor development, emotion, visual perception, audition, multicultural assessment, and the assessment of special populations.

Braden, J. P., Shaw, S., & Grecko, L. (1991). An evaluation of a computer-assisted instructional program for elementary hearing-impaired students. *Volta Review*, 93, 247-252. COMPUTER ASSISTED THERAPY DEAF CHILDREN:

Braden-Harder, L. (1991). Lexicons for broad coverage semantics. In U. Zernik (Ed.), *Lexical Acquisition-Exploiting On-Line Resources to Build a Lexicon*. Hillsdale, NJ: Lawrence Erlbaum Associates. LEXICAL DEVELOPMENT SEMANTIC DEVELOPMENT:

Bradley, Lynette. (1992). Rhyme, rime and learning to read and spell. In C. A. Ferguson, L. Menn, & C. Stoel-Gammon (Eds), *Phonological development: Models, research, implications*. Monkton, MD: York Press. LITERACY WRITTEN LANGUAGE:

Bradshaw, G. (1993). Beyond animal language. In L. M. Herman, H. L. Roitblat, & P. E. Nachtigall (Eds), *Language and communication: Comparative perspectives*. Hillsdale, NJ: Lawrence Erlbaum Associates. NEUROLINGUISTCIS LANGUAGE AND OTHER PRIMATES ANIMAL COMMUNICATIONS:

Bradshaw, John L. (1990). *Hemispheric specialization and psychological function*. New York, NY: Wiley. LATERALIZATION COMMISUROTOMY:

> This book covers the three main sources of evidence on lateralization: brain trauma, commisurotomy, and experimental studies of the undamaged brain's performance. The author presents arguments for: interhemispheric cooperation such as nondominant language processes, gender related differences, handedness issues, and aspects of development and cognitive style.

Brand, Handre J., & Welch, Kim. (1989). Cognitive and social-emotional development of children in different preschool environments. *Psychological Reports*, 65, 480-482. LANGUAGE AND EDUCATION:

> Sixty-two English-speaking preschool children were divided into three groups, a Montessori group (n = 21), a traditional preschool group (n = 21), and a stay at home group (n = 20)

to compare their relative cognitive and social-emotional development. Significant differences in favor of school groups were found for vocabulary, language, comprehension, ability to judge the correctness of figural stimuli, visual memory, and perceptual organization. - From Child Development Abstracts.

Brandt, P. A. (1992). The sources of meaning. *Journal of Pragmatics*, 17(5-6) , 435-440. SEMANTIC DEVELOPMENT LEXICAL DEVELOPMENT SEMANTIC MAPPING CONCEPT DEVELOPMENT:

Bredart, Serge, & Rondal, Jean A. (1981). L'adaption verbale a l'interlocuteur chez l'enfant. Une revue de quelques études récentes. (Children's verbal adaptation to the questioner. A revue of several recent studies.). *Enfance*, 3, 195-206. COMMUNICATIVE COMPETENCE: FRENCH

Bredart, Serge, & Rondal, Jean A. (1982). *L'analyse du langage chez l'enfant. (The analysis of language by the child.).* Bruxelles: Mardaga. METHODOLOGY-ANALYSIS: FRENCH

Bregman, Albert S. (1990). *Auditory scene analysis: The perceptual organization of sound*. Cambridge, MA: MIT/Batsford. SPEECH PERCEPTION AUDITORY DISCRIMINATION AUDITORY LOCALIZATION COMPUTER SIMULATIONS:

Addresses the question of how humans are able to perceive individual sounds in the highly complex and mixed sound environment. Covers speech perception, the perception of musical notes and melodies, and examines computer simulations of the process.

Brent, M. R. (1990). Semantic classification of verbs from their syntactic contexts: Automated lexicography with implications for child language acquisition. In M. Piatelli-Palmarini (Ed.), *Proceedings of the Twelfth Annual Conference of the Cognitive Science Society*. Hillsdale, NJ: Lawrence Erlbaum Associates. SEMANTIC ORGANIZATION VERBS CUES-SYNTACTIC:

Bretherton, Inge. (1991). Intentional communication and the development of an understanding of mind. In D. Frye, & C. Moore (Eds), *Children's theories of mind.* Hillsdale, NJ: Lawrence Erlbaum Associates. THEORY OF MIND INTENTIONALITY:

Brigaudiot, M. (1988). Le plus-que-parfait chez les enfants de 5 à 6 ans (The pluperfect tense in language of 5 to 6 year-old children). *Le français aujourd'hui.*, 83, 41-46. VERBS ASPECT TENSE: FRENCH

Broberg, A. G., Hwang, C. P., Lamb, Michael E., & Bookstein, F. L. (1990). Factors related to verbal abilities in Swedish preschoolers. *British Journal of Developmental Psychology*, 8, 335-349. SWEDISH LANGUAGE PRECURSORS:

Broderick, Victor. (1991). Young children's comprehension of similarities underlying metaphor. *Journal of Psycholinguistic Research*, 20, 65-81. FIGURATIVE LANGUAGE:

> The comprehension of similarity by 3-, 4-, and 5-year-olds was investigated using a set of binary choice tasks. These tasks were composed of contrasting concepts that were to be matched to conceptually related target stimuli on the basis of relationships underlying object/personality metaphor, color/personality metaphor, concrete metaphor, taxonomic similarity, and functional association. The youngest children were able to comprehend each of the metaphoric and nonmetaphoric relationships, and this ability improved with age.

Broderick, Victor. (1992). Incidence of verbal comparisons in beginners' books and in metaphor comprehension research-a search for ecological validity. *Journal of Child Language*, 19, 183-193. FIGURATIVE LANGUAGE:

Brodin, Jane. (1986). *Gravt utvecklingsstorda flerhandikappade barns leksituation. (The play situation of profoundly mentally retarded and multiply handicapped children.)* . Stockholm, Sweden: Handikappinstitutet. RETARDED CHILDREN: SWEDISH

Brodin, Jane. (1987). Foraldraintervjuer om utvecklingsstorda flerhandikappade barns kommunikation. (Interviews with parents about mentally retarded and multiply handicapped childrens' communication.). *Rapport Utvecklingspsykologiska seminariet, Pedagogiska Institutionen*, 25, RETARDED CHILDREN: SWEDISH

About 90% of all profoundly mentally retarded children are speech impaired or have severe disturbances in their communication. A study based on interviews with parents of six severely handicapped children's communication has been done. One of these children is moderately retarded, the others are profoundly retarded. None of them has spoken language or has the ability to point at objects in the environment with their hands. The result of the study shows that it's difficult to understand what these children mean, sometimes even for their parents. Nobody knows for sure how much they really understand and there is a risk to underestimate their abilities. My conclusion from this study is that the best support for these children is an observant and sensitive social environment. The parents are able to interpret their children and must be encouraged to transfer their knowledge to other persons in the child's environment. JB.

Brodin, Jane. (1988). The play situation for children with profound mental retardation and multiple handicaps. In P. Heseltine (Ed.), *Creativity through Play*. Cambridge University Press: New York, NY. RETARDED CHILDREN:

Brodin, Jane. (1989). *Barn med handikapp i forskolan. (Children with disability in preschools.).* Rockneby: WRP International. RETARDED CHILDREN: SWEDISH

Brodin, Jane. (1989). Ett gravt flerhandikappat barns kommunikation-Utprovning av en analysmodell. (Testing a model for analyzing a profoundly mentally retarded child's communication.) *Rapport Utvecklingspsykologiska seminatiet Pedagogiska institutionen*, 34, RETARDED CHILDREN METHODOLOGY-DESIGN METHODOLOGY-ANALYSIS METHODOLOGY-TRANSCRIPTION INTELLIGIBILITY: SWEDISH

A case study of a profoundly mentally retarded and multiply handicapped boy (10:0) which focusses on his communicative interaction during a two hour videotape. The videotape has been transcribed and used to show the communicative interaction of children at an early level of development. A model for transcribing, analyzing and interpreting of videotaped material is elaborated. Transcription, analysis and interpretation were done by the researcher, and the boy's parents interpretated the film as a complement to the researcher's interpretation. This 'double-checking' method will be used for further work with analysis and interpretation of communication in six severely handicapped children. JB.

Brodin, Jane. (1989). Kommunikation och kommunikationshjalpmedel for forstandshandikappade. (Communication and communication aids for the mentally retarded.). In *Utvecklingsstorning och Kommunikation*. Sodertalje: Studieforbundet Vuxenskolan. SWEDISH RETARDED CHILDREN INTERVENTION PROGRAMS: SWEDISH

The article is based on a paper presented at a Swedish national conference arranged by the Swedish Handicap Institute and the Association for the Mentally Retarded in Sweden. The paper discusses the possibilities to compensate the communication ability of mentally retarded children with communication aids. It also gives a brief survey of available communication aids.

Brodin, Jane. (1990). The aids requirements for severely mentally retarded and multiply handicapped adolescents. In E. Chigier (Ed.), *Youth and Disability*. London: Freund Publishing House Ltd. INTERVENTION PROGRAMS RETARDED CHILDREN:

A paper presented in Israel at an international symposium of Youth and Disability in 1985. The paper discusses the aids requirements in general for persons with mental retardation. Part of the paper discusses the requirements of communication and communication aids as a basic need for human beings.

Brodin, Jane, & Bjorck-Akesson, E. (1988). Internationell forskning kring samspel hos barn som anvander alternativ kommunikation. (International research about interaction with children using alternative communication.). In *Rapport nr 2, Seminariet Tidig Interaktion, Pedagogiska institutionen*. Stockholm: Stockholm University. INTERVENTION PROGRAMS: SWEDISH

A report from an international conference on Alternative and Augmentative Communication held in Anaheim, California, USA, 1988.

Brodin, Jane, & Bjorck-Akesson, E. (1990). *Interaction research in Sweden. Report No 7*. Sweden: University College of Jonkoping. COMMUNICATIVE DISORDERS INTERVENTION PROGRAMS:

A survey of Swedish interaction research within the area of disability. The definition of the concept of communication varies between different researchers and this report focusses on the unclear definition of the concept 'communication.'.

Brodin, Jane, & Larsson, L. (1989). Kommunikation for en gravt utvecklingsstord vuxen-en fallstudie. (Communication in a profoundly mentally retarded adult-a case study.). In *Report No 35, Utvecklingspsykologiska seminariet, Pedagogiska institutionen*. Stockholm: Stockholm University. INTERVENTION PROGRAMS RETARDED CHILDREN: SWEDISH

A case study of the communication of a profoundly mentally retarded man, who has moved to a group home after spending 33 years in an institution. Our conclusion is that communication training should not be done in a group home. The best place would probably be in a workshop. The staff working at the workshop are motivated and educated to work with this type of task, and have a higher continuity than staff in group homes.

Brodin, Jane, & Lindberg, M. (1989). *Kom och lat oss leka, lekar och lekmaterial for gravt flerhandikappade barn. (Come and lets play-games and play material for severely handicapped children.).*

Rockneby: WRP International. INTERVENTION PROGRAMS RETARDED CHILDREN: SWEDISH

Broen, Patricia A., & Westman, M. J. (1990). Project parent-a preschool speech program implemented through parents. , 495-502. INTERVENTION PROGRAMS FOR PARENTS:

Bronckart, J. P. (1977). *Théories du langage. (Theories of language.).* Bruxelles: Mardaga. ACQUISITION AND LINGUISTIC THEORY: FRENCH

Bronckart, J. P., & Sinclair, Hermina. (1978). Genfer Untersuchung zur genetischen Psycholinguistik. (Genevan investigation of genetic psycholinguistics.). In *Die Psychologie des 20. Jahrhunderts*. Zurich, Switzerland: Kindler Verlag. PIAGETIAN THEORY: GERMAN

Bronckart, J. P., Sinclair, Hermina, & Berthoud-Papandropoulou, Ioanna. (1976). Semantique et réalite psycholinguistique. (Semantics and psycholinguistic reality.). *Bulletin de Psychologie (Spécial Annuel)*, , 225-231. ACQUISITION AND LINGUISTIC THEORY SEMANTIC DEVELOPMENT OVERVIEW-PSYCHOLINGUISTICS: FRENCH

Brook, S. L., & Bowler, D. M. (1992). Autism by another name-semantic and pragmatic impairments in children. *Journal of Autism and Developmental Disorders*, 22, 61-81. AUTISM SEMANTIC DISORDERS PRAGMATIC DISORDERS:

Brown, B., & Conti-Ramsden, Gina. (1989). Teaching letter formation in handwriting to young pupils with special educational needs. *European Journal of Special Needs Education*, 4, 45-54. WRITTEN LANGUAGE LANGUAGE AND EDUCATION:

Brown, B., & Conti-Ramsden, Gina. (1990). Young pupil's letter formation in handwriting. *Handwriting Review*, 7-11. WRITTEN LANGUAGE LANGUAGE AND EDUCATION:

Brown, Betty Byers, & Edwards, Margaret. (1990). *Developmental disorders of language*. San Diego, CA: Singular Group. DEVELOPMENTAL DISORDERS CLASSIFICATION OF DISORDERS ASSESSMENT PROCEDURES INTERVENTION PROGRAMS:

The identification, assessment and treatment of developmental language disorders.

Bruck, Maggie, & Waters, Gloria. (1990). Effects of reading skill on component spelling skills. *Applied Psycholinguistics*, 11, 425-437. LITERACY:

Sixth-grade good readers-good spellers (Good), good readers-poor spellers (Mixed), and poor readers-poor spellers (Poor) were examined. Good subjects performed consistently better than Mixed and Poor subjects. Mixed and Poor subjects did not differ on measures requiring use and knowledge of sound- spelling, orthographic, and visual information. Mixed subjects performed better than Poor subjects on measures assessing use and knowledge of morphological information.

Brumark, Asa. (1987). The contextual conditions of communicative development in sighted and blind-sighted dyads. In *79 Revised Summaries and 24 Reprinted Abstracts from Posters and Section Papers at the Fourth International Congress for the Study of Child Language. Paper no. 2*. Lund: Department of Linguistics, Lund University. BLIND CHILDREN:

Brumark, Asa. (1989). Routines as context of language acquisition. In R. Soederbergh, et al. (Eds), *Colloquium Paedolinguisticum Lundensis*. Lund, Sweden: Department of Linguistics, Lund University. BLIND CHILDREN SOCIAL INTERACTION PRAGMATIC DEVELOPMENT LEXICAL DEVELOPMENT:

Dyadic communication occuring during the first three years in one sighted and two blind-sighted mother-child pairs (one with a blind mother and one with a blind child) was video-recorded every three months in natural settings. The tapes were analyzed with regard to interactional and communicative 'routines' during play. Not unexpectedly, all three dyads displayed repertoires of recurrent play activities. When compared, they even showed surprising similarities in their choice and development of play routines. However, interesting differences could also be noticed in the performance of such common games as Disappearance-Reappearence and Identification-Naming. Furthermore, a qualitative analysis suggested that such routines are initiated and controlled by the mother play a greater role for the maintenance of communication in the blind-sighted dyads than in the sighted dyad. Finally, such routines as the "Disappearance Reappearance" game appear to assist the child's pragmatic development, whereas others, for instance "Identification Naming" seem to have the additional value of supporting his acquisition of referential skills and lexicon.

Brumark, Asa. (1990). Saying-doing routines in sighted and blind-sighted dyads. In R. Soederbergh, et al. (Eds), *Colloquium Paedolinguisticum Lundensis*. Lund, Sweden: Department of Linguistics, Lund University. BLIND CHILDREN SOCIAL INTERACTION PRAGMATIC DEVELOPMENT LEXICAL DEVELOPMENT :

Brumark, Asa, Hellspong, L., & Junefelt, K. (1983). Blindness and communication. *VISUS*, 4 (43), 12-19. BLIND CHILDREN:

Brumark, Asa, Hellspong, L., & Junefelt, K. (1984). Blindness and expressions of emotions. *VISUS*, 5 (44), 33-44. BLIND CHILDREN LANGUAGE AND AFFECT:

Brumark, Asa, Hellspong, L., & Junefelt, K. (1984). Patterns of communication among the blind. In R. Soderbergh (Ed.), *Proceedings from Child Language Symposium, Lund*. Lund: Department of Linguistics, Lund University. BLIND CHILDREN:

Bruner, Jerome S. (1977). The ontogenesis of speech acts. In M. S. Barbieri (Ed.), *Gli inizi del linguaggio: aspetti cognitivi e comunicativi (The emergence of language: cognitive and communicative aspects)*.. La Nuova, Italy: Firenze. JOINT REFERENCE LANGUAGE PRECURSORS PRELINGUISTICS:

Bruner, Jerome S. (1992). Narrative as the construction of reality. In H. Beilin, & P. B. Pufall (Eds), *Piaget's theory: Prospects and possibilities*. Hillsdale, NJ: Lawrence Erlbaum Associates. NARRATIVES:

Bruner, Jerome S., & Lucariello, Joan. (1989). Monologue as narrative recreation of the world. In K. Nelson (Ed.), *Narratives from the crib*. Cambridge, MA: Harvard University Press. SEQUENCING CONNECTIVES-CAUSAL PERSPECTIVE TAKING CRIB SPEECH NARRATIVES:

The authors compare a child's monologues from two periods, 1:10-1:11 and 2:4-2:9 noting the progression from a focus on temporal sequencing to causal connectives, and the development of perspective taking. A review appears in Language 66(3), pp. 558-562.

Bryant, Peter E., & Bradley, Lynette (Eds). (1991). *Children's reading problems: psychology and education, vol.* (2). Cambridge, MA: Basil Blackwell. READING DISORDERS LANGUAGE AND EDUCATION DYSLEXIA:

Examines the relationships between the awareness of sounds and reading development, and developmental and acquired dyslexia, and their impact upon pedagogical practice.

Bryant, Peter E., Bradley, Lynette, MacLean, M., & Crossland, J. (1989). Nursery rhymes, phonological skills and reading. *Journal of Child Language*, 16(2), 407-428. LITERACY RHYME PHONOLOGICAL PATTERNS:

From Stockholm Bibliographies.

Bryen, D. N. (1982). *Inquiries into child language*. Boston, MA: Allyn and Bacon. OVERVIEW-GENERAL:

Budden, Sarojini, Meek, Merry, & Henighan, Carol. (1990). Communication and oral-motor functioning Rett syndrome. *Developmental Medicine and Child Neurology*, 32, 51-55. RETT SYNDROME LANGUAGE AND MOTOR DEVELOPMENT:

All the subjects (females between the ages of 4:0 and 19:0) showed a regression in speech and language function by the on set of the second stage. Oral-motor function correlated with the progress of the disease in stage two, three and four.

Budwig, Nancy. (1989). The linguistic marking of agentivity and control in child language. *Journal of Child Language*, 16(2), 263-284. SEMANTIC RELATIONS:

Budwig, Nancy. (1990). The linguistic marking of nonprototypical agency-an exploration into children's use of passives. *Linguistics*, 28(6). SEMANTIC RELATIONS RULES-SEMANTIC PASSIVES:

Budwig, Nancy. (1993). *A developmental-functionalist approach to child language*. Hillsdale, NJ: Lawrence Erlbaum Associates. SEMANTIC RELATIONS ACQUISITION THEORIES SELF-CONCEPT DEIXIS-PERSONAL PRONOUNS-PERSONAL REORGANIZATIONAL PROCESSES:

In Part One, Budwig compares functionalist accounts of language development and then turns to an examination of agentivity and control in child language. In Part Two, she addresses the development of self-reference using data from six children, and in Part Three she looks at organizational and reorganizational processes in child language.

Bujdosóné, Arato A. (1989). Siket, nagyothalló és éphallásü tanulók beszéd tempojának összehasonlító vizsgálata. (Comparative study of the speech rate of deaf, hard-of-hearing and normal subjects.). *Magyar Fonetikai Füzetek*, 21, 157-160. DEAF CHILDREN SPEAKING RATE HUNGARIAN: HUNGARIAN

Buky, Béla, Egyéd, András, & Pléh, Csaba. (1984). *Nyelvi képességek, fogalomkincs, megértés. (Linguistic abilities, concepts and understanding.)*. Budapest: Tankönyvkiadó. LANGUAGE AND SOCIAL CLASS HUNGARIAN: HUNGARIAN

Includes introductory chapters on child language and social class differences in child language.

Bullard, C. S., & Schirmer, B. R. (1991). Understanding questions: hearing-impaired children with learning problems. *Volta Review*, 93, 235-245. COMPREHENSION QUESTIONS DEAF CHILDREN:

Bullowa, Margaret (Ed.). (1979). *Before speech*. New York, NY: Cambridge University Press. PRELINGUISTICS ADULT-CHILD INTERACTION:

Burnham, Denis K., Earnshaw, Linda J., & Clark, John E. (1991). Development of categorical identification of native and non-native bilabial stops: infants, children, and adults. *Journal of Child Language*, 18, 231-260. PHONOTACTICS STOPS:

Native English speaking infants, two- and six-year old children, and adults were required to identify sounds in a native and non-native speech continuum. Contrastive perception increased for native sounds and decreased for non-native sounds between 2:0 and 6:0 as a function of age. From Child Development Abstracts.

Butterworth, G., Harris, P., Leslie, A., & Wellman, H. (1991). Perspectives on the childs theory of mind. *British Journal of Developmental Psychology*, 9(2). THEORY OF MIND:

Special issue (June).

Butterworth, G., & Jarrett, N. (1991). What minds have in common is space-spatial mechanisms serving joint visual attention in infancy. *British Journal of Developmental Psychology*, 9, 55-72. JOINT REFERENCE THEORY OF MIND:

Byrne, Brian, & Fielding-Barnsley, Ruth. (1989). Phonemic awareness and letter knowledge in the child's acquisition of the alphabetic principle. *Journal of Educational Psychology*, 81(3), 313-321. PHONEMIC DEVELOPMENT LANGUAGE AND EDUCATION:

From Stockholm Bibliographies.

Byrne, K., Abbeduto, Leonard, & Brooks, P. (1990). The language of children with spina bifida and hydrocephalus-meeting task demands and mastering syntax. *Journal of Speech and Hearing Disorders*, 55, 118-123. ATYPICAL DEVELOPMENT SYNTACTIC DEVELOPMENT:

Byrnes, James P. (1991). Acquisition and development of "if" and "because": Cognitive and linguistic strategies. In S. A. Gelman, & J. Byrnes (Eds), *Perspectives on language and thought*. New York, NY: Cambridge University Press. LANGUAGE AND COGNITION LANGUAGE AND COGNITIVE DEVELOPMENT CONNECTIVES-CONDITIONAL NONLINGUISTIC STRATEGIES:

Byrnes, James P., & Duff, Michelle A. (1989). Young children's comprehension of modal expressions. *Cognitive Development*, 4, 369-387. MODALS AUXILIARIES:

The present study assessed children's knowledge of how speakers use modal auxiliaries such as might and have to indicate their degree of belief in the truth of their statements, and to socially regulate behavior. Children aged 3 to 5 years were given two task: one that assessed comprehension of modal expressions for the epistemic domain, and one that assessed comprehension of such expressions for the deontic domain. Results showed that even 3 year olds comprehend partial aspects of meaning of epistemic expressions considered individually. The results, which show a progressive attainment of the meaning of modals, indicate metacognitive and social cognition ability not usually attributed to preschoolers.-From Child Development Abstracts.

Byrnes, James P., & Gelman, Susan A. (1991). Perspectives on thought and language: Traditional and contemporary views. In S. A. Gelman, & J. Byrnes (Eds), *Perspectives on language and thought*. New York, NY: Cambridge University Press. LANGUAGE AND COGNITION LANGUAGE AND COGNITIVE DEVELOPMENT:

Bzoch, Kenneth R. (1989). *Communicative disorders related to cleft lip and palate (Third Edition)*. San Diego, CA: Singular Group. CLEFT PALATE:

Evaluation, causes, and treatment of cleft lip and palate disorders.

C

Cacciari, Christina, & Levorato, Maria C. (1989). How children understand idioms in discourse. *Journal of Child Language*, 16(2), 387-405. IDIOMS FIGURATIVE LANGUAGE:

From Stockholm Bibliographies.

Cahan, Sorel, & Cohen, Nora. (1989). Age versus schooling effects on intelligence development. *Child Development*, 60, 1239-1249. LANGUAGE AND EDUCATION ASSESSMENT PROCEDURES:

The results unambiguously point to schooling as the major factor underlying the increase of intelligence test scores as a function of age and to the larger effect schooling has on verbal than nonverbal tests. - From Child Development Abstracts.

Caldognetto, E. Magno, Tonelli, L., & Luciani, N. (1987). Problemi di classificazione e distribuzione nell'analisi di parafasie e lapsus fonologici. (A comparison between speech errors and paraphrasies: an analysis of error types and their distribution.). *Acta Phoniatrica Latina*, 9 (1), 51-59. SPEECH ERRORS ITALIAN: ITALIAN

This paper is concerned with the similarities and differences which are seen in the distributional patterns of error types in phonological speech errors and paraphasias. It furthermore discusses them in relation to the issue of phonological disruption vs. disruption of planning mechanisms in both types of errors.

Callanan, Maureen A. (1991). Parent-child collaboration in young children's understanding of categorical hierarchies. In S. A. Gelman, & J. Byrnes (Eds), *Perspectives on language and thought.* New York, NY: Cambridge University Press. LANGUAGE AND COGNITION LANGUAGE AND COGNITIVE DEVELOPMENT CONCEPT DEVELOPMENT CATEGORIZATION ADULT-CHILD INTERACTION:

Calzolari, N. (1991). Lexical databases and textual corpora: Perspectives of integration for a lexical knowledge-base. In U. Zernik (Ed.), *Lexical Acquisition-Exploiting On-Line Resources to Build a Lexicon.* Hillsdale, NJ : Lawrence Erlbaum Associates. LEXICAL DEVELOPMENT:

Camaioni, Luigia. (1978). *Sviluppo del linguaggio e interazione sociale. (Language development and social interaction.).* Bologna, Italy: Il Mulino. SOCIAL INTERACTION HYPOTHESIS SOCIAL INTERACTION: ITALIAN

Camaioni, Luigia. (1985). Piaget's theory and child language research: a reassessment. In L. Camaioni, & C. de Lemos (Eds), *Questions on social explanation: Piagetian themes reconsidered.* Amsterdam, The Netherlands: John Benjamins. PIAGETIAN THEORY LANGUAGE AND COGNITIVE DEVELOPMENT:

Camaioni, Luigia. (1986). From early interaction to language acquisition: which continuity? In J. Cook-Gumperz, W. Corsaro, & J. Streek (Eds), *Children's worlds and children's language.* Berlin: Mouton de Gruyter. SOCIAL INTERACTION:

Camaioni, Luigia, & Bates, Elizabeth. (1976). *La comunicazione nel primo anno de vita. (Communication in the first year of life.)* . Torino, Italy: Boringhieri. PRELINGUISTICS GESTURE LANGUAGE PRECURSORS: ITALIAN

Camaioni, Luigia, de Castro Campos, M. F. P., & de Lemos, C. (1984). On the failure of the interactionist paradigm in language acquisition: a re-evaluation. In W. Dorise, & A. Palmonari (Eds), *Social interaction in individual development.* New York, NY: Cambridge University Press. SOCIAL INTERACTION HYPOTHESIS ACQUISITION THEORIES:

Camaioni, Luigia, & Ercolani, A. P. (1992). Levels of categorization and the development of referential descriptions. *British Journal of Developmental Psychology*, 10, 143-152. LANGUAGE AND COGNITIVE DEVELOPMENT CATEGORIZATION DESCRIPTIONS REFERENTIAL COMMUNICATION:

Campbell, T. F., & Dollaghan, C. A. (1990). Expressive language recovery in severely brain-injured children and adolescents. *Journal of Speech and Hearing Disorders*, 55, 567-581. TRAUMATIC DISORDERS CEREBRAL DISORDERS:

Cannito, Micheal P., Kondraske, George V., & Johns, Donnell F. (1991). Oral-Facial Sensorimotor Function in Spasmodic Dysphonia. In C. A. Moore, K. M. Yorkston, & D. R. Beukleman (Eds), *Dysarthria and Apraxia of Speech*. Baltimore, MD: Paul H. Brookes. MOTOR DISORDERS ARTICULATORY DISORDERS:

Capelli, Carol A., Nakagawa, Noreen, & Madden, Cary M. (1990). How children understand sarcasm: The role of context and intonation. *Child Development*, 61, 1824-1841. COMMUNICATIVE COMPETENCE FIGURATIVE LANGUAGE REGISTER:

Third and sixth graders were able to recognize sarcasm when the speakers used sarcastic intonation but failed without this intonation cue. Young children appeared oblivious to contextually implied sarcasm.

Caplan, David. (1992). *Language: Structure, processing, and disorders*. Cambridge, MA: Bradford Books. APHASIAS ACQUIRED APHASIAS LANGUAGE PROCESSING TRAUMATIC DISORDERS:

Cappelli, Giuseppe, Maccari, Anna, & Pfanner, Lucia. (1990). *Utilizzazione dei sistemi computazionali per lo studio del linguaggio infantile: trattamento automatico con il CHILDES di campini linguistici di un soggetto normale. (Use of computational tools in the study of child language: automatic treatment of linguistic samples of one normal subject with CHILDES.)*. Pisa: Istituto di Linguistica Computazionale del CNR. METHODOLOGY-DESIGN METHODOLOGY-COMPUTERS CHILDES: ITALIAN

After comparing various computational systems created for use with child language data, the authors describe the use of the CHILDES system. The programs were applied to samples of spontaneous speech of one normal Italian speaking child, G.C. (age 26-36 months) to examine errors, omissions and pre-syntactic devices.

Caprez, G., Sinclair, Hermina, & Studer, B. (1971). Entwicklung der Passivform im Schweizerdeutschen. (The development of passives in Swiss-German.). *Archives de Psychologie*, 41, 23-52. PASSIVES SWISS-GERMAN: GERMAN

Carabine, B. (1991). Fuzzy boundaries and the extension of object-words. *Journal of Child Language*, 18, 355-372. PROTOTYPE THEORY SEMANTIC MAPPING LEXICAL DEVELOPMENT:

Caramazza, Alfonso. (1991). *Issues in reading, writing, and speaking.* Hingham, MA: Kluwer Academic Press. LEXICAL DEVELOPMENT AGRAPHIA READING DISORDER DYSLEXIA DEVELOPMENTAL DISORDERS MORPHOLOGICAL DISORDERS SYNTACTIC DISORDERS LANGUAGE PROCESSING:

An exacting account of language and lexical processing as revealed by disruptions of reading, writing and speaking.

Carey, P., & de Boysson-Bardies, Bénédicte. (1974). What is the scope of negation? In F. Bresson & J. Mehler. (Eds). *Problèmes actuels en psycholinguistique*. Paris: Edition CNRS. NEGATION: FRENCH

Carey, Susan. (1978). The child as word-learner. In M. Halle, J. Bresnan, & G. A. Miller (Eds), *Linguistic theory and psychological reality*. Cambridge, MA: MIT Press. LEXICAL DEVELOPMENT SEMANTIC DEVELOPMENT:

Carpenter, K. (1991). Later rather than sooner-extralinguistic categories in the acquisition of Thai. *Journal of Child Language*, 18, 93-113. CLASSIFIERS THAI:

Carroll, Susanne. (1989). Language acquisition studies and a feasible theory of grammar. *The Canadian Journal of Linguistics*, 34(4), 399-418. ACQUISITION THEORIES-SYNTAX:

Casteel, Carolyn, & Isom, Bess. (1989). The effect of school type on prereaders' acquisition of print concepts. *Journal of Research in Reading*, 12, 131-145. LANGUAGE AND EDUCATION LITERACY:

This study was conducted to determine if children enrolled in different types of preschool programs differed in their knowledge of print concepts. The investigation included subjects who were enrolled in programs, ranging in type from rational to early formal reading. Results suggest that children in each type of school program acquire basic prereading concepts about print. The type of program was not a deciding factor in acquiring prereading print knowledge.-From Child Development Abstracts.

Castelfranchi, A. (1989). Understanding causal relations. In M. S. Barbieri (Ed.), *La speigazione nell'interazione sociale*. Torino, Italy: Loescher. CONNECTIVES-CAUSAL CONNECTIVES-CONDITIONAL : ITALIAN

A computational approach to the semantics of 'because' showing that in natural language this term can carry many different meanings-cause, enable, purpose, etc.-and that the unifying feature is the possibility of inferring y from x, given a link such as 'Y' because of 'X'..

Catania, A.C. (1991). The phylogeny and ontogeny of language function. In N. A. Krasnegor, et al. (Eds), *Biological and Behavioral Determinants of Language Development*. Hillsdale, NJ: Lawrence Erlbaum Associates. LANGUAGE FUNCTIONS ACQUISITION THEORIES:

Caycho, L., Gunn, P., & Siegal, M. (1991). Counting by children with Down syndrome. *American Journal of Mental Retardation*, 95, 575-583. DOWN SYNDROME NUMERALS:

No significant differences were observed in the mean task scores for one-to-one, stable order, and cardinal principles between 15 Down syndrome children and 15 normal children matched on the PPVT. From Child Development Abstracts.

Cession, A., Kilen, A., Denhiere, G., & Rondal, Jean A. (1988). Maman, une histoire! Une étude de la structure lexico-syntaxique et semantique des histoires racontées aux enfants par leur mere dans deux classes sociales contrastées. (Mommy, a story! A study of the lexico-syntactic and semantic structure of stories told to children by their mothers from two contrasting social classes.). *Enfance*, -, 341-358. LANGUAGE AND SOCIAL CLASS ADULT-CHILD INTERACTION PARENTAL SPEECH PARENTAL INPUT SOCIAL INTERACTION: FRENCH

Ceytlin, Stella N. (1975). Ne rassmeshyvay menya! (Don't make me laughing!). *Nauka i zchyzn*, 12, 97-92. RUSSIAN ASPECT: RUSSIAN

This article is intended for parents and Russian language teachers. It reveals language operations providing recurring occasionalisms within the framework of perfect/imperfect opposition as built by Russian-speaking children. SNC

Ceytlin, Stella N. (1975). O nekotorykh osobenostyakh imperfektivacii v detskoy rechi. (On some peculiarities of imperfective changes in children's speech). In Vorohezch (Ed.), *The problems of Russian aspectology (Voprosy russkoy aspectologii)*. RUSSIAN ASPECT: RUSSIAN

It has been established that when making choice between perfective and imperfective members of aspectual opposition Russian-speaking children, as distinct from foreign learners, do not err as a rule. At the same time the use of form-building suffixes -iva/ -yva instead of an -a and vice versa causes greater difficulties for a child. Children also tend to build oppositive forms of aspect defective verbs on the analogy with those having the opposition (as if to eliminate this deficiency). SNC

Ceytlin, Stella N. (1976). Zchyl korol so svojey korolicey-Zametki o detskom slovoobrazovanii. (There lived a king and his kingress - Notes on the peculiarities of children's word-building). *Russkaya rech*, 2, 71-76. RUSSIAN MORPHOLOGICAL DEVELOPMENT LEXICAL DEVELOPMENT: RUSSIAN

This article is intended for parents and teachers. It introduces the reader into the realm of children's creativity and makes him/her understand why Russian-speaking children create a great number of neologisms. SNC

Ceytlin, Stella N. (1977). Semantika proizvodnogo slova i detskaja rech. (The semantics of derivatives and children's speech.). In *Slovo kak predmet izuchenia. (The word as a research object).* Leningrad: RUSSIAN LEXICAL DEVELOPMENT SEMANTIC MAPPING CONCEPT DEVELOPMENT: RUSSIAN

Ceytlin, Stella N. (1978). *Vozvratnyie glagoly i detskaya rech: Problemy teorii grammaticheskogo zaloga. (Reflexive verbs in children's speech: The problems of the category of voice theory).* Leningrad: Nauka. VERBS-REFLEXIVE PRONOUNS-REFLEXIVE RUSSIAN: RUSSIAN

This article deals with the semantic types of reflexive verbs formed by Russian-speaking children. Reverse form-building (cases when the reflexive morpheme -sja [-self] is omitted in children's speech) is also under study. SNC

Ceytlin, Stella N. (1978). Vverkh karmashkami! (In a topsy-turvy way or pockets upside down!). *Nauka i zshyzn*, 7, 128-130. RUSSIAN MORPHOLOGICAL DEVELOPMENT SEMANTIC MAPPING LEXICAL DEVELOPMENT: RUSSIAN

This article is one in the series of science popularizing publications on children's speech. It poses the problems of children's attempts to find out how word-nominations are motivated. Special attention is being paid to cases when a word or phraseological unit is modified by a child in an effort (unconscious more often than not) to endow a word with traceable semantic roots or reconstruct its lost conceptual ties. SNC

Ceytlin, Stella N. (1979). Detskiye rechevyje oshibki v oblasti glagolnogo formoobrazovania. (Children's errors in the sphere of verbal form-building.). *Russkiy yazyk v shkole*, 1, 30-31. RUSSIAN MORPHOLOGICAL DEVELOPMENT INFLECTION: RUSSIAN

It is common knowledge that Russian-speaking children tend to build verbal forms which do not correspond to standard

Russian. The reason is that there may be two different stems of one verb: open (vocalic) and closed (consonant). Transition from one to the other is complicated and hardly predictable in each case. That is why children may and often do form an open stem from a closed one and vice versa incorrectly. As to the choice of inflections, due to scanty variety errors in their choice are rare. SNC

Ceytlin, Stella N. (1979). Tipy detskikh rechevykh oshibok. (The types of mistakes made by Russian-speaking children in the use of their mother tongue.). *Russkiy yasyk v shkole*, 4, 62-63. RUSSIAN SPEECH ERRORS LANGUAGE AND EDUCATION

The typology of mistakes made by Russian-speaking children in the use of their native language is presented. The classification of mistakes given in the article echoes the one in the book 'Speech errors and how to prevent them.' Mistakes made by school children are analyzed. The given classification should be turned to and taken into consideration in the process of teaching pupils the Russian language. SNC.

Ceytlin, Stella N. (1980). Kausativnyie oppozicii v detskoy rechi: Funkcionalnyj analiz grammaticheskikh edinic. (Causative oppositions in children's speech: Functional analysis of grammatical units). Leningrad. RUSSIAN INFLECTION MORPHOLOGICAL DEVELOPMENT CAUSATIVES: RUSSIAN

Causative oppositions in the speech of Russian-speaking children are often built by means of adding the morpheme -sja, that is in the simplest possible way, quite common in the Russian grammar. Besides this, children may form causative oppositions by means of conversion, using intransitive verbs incorrectly as if they were transitive. This means of form-building is not used in adult language (standard Russian) with the exception of certain colloquialisms. Evidently in this case a child brings to realization some covert potentialities of the language.SNC

Ceytlin, Stella N. (1980). Narushenije sintaksicheskikh norm v rechi shkolnikov: nenormativnoje upravlenije. (The breach of syntactic norms in the speech of school children: Incorrect government). *Russkiy yazyk v shkole*, 1, 55-58. RUSSIAN NOUNS MORPHOSYNTACTIC DEVELOPMENT INFLECTION: RUSSIAN

The choice of governed form of the noun in the Russian language may prove difficult enough and cannot be accounted for by semantic peculiarities alone. The article presents typological classification of mistakes of this kind. The cases of unification of government in certain semantic groups of words are dealt with as well as the cases of an incorrect variant choice from all those possible.SNC

Ceytlin, Stella N. (1981). Leksicheskije nepravilnosti v detskoy rechi. (Lexical errors in children's speech.). *Russkiy yasyk v shkole*, 4, 51-54. RUSSIAN MORPHOLOGICAL DEVELOPMENT LEXICAL DEVELOPMENT SEMANTIC MAPPING: RUSSIAN

This paper refers to typical mistakes made by children in the use of lexical units: words and phraseologisms. The cases of the use of words in the meanings they do not have virtually. The breach of semantic congruence, the change of the form of phraseological units and literal interpretation of their meaning are dealt with in the article.

Ceytlin, Stella N. (1982). Rechevye oshibki i ikh preduprezchdenie. (Speech errors and how to prevent them.). In *Fremdlingva instruado eksterlande (Vol. 2)*. Moscow: Prosveshenie. RUSSIAN MORPHOLOGICAL DEVELOPMENT LANGUAGE AND EDUCATION: RUSSIAN

The book is designed as an aid for Secondary (higher) school teachers of Russian. The author analyzes typical mistakes generally made by school children in the use of their native (Russian) language. Attention is paid to erroneous form-building of nouns, adjectives and verbs as well as the incorrect use of pronouns. Syntactic mistakes, such as incorrect government and agreement, wrong use of participial and other specifically Russian constructions, wrong patterning of complex sentences are under study. The abuse of words and phraseological units mainly caused by necessity to find motivation of their meaning is considered. The aim of the book, as the author sees it, is to explain the linguistic mechanism of children's errors which is certain to help to anticipate them. In the closing chapter the author speculated on how to prevent possible mistakes of Russian-speaking children, when teaching them their mother tongue and how to correct them. Some chapters are translated into Chinese.

Ceytlin, Stella N. (1985). (Ot dvukh do piati K.I. Chuckovskogo i problemy sovremennoy lingvistiki. (K. Chuckovsky's book 'children aged 2-5 speak' and the problems of contemporary linguistics.). *Russkiy yazyk v shkole*, 6, 56-61. SPEECH ERRORS: RUSSIAN

K. Chuckovsky, a well known translator and critic used to collect the examples of children's speech errors and innovations. Though he wasn't a professional linguist, he made a number of extremely interesting observations and remarks on linguistic and psychological mechanisms of children's errors in the process of acquisition of their mother tongue. SNC.

Ceytlin, Stella N. (1987). Kategoria chisla v ontogeneze. (The ontogenesis of the category of number in the Russian language.). In *Detskaja rech kak predmet lingvisticheskogo izuchenia. (Children's speech as the subject of linguistic investigation.).* Leningrad: RUSSIAN NOUNS NUMBER MORPHOLOGICAL DEVELOPMENT: RUSSIAN

It is common knowledge that nouns possess the category of number. This can be accounted for by their semantics which factor is taken as one of the basis criteria for nouns' reference to contain lexico-grammatical groups or subclasses. Russian-speaking children tend to supergeneralize the ability of the noun to form plural which results in an incorrect plural form-building irrespective of ability/inability of nouns to have this form (for example the unaccountables).SNC

Ceytlin, Stella N. (1987). Tipy detskikh rechevykh oshibok v oblasti slovoismenenia sushestvitelnykh. The types of grammatical mistakes of Russian-speaking children: grammatical categories of the noun.). *Russkiy yazyk v shkole*, 6, 49-534. RUSSIAN INFLECTION NOUNS MORPHOLOGICAL DEVELOPMENT NUMBER CASE: RUSSIAN

The article focuses on two types of errors characteristic of children's speech. The first one is defined as the wrong formation of noun stems which is accounted for by the tendency for unification resulting in the loss of sound-alteration and the shift of stress. The second one is an incorrect choice of inflection which seems difficult due to the fact that there are three types of declension in the Russian language which are only indirectly determined by the gender of the noun. Mistakes in the formation of the nominative plural (the exchange of -i/-ji for-a) and genetive plural (the use of -ov instead of -ei or a zero morpheme) are sepecially frequent.SNC

Ceytlin, Stella N. (1988). Kategoria vida russkogo glagola v ontogeneze. (The ontogenesis of the category aspect of Russian verbs.). In *Funkcionalnyi analiz grammaticheskikh form i konstrukciy. (Functional analysis of Grammatical forms and constructions).* Leningrad: RUSSIAN ASPECT INFLECTION: RUSSIAN

Typical pecularities of aspectual form-building are described. The cases of incorrect use of one member of the opposition instead of the other also the facts of incorrect form-building of dual verbs are under analysis.SNC

Ceytlin, Stella N. (1988). Obratnoje slovoobrazovanie v detskoy rechi. (Reverse word formation in children's speech.). In *Psyholingvisticheskie issledovania. Rechevoe razvitie i obuchenie yazyku. (Psycholinguistic research. Speech development and language teaching.)* Moscow: RUSSIAN INFLECTION LEXICAL DEVELOPMENT LANGUAGE CHANGE: RUSSIAN

A description of the ways in which Russian-speaking children create lexical innovations in their mother tongue by means of eliminating prefixes, suffixes, and affixes.SNC

Ceytlin, Stella N. (1988). *Okkazionalnyje morfologicheskie formy v detskoy rechi. (Occasional morphological forms in children's speech.)* Leningrad. RUSSIAN INFLECTION NOUNS VERBS ADJECTIVES MORPHOLOGICAL DEVELOPMENT OVERGENERALIZATION-MORPHOLOGICAL: RUSSIAN

The author investigates typical speech errors characteristic of a child's language acquisition especially in the sphere of Russian (the native language) morphology. Having acquired the most general morphological rules and having no notion of exceptions to them imposed on grammar by the semantics of the child makes a lot of incorrect forms all of which either fill in the language gaps or are built on the anology with the possible unrestricted forms. In comparison with the normative (correct) grammatical forms of children's formations are characterized by a greater degree of simplicity and semantic transparence. The preferred form-markers are: inflexions, the shift of stress and sound-alteration (optional means often used shift of stress and sound- alteration (optional means often used by adults in standard Russian are less frequent in children's speech). The undertaken investigation concerns Nouns, Adjectives and Verbs.SNC

Ceytlin, Stella N. (1989). Innovacii kak produkt rechevoy deyatelnosti. (Innovations as the result of children's verbalcommunication.). In *Detskaya rech: problemy i nabludenia. (Children's speech: problems and observations.)* Leningrad: RUSSIAN LEXICAL DEVELOPMENT LEXICAL GAPS OVERGENERALIZATION-MORPHOLOGICAL OVERGENERALIZATION-SYNTACTIC: RUSSIAN

Children's speech is creative rather than formal. More often a child creates words and forms basing his activity on the acquired rules and less frequently he reproduces the set forms. When the word or the grammatical form used by the child coincides with the accepted norms of the language we fail to recognize it as creative work. The basic mechanisms of word and form-building is regulated by the law of analogy. If words and grammatical forms of the language we use were built on the analogy (if all means of word-formation were unified) the units created by children would have coincided with them.SNC

Ceytlin, Stella N. (1989). Osnovnyje osebennosti detskoy prakticheskoy grammatiki. (General peculiarities of children's practical grammar.). In *Sovershenstvovanie metodov diagnostiki i preodolenia narusheniy rechi. (The improvement of diagnosis methods and measures preventing speech errors.)* Leningrad: RUSSIAN GRAMMATICALITY SYNTACTIC DEVELOPMENT SYNTACTIC CATEGORIES: RUSSIAN

The reasons leading to children's early or late acquisition of certain grammatical forms are revealed. The ways in which a child acquires the meaning of the category and the means of expressing this meaning are exposed. The peculiarities of children's grammar (form-building and sentence patterning) to the language of adults (standard Russian grammar) are speculated on. Basing the investigation on the conception adhered to by E. Coseriu and enlarging on the posed problems the author proves the fact that a child primarily acquires the system of the language and only after it he masters the norm. The greater the gap between the system and the norm of the language the more difficult is the process of learning to use it.SNC

Chafetz, J., Feldman, Heidi M., & Wareham, N. L. (1992). There car-ungrammatical. *Journal of Child Language*, 19, 473-480. PARENTAL SPEECH-STYLE:

Chambers, J. K. (1992). Dialect acquisition. *Language*, 68, 673-705. NONSTANDARD DIALECTS SOCIOLINGUISTIC FACTORS:

Chamot, Anna Uhl, & O'Malley, J. Michael. (1990). *Learning strategies in second language acquisition*. New York, NY: Cambridge University Press. L2 ACQUISITION STRATEGIES L2 EDUCATION LANGUAGE AND EDUCATION:

Chandler, Michael, & Chapman, Michael (Eds). (1993). *Criteria for competence: Controversies in the conceptualization and assessment of children's abilities, vol.*. Hillsdale, NJ: Lawrence Erlbaum Associates. PIAGETIAN THEORY NEOPIAGETIAN THEORY ASSESSMENT PROCEDURES LANGUAGE AND COGNITIVE DEVELOPMENT:

An examination of the diversity of research that has concentrated on attempting to establish a schema for developmental milestones. Approximately half of the book deals with Piagetian theory and its development into NeoPiagetian theory.

Chaney, Carolyn. (1989). I pledge a legiance tothe flag: Three studies in word segmentation. *Applied Psycholinguistics*, 10, 261-281. SEGMENTATION WORD BOUNDARIES:

Children used several strategies: segment-by-phrase, segment-by-syllable, and segment-by-word. Children were less successful in segmenting the more abstract piece. They tended to revert to a phrase strategy and/or to change abstract words into more common vocabulary. When preschoolers and kindergartners segmented phrases using the functors 'a, an, my, ' or 'and' phrases using phonetically similar embedded syllables, scores increased with age. Children who had begun to read performed better than their same-age peers. - From Child Development Abstracts.

Chaney, Carolyn. (1992). Language development, metalinguistic skills, and print awareness in 3-year-old-children. *Applied Psycholinguistics*, 13, 485-514. METALINGUISTICS LITERACY:

Chapman, Kathy L., & Mervis, Carolyn B. (1989). Patterns of object-name extension in production. *Journal of Child Language*, 16, 561-571. CATEGORIZATION OVERGENERALIZATION LABELING MUTUAL EXCLUSIVITY:

Four children (initially 1:1 to 1:3) were visited twice a week for a four-to-six month period until they were 1:7. In play sessions, the children were asked to label specially chosen objects. The results showed that there were four periods of category formation resulting from the intersection of the overlap- mutual exclusivity continuum with the first separate and first joint reassignment continuum.

Chapman, Michael. (1988). *Constructive evolution.* New York, NY: Cambridge University Press. OVERVIEW-PIAGET PIAGETIAN THEORY:

Piaget sought to elucidate human knowledge by studying its origins and development. In this book, Michael Chapman applies the same method to Piaget's own thinking. He shows that some of the Swiss psychologist's essential ideas originated in adolescent philosophical speculations about the relation between science and value. These same ideas were then developed step by step in Piaget's investigations of children's cognitive development. According to the author, Piaget's use of developmental psychology as a means for addressing questions about the evolution of knowledge has been misunderstood by psychologists who have approached his work exclusively from the perspectives of their own discipline.

Chapman, Michael, & Skinner, Ellen A. (1989). Children's agency beliefs, cognitive performance and conceptions of effort and ability: Individual and developmental differences. *Child Development*, 60, 1229-1238. SEMANTIC RELATIONS:

Fourth and sixth graders were given the following assessments: (a) agency beliefs, including effort, ability, powerful others, and luck, (b) intelligence test scales, including figural patterns, letter series, arithmetic, and spelling, (c) an interview designed to assess conceptions of effort and ability. Correlations between intelligence and agency beliefs for ability increased with increasing levels of reasoning.-From Child Development Abstracts..

Chapman, Robin S. (1992). *Processes in language acquisition and disorders.* St. Louis, MO: Mosby Year Book. LANGUAGE DISORDERS DEVELOPMENTAL DISORDERS LANGUAGE PROCESSING:

Chapman, Robin S., Bird, E. K. R., & Schwartz, S. E. (1990). Fast mapping of words in event contexts by children with Down syndrome. *Journal of Speech and Hearing Disorders*, 55, 761-770. DOWN SYNDROME FAST MAPPING:

Chapman, Robin S., Schwartz, S. E., & Bird, E. K. R. (1991). Language skills of children and adolescents with Down syndrome: 1. Comprehension. *Journal of Speech and Hearing Research*, 34, 1106-1120. DOWN SYNDROME COMPREHENSION:

Charles, Walter G., & Miller, George A. (1989). Contexts of antonymous adjectives. *Applied Psycholinguistics*, 10, 357-375. ADJECTIVES ANTONYMS:

Contexts of directly antonymous adjectives are highly discriminable, both with sentential and phrasal contexts. These results are used to argue that the cue for learning to associate direct antonyms is not their substitutability, but rather their relatively frequent co-occurrences.-From Child Development Abstracts.

Charles-Luce, Jan, & Luce, Paul A. (1990). Similarity neighborhoods of words in young children's lexicons. *Journal of Child Language*, 17, 205-215. LEXICAL DEVELOPMENT SEMANTIC ORGANIZATION SPREADING-ACTIVATION NETWORK:

Computerized databases, representative of 5 and 7 year olds and adults, were used to examine the similarity neighborhoods in the lexica of the age groups. The lexical organization of the children proved to be simpler in that it had a much smaller number of similarity neighborhoods than the organization of the adult lexicon.

Charvillat, Agnés, & Kail, Michéle. (1991). The status of canonical SVO sentences in French-a developmental study of the on-line processing of dislocated sentences. *Journal of Child Language*, 18, 591-608. LANGUAGE PROCESSING SYNTACTIC STRUCTURES GRAMMATICAL RELATIONS FRENCH:

Chengappa, Shyamala. (1984). Code-alteration in an early bilingual. *Psycho-lingua*, 14, No. 1, 55-62. CODE-SWITCHING:

This paper deals with the phenomenon of code-alteration observed in an early bilingual. A comparison of constraints both linguistic and extra- linguistic, crucial to code-choice in adults and children is presented. The social, psychological, individualistic and situational variables contributing to the code-choice are discussed. The variables such as the interlocutors, setting. form and function are examined in detail in the light of present evidence. The illustrations from speech sample of a 3 year old with Kannada- Kodava bilingual exposure from birth are cited to supplement the observations. The developmental process of mastering bilingual competence vis-avis the conscious and unconscious process of code-switching are examined in the present context of bilingual language situation. Results showed that elements of code-switching are evident in the bilingual's speech behaviour at this age itself. The distinctive use of the two languages were facilitated by the consistently differentiated use of two languages by parents in the beginning at home and later, outside the home.

Chien, Yu-Chin, & Wexler, Kenneth. (1990). Children's knowledge of locality conditions in binding as evidence for the modularity of syntax and pragmatics. *Language Acquisition*, 1, 225-295. MODULARITY PRAGMATIC DEVELOPMENT SYNTACTIC DEVELOPMENT ANAPHORA PRONOUNS:

The authors report four experiments which indicate that six-year-old children may understand local pronominal and reflexive binding, but they do not understand 'long-distance' binding. They offer the fact that children lack a pragmatic principle, rather than lack binding Principle B, as an explanation of this phenomenon.

Chin, S. B., & Dinnsen, Daniel A. (1992). Consonant clusters in disordered speech-constraints and correspondence patterns. *Journal of Child Language*, 19, 259-285. PHONOLOGICAL DISORDERS CONSTRAINTS-PHONOLOGICAL CONSONANTS-CLUSTERS:

Chipman, Harold H., & Imperiali di Francavilla, Margherita. (1989). His or hers? How young English and Algerian Arabic speaking children understand third person possessive pronouns in object position. *Folia Linguistica*, 23, 157-180. CROSSLINGUISTIC STUDY-MORPHOSYNTAX ARABIC PRONOUNS-POSSESSIVE CASE PRONOUNS-PERSONAL POSSESSIVES:

Choi, Soonja. (1991). Early acquisition of epistemic meaning in Korean: A study of sentence- ending suffixes in the spontaneous speech of three children. *First language*, 11, 93-119. MOOD AFFIXATION KOREAN LANGUAGE FUNCTIONS TRUTH VALUES:

The study investigates the form and function of three sentence- ending suffixes in Korean: -ta, -e, and -ct, which indicate the state of the speaker's knowledge of the truth value of the utterance. The paper also relates to the acquisition of grammatical mood, and specifically addresses the development of epistemic meaning in relation to deontic meaning. The author reports that in Korean epistemic meanings appear before deontic meaning whereas in the majority oflanguages studied to date the reverse is true, i.e deontic appears before epistemic meaning.

Christie, James F. (1991). *Play and early literacy development*. Albany, NY: SUNY Press. LANGUAGE AND PLAY LITERACY:

Chung, S. Y., Luk, S. L., & Lee, P. W. (1990). A follow-up study of infantile autism in Hong Kong. *Journal of Autism and Developmental Disorders*, 20, 177-187. AUTISM CROSSCULTURAL STUDY CROSSLINGUISTIC STUDY CHINESE:

Authors believe that there is no difference in the way in which autism manifests itself in Hong Kong and its symptoms in other countries.

Church, K., Gale, W., Hanks, P., & Hindle, D. (1991). Using statistics in lexical analysis. In U. Zernik (Ed.), *Lexical Acquisition-Exploiting On-Line Resources to Build a Lexicon*. Hillsdale, NJ : Lawrence Erlbaum Associates. LEXICAL DEVELOPMENT METHODOLOGY-ANALYSIS:

Clahsen, Harald. (1989). The grammatical characterization of developmental dysphasia. *Linguistics*, 27-5(303), 897-920. SYNTACTIC DISORDERS DEVELOPMENTAL DISORDERS:

From Stockholm Bibliographies.

Clahsen, Harald. (1991). Constraints on parameter seting: A grammatical analysis of some acquisitonal stages in German child language. *Language Acquisition*, 1, 361-391. PARAMETER SETTING GERMAN CONSTRAINTS-SYNTACTIC AGREEMENT NULL SUBJECTS VERBS NEGATION:

Clahsen argues that three syntactic constraints are needed to make the parameter setting model of language acquisition functional. He draws upon empirical studies of German to demonstrate the operation of these constraints in: subject-verb agreement, verb-placement, null subjects, and negation.

Clahsen, Harald. (1991). Learnability theory and the problem of development in language acquisition. In J. Weissenborn, H. Goodluck, & T. Roeper (Eds), *Theoretical Issues in Language Acquisition-Continuity and Change in Development*. Hillsdale, NJ: Lawrence Erlbaum Associates. LEARNABILITY:

Clahsen, Harald. (1991). *Normale und gestorte Kindersprache. (Child language and developmental dysphasia-Linguistic studies of the acquisition of German.)*. Amsterdam, The Netherlands: John Benjamins. LEARNABILITY DEVELOPMENTAL DISORDERS GERMAN SYNTACTIC DISORDERS MORPHOLOGICAL DISORDERS SYNTACTIC DEVELOPMENT MORPHOLOGICAL DEVELOPMENT LANGUAGE ACQUISITION DEVICE: GERMAN

The subject of this two part work is the acquisition of language in which the development of syntax and morphology is examined by investigations on children without language problems and on children with developmental dysphasia. The author uses a comparative acquisition study to provide insights into the structure and development of the language acquisition device, which cannot be obtained by isolated analysis of only one type of learning. The theoretical framework used for the investigations is the learnability theory, in which acquisition models are proposed which are heavily influenced by theoretical linguistics. Part I shows how child grammar acquisition can be explained in the framework of learnability theory and Part II deals with deficiencies in normal grammar acquisition using the learnability theory. Also available in an English translation from Benjamins.

Clancy, Patricia M. (1989). A case study in language socialization: Korean wh-questions. *Discourse Processes*, 12(2), 161-191. KOREAN QUESTIONS-WH LANGUAGE SOCIALIZATION:

From Stockholm Bibliographies.

Clancy, Patricia M. (1989). Form and function in the acquisition of Korean wh-questions. *Journal of Child Language*, 16(2), 323-347. KOREAN QUESTIONS-WH:

From Stockholm Bibliographies.

Clark, Eve V. (1990). Speaker perspective in language acquisition. *Linguistics*, 28(6), 1201-122. PERSPECTIVE TAKING PRAGMATIC DEVELOPMENT:

Clark, Eve V. (1991). Acquisition principles in lexical development. In S. A. Gelman, & J. Byrnes (Eds), *Perspectives on language and thought*. New York, NY: Cambridge University Press. LANGUAGE AND COGNITION LANGUAGE AND COGNITIVE DEVELOPMENT LEXICAL DEVELOPMENT:

Clark, M. Diane. (1991). When the same is different-a comparison of the information processing strategies of deaf and hearing people. *American Annals of the Deaf*, 136, 349-353. RELATIONAL TERMS DEAF CHILDREN:

Clark, Robin. (1992). The selection of syntactic knowledge. *Language Acquisition*, 2, 83-149. PARAMETER SETTING LEARNABILITY ACQUISITION THEORIES:

Clark proposes that contrary to the standard assumption, parameter setting is not a deductive process and argues that if it were a deductive process then the cost of processing would make it prohibitive. An alternative, nondeductive, process is proposed as an explanation and model of language acquisition.

Cleeremans, A., & McClelland, James L. (1990). Learning the structure of event sequences. In M. Piatelli-Palmarini (Ed.), *Proceedings of the Twelfth Annual Conference of the Cognitive Science Society*. Hillsdale, NJ: Lawrence Erlbaum Associates. EVENTS/SCRIPTS CONNECTIONISM:

Code, Christopher. (1989). *The characteristics of aphasia.* Hillsdale, NJ: Lawrence Erlbaum Associates. APHASIAS INTERVENTION PROGRAMS CLASSIFICATION OF DISORDERS:

A survey of the main behavioral characteristics of various aphasias and their history and research bases. Includes information on current rehabilitation and recovery programs.

Code, Christopher. (1991). *Aphasia therapy.* San Diego, CA: Singular Group. APHASIAS AGRAPHIA ALEXIA TRAUMATIC DISORDERS CLASSIFICATION OF DISORDERS INTERVENTION PROGRAMS BLISS SYMBOLS SPLINK:

Includes agraphia, alexia and other forms of aphasia and their treatment. Includes treatment programs using Bliss symbols and other artificial language systems, and a report on the clinical trial of Splink.

Code, Christopher, & Ball, Martin J. (1982). Fricative production in Broca's aphasia: a spectrographic analysis. *Journal of Phonetics*, 10, 325-331. BROCA'S APHASIA FRICATIVES ACOUSTIC PHONETICS:

Code, Christopher, & Ball, Martin J. (1984). *Experimental clinical phonetics (U.S.: Instrumentation in speech language pathology).* San Diego, CA: College Hill. ASSESSMENT PROCEDURES PHONOLOGICAL DISORDERS:

Code, Christopher, & Ball, Martin J. (1988). Apraxia of speech. In M. J. Ball (Ed.), *Theoretical linguistics and disordered language.* London: Croom Helm. APRAXIA:

Coe, David A., Matson, Johnny L., Fee, Virginia E., Manikam, Ramasamy, & Linarello, Christine. (1990). Training nonverbal and verbal play skills to mentally retarded and autistic children. *Journal of Autism and Developmental Disorders*, 20, 177-187. DOWN SYNDROME AUTISM RETARDED CHILDREN INTERVENTION PROGRAMS:

Two autistic boys and a girl with Down syndrome (all mentally retarded) were taught to initiate and play a ball game using physical and verbal prompts and reinforcement techniques.

Cole, Kevin N., Dale, Philip S., & Mills, Paulette E. (1991). Individual differences in language delayed children's responses to direct and interactive preschool instruction. *Topics in Early Childhood Special Education*, 11, 99-124. LANGUAGE AND EDUCATION LANGUAGE DELAY INTERVENTION PROGRAMS:

This study examined the relative effects of two highly contrasting preschool curricula on language development for children with delayed language. No main effect differences were found between Direct Instruction and Mediated Learning.

Cole, M. (1992). Context, modularity, and the cultural constitution of development. In L. T. Winegar, & J. Valsiner (Eds), *Children's development within a social context, (Vol. 2).* Hillsdale, NJ: Lawrence Erlbaum Associates. MODULARITY CONTEXT:

Coley, John D., & Gelman, Susan A. (1989). The effects of object orientation and object type on children's interpretation of the word 'big'. *Child Development*, 60(2), 372-380. DIMENSIONAL ADJECTIVES SEMANTIC MAPPING:

From Stockholm Bibliographies.

Collins, Michael. (1991). *Diagnosis and treatment of global aphasias.* San Diego, CA: Singular Group. APHASIAS CLASSIFICATION OF DISORDERS:

Colombo, John, & Fagen, Jeffrey W. (Eds). (1990). *Individual differences in infancy: Reliability, stability, and prediction.* Hillsdale, NJ: Lawrence Erlbaum Associates. INDIVIDUAL VARIATION:

A collection of papers discussing individual differences and variations in child development. Specific chapters are included on: learning and memory, visual attention, neurobehavioral development, and socioemotional development.

Colombo, John, Mitchell, D. Wayne, Coldren, Jeffrey T., & Atwater, Jay D. (1990). Discrimination learning during the first year: Stimulus and positional cues. *Journal of Experimental Psychology*, 16, 98-109. METHODOLOGY-DESIGN INFANT PERCEPTION:

In four studies, 3, 6, and 9-month-old human infants were tested in a discrimination learning task in which visual fixation to a particular stimulus or lateral position was reinforced with an auditory stimulus. In experiment 1, all age groups exhibited acquisition, extinction, and reinstatement of fixation to the reinforced target or position. Experiment 2 revealed that 3-month-olds retained the positional discrimination but not the stimulus discrimination after a 5-minute delay between acquisition and extinction. In experiments 3 and 4, we investigated a possible developmental shift in the dominance of positional versus stimulus cues by training the infants on displays in which stimulus and position were confounded and then by dissociating the cues on test trials. Results from both experiments indicated positional cue dominance for young infants and stimulus cue dominance for older infants.-From Child Development Abstracts.

Colson, J. P. (1989). *Krashens Monitortheorie: een experimentele studie van het Nederlands als vreemde taal (Krashen's monitor theory: A Dutch experimental study.).* The Netherlands: Peeters. DUTCH
L2 ACQUISITION THEORIES MONITORING: DUTCH

Comblain, A., & Rondal, Jean A. (1990). L'apprentissage des langues étrangeres: aspects psycholinguistiques. (Learning foreign languages: psycholinguistic aspects.). *Langes Étrangeres.* L2 EDUCATION: FRENCH

Comeau, Judith, & Therrien, Marie-Claude. (1990). Conversational exchange between a 5- to 6 year old and the mother in a playroom situation. In M. A. K. Halliday, J. Gibbons, & H. Nicholas (Eds), *Learning, keeping and using language.* Amsterdam, The Netherlands: John Benjamins. ADULT-CHILD INTERACTION LANGUAGE AND PLAY SOCIAL INTERACTION INTERSUBJECTIVITY:

Compernol-Bredart, C., Rondal, Jean A., & Perée, F. (1981). More about maternal and paternal speech to language-learning children in various dyadic and tryadic contexts. *International Journal of Psycholinguistics*, 8 (4), 149-168. PARENTAL SPEECH-SEX DIFFERENCES:

Comrey, Andrew L., & Lee, Howard B. (1992). *A first course in factor analysis*. Hillsdale, NJ: Lawrence Erlbaum Associates. METHODOLOGY-ANALYSIS:

An introductory text which explains the theoretical basis and the application and interpretation of factor analysis techniques. The second edition includes later developments of the factor analysis technique. A set of diskettes that enable the user to run factor analyses on the PC and/or a FORTRAN reading mainframe is available from the publisher.

Connell, P. J., & Stone, C. A. (1992). Morpheme learning of children with specific language impairment under controlled instructional conditions. *Journal of Speech and Hearing Research*, 35, 844-852. MORPHOLOGICAL DEVELOPMENT MORPHOSYNTACTIC DEVELOPMENT SPECIFIC LANGUAGE IMPAIRMENT:

Conrad, R. (1972). The developmental role of vocalizing in STM. *Journal of Verbal Learning and Verbal Behavior*, 11, 521-533. VOCALIZATIONS LANGUAGE AND MEMORY LANGUAGE AND COGNITIVE DEVELOPMENT:

Conti-Ramsden, Gina. (1984). Situational variability in nother-child dialogues with normal and language-impaired children. *Proceedings of the XIX Congress of the International Association of Logopaedics and Phoneatrics*, 1, 457-462. PARENTAL SPEECH-ATYPICAL CHILDREN:

Conti-Ramsden, Gina. (1985). Mothers in dialogue with language-impaired children. *Topics in Language Disorders*, 5, 58-68. LANGUAGE DISORDERS PARENTAL SPEECH-ATYPICAL CHILDREN:

Conti-Ramsden, Gina. (1986). Scriptedness: a factor in children's variation in language use? *Proceedings of the Child Language Seminar,* 88-96. EVENTS/SCRIPTS INDIVIDUAL VARIATION:

Conti-Ramsden, Gina. (1986). Share knowledge with parents. *Speech Therapy in Practice*, 2, 24. INTERVENTION PROGRAMS FOR PARENTS:

Conti-Ramsden, Gina. (1987). Mother-child talk with language-impaired children. *Proceedings of the First International Symposium on Specific Speech and Language Disorders in*

Children. PARENTAL SPEECH-ATYPICAL CHILDREN PARENTAL SPEECH-STYLE:

Conti-Ramsden, Gina. (1989). Developmental language disorders. In K. Grundy (Ed.), *Linguistics in clinical practice.* London: Taylor & Francis. DEVELOPMENTAL DISORDERS:

Conti-Ramsden, Gina. (1989). *Language and communication in mentally handicapped people.* London: Chapman & Hall. ATYPICAL DEVELOPMENT RETARDED CHILDREN PARENTAL SPEECH-STYLE ADULT-CHILD INTERACTION:

An evaluation of parent-child interaction and mental handicap.

Conti-Ramsden, Gina. (1989). Proper name usage: mother-child interactions with language-impaired and non-language-impaired children. *First Language*, 9, 271-284. LANGUAGE DISORDERS NOUNS-PROPER PARENTAL SPEECH-VOCABULARY PARENTAL SPEECH-ATYPICAL CHLDREN:

Conti-Ramsden, Gina. (1990). Recasts and other contingent replies to language-impaired children. *Journal of Speech and Hearing Disorders*, 55, 262-274. PARENTAL INPUT PARENTAL SPEECH-ATYPICAL CHILDREN RECASTS:

Conti-Ramsden, Gina, & Beveridge, Michael. (1987). Context and sequence in language teaching. *Bulletin (College of Speech Therapists)*, 427, 1-2. LANGUAGE AND EDUCATION INTERVENTION PROGRAMS:

Conti-Ramsden, Gina, & Dykins, J. (1991). Mother-child interactions with language-impaired children and their siblings. *British Journal of Disorders of Communication,* 26. PARENTAL SPEECH-ATYPICAL CHILDREN PARENTAL INPUT SIBLING EFFECTS:

Conti-Ramsden, Gina, & Friel-Patti, Sandy. (1983). Mothers' discourse adjustments to language-impaired and non-language-impaired children. *Journal of Speech and Hearing Disorders*, 48, 360-367. PARENTAL SPEECH-STYLE PARENTAL SPEECH-ATYPICAL CHILDREN LANGUAGE DISORDERS:

Conti-Ramsden, Gina, & Friel-Patti, Sandy. (1984). Mother-child dialogues: a comparison of normal and language-impaired children. *Journal of Communication Disorders*, 17, 19-35. LANGUAGE DISORDERS PARENTAL SPEECH-STYLE PARENTAL SPEECH-ATYPICAL CHILDREN:

Conti-Ramsden, Gina, & Friel-Patti, Sandy. (1986). Mother-child dialogues: considerations of cognitive complexity for young language learning children. *British Journal of Disorders of Communication*, 21, 245-255. PARENTAL SPEECH-ATYPICAL CHILDREN:

Conti-Ramsden, Gina, & Friel-Patti, Sandy. (1987). Situational variability in mother-child conversations. In K. Nelson, & A. van Kleeck (Eds), *Children's language*, vol. 6. New Jersey: Lawrence Erlbaum. PARENTAL SPEECH-STYLE ADULT-CHILD INTERACTION:

Conti-Ramsden, Gina, & Gunn, M. (1986). The development of conversational disability: a case study. *British Journal of Disorders of Communication*, 21, 339-351. CONVERSATIONAL DISORDERS METHODOLOGY-DIARY/CASE STUDY:

Conti-Ramsden, Gina, Hensey, O., & Rosenbloom, L. (1985). Management of severe language disorders: a multidisciplinary approach. *Bulletin (College of Speech Therapists)*, 397, 8-9. INTERVENTION PROGRAMS:

Conti-Ramsden, Gina, & Snow, Catherine E. (1990). *Children's language*, vol. 7. Hillsdale, NJ: Lawrence Erlbaum Associates. LITERATURE COLLECTION PRAGMATIC DEVELOPMENT LITERACY QUESTIONS LEXICAL DEVELOPMENT BILINGUALISM PRONOUNS-PERSONAL INTONATION FAST MAPPING PARENTAL SPEECH METALINIGUISTICS CHILDREN'S EXPLANATIONS SOCIAL SPEECH SPEECH ACTS:

Proceedings of the Fourth Child Language Congress, Austin, TX.

Conti-Ramsden, Gina, & Taylor, J. (1990). Teacher-pupil talk: integrated versus segregated environments for children with severe learning difficulties. *British Journal of Disorders of Communication*, 25, 1-15. LANGUAGE AND EDUCATION:

Conway, David F. (1990). Semantic relationships in the word meanings of hearing-impaired children. *Volta Review*, 92, 339-349. DEAF CHILDREN SEMANTIC RELATIONS:

The amount, type, and complexity of the semantic relationships expressed in the word meanings of hearing-impaired children was examined. Profoundly hearing-impaired subjects between six and eleven years of age were divided equally into a younger group (<9.0 years). Semantic relationships were identified using a case grammar analysis scheme. The groups did not differ significantly on the types or complexity of relationships expressed.

Conway, David F. (1992). Literacy, learning, and interaction. *Volta Review*, 94 , 343-344. LITERACY:

Conway, David F. (1992). Speech production and language understanding. *Volta Review* , 94, 239-240. COMPREHENSION SPEECH PRODUCTION:

Conway, David F. (1992). Understanding and improving speech production. *Volta Review* , 94, 241-242. SPEECH PRODUCTION INTELLIGIBILITY COMPREHENSION:

Cook, Vivian. (1991). *Second language learning and language teaching..* New York, NY: Edward Arnold. L2 EDUCATION L2 ACQUISITION L2 SYNTAX L2 VOCABULARY L2 PHONOLOGY L2 COMMUNICATIVE COMPETENCE L2 VARIATION:

Topics covered include: the acquisition of grammar, pronunciation, vocabulary, and conversation, and processes of language use and memory. The author also examines: individual variation, and aspects of language pedagogy.

Cooper, B., & Conti-Ramsden, Gina. (1989). Entry with little reward: less-able pupils and GCSE (General Certificate of Secondary Education) English. *Education*, 173, 237-238. LANGUAGE AND EDUCATION:

Cooper, Robin Panneton, & Aslin, Richard N. (1990). Preference for infant-directed speech in the first month after birth. *Child Development*, 61, 1584-1595. PARENTAL SPEECH-PROSODY INFANT PERCEPTION NEONATES:

Both 1-month olds and newborns preferred ID (infant-directed) over AD (adult-directed) speech. These results suggest that infants' preference for the exaggerated prosodic features of ID speech is present from birth.

Cooreman, A., & Kilborn, K. (1991). Second language acquisition and functional linguistics. In T. Huebner, & C. A. Ferguson (Eds), *Cross-currents in second language acquisition and linguistic theory*. Amsterdam: John Benjamins. L2 ACQUISITION THEORIES L2 RESEARCH DESIGN:

Coppieters, Rene. (1990). Review of 'Variation theory and second language acquisition' by H. D. Adamson. *Language*, 66(1), 163. BOOK REVIEW L2 VARIATION L2/L1 ACQUISITION PIDGINS/CREOLES L2 ACQUISITION THEORIES MONITORING:

The basic issue tackled by A is how to analyze variation in the speech of second language learners. The unifying theme is methodology. Within the constraints mentioned above, A's discussion is informative and well organized. It includes a review of the early first-and second-language morpheme acquisition studies, an overview of the techniques developed by sociolinguists for the analysis of variation, an outline of the possible similarities between the speech of second-language learners and pidgins and creoles, an essay on the psychological reality of linguistic rules, in particular variable rules, a discussion of the variable rule notation to express the results of 'prototype' studies, and a short discussion of Krashen's monitor model (see, for instance, Krashen 1981) in relation to variation theory. - From Language.

Corballis, Michael C. (1991). *The lop-sided ape*. New York, NY: Oxford University Press. LATERALIZATION PHYLOGENETIC ORIGINS:

Corballis takes us on a fascinating tour of the origins and implications of the two halves of the brain-known as laterality-in human evolution. He begins by surveying current views of evolution, ranging from the molecular level to the tremendous implications of such physical changes as walking on two feet. He goes on to look at the structure of language, following the work of Noam Chomsky and others, showing how grammar allows us to create an infinite variety of messages. He demonstrates that only humans have this unlimited ability for expression. Both a detailed account of human language and evolution and a convincing argument for a new view of the brain, the book provides fascinating insight into our origins and the nature of human thought itself.

Cordes, A. K., Ingham, R. J., Frank, P., & Ingham, J. C. (1992). Time-interval analysis of interjudge and intrajudge agreement for stuttering event judgments. *Journal of Speech and Hearing Research*, 35, 483-494. STUTTERING:

Coren, Stanley. (1992). *The left-hander syndrome: The causes and behavioral consequences of left-handedness*. New York, NY: The Free Press. LANGUAGE AND HANDEDNESS LANGUAGE AND COGNITIVE DEVELOPMENT:

Author reviews the causes and consequences of left-handedness and suggests that there are physical, cognitive, and other psychological effects of left-handedness that need to be considered.

Cormier, Pierre, & Tomlinson-Keasey, Carol. (1991). The development of hemispheric specialization of letter matching. *Developmental Neuropsychology*, 7, 161-176. LATERALIZATION LANGUAGE AND EDUCATION:

Differences between kindergarteners, first- and second-graders were observed in the normal development of hemispheric specialization for letter matching. Kindergarteners treated the skills involved as linguistic, whereas second graders approached the task as a test of speed. From Child Development Abstracts.

Corradini, S. (1990). La réflexion métalinguistique chez des schizophrènes. (Metalinguistic reflection in schizophrenics.). *Bulletin CILA*, 51, 92-101. METALINGUISTICS PSYCHOPATHOLOGICAL CHILDREN: FRENCH

Corrigan, Roberta L., Eckman, Fred R., & Noonan, Michael (Eds). (1989). *Linguistic categorization.* Amsterdam, The Netherlands: Benjamins. CATEGORIZATION PROTOTYPE THEORY CROSSLINGUISTIC STUDY-CATEGORIZATION CONCEPT DEVELOPMENT SEMANTIC DEVELOPMENT:

A collection of essays, from an international symposium held in Madison, Wisconsin in 1987. The volume is divided into three sections: prototype effects in language, categorization processes, and crosslinguistic categorization.

Cosnier, Jacques, & Jisa, Harriet. (1988). Le développement de la fonction langagière. (The development of the language function). *Cahier de l'audition*, 12, 17-25. INTERSUBJECTIVITY ADULT-CHILD INTERACTION PARENTAL INPUT: FRENCH

Recent developments in child language research have shown that communicative competence is built upon communicative foundations. Functional communication appears long before the child's first uses of meaning-bearing sound sequences. Everyday conversation during prelinguistic and early linguistic stages provide the essential framework upon which verbal communication is based.

Costello, Janis M. (1984). *Speech disorders in children.* San Diego, CA: Singular Group. DEVELOPMENTAL DISORDERS CONGENITAL DISORDERS:

Coster, Wendy J., Gersten, Michelle S., Beeghly, Marjorie, & Cicchetti, Dante. (1989). Communicative functioning in maltreated toddlers. *Developmental Psychology*, 25(6), 1020-1029. SOCIOLINGUISTIC FACTORS ABUSED CHILDREN:

From Stockholm Bibliographies.

Cottrell, Gary W., & Plunkett, Kim. (1991). Learning the past tense in a recurrent network: acquiring the mapping from meaning to sounds. In K. Hammond, & D. Gentner (EdS), *Proceedings of the Thirteenth Annual Conference of the Cognitive Science Society*. Hillsdale, NJ: Lawrence Erlbaum Associates. TENSE CONNECTIONISM:

Coudry, M.I., & Scarpa, Ester M. (1986). De como a avaliacao dalinguagem pode contribuir parainaugurar ou sistematizar odeficit. (On how language assessment may contribute to install or systematize the deficit). *Revista Disturbios dacomunicacao (PUC, SP)*, , 117-136. ASSESSMENT PROCEDURES CLASSIFICATION OF DISORDERS DYSLEXIA PORTUGUESE APHASIAS: PORTUGUESE

A paper which describes the use of linguistic and pragmatic information to assess language disability in dyslexia and aphasia. EMS.

Coulter, Geoffrey R. (1992). *Current issues in ASL phonology*. San Diego, CA: Academic Press. SIGNING-ASL:

A description of the forms and patterns used in signing ASL.

Courchene, Robert J., et al. (1992). *Comprehension-based second language teaching. (L'enseignement des langues seçondes axe sur la compréhension.)*. Ottawa, Canada: University of Ottawa Press. BILINGUALISM-EDUCATION LANGUAGE AND EDUCATION L2 EDUCATION: FRENCH

Text available in in English and French editions. A collection of selected papers on comprehension-based second language teaching, most of which were presented at the International Conference on Comprehension-Based Second Language Teaching hosted by the Second Language Institute of the University of Ottawa in May, 1989.

Cowan, Nelson. (1989). Acquisition of Pig Latin: a case study. *Journal of Child Language*, 16(2), 365-386. SLANG LANGUAGE GAMES RULES:

From Stockholm Bibliographies.

Cox, Maureen V. (1991). *The child's point of view, 2nd ed.* New York, NY: Guilford Press. COMPREHENSION SOCIAL SPEECH SOCIAL INTERACTION LANGUAGE AND COGNITIVE DEVELOPMENT CHILDREN'S DISCOURSE:

Cox, Maureen V., & Isard, Sarah. (1990). Children's deictic and non deictic interpretations of the spatial locatives in front of and behind. *Journal of Child Language*, 17, 481-488. SPATIAL TERMS DEIXIS-SPATIAL LOCATIVES RELATIONAL TERMS DECENTRATION EGOCENTRISM:

> Two groups of children (mean ages 5:10 and 9:11) were asked to place a toy man in front of or behind a car which either faced away from them or faced sideways. When the observer's viewpoint was not emphasized in the instructions, or was merely implied, both age groups responded in a nondeictic way. When the viewpoint of the observer was an essential component of the task and the spatial term was omitted, both age groups selected a deitic location. When the viewpoint was emphasized but when the spatial term was also included the responses were split between deictic and nondeictic locations.

Crago, Martha B., & Cole, Elizabeth B. (1991). Using ethnography to bring children's communicative and cultural worlds into focus. In T. M. Gallagher, & N. Rees (EdS), *Pragmatics of language: Clinical practice issues..* San Diego, CA: Singular Group. ETHNOGRAPHIC APPROACHES SOCIAL TRANSMISSION COMMUNICATIVE COMPETENCE CROSSLINGUISTIC STUDY-PRAGMATICS:

> A review of language socialization processes, ethnography, and crosscultural perspectives on communicative competence.

Craig, A. (1990). An investigation into the relationship between anxiety and stuttering. *Journal of Speech and Hearing Disorders*, 55, 290-294. STUTTERING:

Craig, Holly K. (1991). Pragmatic characteristics of the child with specific language impairment: An interactionist perspective. In T. M. Gallagher, & N. Rees (Eds), *Pragmatics of language: Clinical practice issues..* San Diego, CA: Singular Group. SPECIFIC

LANGUAGE IMPAIRMENT INTERVENTION PROGRAMS PRAGMATIC DISORDERS:

A review of the characteristics of SLI and a discussion of the methodological implications of the literature on the treatment of the pragmatic disorders of SLI.

Craig, Holly K., & Evans, J. L. (1991). Turn exchange behaviors of children with normally developing language-the influence of gender. *Journal of Speech and Hearing Research*, 34, 866-878. TURN TAKING SEX DIFFERENCES:

Crain, Stephen, & Shankweiler, Donald P. (1990). Modularity and learning to read. In I. G. Mattingly, & M. Studdert-Kennedy (Eds), *Modularity and the motor theory of speech perception*. Hillsdale, NJ: Lawrence Erlbaum Associates. LITERACY:

Crain, Stephen, & Thornton, R. (1991). Recharting the course of language acquisition: studies in elicited production. In N. A. Krasnegor, et al. (Eds), *Biological and behavioral determinants of language development*. Hillsdale, NJ: Lawrence Erlbaum Associates. ACQUISITION THEORIES SPEECH PRODUCTION METHODOLOGY-DESIGN:

Craton, Lincoln G., Elicker, James, Plumert, Jodie M., & Pick, Herber L., Jnr. (1990). Children's use of frames of reference in communication of spatial location. *Child Development*, 61, 1528-1543. LOCATIVES SPATIAL TERMS DEIXIS-SPATIAL RELATIONAL TERMS:

Children, 4, 6, and 8 were asked to specify verbally the location of a toy hidden under one of several identical cups. Communication about the left- right dimension was particularly difficult for 4-year-old children and showed a higher rate of improvement with age than communication about the front-back dimension and, the frames of reference changed with age and differed for directions about the front-back and left-right dimensions. Children used person references to specify front-back relations, but only 6-year-olds were able to use landmarks to specify the left-right dimension.

Eight-year-olds used a combination of person and landmark references in both dimensions.

Cromer, Richard F. (1991). *Language and thought in normal and handicapped children*. Oxford, UK: Blackwell. COGNITION HYPOTHESIS LANGUAGE AND COGNITION LANGUAGE AND COGNITIVE DEVELOPMENT ACQUISITION STRATEGIES ACQUISITION THEORIES ATYPICAL DEVELOPMENT:

In this book Richard Cromer sets out the crucial issues in the field of language acquisition. Consisting of a series of comprehensive reviews of various aspects of of the topic, this volume is speculative and provocative, backing its theoretical statements with experimental and observational evidence. The book opens with Cromer's classic statement of the cognition hypothesis of language acquisition. Following that is a reassessment of this hypothesis in the light of later findings which call for important modifications to the original theory. He then explores the strategies children use in acquiring language, and suggests much needed reconceptualizations of language acquisition and cognitive development more generally. The final part of the book examines recent important research into language handicap to theories of linguistic and cognitive development.

Cromer, Richard F. (1993). A case study of dissociations between language and cognition. In H. Tager-Flusberg (Ed.), *Constraints on language acquisition: Studies of atypical children*. Hillsdale, NJ: Lawrence Erlbaum Associates. ATYPICAL DEVELOPMENT LANGUAGE AND COGNITION LANGUAGE AND COGNITIVE DEVELOPMENT:

Crowder, Robert G., & Wagner, Richard K. (1991). *The psychology of reading,* 2nd Ed. New York, NY: Oxford University Press. LITERACY:

Cognitive psychologists have discovered that reading represents a natural laboratory for studying almost all cognitive processes-from sensation and perception to comprehension and reasoning. This introductory textbook examines the important principles of cognitive psychology that pertain to reading, but it is not written for the cognitive psychologist. Though grounded in the latest research, this revision maintains the objective of the first edition-to provide a highly accessible introduction to students approaching the subject for the first time.

Cruttenden, Alan. (1970). A phonetic study of babbling. *British Journal of Disorders of Communication*, 5, 110-7. BABBLING BABBLING DRIFT HYPOTHESIS:

The babbling of a pair of twins from birth to 1:3 was transcribed at approximately monthly intervals. The onset of babbling at around three months was marked by the first occurance of pulmonic-lingual segments and by the playful use of sounds. The inventory of sounds used in babbling was not as all- embracing as previously claimed but was limited to plosives, nasals and an open vowel, together with temporary 'rogue' sounds. There was considerable difference in the quantity of babbling between the twins. There was clear non-language specific babbling drift. The first words took over the sounds of late babbling. Phonemic analysis was not relevant to the first words.AC

Cruttenden, Alan. (1972). Phonological procedures for child language. *British Journal of Disorders of Communication*, 7, 30-7. ACQUISITION THEORY-PHONOLOGY:

Attempting to analyze children's sounds as having their own system does not work as a procedure: even those analyses which claim to do so are in fact using the adult system as a basis of comparison.AC

Cruttenden, Alan. (1974). The acquisition of pronouns and language simplification. *Language and Speech*, 20, 191-7. PRONOUNS CROSSLINGUISTIC STUDY PIDGINS/CREOLES FRENCH ARABIC:

The order of acquisition of pronouns in English (together with common confusions) is surveyed, using evidence from published studies and from two new sets of data. Perceptual reasons are advanced for the order of acquisition: end saliency and syllabicity (together with a preference for animate subjects and inanimate objects). Comparison is made with acquisition in Arabic and French, and with simplification in creole languages.AC

Cruttenden, Alan. (1978). Assimilation in child language and elsewhere. *Journal of Child Language*, 5, 373-8. PHONOLOGICAL PROCESSES:

Apicals probabilistically precede velars in acquisition, yet once both have been acquired apicals continue to be assimilated to velars in assimilation. This type of assimilation, commonly regressive, is also most common in historical and contectual change. Apicals probably develop first because they are maximally different from labials in both noise burst and in format transitions, i.e. for perceptual reasons: wheras apicals change to velars in assimilation because of productive reasons.AC

Cruttenden, Alan. (1979). *Language in infancy and childhood: a linguistic introduction to language acquisition*. Manchester/New York: Manchester University Press/St. Martin's Press. OVERVIEW-GENERAL PHONOLOGICAL DEVELOPMENT BABBLING SYNTACTIC DEVELOPMENT LEXICAL DEVELOPMENT:

A textbook for postgraduates, advanced undergraduates, and speech therapists, with special emphasis on phonology and on the detailed order of development in babbling, phonology, grammar and lexis.AC

Crystal, David. (1981). *Clinical linguistics*. San Diego, CA: Singular Group. ASSESSMENT PROCEDURES CLINICAL LINGUISTICS INTERVENTION PROGRAMS NONLINEAR PHONOLOGY OVERVIEW-PHONOLOGY OVERVIEW-SYNTAX:

A description of the application of linguistics to the treatment of speech and language disorders.

Crystal, David. (1988). *Introduction to language pathology, 2nd Ed.* San Diego, CA: Singular Group. CLASSIFICATION OF DISORDERS LANGUAGE DISORDERS INTERVENTION PROGRAMS:

Crystal, David, Fletcher, Paul, & Garman, Michael A. (1990). *The grammatical analysis of language disability, 2nd Ed.* San diego, CA: Singular. ASSESSMENT PROCEDURES LARSP SYNTACTIC DISORDERS INTERVENTION PROGRAMS SYNTACTIC DEVELOPMENT:

This book introduces, justifies, and describes procedures for the grammatical analysis, and remediation of syntactic abnormalities in both adults and children. This new edition also includes a section on the development of LARSP from 1975 to 1990.

Csányi, Yvonne. (1974). Siketek irásbeli kifejezökészségének vizsgálata formai és tartalmi szempontból a Myklebust féle PSL teszt felhasználásával. (Formal and content analysis of the written communication of deaf subjects with the use of the Mykebust test.). *Gyógypedagógia*, 1, DEAF CHILDREN WRITTEN LANGUAGE HUNGARIAN: HUNGARIAN

Csányi, Yvonne. (1974). Szövegmegertési vizsgálatok hallási fogyatékosoknál (Text understanding in hearing deficient children). In *Kommunikáció -- hallásserülés*. Budapest: DEAF CHILDREN HUNGARIAN COMPREHENSION DISCOURSE COMPREHENSION: HUNGARIAN

Csányi, Yvonne. (1975). Gondolatok súlyos fokban hallássérult gyermekek anyanyelvi fejlesztéséröl egy informació elmeleti kommunikációs séma tükrében. (Thoughts on first language acquisition of seriously hearing-impaired children in the framework of information communication theory). *Gyógypedagógiai Szemle*, 2, LANGUAGE AND EDUCATION DEAF CHILDREN HUNGARIAN: HUNGARIAN

Csányi, Yvonne. (1976). A Peabody-szókincsvizsgálat hazai alkalmazásának elsö tapasztalatai siket és halló gyermekeknél (First Hungarian experiences with the use of the Peabody Picture Vocabulary Test in hearing and deaf children). *Magyar Pszichológiai Szemle*, 33, HUNGARIAN PEABODY PICTURE VOCABULARY TEST DEAF CHILDREN: HUNGARIAN

Csányi, Yvonne. (1978). Tapasztalatok a hallássérültek kiejtésének felméréséröl. (Experiences in measuring pronunciation in hearing disordered children). *Gyógypedagógiai Szemle*, 5, DEAF CHILDREN ARTICULATION ARTICULATION DISORDERS HUNGARIAN: HUNGARIAN

Csányi, Yvonne. (1980). Verbal testing of deaf persons and its consequences for remedial education methods. *International Foundation of Rehabilitation Research*, 3, DEAF CHILDREN LANGUAGE AND EDUCATION HUNGARIAN:

Csányi, Yvonne. (1981). Beszéd és nyelvtananulási nehézségek épértelmü dysphásiás gyermekeknél (Speech and language problems of intellectually non-retarded dysphasic children). *Gyógypedagógia*, 3, LANGUAGE DISORDERS APHASIAS HUNGARIAN: HUNGARIAN

Csányi, Yvonne. (1982). *Sprachuntersuchungen bei Gehörlosen und ihre pädagogischen Folgerungen. (Speech comprehension by the deaf and its educational implications.).* Giessen: LANGUAGE AND EDUCATION DEAF CHILDREN HUNGARIAN COMPREHENSION: GERMAN

Csányi, Yvonne. (1987). Die Förderung der Sprachverständlichkeit in den Ungarischen Gehörlosenschulen. (The improvement of language comprehension in Hungarian deaf students.). In Stranbeig (Ed.), *Spracherziehungnoch gefragt*. DEAF CHILDREN ARTICULATION HUNGARIAN COMPREHENSION: GERMAN

Culbert, James P., Hamer, Robert, & Klinge, Valerie. (1989). Factor structure of the Wechsler Intelligence Scale for Children-revised, Peabody Picture Vocabulary Test, and Peabody Individual Achievement Test in a psychiatric sample. *Psychology in the Schools*, 26, 331-336. ASSESSMENT PROCEDURES PEABODY PICTURE VOCABULARY TEST WECHSLER SCALES:

> This study analyzed the factor structure of the Wechsler Intelligence scale for Children Revised (WISC-R), the Peabody Picture Vocabulary Test (PPVT), and the Peabody Individual Achievement Test (PIAT) in psychiatric sample (n = 329) that ranged in age from 6 to 16 years. The resultant factor structure of this sample was compared with patterns reported on normal and learning-disabled children. The results were

similar to previous factor analytic studies of the WISC-R and PIAT showing four factors: verbal comprehension, verbal achievement, perceptual organization, and number facility. - From Child Development Abstracts.

Curtiss, Susan R. (1980). The critical period and feral children. *UCLA Working papers in Cognitive Linguistics*, 2. CRITICAL PERIOD FERAL AND ISOLATED CHILDREN:

An extensive and comprehensive survey of all the known studies on feral and isolated children and their ability to develop language. The data is related to the critical period theory. The studies covered range from anecdotal studies such as Casper Hauser to scientific studies such as Genie.

Curtiss, Susan R., Katz, W. F., & Tallal, Paula. (1992). Delay versus deviance in the language acquisition of language-impaired children. *Journal of Speech and Hearing Research*, 35, 373-383. ATYPICAL DEVELOPMENT LANGUAGE DELAY:

Curtiss, Susan R., Kempler, D., & Yamada, Jeni E. (1981). The relationship between language and cognition in development: Theoretical framework and research design. *UCLA Working Papers in Cognitive Linguistics*, 3. LANGUAGE AND COGNITIVE DEVELOPMENT METHODOLOGY-DESIGN:

Cuvelier, Pol. (1986). Situational properties of early verb meaning. *Papers and Reports on Child Language Development*, 25, 17-24. VERBS PRAGMATIC DEVELOPMENT SPEECH ACTS:

Based on data from Cuvelier's 1985 dissertation, the influence of illocutionary aspects in verb meaning is discussed in detail. PC.

Cuvelier, Pol. (1988). The prototypical background in the acquisition process of relational verb meaning. In F. van Besien (Ed.), *First Language Acquisition (ABLA Papers n.12)*. VERBS SEMANTIC DEVELOPMENT LEXICAL DEVELOPMENT EVENTS/SCRIPTS:

Data taken from Cuvelier's 1985 dissertation are analyzed. They provide evidence in favor of the hypothesis that verb meaning may be based to a large extent on the existence of structured event representations (e.g. Nelson 1986) rather than on the relation between learning verbs and learning the basic structure of sentences (Bloom 1981). PC.

Cyrulnik, Boris. (1991). *La naissance du sens. (The birth of thought).* Paris, France: Hachette. LANGUAGE AND COGNITIVE DEVELOPMENT SEMANTIC DEVELOPMENT: FRENCH

Cziko, Gary A. (1989). A review of the state-process and punctual-nonpunctual distinctions in children's acquisitions of verbs. *First Language*, 9, 1-31. VERBS-STATIVE VERBS-PUNCTUAL CROSSLINGUISTIC STUDY:

Approximately 60 empirical studies were initially reviewed with 13 reporting findings relevant to the state-process and/or punctual-nonpunctual distinctions involving the languages of English, French, Greek, Hebrew, Italian, Japanese, Polish, Serbo-Croatian, and Turkish. It was found that these studies in general provide support for the hypothesis that children universally distinguish stative from process verbs. - From Child Development Abstracts.

D

D'Odorico, Laura, & Franco, F. (1991). Selective production of vocalization types in different communication contexts. *Journal of Child Language*, 18, 475-499. SELECTION/AVOIDANCE:

Dagenais, P. A., & Critz-Crosby, P. (1992). Comparing tongue positioning by normal-hearing and hearing-impaired children during vowel production. *Journal of Speech and Hearing Research*, 35, 35-44. DEAF CHILDREN VOWELS ARTICULATION:

Dale, Philip S. (1991). The validity of a parent report measure of vocabulary and syntax at 24 months. *Journal of Speech and Hearing Research*, 34, 565-571. METHODOLOGY-DESIGN ASSESSMENT PROCEDURES VOCABULARY DEVELOPMENT SYNTACTIC DEVELOPMENT MACARTHUR COMMUNICATIVE DEVELOPMENT INVENTORIES:

Dale, Philip S., Bates, Elizabeth, Reznick, J. Steven, & Morisset, Colleen E. (1989). The validity of a parent report instrument of child language at twenty months. *Journal of Child Language*, 16(2), 239-249. ASSESSMENT PROCEDURES METHODOLOGY MACARTHUR COMMUNICATIVE DEVELOPMENT INVENTORIES:

Dalton, Peggy, & Hardcastle, W. (1989). *Disorders of fluency, 2nd Ed.* San Diego, CA: Singular Group. STUTTERING DISFLUENCIES:

Development and treatment of disfluency disorders, including: stuttering, cluttering and other organic disorders.

Daniloff, Raymond G. (1985). *Speech science*. San Diego, CA: Singular Group. SPEECH PRODUCTION SPEECH PERCEPTION VOWELS ARTICULATION AUDIOLOGY LANGUAGE AND MOTOR DEVELOPMENT:

Includes discussions of many aspects of speech science pertaining to speech production and perception.

Dart, S. N. (1992). Narrative style in the 2 languages of a bilingual child. *Journal of Child Language*, 19, 367-387. NARRATIVES BILINGUALISM-DISCOURSE ANALYSIS:

Davidson, Natalie S., & Gelman, Susan A. (1990). The role of language and conceptual structure. *Cognitive Development*, 5, 151-176. CONTRAST-SEMANTIC MUTUAL EXCLUSIVITY CONCEPT DEVELOPMENT CATEGORIZATION LEXICAL DEVELOPMENT SEMANTIC MAPPING:

When category labels and appearances were completely independent of one another, children drew inferences based on appearances rather than novel category labels. However, when the same pictures received familiar labels instead of novel labels children drew inferences based on category levels as well as appearances.

Davidson, R. J., & Saron, C. D. (1992). Evoked potential measures of interhemispheric transfer time in reading disabled and normal boys. *Developmental Neuropsychology*, 8, 261-277. READING DISORDERS LATERALIZATION:

Dawson, Geraldine, & Galpert, Larry. (1990). Mothers' use of imitative play for facilitating social responsiveness and toy play in young autistic children. *Development and Psychopathology*, 2, 151-162. AUTISM INTERVENTION PROGRAMS:

The effectiveness of imitating an autistic childs' actions as a means for promoting social responsiveness and creative toy play was explored. Significant cumulative increases in duration of gaze at mother's face and creative toy play were found.

Dawson, Peter M., Robinson, JoAnn L., Butterfield, Perry M., van Doornick, William J. , Gaensbauer, Theodore J., & Harmon, Robert J. (1990). Supporting new parents through home visits:

Effects on mother-infant interaction. *Topics in Early Childhood Special Education*, 10, 29-44. ADULT-CHILD INTERACTION AT-RISK CHILDREN:

In a study of family support through home visiting, paraprofessionals provided informal social support to low income parents during pregnancy and for 1 year afterward. Mother-infant interaction was better at 4 months in home-visited families than in controls, especially with teen and Hispanic mothers and other subgroups.

Day, D., & Stromqvist, Sven. (1989). The Development of Discourse Cohesion: An Asymmetry Between Child L1 and Adult L2 Acquisition. *Gothenburg Papers in Theoretcial Linguistics*, 56, DISCOURSE COHERENCE L2 DISCOURSE BILINGUALISM-DISCOURSE ANALYSIS:

de Acedo, B. (1993). The acquisition of specific grammatical morphemes in Spanish. In J. L. Sokolov, & C. E. Snow (Eds), *Handbook of research in language development using CHILDES*. Hillsdale, NJ: Lawrence Erlbaum Associates. SPANISH CHILDES MORPHOSYNTACTIC DEVELOPMENT METHODOLOGY-DESIGN METHODOLOGY-COMPUTERS:

de Boysson-Bardies, Bénédicte. (1970). Syntax and semantics in memorisation of negation. In G. B. Flores d'Arcais, & W. J. Levelt (Eds), *Advances in psycholinguistics*. Amsterdam, The Netherlands: North-Holland/Elsevier. SEMANTICS AND SYNTAX NEGATION LANGUAGE AND MEMORY:

de Boysson-Bardies, Bénédicte. (1971). L'acquisition du langage. (The acquisition of language). *L'Année Psychologique*, 2, 562-596. OVERVIEW-GENERAL: FRENCH

de Boysson-Bardies, Bénédicte. (1976). *Négation et performance linguistique. (Negation and linguistic performance.)*. The Hague, The Netherlands: Mouton. NEGATION: FRENCH

de Boysson-Bardies, Bénédicte. (1980). Interdépendence de la perception et de la production chez les bébés et les jeunes enfants. (Interdependence of perception and production in babies and young children.). In *La percezione del linguaggio*. Florence, Italy: PRODUCTION/PERCEPTION: FRENCH

de Boysson-Bardies, Bénédicte. (1981). Les dispositions pour la parole chez le bébé: processus d'encodage et de décodage phonétique. (The infant's predisposition for language: Phonetic encoding and decoding processes.). In *Actes du Seminaire*. Toulouse, France: PHONOLOGICAL PROCESSES PRELINGUISTICS LANGUAGE PRECURSORS SPEECH PERCEPTION PRODUCTION/PERCEPTION: FRENCH

de Boysson-Bardies, Bénédicte. (1982). Balbucean los bebes en su lengua materna. (Infant babbling in their mother tongue.). *Mundo Scientifico*, 12, BABBLING: SPANISH

de Boysson-Bardies, Bénédicte. (1982). Do babies babble as speakers speak? *Infant Behavior & Development*, 5, BABBLING:

de Boysson-Bardies, Bénédicte. (1982). La perception chez le nourrisson. (Perception in the infant.). *Bulletin de l'Institut de Phonétique de Grenoble*, X-XI, INFANT PERCEPTION: FRENCH

de Boysson-Bardies, Bénédicte. (1982). Les bébés babillent-ils dans leur langue naturelle? (Babies, do they babble in their natural language?). *La Recherche*, 129, 102-104. BABBLING: FRENCH

de Boysson-Bardies, Bénédicte. (1984). Influence des langues-cibles sur le développement de la parole: Études comparatives sur les enfants de 6 à 10 mois. (Influence of the target language on language development.). In M. Moscate, & G. Pierraut-Le Bonniec (Eds), *Le langage, construction èt actualisation*. Rouen, France: Presse Universitaires Français. BABBLING VOCALIZATIONS PHONOLOGICAL DEVELOPMENT: FRENCH

See also a paper in English with a similar title in G. Pierraut-Le Bonniec and M. Dolitsky (Eds.) (1990) From basic language to discourse bases. Amsterdam: Benjamins.

de Boysson-Bardies, Bénédicte. (1990). Capacités des jeunes enfants pour la parole: Que nous apprennent les productions prelinguistique? (Young children's capacities for language: What do we learn from prelinguistic productions?). In N. Zavialoff (Ed.),

La Lecture I: De la neurobiologie à la pedagogie. Paris, France: L'Harmattan. BABBLING VOCALIZATIONS PROSODY PRELINGUISTCIS: FRENCH

de Boysson-Bardies, Bénédicte. (1990). Les mots naissent de ce qu'ils ont été entendus. (Words born from those that have been heard.). In N. Zavialoff (Ed.), *La lecture 1: De la neurobiologie à la pedagogie.* Paris, France: L'Harmattan. PRODUCTION/PERCEPTION LEXICAL DEVELOPMENT: FRENCH

de Boysson-Bardies, Bénédicte. (1990). Some reflections on the sensorimotor organisation of speech during the first year of life. In H. Bloch, & B. I. Bertenthal (Eds), *Sensory motor organisations of development.* Dordrecht, The Netherlands: Kluwer Academic. LANGUAGE AND COGNITIVE DEVELOPMENT:

de Boysson-Bardies, Bénédicte. (1990). Target language influences on prespeech. In G. Pierraut-Le Bonniec, & M. Dolitsky (Eds), *From basic language to discourse bases.* Amsterdam, The Netherlands: John Benjamins. PRELINGUISTICS PROSODY BABBLING VOCALIZATIONS:

de Boysson-Bardies, Bénédicte. (1991). La perception du langage. Une activité preformée? (The perception of language: A preformed activity?). In F. Jouen, & V. Pouthas (Eds), *Les comportements du nourrisson: Expression de son savoir?.* Mardaga. SPEECH PERCEPTION INFANT PERCEPTION NEONATES NATIVISM: FRENCH

de Boysson-Bardies, Bénédicte, & Bacri, N. (1977). The interpretation of negative sentences. *International Journal of Psycholinguistics*, 4 (2), 73-81. NEGATION:

de Boysson-Bardies, Bénédicte, & O'Regan, K. (1973). What children do in spite of adults' hypotheses. *Nature*, 246, 5434. PARENTAL INPUT:

de Boysson-Bardies, Bénédicte, & Vihman, Marilyn May. (1991). Adaptation to language: evidence from babbling and first words in four languages. *Language*, 67(2), 297-319. BABBLING FIRST WORDS LINGUISTIC ENVIRONMENT ENVIRONMENTAL INFLUENCES:

Differences among languapes offer a way of studying the process of infant adaption from broad initial capaacities to language-specifc phonetic production. We designed analyses of the distribution of consonantal place and manner categories in French, English, Japanese, and Swedish to determine (1) whether systematic differences can be found in the babbling and first words of infants from different language backgrounds, and, (2) whether these differences are relaled to the phonetic structure of the language spoken in the environment. Five infants from each linguistic environment were recorded under similar conditions from babbling only to the production of 25 words in a session. Although all of the infants generally made greater use of labials, dentals, and stops than of other classes of sounds, a clear phonetic selection could already be discerned in babbling, leading to statistically significant differences among the groups. This selection can be seen to arise from phonetic patterns of the ambient language. Comparison of the babbling and infant word repertoires reveals differences reflecting the motoric consequences of sequencing constraints. From-Language.

de Boysson-Bardies, Bénédicte, Vihman, Marilyn May, Roug-Hellichius, Liselotte, Durand, Catherine, Landberg, Ingrid, & Arao, Fumiko. (1992). Evidence of infant selection from target language: A crosslinguistic phonetic study. In C. A. Ferguson, L. Menn, & C. Stoel-Gammon (Eds), *Phonological development: Models, research, implications*. Monkton, MD: York Press. BABBLING VOCALIZATIONS CROSSLINGUISTIC STUDY-PHONOLOGY PRELINGUISTICS LINGUISTIC ENVIRONMENT:

de Groot, A. M. B., & Barry, C. (Eds). (1993). *The multilingual community*. Hillsdale, NJ: Lawrence Erlbaum Associates. L2 ACQUISITION L2 EDUCATION BILINGUALISM-NEUROLINGUISTICS BILINGUALISM-LEXICAL DEVELOPMENT:

A special issue of the *European Journal of Cognitive Psychology* containing seven articles on bilingualism pertaining to the question of whether bilingualism involves a single intergrated lexicon, or two separate lexica, and two on second language acquisition.

de Groot, A. M. B., & Barry, C. (1993). The multilingual community: Introduction. In A. M. B. de Groot, & C. Barry (Eds), *The multilingual community*. Hillsdale, NJ: Lawrence Erlbaum Associates. BILINGUALISM:

De Hart, G. B. (1993). Placing affect and narrative in developmental and cultural context. In C. A. Nelson (Ed.), *Memory and affect in development*. Hillsdale, NJ: Lawrence Erlbaum Associates. NARRATIVES LANGUAGE AND AFFECT LANGUAGE ANDMEMORY:

De Houwer, Annick. (1982). Second language acquistion: A survey of recent literature. *ITL*, 55, 39-68. BILINGUALISM L2 ACQUISITION:

De Houwer, Annick. (1983). Some aspects of the simultaneous acquisition of Dutch and English by a three-year old child. *Nottingham Linguistic Circular*, 12, 106-129. BILINGUALISM-SIMULTANEOUS DUTCH-ENGLISH ENGLISH-DUTCH:

De Houwer, Annick. (1984). The development of the verb phrase in a bilingual child. In Singelton, et al. (Eds), *Language learning in formal and informal contexts*. Dublin, Ireland: IRAAL. BILINGUALISM-SYNTACTIC DEVELOPMENT SYNTACTIC STRUCTURES:

De Houwer, Annick. (1984). Mezcla de códigos en el habla de una niña de tres años bilingue de inglés y holandés. (Code-mixing in the speech of a three-year-old Dutch-English bilingual girl.). In M. Siguan (Ed.), *Adquisición precoz de una segunda lengua*. Barcelona: Publicacions i ediciōns de la Universitat de Barcelona. CODE-SWITCHING BILINGUALISM-SIMULTANEOUS DUTCH-ENGLISH ENGLISH-DUTCH: SPANISH

De Houwer, Annick. (1984). Repairs and the use of the monitor in early second language acquisition. In Krenn, & Niemeyer, et al. (Eds), *Sprache und gesellschaft: Akten des 18. Linguistischen Kolloquiums, Linz*. Tubingen: Max Niemeyer Verlag. MONITORING CONVERSATIONAL REPAIRS L2 MONITORING:

De Houwer, Annick. (1984). Repetition in the speech of a three-year-old bilingual. In D. Haese, et al. (Eds), *Proceedings of AILA*. Brussels: Free University of Brussels. IMITATION L2 IMITATION:

De Houwer, Annick. (1985). The simultaneous acquisition of English and Dutch: A case study. In F. Spoelders, F. van Besien, F. Lowenthal, & F. van Damme (Eds), *Language acquisition and learning. Essays in educational pragmatics 2.* Ghent: Communication and Cognition Publishers. BILINGUALISM-SIMULTANEOUS DUTCH-ENGLISH ENGLISH-DUTCH:

De Houwer, Annick. (1985). Some features of the verb phrase in the speech of a three-year-old bilingual. In Dominicy, & Baetens, et al. (Eds), *Linguistics in Belgium 7.* Brussels, Belgium: Free University of Brussels. BILINGUALISM-SYNTACTIC DEVELOPMENT SYNTACTIC STRUCTURES:

De Houwer, Annick. (1987). Gender marking in a young Dutch-English bilingual child. In *Proceedings of the Child Language Seminar.* York, United Kingdom: University of York. BILINGUALISM-MORPHOLOGICAL DEVELOPMENT GENDER DUTCH-ENGLISH ENGLISH-DUTCH:

De Houwer, Annick. (1987). Nouns and their companions or how a three-year-old handles the Dutch gender system. *Belgian Journal of Linguistics*, 2, 55-73. GENDER DUTCH NOUNS:

De Houwer, Annick. (1988). Word order patterns in the speech productions of a three-year-old. *ABLA Papers*, 2, 189-206. WORD ORDER:

De Houwer, Annick. (1990). *The acquisition of two languages from birth: A case study.* New York, NY: Cambridge University Press. BILINGUALISM-SIMULTANEOUS BILINGUALISM-OVERVIEW DUTCH-ENGLISH ENGLISH-DUTCH METHODOLOGY-DIARY/CASE STUDY BILINGUALISM-MORPHOLOGICAL DEVELOPMENT BILINGUALISM-SYNTACTIC DEVELOPMENT:

> De Houwer examines the simultaneous acquisition of Dutch and English and pays specific attention to morphological and syntactic development. She also provides a comprehensive review of former studies of simultaneous bilingualism.

De Houwer, Annick, & Gillis, Steven. (1985). Language and communication during the second year of life. *Journal of Pragmatics*, 9, 683-704. SINGLE-WORD SPEECH SPEECH ACTS:

De Houwer, Annick, & Gillis, Steven. (1987). Perspectives on child language. *Belgium Journal of Linguistics*, 2. OVERVIEW-THEORY:

Special issue dealing with 'Perspectives on Child Language.'.

de Loache, J. S.. (1989). The development of representation in young children. In H. W. Reese (Ed.), *Advances in child development and behavior*. New York, NY: Academic Press. REPRESENTATIONS:

de Villiers, Jill. G., de Villiers, Peter A., & Hoban, A. (1993). The central problem of functional categories in the English syntax of oral deaf children. In H. Tager-Flusberg (Ed.), *Constraints on language acquisition: Studies of atypical children*. Hillsdale, NJ: Lawrence Erlbaum Associates. ATYPICAL DEVELOPMENT DEAF CHILDREN SYNTACTIC STRUCTURES:

de Villiers, Peter A., & de Villiers, Jill. G. (1992). Language development. In M. H. Bornstein, & M. E. Lamb (Eds), *Developmental psychology: An advanced textbook, 3rd Ed.* Hillsdale, NJ: Lawrence Erlbaum Associates. OVERVIEW:

de Villiers, Peter A., & Pomerantz, S. B. (1992). Hearing-impaired students learning new words from written context. *Applied Psycholinguistics* , 13 , 409-431. LEXICAL DEVELOPMENT CONTEXT WRITTEN LANGUAGE DEAF CHILDREN SEMANTIC MAPPING:

de Zuani, E., & Levorato, Maria C. (1988). La comprensione di testi procedurali e descrittivi nei bambini. (The comprehension of procedural and descriptive texts by children.). *Giornale Italiano di Psicologia*, 15, 427-446. LANGUAGE AND MEMORY DISCOURSE ANALYSIS TEXT/STORY GRAMMARS: ITALIAN

A comparison of children's recall of texts with the same semantic content but different structural characteristics.MCL

Dechert, Hans W. (1990). *Current trends in European second language acquisition research*. Philadelphia, PA: Multilingual Matters. L2 ACQUISITION L2 EUROPEAN RESEARCH:

Papers originating from a workshop held July 27-28, 1985 at Georgetown University in conjunction with the 1985 LSA/TESOL Summer Institute.

Dechert, Hans W., & Raupach, Manfred (Eds). (1989). *Transfer in language production, vol.*. Norwood, NJ: Ablex. TRANSFER SPEECH PRODUCTION:

del Rio, M. J., & Vilaseca-Momplet, Rosa M. (1988). Algunos comentarios sobre la adquisición y el desarrollo del lenguaje (Some comments on the acquisition and development of language). In J. Pena (Ed.), *Manual de logopedia*. Barcelona, Spain: Masson. SPANISH OVERVIEW-THEORY: SPANISH

Demuth, Katherine. (1984). Modified self-repetitions and the development of focus constructions in Sesotho. *Papers and Reports on Child Language Development.*, 23, 33-40. SESOTHO SYNTACTIC STRUCTURES TOPIC-COMMENT SPEECH MODIFICATIONS REPETITIONS:

Demuth, Katherine. (1987). Discourse functions of word order in Sesotho acquistion. In R. Tomlin (Ed.), *Coherence and grounding in discourse. Proceedings of a symposium on discourse, cognition, and syntax.*. Amsterdam: SESOTHO WORD ORDER DISCOURSE FUNCTIONS:

Demuth, Katherine. (1987). Prompting routines in the language socialization of Basotho children. In B. Schieffelin, & E. Ochs (Eds), *Language socialization across cultures*. New York, N.Y.: Cambridge University Press. SESOTHO LANGUAGE AND SOCIAL TRANSMISSION LANGUAGE SOCIALIZATION:

Demuth, Katherine. (1988). Noun classes and agreement in Sesotho acquisition. In M. Barlow, & C. Ferguson (Eds), *Agreement in natural languages: Approaches, theories, and descriptions*. Stanford, CA: SESOTHO GENDER AGREEMENT:

Demuth, Katherine. (1989). Problems in the acquisition of grammatical tone. *Papers and Reports on Child Language Development.*, 28, 81-88. TONE:

Demuth, Katherine. (1990). Subject, topic, and the Sesotho passive. *Journal of Child Language.*, 17(1), 67-84. SESOTHO PASSIVES TOPIC-COMMENT SUBJECTIVITY:

Demuth, Katherine. (1992). The acquisition of Sesotho. In D. I. Slobin (Ed.), *The crosslinguistic study of language acquisition (Vol. 3).* Hillsdale, NJ: Lawrence Erlbaum Associates. SESOTHO CROSSLINGUISTIC STUDY:

Demuth, Katherine, Faraclas, N., & Marchese, L. (1986). Niger-Congo noun class and agreement systems in language acquisition and historical change. In C. Craig (Ed.), *Noun class and categorization.* Amsterdam: John Benjamins. LANGUAGE CHANGE AGREEMENT GENDER NIGER-CONGO:

Denil, L. F., & Brutten, G. J. (1991). Speech-associated attitudes of stuttering and nonstuttering children. *Journal of Speech and Hearing Research*, 34, 60-66. STUTTERING:

Dennis, Maureen. (1988). Language and the young damaged brain. In T. Boll, & B. K. Bryant (Eds), *Clinical neuropsychology and brain function: Research, measurement, and practice.* Hyattsville, MD: American Psychological Association. TRAUMATIC DISORDERS CEREBRAL DISORDERS:

Dennis, Maureen. (1990). Scenes from childhood-visual metaphors in the developmental neuropsychology of language. *Developmental Neuropsychology*, 6, 351-370. NEUROLINGUISTICS:

Dent, Cathy H. (1990). An ecological approach to language development: An alternative functionalism. *Developmental Psychobiology*, 23(7), NATIVISM:

Dent, Cathy H., & Rosenberg, Lois. (1990). Visual and verbal metaphors: Developmental interactions. *Child Development*, 61, 983-994. FIGURATIVE LANGUAGE:

Five, 7- and 10-year-old children and adults described objects ordered in pairs. Half described standard objects and the other half corresponding compound objects (half stationary, half moving, e.g., spinning). Metaphoric descriptions reached the adult frequency by age 7 for compound objects, but increased from 5 to 10 to adult for standard objects. Moving objects were more likely to be described using action vehicles after five.

Dent, Cathy H., & Zukow, Patricia G. (1990). The idea of innateness: Effects on language and communication research. *Developmental Psychobiology*, 23(7), NATIVISM:

A special issue of the journal with guest editors Dent and Zukow. Includes commentaries by Oyama, Alberts, Wexler, Locke, and Dent.

Deutsch, Werner. (1989). William Stern-50 Jahre nach seinem Tode. (Wm. Stern-50 years after his death.). In W. Schonplug (Ed.), *Bericht über den 36. Kongress der Deutschen Gesellschaft für Psychologie in Berlin 1988* (vol. 2,). Gottingen: Hogrefe. OVERVIEW-GENERAL: GERMAN

Devescovi, A., Orsolini, Margherita, & Pace, C. (1989). Consapevolezza linguistica nei bambini in eta prescolare. (Preschoolers' metalinguistic awareness.). *Rassegna di Linguistica Applicata*, 1 (2), 153-178. METALINGUISTICS GRAMMATICALITY CHILDREN'S JUDGMENTS NARRATIVES ANAPHORA: ITALIAN

In this study different metalinguistic tasks were used: identification of morphemes, syllables and phonemes in the word, judgements on sentences acceptability, judgements on stories' coherence. 60 subjects were observed, 15 for each of the following mean-age groups: 4.7, 5.5, 6.2, 6.7. Subjects of the last group were attending the primary school. Subjects of the third group were attending the Italian preschool ('scuola materna'). Children's performance at every task shows significant developmental trends. Children who were exposed to a systematic teaching of reading and writing (the fourth group) show a discontinuity in the performance in some tasks, which can be related to the 'literacy' factor. For example, they do significantly better than the preschoolers in identification of syllables located in the final position. Conversely, 5-year and 6-year old children (both attending the preschool) are significantly more able than the 4-year old children in identifying syllables located in initial position. The 6-year old children attending primary school are also significantly more able than the preschoolers in detecting story incoherences conveyed by anaphoric pronouns. Conversely, judgements on sentences acceptability do not seem to be affected by the 'literacy' factor. The 6-year old children (attending either the preschool or the primary school) have a significantly better performance than the fours and the fives, and their mean score does not differ from that of group of adults. MO.

Devi, A. Usha. (1990). *Acquisition of syntax : a case study in Telugu.* New Delhi, India: Bahri Publications. TELUGU SYNTACTIC DEVELOPMENT:

Devine, Monica. (1991). *Baby talk: The art of communicating with infants and toddlers.* New York, NY: Plenum. INTERVENTION PROGRAMS PARENTAL SPEECH TEACHABILITY:

A popular psychology trade book which provides 'a parent's journey through a child's early years'. Provides games and activities for caregivers to engage in with children to enhance their language skills. Also provides quarterly overviews of stages of infant development.

Dezsö, László. (1967). Szórend és mondathangsúly. (Word order and sentence stress patterns.). *Altalános Nyelvészeti Tanulmányok*, 5, 79-121. HUNGARIAN WORD ORDER INTONATION STRESS PROSODY: HUNGARIAN

Dezsö, László. (1970). A gyermeknyelv mondattanivizsgálatának elvi-módszertani kérdései (Principal-methodological issues in the syntactic study of child language). *Altalános Nyelvészeti Tanulmányok*, 7, 77-99. METHODOLOGY-ANALYSIS METHODOLOGY-DESIGN HUNGARIAN: HUNGARIAN

Dezsö, Lásló. (1976). Universals in child language: comments by a typologist. In *Akten des Erste Salzburger Kolloquium uber Kindersprache.* Tubingen, Germany: Gunter Narr. LANGUAGE UNIVERSALS ACQUISITION THEORIES DEVELOPMENTAL UNIVERSALS HUNGARIAN:

Di Pietro, Roberto J. (1990). Interactive discourse in the L2 classroom. In M. A. K. Halliday, J. Gibbons, & H. Nicholas (Eds), *Learning, keeping and using language*. Amsterdam, The Netherlands: John Benjamins. L2 EDUCATION:

Selected paper from the proceedings of the Eighth World Congress of Applied Linguistics, Sydney, 1987.

Diachenko, Olga M. (1986). Formirivaniye sposobnosty k nagliadnomu modelirovaniyu pri ozakomlenii s detskoy hudozhestvennoy literaturoy (Formation of ability for visual modelling in the process of children's familiarizing with child's fiction). In M. Pedagogika (Ed.), *Razvitie poznavatelnieh sposobnostey v protsesse doshkolnogo vosptaniya (Development of congnitive abilities in preschool education).*. Venger L.A. LITERACY TEXT/STORY GRAMMARS DISCOURSE COMPREHENSION LANGUAGE AND EDUCATION: RUSSIAN

The problem of verbal and cognitive development in the process of acquisition of child's literature is considered. The data about the use of different types of models by preschoolers was used for elaboration of an educational program capable of stimulating verbal creative behavior in 3-7 year-old children.OMD.

Diachenko, Olga M. (1988). O sootnoshenii rechevykh i obraznykh sredstv pri reshenii zadzch na voobrazheniye (On connections of verbal and visual means in creative tasks solution). *Noviye issledovaniya v psykhologicheskykh naukakh*, 2, LANGUAGE AND COGNITIVE DEVELOPMENT: RUSSIAN

The connections between preschoolers' use of verbal and visual means at different stages of the imagination process are considered. The specific functions of language acquistion both at the stage of generating creative ideas and at the stage of planning the realization of such ideas are shown.OMD

Diaz, Rafael M., & Berk, Laura E. (1991). *Private speech: From social interaction to self-regulation*. Hillsdale, NJ: Lawrence Erlbaum Associates. VYGOTSKYAN THEORY PRIVATE SPEECH INDIVIDUAL

VARIATION BIBLIOGRAPHY REGULATIVE FUNCTION OF SPEECH PIAGETIAN THEORY INNER SPEECH:

This text is an extension of the basic premise of Vygotskyan theory. It examines the role of private speech in development, and its variation from individual to individual. The book also includes recent research on Piagetian language theory, and an extensive bibliography.

Dickinson, David R. (1990). Teaching agenda and setting: Constraints on conversation in preschools. In A. McCabe, & C. Peterson (Eds), *Developing narrative structure.* Hillsdale, NJ: Lawrence Erlbaum Associates. NARRATIVES LANGUAGE AND EDUCATION CONVERSATIONAL SKILLS:

Dickson, David R., & Maue-Dickson, Wilma. (1982). *Anatomical and physiological bases of speech.* San Diego, CA: Singular Group. BIOLOGICAL FOUNDATIONS NEUROLINGUISTICS:

Dieck, Marianne. (1989). *Der Erwerb der Negation bei bilingualen Kinder (Französisch-Deutsch). Eine Fallstudie. (The acquisition of negation by French/German bilingual children -- A case study).* Hamburg, Germany: Universität Hamburg. NEGATION FRENCH-GERMAN GERMAN-FRENCH BILINGUALISM-SYNTACTIC DEVELOPMENT: GERMAN

Diehl, Erika, Albrecht, Helga, & Zoch, Irene. (1991). *Lernerstrategien im Fremdsprachenerwerb : Untersuchungen zum Erwerb des deutschen Deklinationssystems. (Learning strategies for foreign language acquisition: Investigations of the acquisition of the German declension system.).* Tübingen, Germany: Niemeyer. MORPHOSYNTACTIC DEVELOPMENT AGREEMENT GERMAN GENDER CASE NUMBER: GERMAN

Dijkstra, A. (1989). "PROTEIN", a Turbo-Pascal program for micro-analysis of video-recordings. In *Report, Instituut voor Fonetische Wetenschappen.* Amsterdam, The Netherlands: University of Amsterdam. METHODOLOGY-COMPUTERS METHODOLOGY-ANALYSIS: DUTCH

Dimitracopoulou, Ioanna. (1990). *Conversational competence and social development.* New York, NY: Cambridge University Press. CONVERSATIONAL SKILLS SOCIAL INTERACTION COMMUNICATIVE COMPETENCE:

> This book provides new insight into the development of the child's ability to become a competent participant in conversation. The author combines a pragmatic analysis of the functions language can perform with an innovative and extensive empirical investigation of the development of young children's language use and sociocognitive skills. She gives a detailed description of the development of children's language between the ages of three-and-a-half and seven, broadens the scope of theorizing about language development by placing it in relation to the development of social understanding, and provides a new framework for understanding speech problems and designing ways to solve them. It is the first study to find a strong link between language, sociocognitive development, and social development.

Dinnsen, Daniel A. (1992). Variation in developing and fully developed phonetic inventories. In C. A. Ferguson, L. Menn, & C. Stoel-Gammon (Eds), *Phonological development: Models, research, implications.* Monkton, MD: York Press. PHONETIC INVENTORIES:

Dinnsen, Daniel A., Chin, S. B., & Elbert, Mary F. (1992). On the lawfulness of change in phonetic inventories. *Lingua*, 86(2-3), 207-222. PHONETIC INVENTORIES:

Dinsmore, John. (1992). *The symbolic and connectionist paradigms.* Hillsdale, NJ: Lawrence Erlbaum Associates. CONNECTIONISM LANGUAGE AND COGNITION:

> A collection of essays which seek to bridge the gaps betwen symbolic and connectionist accounts of cognition.

Dobrich, W., & Scarborough, Hollis S. (1992). Phonological characteristics of words young children try to say. *Journal of Child Language*, 19, 597-616. PHONETIC INVENTORIES FIS-PHENOMENON REPRESENTATIONS-PHONOLOGICAL:

Doehring, Donald G. (1988). *Research strategies in human communication disorders*. San Diego, CA: Singular Publishing Group. LANGUAGE DISORDERS METHODOLOGY-DESIGN METHODOLOGY-ANALYSIS:

Introduction. The sequence of events in research. Aspects of human communication disorders studied by reseachers. Basic principles of research design. Simple group research design. Complex group research designs. Advantages and disadvantages of group research designs. Procedures. Data reduction and descriptive statistics. Basic principles of statistical analysis. Statistical analysis of simple group designs. Statistical analysis of complex group designs. Statistical analysis of relationships. Analysis of data obtained with other designs. Interpretation of research. Research strategies. How to read and evaluate HCD research. How to plan, carry out, and interpret HCD research. How to write research reports. Answers to exercises. References. Subject index.

Doepke, Susanne. (1990). Are mothers really the main mediators of language? In M. A. K. Halliday, J. Gibbons, & H. Nicholas (Eds), *Learning, keeping and using language* . Amsterdam, The Netherlands: John Benjamins. INPUT FACTORS PARENTAL SPEECH:

Selected paper from the proceedings of the Eighth World Congress of Applied Linguistics, Sydney, 1987.

Dolley, Diane, Glynn, Ted, & Wheldall, Kevin. (1989). Increasing pre-schoolers' language use through incidental teaching. *New Zealand Journal of Educational Studies*, 24, 65-76. LANGUAGE AND EDUCATION INTERVENTION PROGRAMS:

A kindergarten teacher was introduced to and instructed in the use of incidental teaching procedures designed to increase the frequency of child initiated language sequences in an ABAB design. In addition, the teacher was requested to arrange the environment so that children were required to request access to certain materials. The teacher wore a radio microphone during the sessions so that all child language addressed to her together with all teacher responses could be accurately recorded. After the implementation of the procedures the number of child initiations, the teacher's use of incidental teaching and the number of words spoken by the children to the teacher increased. - From Child Development Abstracts.

Donin, J., Doehring, Donald G., & Browns, F. (1991). Text comprehension and reading achievement in orally educated hearing-impaired children. *Discourse Processes*, 14, 307-337. DEAF CHILDREN COMPREHENSION LITERACY:

Dopke, Susanne. (1992). *One parent, one language : an interactional approach*. Amsterdam, The Netherlands: John Benjamins. BILINGUALISM-SIMULTANEOUS:

Dore, John. (1977). Holophrases, speech acts, and language universals. In M. S. Barbieri (Ed.), *Gli inizi del linguaggio: aspetti cognitivi e comuncativi (The emergence of language: cognitive and communicative aspects)*.. La Nuova, Italy: Firenze. SINGLE-WORD SPEECH SPEECH ACTS: ITALIAN

Dore, John. (1977). Oh them sherriff: A pragmatic analysis of children's responses to questions. In C. Mitchell-Kernan, & S. Ervin-Tripp (Eds), *Children's discourse*. New York, NY: Academic Press. CHILDREN'S RESPONSES CHILDREN'S DISCOURSE:

Dore, John. (1978). Requestive systems in nursery school conversations: Analysis of talk in its social context. In R. N. Campbell, & P. T. Smith (Eds), *Recent advances in the psychology of language*. New York, NY: Plenum. REQUESTS SOCIAL SPEECH:

Dore, John. (1989). Monologue as re-envoicement of dialogue. In K. Nelson (Ed.), *Narratives from the crib*. Cambridge, MA: Harvard University Press. CRIB SPEECH NARRATIVES PARENTAL SPEECH:

Dore describes the relationships between the child's monologues and her dialogues with her father.

Dorr, B. (1991). Conceptual basis of the lexicon in machine translation. In U. Zernik (Ed.), *Lexical Acquisition-Exploiting On-Line Resources to Build a Lexicon*. Hillsdale, NJ : Lawrence Erlbaum Associates. LEXICAL DEVELOPMENT:

Dowker, A. D. (1991). Modified repetition in poems elicited from young children. *Journal of Child Language*, 18, 625-639. IMITATION:

Drash, Philip W., Raver, Sharon A., Murrin, Mary R., & Tudor, Roger M. (1989). Three procedures for increasing vocal response to therapist prompt in infants and children with Down Syndrome. *American Journal on Mental Retardation*, 94, 64-73. DOWN SYNDROME INTERVENTION PROGRAMS:

> The relative effectiveness of three procedures for increasing vocal response to prompts in 15 preschool children with Down syndrome was compared. The procedures were positive reinforcement only, positive reinforcement combined with light- dimming, and positive reinforcement combined with visual screening. All procedures produced a significant increase in percentage of response to prompt over baseline.-From Child Development Abstracts.

Dressler, W. W., Caldognetto, E. Magno, & Tonelli, L. (1986). Phonologische fehlleistungen und paraphasien im Deutschen und Italienischen. (Phonological speech errors and paraphasias in German and Italian.). *Gräzer Linguistische Studien*, 26, 43-57. CROSSLINGUISTIC STUDY-PHONOLOGY GERMAN ITALIAN SPEECH ERRORS: GERMAN

> The study is concerned with some relevant aspects of a comparison between speech errors and paraphasias in German and in Italian. It is shown that: 1) both types of errors are characterized by important quantitative as well as qualitative differences, and 2) different language structures, in particular different syllable structures, are responsible for differences between paraphasias in German and Italian.

Dressler, W. W., Tonelli, L., & Caldognetto, E. Magno. (1990). Phonological paraphasias vs. slips of the tongue in German and Italian. In J. Nespoulous, & P. Villard (Eds), *Morphology, phonology, and aphasia*. New York, NY: Springer. SPEECH ERRORS GERMAN ITALIAN CROSSLINGUISTIC STUDY-PHONOLOGY:

> In this paper we briefly discuss two aspects of our ongoing contrastive project of contrasting 1) speech errors (lapsus, slips

of the tongue) and phonological paraphasias in general, and 2) in German vs. Italian in particular. The first aspect is the different distribution of simplification and complication of syllable structure in slips and paraphasias, the second concerns phenomena of repair (successive approximations) and the liklihood of their occurence.

Duchan, Judith F. (1991). Everyday events: Their role in language assessment and intervention. In T. M. Gallagher, & N. Rees (Eds), *Pragmatics of language: Clinical practice issues.*. San Diego, CA: Singular Group. EVENTS/SCRIPTS PRAGMATIC DEVELOPMENT ASSESSMENT PROCEDURES INTERVENTION PROGRAMS:

The representation of events and scripts in language and the application of research literature on events/scripts to language assessment and intervention programs.

Duckworth, M., Allen, George D., Hardcastle, W., & Ball, Martin J. (1991). Extensions to the International Phonetic Alphabet for the transcription of atypical speech. *Clinical Linguistics and Phonetics*, 4, METHODOLOGY-TRANSCRIPTION ATYPICAL DEVELOPMENT:

Duckworth, M., & Ball, Martin J. (1988). Problems in the transcription of dysfluent speech. *Journal of the International Phonetic Association*, 18, 152-155. METHODOLOGY-TRANSCRIPTION DISFLUENCIES:

Dunlea, Anne. (1990). *Vision and the emergence of meaning: blind and sighted children's early language.* New York, NY: Cambridge University Press. ATYPICAL DEVELOPMENT BLIND CHILDREN LANGUAGE AND COGNITIVE DEVELOPMENT SEMANTIC DEVELOPMENT PRAGMATIC DEVELOPMENT:

Dunlea's examination of the relationship between language and conceptual development is based on her analysis of the early language in a group of blind, partially sighted, and fully sighted children who participated in a pioneering longitudinal study at the University of Southern California. In particular, the study reveals a convergence of early language and conceptual development. By focusing on the processes of development rather than merely describing the end products of language acquisition, the author not only identifies significant differences in blind and sighted children, but also offers new insights on semantic and pragmatic development in general.

Dunn, Judy. (1991). Young children's understanding of other people: Evidence from observations within the family. In D. Frye, & C. Moore (Eds), *Children's theories of mind.* Hillsdale, NJ: Lawrence Erlbaum Associates. THEORY OF MIND SELF-CONCEPT PERSPECTIVE TAKING:

Dunn, Judy, & Brown, J. (1991). Becoming American or English? Talking about the social world in England and the United States. In M. H. Bornstein (Ed.), *Cultural approaches to parenting.* Hillsdale, NJ: Lawrence Erlbaum Associates. CROSSLINGUISTIC STUDY-PARENTAL SPEECH LANGUAGE SOCIALIZATION:

Dunn, Judy, & Shatz, Marilyn. (1989). Becoming a conversationalist despite (or because of) having an older sibling. *Child Development,* 60(2), 399-410. SIBLING EFFECTS:

Dyer, M. (1991). Lexical acquisition through symbol recirculation. In U. Zernik (Ed.), *Lexical Acquisition-Exploiting On-Line Resources to Build a Lexicon.* Hillsdale, NJ : Lawrence Erlbaum Associates. LEXICAL DEVELOPMENT:

Dziubalska-Kolaczyk, Katarzyna. (1990). *A theory of second language acquisition within the framework of natural phonology : a Polish-English contrastive study.* Poznan, Poland: Uniwersytet im. Adama Mickiewicza. L2 ACQUISITION THEORIES POLISH-ENGLISH ENGLISH-POLISH L2 PHONOLOGY:

E

Echols, Catherine H., & Newport, Elissa L. (1992). The role of stress and position in determining first words. *Language Acquisition*, 2, 189-220. FIRST WORDS STRESS SYLLABLES SINGLE-WORD SPEECH ACQUISITION STRATEGIES:

The authors examined the production of 616 multisyllabic words by three children in the single-word stage. They report that stressed syllables and word final syllables were least likely to be omitted in the children's productions, and were produced more accurately than unstressed or nonfinal position syllables. This is consistent with Slobin's acquisition strategies.

Eckman, Fred R., & Hastings, A. J. (Eds). (1979). *Studies in first and second language acquisition, vol.*. Rowley, MA: Newbury House. L2/L1 ACQUISITION L2 ACQUISITION ACQUISITION THEORIES:

Edwards, Jane A. (1992). Computer methods in child language research-4 principles for the use of archived data. *Journal of Child Language*, 19, 435-458. METHODOLOGY-COMPUTERS CHILD LANGUAGE CORPORA METHODOLOGY-ANALYSIS:

Edwards, Jane A., & Lampert, Martin D. (Eds). (1992). *Talking data: Transcription and coding in discourse research*. Hillsdale, NJ: Lawrence Erlbaum Associates. METHODOLOGY-TRANSCRIPTION METHODOLOGY-COMPUTERS DISCOURSE ANALYSIS:

Discusses all aspects of language transcription. Includes chapters by Bloom, Ervin-Tripp and Slobin which specifically address child language data. The final chapter is a compendium of computerized language corpora databases and informational sources.

Edwards, John. (1989). *Language and disadvantage.* San Diego, CA: Singular Group. LANGUAGE AND EDUCATION LANGUAGE AND SOCIAL CLASS ETHNICITY ACCULTURATION NONSTANDARD DIALECTS BILINGUALISM-EDUCATION:

A review of all aspects of the debate revolving around language and disadvantage: difference, deficiency, nonstandard dialects and education, acculturation, ethnicity, and bilingualism.

Edwards, Margaret, Cape, Julie, & Brown, Darrel. (1989). Patterns of referral for children with speech disorders. *Child: Care, Health and Development*, 15, 417-424. CLASSIFICATION OF DISORDERS ASSESSMENT PROCEDURES:

This paper presents information about a sample of 200 children aged 3-6 years in four Health Authorities who were referred routinely for speech therapy.-From Child Development Abstracts.

Efron, Robert. (1990). *The decline and fall of hemispheric specialization.* Hillsdale, NJ: Lawrence Erlbaum Associates. LATERALIZATION:

A comprehensive review of the literature on lateralization and hemispheric specialization which presents arguments from both sides of the debate on hemisphericity. This is an expanded text version of the 1989 MacEachran Lecture Series given at the University of Alberta.

Eichhorn, Renate, & Reimann, Bernd. (1985). Leistungsdiagnostisches Verfahren zur Ermittlung des kognitiven Entwicklungsstandes bei hörgeschädigten Kindern im Alter von 5-9 Jahren. (Diagnostic achievement procedure from the investigation of cognitive development stages in hearing impaired children between the ages of 5-9 years.). *Scienta Pädagogica Experimentalis, Belgien (Gent)*, 22 (1), 30-39. DEAF CHILDREN ASSESSMENT PROCEDURES LANGUAGE AND COGNITIVE DEVELOPMENT COGNITIVE DEVELOPMENT: GERMAN

Eilers, Rebecca E., Oller, D. Kimbrough, Urbano, Richard, & Moroff, Debra. (1989). Conflicting and cooperating cues: Perception of cues to final consonant voicing by infants and adults. *Journal of Speech and Hearing Research*, 32, 307-316. CUES-PHONOLOGICAL CONSONANTS-FINAL CONTRAST-VOICE:

Three experiments were conducted to ascertain the relative salience of two cues for consonant voicing in infants and adults. Results indicate that in adults and infants combined cues facilitate discrimination of the phonemic contrast regardless of whether the cues cooperate or conflict.-From Child Development Abstracts.

Eimas, Peter D. (1991). Comment: some effects of language acquisition on speech perception. In I. G. Mattingly, & M. Studdert-Kennedy (Eds), *Modularity and the motor theory of speech perception*. Hillsdale, NJ : Lawrence Erlbaum Associates. SPEECH PERCEPTION:

Eisenmajer, R., & Prior, M. (1991). Cognitive linguistic correlates of theory of mind ability in autistic children. *British Journal of Developmental Psychology*, 9, 351-364. AUTISM THEORY OF MIND LANGUAGE AND COGNITION:

Eiser, Christine, Eiser, John R., & Lang, James. (1989). Scripts in children's reports of medical events. *European Journal of Psychology of Education*, 4, 377-384. EVENTS/SCRIPTS:

Descriptions provided by 20 five-year-olds and 20 eight-year-olds of what happens in five medical contexts (when visiting a doctor, dentist, not feeling well, going to the hospital, having an operation) were assessed for their degree of sequential structure. Subjects' descriptions conformed closely to conventional ordering of events, with almost no descriptions containing implausible reversals of sequence. However, whereas younger children tended to list events, older children provided descriptions of greater complexity and sequential organization.-From Child Development Abstracts.

Elbers, Loekie, & Wijnen, Frank. (1992). Effort, production skill, and language learning. In C. A. Ferguson, L. Menn, & C. Stoel-Gammon (Eds), *Phonological development: Models, research, implications*. Monkton, MD: York Press. ARTICULATION PHONOLOGICAL DEVELOPMENT:

Elbert, Mary F., Dinnsen, Daniel A., Swartzlander, P., & Chin, S. B. (1990). Generalization to conversational speech. *Journal of Speech and Hearing Disorders*, 55, 694-699. TREATMENT GENERALIZATION:

Elbert, Mary F., & Gierut, Judith A. (1986). *Handbook of clinical phonology: Approaches to assessment and treatment*. San Diego, CA: Singular Group. CLINICAL LINGUISTICS PHONOLOGICAL DISORDERS INTERVENTION PROGRAMS ASSESSMENT PROCEDURES TREATMENT GENERALIZATION:

> Topics covered include: the development of normal and disordered phonology, assessment of productive knowledge, analysis of disordered speech, and treatment generalization.

Elbert, Mary F., Powell, T. W., & Swartzlander, P. (1991). Toward a technology of generalization-how many exemplars are sufficient. *Journal of Speech and Hearing Research*, 34, 81-87. TREATMENT GENERALIZATION:

Elias, Gordon, & Broerse, Jack. (1989). Timing in mother-infant communications: a comment on Murray and Trevarthen. *Journal of Child Language*, 16, 703-706. INTERSUBJECTIVITY PRELINGUISTICS ADULT-CHILD INTERACTION:

Elias, Gordon, Broerse, Jack, Hayes, Alan, & Jackson, K. (1984). Comments on the use of conversational features in studies of the vocalization behaviours of mothers and infants. *International Journal of Behavioural Development*, 7, 177-191. INTERSUBJECTIVITY METHODOLOGY-DESIGN METHODOLOGY-ANALYSIS PRELINGUISTICS ADULT-CHILD INTERACTION:

Eliason, Michele J., & Richman, Lynn C. (1990). Language development in preschoolers with cleft. *Developmental Neuropsychology*, 6, 173-182. CLEFT PALATE:

Elliott, Marietta. (1990). The development of genre in the writing of two adolescent Lebanese students of English as a second language. In M. A. K. Halliday, J. Gibbons, & H. Nicholas (Eds), *Learning, keeping and using language* . Amsterdam, The Netherlands: John Benjamins. WRITTEN LANGUAGE L2 DISCOURSE L2 EDUCATION:

Selected paper from the proceedings of the Eighth World Congress of Applied Linguistics, Sydney, 1987.

Ellis, Rod. (1990). *Instructed second language acquisition: Learning in the classroom.* Oxford, UK : Basil Blackwell. L2 EDUCATION:

Ellis, Rod. (1992). *Second language acquisition and language pedagogy*. Philadelphia, PA: Multilingual Matters. L2 ACQUISITION L2 EDUCATION:

Emblem, B., & Conti-Ramsden, Gina. (1991). Working towards Level I: reality or illusion? *British Journal of Special Education*. LANGUAGE AND EDUCATION:

Emde, Robert N., Plomin, R., Robinson, J., & Corley, R., et al. (1992). Temperament, emotion, and cognition at 14 months-the Macarthur Longitudinal Twin Study. *Child Development*, 63, 1437-1455. MULTIPLE BIRTHS:

Emmorey, K. (1991). Repetition priming with aspect and agreement morphology in American Sign Language. *Journal of Psycholinguistic Research*, 20, 365-388. SIGNING-ASL MORPHOLOGICAL DEVELOPMENT ASPECT AGREEMENT:

Engstrand, Olle, Landberg, Ingrid, & Roug-Hellichius, Liselotte. (1990). When do Swedish children acquire accent? In E. Strangert, & P. Czigler (Eds), *Papers from FONETIK-90. The Fourth Swedish Phonetic Conference*. Umea, Sweden: Department of Phonetics, University of Umea. STRESS SWEDISH:

Erbaugh, Mary S. (1992). The acquisition of Mandarin. In D. I. Slobin (Ed.), *The crosslinguistic study of language acquisition (Vol. 3)*. Hillsdale, NJ: Lawrence Erlbaum Associates. MANDARIN CHINESE:

Eriksson, A. S., & de Chateau, P. (1992). A girl aged 2 years and 7 months with autistic disorder videotaped from birth. *Journal of Autism and Developmental Disorders*, 22, 127-129. AUTISM:

Eriksson, Marten. (1989). Development of decontextualization in object naming. *Cognitive Development*, 4, 389-405. LABELING FUNCTIONAL CORE HYPOTHESIS:

Three experiments are described. The first experiment investigated environemntal influences on children's (ages 2-6 years) naming practices and showed that the environmental context does effect children's naming behavior, sometimes to a such a high degree that it overwhelmed the perceptual input. The importance of environmental effects was standard over the period 2-5 years but significantly decreased at age 6. The second experiment examined the environmental effects on adults' naming behavior and found them to be at about the same level as the oldest of the child subjects. The third experiment validate the other two. The results were interpreted as a support for Nelson's functional theory of concept formation, both regarding the importance of the functional relationships in which objects take part, as well as to the age of when decontextualization of these terms are to be expected.ME

Eriksson, Marten, & Berglund, E. (1990). Vocabulary acquisition in two modalities: the case for partial- signing children with Down's syndrome. In *Uppsala Psychological Reports, No. 426.* Uppsala, Sweden: Department of Psychology, Uppsala University. DOWN SYNDROME VOCABULARY DEVELOPMENT INTERVENTION PROGRAMS SIGNING:

Simultaneous teaching of signed and oral language to mentally delayed children often result in a productive vocabulary of both manual signs and spoken words. The first question addressed in this study, is whether a mixed lexicon of this kind in a group of children with Down's syndrome (referred to as partial signing), is composed differently from that of oral, non-retarded children. The active vocabularies of two such groups were investigated by an object naming task. The groups were matched with regard to a mean performance. Frequencies of known labels to target objects between the groups were highly correlated, indicating no difference in vocabulary composition. A second question was if the data of the parital-signing group would reveal any consistent modality preferences in naming particular objects. However, no object modality interaction in naming was found.ME

Eubank, Lynn. (1991). *Point counterpoint: universal grammar in the second language.* Philadelphia, PA: Language acquisition and language disorder. PARAMETER SETTING ACQUISITION AND LINGUISTIC THEORY L2 LINGUISTIC THEORY:

This adversarial set of papers/replies originated at a special session of the Second Language Research Forum, UCLA. March 1989. With the invited speakers premeditatedly chosen for their clashing views, the conference focused on the role of Universal Grammar in second language acquisition with side forays into the explanatory potential of linguistic theory in native-language development.

Evans, J. L., & Craig, Holly K. (1992). Language sample collection and analysis-interview compared to freeplay assessment contexts. *Journal of Speech and Hearing Research*, 35, 343-353. ASSESSMENT PROCEDURES METHODOLOGY-ANALYSIS METHODOLOGY-DESIGN:

Evans, Mary Ann, & Schmidt, Fred. (1991). Repeated maternal book reading with two children: language-normal and language-impaired. *First Language*, 11, 269-287. PARENTAL SPEECH-STYLE ADULT-CHILD INTERACTION:

Two mother-child dyads were observed, one child from a normal group, and one from the language impaired population: both children were matched for MLU and expressive vocabulary. Different dynamics were observed for the dyads: the impaired dyad being characterized by a greater use of maternal obliges, and more incorrect child responses, whereas the language normal dyad showed a more equally balance distribution of power between the mother and the child. From Child Development Abstracts.

Everitt, Brian, & Hay, Dale. (1992). *Talking about statistics: A psychologist's guide to design and analysis*. New York, NY: John Wiley & Sons. METHODOLOGY-ANALYSIS METHODOLOGY-DESIGN:

Introductory explanantion of the use of statistics in behavioral science which includes recent advances in statistical analysis. The authors use a case study model to illustrate the techniques.

Ezell, H. K., & Goldstein, Howard. (1991). Comparison of idiom comprehension of normal children and children with mental retardation. *Journal of Speech and Hearing Research*, 34, 812-819. FIGURATIVE LANGUAGE RETARDED CHILDREN:

Ezell, H. K., & Goldstein, Howard. (1991). Observational learning of comprehension monitoring skills in children who exhibit mental retardation. *Journal of Speech and Hearing Research*, 34, 141-154. RETARDED CHILDREN MONITORING COMPREHENSION:

F

Falmagne, Rachel J., Mawby, Ronald A., & Pea, Roy D. (1989). Linguistic and logical factors in recognition of indeterminacy. *Cognitive Development*, 4, 141-176. LANGUAGE AND COGNITIVE DEVELOPMENT LOGICAL ABILITIES:

This article examines the contribution of logical and linguistic factors to recognition cases of logical indeterminacy.-From Child Development Abstracts.

Farkas, Zsolt, Gosy, Mária, & Hirschberg, Jenö. (1983). Kisgyermekkori beszéd-audiometria (Speech Audiometry in young children). *Fül-orr-gege Gyógyászat*, 29, 93-102. AUDIOLOGY AUDIOMETRY HUNGARIAN: HUNGARIAN

Farran, Dale C., & Kasari, Connie. (1990). A longitudinal analysis of the development of synchrony in mutual gaze in mother-child dyads. *Journal of Applied Developmental Psychology*, 11, 419-430. GAZE:

Dyads were observed at 6, 20, and 36 months in free play situations. Children tended to increase the duration and frequency of looking at their mothers, and also engaged in more independent gazing. Mothers decreased, and became more likely to break off mutual gaze as the child grew. From Child Development Abstracts.

Farrar, M. J., Raney, G. E., & Boyer, M. E. (1992). Knowledge, concepts, and interferences in childhood. *Child Development*, 63, 673-691. CONCEPT DEVELOPMENT LANGUAGE AND COGNITIVE DEVELOPMENT:

Fayol, M. (1982). Le plus-que-parfait: Étude génétique en comprehension et production chez l'enfant de quartre à dix ans (Comprehension and production of pluperfect in four to ten year-old children.). *Archives de psychologie*, 50, 261-283. VERBS FRENCH VERBS-ASPECT: FRENCH

Fayol, M. (1985). *Le réciter sa construction. (The construction of narration in child language).* Paris: Neuchatel. NARRATIVES: FRENCH

Fazio, B., Johnston, Judith R., & Brandl, L. (1993). Relationship between mental age and the development of vocabulary consisting of labels versus relational terms among mildly mentally handicapped children. *American Journal of Mental Retardation*, 97. RELATIONAL TERMS HYPERLEXIA RETARDED CHILDREN VERBS NOUNS LABELING LANGUAGE AND COGNITION LANGUAGE AND COGNITIVE DEVELOPMENT:

This study used standardized tests (PPVT and Boehm) to examine the use of relational terms and object/action terms. It was found that there was a closer correlation between mental age and relational terms than there was between mental age and object/action terms.JRJ

Feenstra-Ikink, G. G. J., & Jansonius-Schultheiss, Kino. (1986). Developments in the treatment of cleft lip and palate children (in Dutch). *Logopedie en Foniatrie*, 58, 175-181. CLEFT PALATE: DUTCH

Comparisons with and reflections on outcomes of former and modern international studies concerning speech and language (developmental problems), assessment, medical intervention and logopedic treatment in cleft lip and palate children.KJS

Feilberg, Julie, Hagtvet, Bente, Smith, Lars, Martinsen, Harald, Simonsen, Hanne G., Mjaavatn, Per E., & von Tetzchner, Stephen. (1988). *Barns sprak. (Children's language).* Oslo: Gyldendal. NORWEGIAN OVERVIEW-GENERAL: NORWEGIAN

Textbook written in cooperation between psychologists, educators, and linguists, illustrated where possible with material from Norwegian children.HGS

Feldman, -. (1993). The course of language development after early brain damage. In H. Tager-Flusberg (Ed.), *Constraints on language acquisition: Studies of atypical children*. Hillsdale, NJ: Lawrence Erlbaum Associates. ATYPICAL DEVELOPMENT TRAUMATIC DISORDERS NEUROLINGUISTICS:

Feldman, Carol F. (1989). Monologue as problem-solving narrative. In K. Nelson (Ed.), *Narratives from the crib*. Cambridge, MA: Harvard University Press. NARRATIVES CRIB SPEECH:

Feldman argues that the subject makes use of presleep monologues to resolve problems she has encountered during the day which were difficult to understand.

Felix, Sascha W. (1991). Language acquisition as a maturational process. In J. Weissenborn, H. Goodluck, & T. Roeper (Eds), *Theoretical issues in language acquisition: Continuity and change in development*. Hillsdale, NJ: Lawrence Erlbaum Associates. ACQUISITION THEORIES CONTINUITY/DISCONTINUITY BIOLOGICAL FOUNDATIONS:

Ferguson, Charles A. (1978). Fricatives in child language acquisition. *Papers and Reports on Child Language Development*, 6, 61-85. FRICATIVES:

Ferguson, Charles A. (1978). Learning to pronounce. In F. Minifie, & L. Lloyd (Eds), *Communicative and cognitive abilities: Early behavioral assessment*. Baltimore, MD: University Park Press. PHONOLOGICAL DEVELOPMENT:

Ferguson, Charles A. (1992). Implications of models and research. In C. A. Ferguson, L. Menn, & C. Stoel-Gammon (Eds), *Phonological development: Models, research, implications*. Monkton, MD: York Press. ACQUISITION THEORIES-PHONOLOGY ACQUISITION AND LINGUISTIC THEORY PHONOLOGICAL DEVELOPMENT:

Ferguson, Charles A., Menn, Lise, & Stoel-Gammon, Carol. (1992). *Phonological development: Models, research, implications*. Monkton, MD: York Press. PHONOLOGICAL DEVELOPMENT PROSODY PHONOLOGICAL DISORDERS L2 PHONOLOGY BILINGUALISM-PHONOLOGICAL DEVELOPMENT ANIMAL COMMUNICATIONS:

A collection of papers dealing with phonological acquisition theory and its implications when applied to phonological disorders, second language acquisition, reading development, and animal communication. The results of an international conference held at Stanford University in 1989; a ten year follow-up to the two volume results of the 1978 conference on child phonology. (q.v. Yeni-Komshian, Kavanagh, & Ferguson, [1980], *Child phonology*. New York, NY: Academic Press.)

Ferland, Mark B., & Mendelson, Morton J. (1989). Infants' categorization of melodic contour. *Infant Behavior and Development*, 12, 341-355. INTONATION INFANT PERCEPTION METHODOLOGY:

Categorization of auditory patterns on the basis of melodic contour was demonstrated in 10-month-old infants with an operant-fixation preference technique. Study 1 established the usefulness of the preference paradigm for assessing discrimination of auditory patterns whose tones differed in frequency, wave form, or both. Study 2 used the same procedure to show that infants can treat as equivalent different auditory sequences that have the same melodic contour. Infants preferred the novel- contour test patterns. The discussion both addresses the implications of 10-month-olds spontaneously equating sequences on the basis of melodic contour and raises methodological issues relevant to auditory categorization. - From Child Development Abstracts.

Fernald, Anne. (1989). Intonation and communicative intent in mothers' speech to infants: Is the melody the message? *Child Development*, 60, 1497-1510. INTONATION PARENTAL SPEECH-PROSODY:

Twenty five infant-directed and 25 adult-directed vocalizations were electronically filtered to eliminate linguistic content and presented to experienced parents and students inexperienced with infants. Listeners were able to use intonation to identify speaker's intent with higher accuracy in infant-directed speech than in adult-directed speech. - From Child Development Abstracts.

Fernald, Anne. (1990). Prosody in speech to children: prelinguistic and linguistic functions. *Annals of Child Development*, 8, PARENTAL SPEECH-PROSODY:

Fernald, Anne, Taeschner, Traute, Dunn, Judy, Papoušek, Mechthild, de Boysson-Bardies, Bénédicte, & Fukui, Ikuko. (1989). A cross-language study of prosodic modifications in mothers' and fathers' speech to preverbal infants. *Journal of Child Language*, 16(3), 477-501. CROSSLINGUISTIC STUDY-PARENTAL SPEECH FRENCH PROSODY:

Ferreiro, Emilia, Othenin-Girard, C., Chipman, Harold H., & Sinclair, Hermina. (1976). How do children handle relative clauses? *Archives de Psychologie*, 44, 229-266. RELATIVIZATION:

Ferreiro, Emilia, & Sinclair, Hermina. (1971). Temporal relationship in language. *Journal of International Psychology*, 6, 39-47. TEMPORAL RELATIONS TEMPORAL TERMS:

Ferreiro, Emilia, & Sinclair, Hermina. (1979). L'enfant et l'écrit. (The child and writing.). *Médecine et Hygiène*, 37, 3530-3536. WRITTEN LANGUAGE LITERACY: FRENCH

Ferreiro, Emilia, & Teberosky, A. (1979). *Los sistemas de escritura en el desarollo del niño*. Mexico: Siglo XXI. WRITTEN LANGUAGE: SPANISH

Fewell, Rebecca R., & Oelwein, Patricia L. (1991). Effective early intervention: Results from the model preschool program for children with Down syndrome and other developmental delays. *Topics in Early Childhood Special Education*, 11, 56-68. DOWN SYNDROME DEVELOPMENTAL DISORDERS INTERVENTION PROGRAMS:

The effectiveness of an intervention program for young children with Down syndrome was investigated. The rate of development during intervention was significantly greater than the rate of development at pretest across all developmental domains of the Classroom Assessment of Developmental Skills. Significant differences were found on six of the seven domains on the Battelle Developmental Inventory.

Fiese, Barbara H. (1990). Playful relationships: A contextual analysis of mother-toddler interaction and symbolic play. *Child Development*, 61, 1648-1656. ADULT-CHILD INTERACTION LANGUAGE AND PLAY TURN TAKING:

Toddlers 15 to 24 months, were observed under 4 conditions: child play along, child play with mother, child modeling mother, and, child play with mother following modeling. More complex play was observed when children were playing with their mothers than when playing by themselves. Maternal intrusions and questioning were negatively related to symbolic play. Turn-taking was more likely to precede symbolic play, and maternal intrusiveness was more likely to precede simple exploratory play.

Fivush, R., Kuebli, J., & Clubb, Patricia A. (1992). The structure of events and event representations: A developmental analysis. *Child Development*, 63, 188-201. EVENTS/SCRIPTS:

Flax, J., Lahey, Margaret, Harris, K., & Boothroyd, A. (1991). Relations between prosodic variables and communicative functions. *Journal of Child Language*, 18, 3-19. COMMUNICATIVE FUNCTIONS DISCOURSE FUNCTIONS PROSODY:

Flege, James E. (1992). Speech learning in a second language. In C. A. Ferguson, L. Menn, & C. Stoel-Gammon (Eds), *Phonological development: Models, research, implications*. Monkton, MD: York Press. L2 PHONOLOGY:

Fletcher, Paul, & Hall, D. (1992). *Specific speech and language disorders in children*. London: Whurr. LANGUAGE DISORDERS DEVELOPMENTAL DISORDERS APHASIAS:

Fogel, A. (1990). The process of developmental change in infant communicative action: Using dynamic systems theory to study individual ontogenies. In J. Colombo, & J. Fagen (Eds), *Individual differences in infancy: Reliability, stability, and prediction*. Hillsdale, NJ: Lawrence Erlbaum Associates. INDIVIDUAL VARIATION COMMUNICATIVE DEVELOPMENT:

Foley, J. A. (1985). A study of the development of language among pre-school children in Singapore with particular reference to English. In P. Larson, E. Judd, & D. Messerschmitt (Eds), *A Brave New World for TESOL*. Washington, DC: Georgetown University. BILINGUALISM-EDUCATION L2 EDUCATION:

Part one of this paper considers the development of English in Singapore between 1970 and 1980 census. Part two looks at the English syllabus in the primary school: part three shows how the findings from a study of pre school children whose parents are English-medium educated may warrent other alternatives to the present English languages programs in primary schools.JAF

Foley, J. A. (1988). Bilingualism and cognitive development. *Singapore Psychologist*, 3 (3), 4-18. BILINGUALISM-COGNITIVE DEVELOPMENT:

This paper looks briefly at recent studies of bilingualism and cognitive development which although showing some confusion in terminology, indicates a positive relationship between bilingualism and cognition within given parameters. Secondly, a survey is done of studies undertaken in Singapore and Malaysia, countries with official multi-lingual education policies but interpreted very differently.JAF

Foley, J. A. (1988). Multilingual settings and the cognitive development of children: studies from the Singapore-Malaysian context. In V. Bickley (Ed.), *Languages in education in a bilingual or multilingual setting*. Hong Kong: Institute of Language in Education, Education Department. BILINGUALISM-COGNITIVE DEVELOPMENT LANGUAGE AND EDUCATION:

The purpose of this paper is to review recent studies which have investigated the relationships between bilingualism and cognitive development and to outline the implications of these research findings for the education system in both Singapore and Malaysia.JAF

Foley, J. A. (1989). Bilingual early reading. *Commentary*, Nov/Dec,
L2 READING PROFICIENCY LANGUAGE AND EDUCATION LITERACY BIDIALECTISM ENGLISH-MALAY ENGLISH-TAMIL ENGLISH-CHINESE CHINESE-ENGLISH MALAY-ENGLISH TAMIL-ENGLISH:

> The case is argued for a conscious approach to the development of bilingual reading (English-Mandarin, English-Malay, English-Tamil) within the context of Singapore. Recent studies are reviewed to show the positive effects of getting a head-start in more than one language. It is further argued that this will not over-tax the child if the right sort of language approach to reading is taken. In particular the author advocates a development of reading similar to the Initial Literacy Programme (University College London, 1964-71), which is highly relevant today.JAF

Foley, J. A. (1990). Developmental features of children's writing in Singapore. In A. Kwan-Terry (Ed.), *Language development in Singapore and Malaysia.* Singapore: Singapore University Press.
WRITTEN LANGUAGE BILINGUALISM-EDUCATION:

> This study examines children's writing in English in the formal system of education in Singapore. Three issues are considered: 1) How the development of the writing of Singapore children compares with children who use English as their mother tongue, 2) How other languages and other forms of English in a multilingual environment influence the development of language, in particular writing, 3) How the teaching of writing especially with regards to genre (a staged goal-oriented social process) is part of the basic encoding skills required in language development.JAF

Foley, J. A. (1990). The lexico-grammatical development of Chinese-speaking children's writing in the multilingual setting of Singapore. In T. Le, T. D. Hien, & J. Hepburn (Eds), *Language and learning: Theory in practice.* Tasmania, Australia: TSIT.
WRITTEN LANGUAGE VYGOTSKYAN THEORY BILINGUALISM-COGNITIVE DEVELOPMENT LANGUAGE AND COGNITION CHINESE LEXICAL DEVELOPMENT:

It has been suggested that in the process of child language development we can identify a number of stages: primary and secondary intersubjectivity out of which protolanguage develops, the holophrastic stage, and the eventual development of the lexico-grammar of the adult system. Vygotsky believed that mastery of the written language (learning to read and write), has a profound effect upon the achievement of abstract thinking. This paper focuses on that period of child language development where the child is gaining a degree of control such that the constancy of the written word, grafted upon the immediacy of the spoken language, enables the child to reflect upon meanings and by so doing, acquire a new level of control. We will argue that by a detailed study of the elements of language which make up cohesion and coherence in a text, one can assess a child's development in the written language.JAF

Foley, J. A. (1991). A psycho-socio-linguistic framework for language development in Singapore and Mauritius. In *Yearbook 1991, Mother Tongue Education*. The Hague, The Netherlands: Foris. LANGUAGE AND EDUCATION WRITTEN LANGUAGE BILINGUALISM-EDUCATION:

This study sets out to show how a framework based on psycho-socio- linguistics theories can help us understand the development of child language. Specifically, this study looks at the development of language at the end of primary school. The multilingual and cultural settings of Singapore and Mauritius were chosed as they have a number of factors in common. What the data shows is that language development of the child, as far as writing is concerned, (and that is the main use of English in Mauritius) is being arrested by a too tightly controlled approach to language development within the classroom.JAF

Folkins, J. W., & Bleile, Kenneth M. (1990). Taxonomies in biology, phonetics, phonology, and speech motor control. *Journal of Speech and Hearing Disorders*, 55, 596-611. PHONOLOGICAL DEVELOPMENT ARTICULATION ASSESSMENT PROCEDURES:

Fonagy, Ivan. (1972). À propos de la genèse de la phrase enfantine. (On the origins of the infantile phrase.). *Lingua*, 30, 31-71. SYNTACTIC DEVELOPMENT HUNGARIAN PROSODY: FRENCH

Fonagy, Ivan. (1975). Prélangage et régressions syntaxiques. (Prelinguistics and syntactic regressions.). *Lingua*, 36, 163-208. PRELINGUISTICS SYNTACTIC DEVELOPMENT HUNGARIAN UNLEARNING: FRENCH

Forman, E. A. (1992). Discourse, intersubjectivity, and the development of peer collaboration: a Vygotskyan approach. In L. T. Winegar, & J. Valsiner (Eds), *Children's development within social context, vol. 1.*. Hillsdale, NJ: Lawrence Erlbaum Associates. SOCIAL SPEECH VYGOTSKYAN THEORY INTERSUBJECTIVITY:

Forrest, Karen, Adams, Scott, & McNeil, Malcom R. (1991). Perioral EMG activity in aphasic, apraxic, and dysarthric speakers. In C. A. Moore, K. M. Yorkston, & D. R. Beukleman (Eds), *Dysarthria and apraxia of speech*. Baltimore, MD: Paul H. Brookes. APRAXIA DYSARTHRIA APHASIAS:

Fortescue, Michael, & Olsen, L. L. (1992). The acquisition of West Greenlandic. In D. I. Slobin (Ed.), *The crosslinguistic study of language acquisition (Vol. 3)*. Hillsdale, NJ: Lawrence Erlbaum Associates, Inc. GREENLANDIC:

Foster, Susan H. (1990). *The communicative competence of young children*. Cambridge, MA: Longmans. COMMUNICATIVE COMPETENCE PRELINGUISTICS LEXICAL DEVELOPMENT ACQUISITION THEORIES-OVERVIEW PRAGMATIC DEVELOPMENT SYNTACTIC DEVELOPMENT MORPHOLOGICAL DEVELOPMENT SEMANTIC DEVELOPMENT SOCIAL INTERACTION HYPOTHESIS:

Foster examines the processes underlying preschool language development from a pragmatic viewpoint. She draws on research in developmental psychology, anthropology, sociology, and linguistics. She provides an introduction to the terminology of acquisition, followed by accounts of prelinguistic and early lexical development, and then accounts of syntactic, morphological, semantic and pragmatic development. She concludes by outlining the behaviorist, rationalist, cognitivist, and social interactionist approaches to acquisition. After Hakuta - Child Development Abstracts.

Foster, W., & Rondal, Jean A. (1976). Translation of Marc Richelle's 'Analyse formelle et analyse fonctionnelle du comportement verbal: notes sur le débat entre Chomsky et Skinner'. (Formal and functional analysis of verbal behavior: notes on the debate between Chomsky and Skinner). *Bulletin de Psychologie (Behaviorism)*, 26(4), 252-259 (209-221). LANGUAGE AND BEHAVIORISM LANGUAGE AND COGNITION: FRENCH

Fowler, A. (1993). Language learning in children with Down syndrome. In H. Tager-Flusberg (Ed.), *Constraints on language acquisition: Studies of atypical children*. Hillsdale, NJ: Lawrence Erlbaum Associates. ATYPICAL DEVELOPMENT DOWN SYNDROME:

Fowler, C. A., & Rosenblum, L. D. (1991). The perception of phonetic gestures. In I. G. Mattingly, & M. Studdert-Kennedy (Eds), *Modularity and the motor theory of speech perception*. Hillsdale, NJ : Lawrence Erlbaum Associates. PHONETIC GESTURES SPEECH PERCEPTION:

Fowler, William. (1990). *Talking from infancy: How to nurture & cultivate early language development*. Cambridge, MA : Brookline Books. INTERVENTION PROGRAMS FOR PARENTS:

Fox, M. J. (1975). *Language and development: A retrospective survey of Ford Foundation language projects*. New York, NY: Ford Foundation. OVERVIEW-PSYCHOLINGUISTICS:

Fox, R. (1991). Developing awareness of mind reflected in children's narrative writing. *British Journal of Developmental Psychology*, 9, 281-298. THEORY OF MIND NARRATIVES WRITTEN LANGUAGE:

Fradd, Sandra H., & Tikunoff, William J. (1987). *Bilingual education and bilingual special education: A guide for administrators*. San Diego, CA: Singular Group. LANGUAGE AND EDUCATION BILINGUALISM-EDUCATION:

Fradd, Sandra H., & Weismantel, M. J. (1989). *Meeting the needs of culturally and linguistically different students*. San Diego, CA:

Singular Group. ACCULTURATION BILINGUALISM-EDUCATION LANGUAGE AND EDUCATION NONSTANDARD DIALECTS BIDIALECTISM:

François, F. (1977). *La syntaxe de l'enfant avant 5 ans. (The child syntax before 5).* Paris: Larousse. EARLY SYNTACTIC DEVELOPMENT: FRENCH

Frank, R. E., & Hall, William S. (1991). Polysemy and the acquisition of the cognitive internal state lexicon. *Journal of Psycholinguistic Research*, 20, 283-304. POLYSEMY LEXICAL DEVELOPMENT:

Fraysse, Jean Claude, & Desprels-Fraysse, Annie. (1990). The influence of experimenter attitude on the performance of children of different cognitive levels. *Journal of Genetic Psychology*, 151, 169-179. METHODOLOGY-DESIGN:

Children's performance was superior when the experimenter was caring even though they did not seem to notice the difference between the two attitudes. P-level children clearly distinguished the experimenter attitudes, but their performance remained the same.

Frazier, Lyn, & de Villiers, Jill. G. (Eds). (1990). *Language processing and language acquisition*. Dordrecht, The Netherlands : Kluwer Academic Publishers. LANGUAGE PROCESSING:

Papers presented at the University of Massachusetts Conference on 'Language Processing and Language Acquisition', held in Amherst, on May 7-8, 1989.

Frederick, Martin N. (1984). *Principles of audiology: a study guide.* San Diego, CA: Singular Publishing Group. AUDIOLOGY AUDIOMETRY:

Review units: Acoustic immittance. Audiogram interpretation. The auditory nerve and central pathways. Aural rehabilitation. Behavioral tests for site of lesion ASLB, SISI, tone decay, Bekesy audiometry, bone conduction. Education of hearing-impaired children. Tests of hearing aids. Hearing aids. The inner ear. Masking for pure tones. Masking for speech tests. The middle ear. Noise. The outer ear. Pediatric audiology. Physics of sound. Pseudohypacusis. Speech audiometry. Tuning forks. Disorders described in case studies.

Freeman, Roger D., Carbin, Clifton F., & Boese, Robert J. (1981). *Can't your child hear? A guide for those who care about children.* San Diego, CA: Singular Publishing Group. INTEVENTION PROGRAMS FOR PARENTS DEAF CHILDREN READING DISORDERS LANGUAGE AND EDUCATION SIGNING:

What is it like to be deaf? Suspicion, delay, and diagnosis. How can you be sure? Why does deafness happen? Can deafness be cured? Associated problems. The parent's dilemma. Early two-way communication. Speech, speech reading, and auditory training. Sign languages. Total communication. Raising a deaf child. Deaf culture. Early intervention programs. Learning vocations. Schools. Parents and professionals as parents. Interpreters. Technical aids. Deafness with other disabilities.

Freeman, Yvonne S., & Freeman, David A. (1992). *Whole language for second language learners*. Portsmouth, NH: Heinemann. L2 EDUCATION BILINGUALISM-EDUCATION LANGUAGE AND EDUCATION:

French, Lucia A. (1989). The systematic acquisition of word forms by a child during the first-fifty-word stage. *Journal of Child Language*, 16(1), 69-90. LEXICAL DEVELOPMENT REPRESENTATIONS-PHONOLOGICAL FIRST WORDS :

French, Lucia A. (1989). Young children's responses to 'When' questions: issues of directionality. *Child Development*, 60(1), 225-236. CHILDREN'S RESPONSES CONNECTIVES-TEMPORAL ADVERBS:

French, Lucia A., Boynton, Marylou, & Hodges, Rosemary. (1991). Beginning to talk with peers: The roles of setting and knowledge. In S. A. Gelman, & J. Byrnes (Eds), *Perspectives on language and thought*. New York, NY: Cambridge University Press. LANGUAGE AND COGNITION LANGUAGE AND COGNITIVE DEVELOPMENT SOCIAL SPEECH SOCIAL INTERACTION PRAGMATIC DEVELOPMENT:

Freund, Lisa S. (1990). Maternal regulation of children's problem-solving behavior and its impact on children's performance. *Child Development*, 61, 113-126. PARENTAL SPEECH-CONTROL:

Sixty 3 and 5-year-olds either worked with their mothers or practiced alone and were given corrective feedback on a sorting task in which miniature furniture was placed in a doll house. Children who interacted with their mothers subsequently created more correct adult-like groupings independently than children who received corrective feedback. Mothers displayed more task responsibility and regulation with younger children and when task demands on children of both age groups increased. Maternal verbal content became less specific when task demands decreased. Child performance was related to (1) variation in maternal regulation of the child, and (2) degree of specificity of maternal verbal content. - From Child Development Abstracts.

Frew, B., & Conti-Ramsden, Gina. (1989). Joint action routines in teaching. *Bulletin (College of Speech Therapists)*, 443, 3-4. INTERVENTION PROGRAMS:

Friederici, Angela D., Weissenborn, Jürgen, & Kail, Michéle. (1990). Phonological and syntactic aspects in aphasics' pronoun comprehension: A crosslinguistic analysis. In E. Bates (Ed.), *Crosslinguistic studies of aphasia*. PRONOUNS COMPREHENSION DISORDERS CROSSLINGUISTIC STUDY-DISORDERS:

A special issue of *Brain and Language.*

Friederici, Angela D., Weissenborn, Jürgen, Lewandowski, C., & Stralka, R. (1991). Über den Einfluss perzeptueller Defizite auf den Erwerb von Raumausdrucken. (On the influence of perceptual deficit on the acquisition of spatial expressions.). *Zeitschrift für Entwicklungs- und Pädagogische Psychologie*, 23, 48-65. LANGUAGE AND PERCEPTION SPATIAL TERMS: GERMAN

Friedrich, Beate. (1976). *Entwicklung des sprachlichen Ausdrucks in der Unterstufe und in Klasse 4. (Development of linguistic expressions in the lower classes).* LANGUAGE AND EDUCATION DISCOURSE DEVELOPMENT DISCOURSE STRUCTURE: GERMAN

In this monograph the pedagogical objectives, tasks and methods of the development of competence in text production in the early school-age are described as types of tasks; narratives, descriptions and reports are differentiated.BF

Friedrich, Beate. (1988). Sprache und Lernen in der Unterstufe - Untersuchungen zum Zusammenhang von begrifflicher und sprachlicher Strukturbildung beim Wissenserwerb. (Language and learning in the lower classes: research in the conceptual and linguistic formation of structures by the acquisition of knowledge.). *Linguistische Studien*, 175, LANGUAGE AND EDUCATION DISCOURSE DEVELOPMENT DISCOURSE STRUCTURE: GERMAN

This paper presents the results of a five year study of language development in the early school years. It concentrates on the acquisition of conceptual knowledge and concept names and describes a method for analyzing coherence in children's discourse and methods for improving it.BF

Friedrich, Beate. (1988). Untersuchungsergebnisse zur Determination der sprachlichen Entwicklung der Kinder im jüngeren Schulalter durch den Unterricht. (Results concerning studies on Determination of Language development in children at early school-age by teaching.). In *Psycholgie für die Praxis*. LANGUAGE AND EDUCATION DISCOURSE DEVELOPMENT DISCOURSE COHERENCE: GERMAN

The connection between learning and language development in age of 6.0 to 11.0 is shown by: development of naming concepts and features, development of structuring texts, development of text-coherence. Tendencies of text-descriptions are deduced.BF

Friedrich, Bodo. (1985). Die Entwicklung des Könnens der Schüler zum komplexen Darstellen. (Development of pupils competence to elaborate complex states of affairs.). *Der Deutschunterricht*, 9, 411-422. DISCOURSE DEVELOPMENT COMPLEX SENTENCES LANGUAGE AND EDUCATION: GERMAN

The modular conception of language learning is illustrated by the components of knowledge and by communicative situations in application.BF

Friedrich, Bodo. (1985). Thesen zu Tendenzen, Linien und Phasen sprachlich-kommunikativer Entwicklung. (Thesis towards tendencies, lines and phases of language development.). *Schriften der Pädegogischen Hochschule Gustrow*, , 60-72. LANGUAGE AND EDUCATION WRITTEN LANGUAGE SYNTACTIC DEVELOPMENT LEXICAL DEVELOPMENT: GERMAN

Tendencies, lines and phases of development of the communicative behavior in school-age is differentiated in the fields of lexik, grammar and text production.BF

Friedrich, Bodo. (1986). Zur Komplexität sprachlich-kommunikativen Verhalterns. (The complexity of communicative behavior.). In *Jahrbuch der APW der DDR*. Berlin: LANGUAGE AND EDUCATION LANGUAGE AND COGNITIVE DEVELOPMENT: GERMAN

The complexity of communicative behavior is interpreted as the contribution of partial systems. The connection between communicative and cognitive (i.e. conceptual) behavior is explained and pedagogical consequences are derived from it.BF

Friedrich, Bodo, & Friedrich, Beate. (1988). Erzählen im Unterricht - Konzentration oder Verengung? (The use of narration in lessons: concentration or narrowing?). *Potsdamer Forschungen*, 77, 11-34. LANGUAGE AND EDUCATION: GERMAN

The use of narrations in teaching, which has been used in German schools for the last 100 years, is questioned from a historical view point with respect to its theoretical background.BF

Friel-Patti, Sandy, & Conti-Ramsden, Gina. (1988). Intervention tactics for learning disabled children with oral language impairments. In D. K. Reid (Ed.), *Teaching the learning disabled.* Boston: Allyn & Bacon, Inc. INTERVENTION PROGRAMS LANGUAGE DISORDERS:

Friel-Patti, Sandy, Finitzo-Heiber, Terese, Conti, Gina, & Brown, K. (1982). Language delay in infants associated with middle ear disease and mild, fluctuating hearing impairment. *Pediatric*

Infectious Diseases, 1, 104-109. LANGUAGE DELAY DEAF CHILDREN AUDIOLOGY:

Frith, Uta. (1991). *Autism and Asperger syndrome.* New York, NY: Cambridge University Press. AUTISM:

Asperger syndrome is defined as a combination of mental handicap and apparent intellectual giftedness -- the idiot-savant. In this text Frith contends that Asperger syndrome is a special type of autism.

Froem-Loeb, Diane, & Leonard, Laurence B. (1991). Subject case marking and verb morphology in normally developing and specifically language-impaired children. *Journal of Speech and Hearing Research*, 34, 340-346. CASE MORPHOLOGICAL DEVELOPMENT VERBS AGREEMENT SPECIFIC LANGUAGE IMPAIRMENT:

Froem-Loeb, Diane, & Schwartz, Richard G. (1990). Language characteristics of a linguistically precocious child. *First Language*, 10, 1-18. RETICENCE-TALKATIVENESS LINGUISTIC PRECOCITY:

This study investigated the language skills of a two-year-old child who displayed apparently advanced communication skills. Analysis of 1,258 utterances in relation to surrounding discourse structures indicated a high functioning level of contingent forms. - From Child Development Abstracts.

Fry, D. B. (1966). Development of the phonological system. In F. Smith, & G. A. Miller (Eds), *The genesis of language.* Cambridge, MA: MIT Press. PHONOLOGICAL DEVELOPMENT PHONEMIC DEVELOPMENT:

Frye, Douglas. (1991). The origins of intention in infancy. In D. Frye, & C. Moore (Eds), *Children's theories of mind.* Hillsdale, NJ: Lawrence Erlbaum Associates. THEORY OF MIND INTENTIONALITY:

Frye, Douglas, Braisby, Nicholas, Lowe, John, Maroudas, Celine, & Nicholls, Jon. (1989). Young children's understanding of counting and cardinality. *Child Development*, 60, 1158-1171. NUMERALS:

Different forms of the cardinality question were given before, after, and before and after the child counted. Both type and time of question had large effects. Children were good at recognizing a standard counting procedure as correct. They had only limited success at treating procedures that violated the stable order of count words or violated the one-on-one correspondence between count words and object as correct. - From Child Development Abstracts.

Frye, Douglas, & Moore, Chris (Eds). (1991). *Children's theories of mind: Mental states and social understanding, vol.*. Hillsdale, NJ: Lawrence Erlbaum Associates. INTENTIONALITY SELF-CONCEPT IMITATION THEORY OF MIND:

The contributors examine the child's theories of mind from various vantage points: cognitive, language, and social development. An explanation of the development of a theory of mind is offered.

Fujiki, Martin, Brinton, Bonnie, & Sonnenberg, Esther A. (1990). Repairs of overlapping speech in the conversations of specifically language-impaired and normally developing children. *Applied Psycholinguistics*, 11, 201-215. CONVERSATIONAL REPAIRS SPECIFIC LANGUAGE IMPAIRMENT:

The proportional occurrence of conversational overlap repairs was relatively similar for children with SLI and their matched group peers.

Furrow, David, Moore, Chris, Davidge, Jane, & Chiasson, L. (1992). Mental terms in mother's and children's speech-similarities and relationships. *Journal of Child Language*, 19, 617-631. VERBS-MENTAL PARENTAL SPEECH:

Furrow, David, Podrouzek, Wayne, & Moore, Chris. (1989). The acoustical analysis of children's use of prosody in assertive and directive contexts. *First Language*, 10, 37-49. ACOUSTIC PHONETICS PROSODY:

In order to determine how acoustical properties of speech are used for communication, prosodic features of children's utterances were compared across assertive directive tasks. Four children aged 1:11, were audiotaped while in contexts designed to elicit assertive or directive utterances to an adult. The children's utterances were analyzed for intensity and duration as well as beginning, end, peak, and low frequencies, frequency range, and contour changes. Results showed that in the directive context intensity was increased overall. - From Child Development Abstracts.

G

Gagné, J. P., Dinon, D., & Parsons, J. (1991). An evaluation of CAST - a computer-aided speechreading training program. *Journal of Speech and Hearing Research*, 34, 213-221. COMPUTER ASSISTED THERAPY INTERVENTION PROGRAMS:

Gaines, N. D., Runyan, C. M., & Meyers, S. C. (1991). A comparison of young stutterers fluent versus stuttered utterances on measures of length and complexity. *Journal of Speech and Hearing Research*, 34, 37-42. STUTTERING:

Galambos, Sylvia J., & Goldin-Meadow, Susan. (1990). The effects of learning two languages on levels of metalinguistic awareness. *Cognition*, 34, 1-56. BILINGUALISM-METALINGUISTIC DEVELOPMENT BILINGUALISM-SIMULTANEOUS SPANISH-ENGLISH ENGLISH-SPANISH BILINGUALISM-PROBLEMS/EFFECTS:

Three groups of children aged 4:0 to 8:0 (32 Spanish monolinguals, 32 English monolinguals, and 32 Spanish-English simultaneous bilinguals) were examined to determine whether the simultaneous acquisition of two languages enhanced the speaker's metalinguistic awareness. No significant differences were found between the groups. They all progressed from a content to a form based orientation to language at approximately the same rate.

Gallagher, Tanya M. (1991). Language and social skills: Implications for clinical assessment and intervention. In T. M. Gallagher, & N. Rees (Eds), *Pragmatics of language: Clinical practice issues.*. San Diego, CA: Singular Group. COMMUNICATIVE DEVELOPMENT SOCIAL SPEECH LANGUAGE FUNCTIONS CONVERSATIONAL SKILLS:

Gallagher, Tanya M. (1991). A retrospective look at clinical pragmatics. In T. M. Gallagher, & N. Rees (Eds), *Pragmatics of language: Clinical practice issues.*. San Diego, CA: Singular Group. INTERVENTION PROGRAMS PRAGMATIC DISORDERS ASSESSMENT PROCEDURES:

Gallagher, Tanya M., & Rees, Norma. (Eds). (1991). *Pragmatics of language: Clinical practice issues*. San Diego, CA: Singular Group. PRAGMATIC DEVELOPMENT PRAGMATIC DISORDERS INTERVENTION PROGRAMS:

Garcia, Ofelia. (Ed.) (1991). *Focus on bilingual education*. Amsterdam, The Netherlands: John Benjamins. BILINGUALISM-EDUCATION:

An interdisciplinary collection of essays dealing with bilingual education and covering such areas as: language policy, curricular issues, language maintenance and revitalization, and social issues. This is the first volume of a three volume set written to honor Fishman. The other volumes deal with language and ethnicity (volume 2, edited by James Dow), and language planning (volume 3, edited by David F. Marshall).

Gardner-Chloros, Penelope. (1991). *Language selection and switching in Strasbourg*. New York, NY: Oxford University Press. CODE-SWITCHING FRENCH-GERMAN GERMAN-FRENCH:

A description of the code-switching behavior of French-German speaking bilinguals in Strasbourg.

Garfin, Deborah G., McCallon, Denise, & Cox, Roger. (1988). Validity and reliability of the Childhood Autism Rating Scale with autistic adolescents. *Journal of Autism and Developmental Disorders*, 18, 367-378. AUTISM ASSESSMENT PROCEDURES CHILDHOOD AUTISM RATING SCALE:

The ability of the CARS to discriminate between autistic and nonautistic retarded adolescents was tested and CARS proved to be an adequate measure of autism in adolescence.

Garman, Michael A. (1990). *Psycholinguistics*. New York, NY: Cambridge University Press. APHASIAS LANGUAGE PROCESSES OVERVIEW-PSYCHOLINGUISTICS WRITTEN LANGUAGE:

An overview text which provides an introduction to the psychological processing of both spoken and written language. The final chapter looks at aphasic language processing.

Garrison, W., Dowaliby, F., & Long, G. (1992). Reading comprehension test item difficulty as a function of cognitive processing variables. *American Annals of the Deaf*, 137, 22-30. READING DISORDERS LITERACY:

Garton, Alison F. (1992). *Social interaction and the development of language and cognition*. Hillsdale, NJ: Lawrence Erlbaum Associates. LANGUAGE AND COGNITIVE DEVELOPMENT SOCIAL INTERACTION SOCIAL INTERACTION HYPOTHESIS PARENTAL SPEECH SEMANTICS AND SYNTAX ACQUISITION THEORIES PARAMETER SETTING PIAGETIAN THEORY VYGOTSKYAN THEORY CONSTRAINTS-COGNITIVE LANGUAGE AND PLAY:

Garton synthesizes a variety of theories (Chomsky, Bruner, Piaget, and Vygotsky) into a unified approach based upon social interaction.

Garton, Alison F., & Pratt, Chris. (1990). Children's pragmatic judgements of direct and indirect requests. *First Language*, 10, 51-59. REQUESTS INDIRECT SPEECH ACTS COMMUNICATIVE COMPETENCE:

Twelve request forms were rated along the three dimensions of politeness, effectiveness and likelihood of use by 216 12-year-old primary school children. There were positive correlations between the three dimensions regardless of the age of the addressee to whom the request was directed. There was no developmental trend in the ratings, although ratings tended to be higher for politeness and likelihood of use than for effectiveness. - From Child Development Abstracts.

Garvey, Catherine. (1990). *Play*. Cambridge, MA: Harvard University Press. LANGUAGE AND PLAY:

Garvey describes the development of five types of play: play with motion, play with objects, play with language, play with social relations, and play with rules in terms acceptable to both lay and professional readers.

Garvey, Catherine, & Kramer, Thayer L. (1989). The language of social pretend play. *Developmental Review*, 9(4), 364-382. LANGUAGE AND PLAY:

Gass, Susan M., et al. (Eds). (1989). *Variation in second language acquisition, 2 volumes, vol.*. New York, NY: Multilingual Matters. L2 VARIATION L2 DISCOURSE L2 PRAGMATICS L2 PSYCHOLINGUISTICS:

Volume 1 deals with L2 discourse and pragmatics, and volume 2 with L2 psycholinguistics.

Gassin, June. (1990). The notion of synchrony in second language learning. In M. A. K. Halliday, J. Gibbons, & H. Nicholas (Eds), *Learning, keeping and using language* . Amsterdam, The Netherlands: John Benjamins. L2 ACQUISITION L2 ACQUISITION THEORIES:

Selected paper from the proceedings of the Eighth World Congress of Applied Linguistics, Sydney, 1987.

Gathercole, Susan E., & Baddeley, Alan D. (1989). Evaluation of the role of phonological STM in the development of vocabulary in children: a longitudinal study. *Journal of Memory and Language*, 28(2), 200-213. LEXICAL DEVELOPMENT LANGUAGE AND MEMORY VOCABULARY DEVELOPMENT:

Gathercole, Susan E., & Baddeley, Alan D. (1993). *Working memory and language processing*. Hillsdale, NJ: Lawrence Erlbaum Associates. LANGUAGE AND MEMORY LITERACY VOCABULARY DEVELOPMENT SPEECH PRODUCTION LANGUAGE PROCESSING:

The authors draw from a variety of sources including language development, psycholinguistics, and neurolinguistics to examine the role played by working memory in: vocabulary acquisition, speech production, reading, and comprehension.

Gathercole, Susan E., Willis, C., & Baddeley, Alan D. (1991). Nonword repetition, phonological memory, and vocabulary - a reply to Snowling, Chiat, and Hulme. *Applied Psycholinguistics* , 12, 375-379. LANGUAGE AND MEMORY VOCABULARY DEVELOPMENT PHONOLOGICAL PROCESSES METHODOLOGY-DESIGN SYLLABLES METALINGUISTICS:

Gathercole, Susan E., Willis, C., Emslie, H., & Baddeley, Alan D. (1991). The influences of number of syllables and wordlikeness on children's repetition of nonwords. *Applied Psycholinguistics*, 12, 349-367. METHODOLOGY-DESIGN PHONOLOGICAL PROCESSES LANGUAGE AND MEMORY VOCABULARY DEVELOPMENT SYLLABLES METALINGUISTICS:

Gathercole, Virginia C. (1989). The acquisition of sex-neutral uses of masculine forms in English and Spanish. *Applied Psycholinguistics*, 10, 401-427. SPANISH LANGUAGE AND GENDER ROLES GENDER CROSSLINGUISTIC STUDY:

The acquisition of sex-neutral uses of masculine terms by English and Spanish-speaking children was examined. Data failed to confirm the hypothesis that Spanish-speaking children might discover the neutral, unmarked interpretations of masculine terms earlier than their English-speaking counterparts, who might have difficulty in moving away from an early sex-based interpretation of such forms to their sex-neutral application. Subjects from both language groups appeared to pay little attention to gender marking outside the noun, and they both paid less attention to masculine gender markers than to feminine gender markers outside the noun. - From Child Development Abstracts.

Gathercole, Virginia C. (1989). Contrast: a semantic constraint? *Journal of Child Language*, 16(3), 685-702. CONSTRAINTS-SEMANTIC MUTUAL EXCLUSIVITY:

Gauvain, Mary, & Rogoff, Barbara. (1989). Ways of speaking about space: The development of children's skill in communicating spatial knowledge. *Cognitive Development*, 4, 295-307. SPATIAL TERMS DEIXIS-SPATIAL LANGUAGE AND MEMORY ORIENTATIONAL TERMS:

This study presents data on the development of children's use of a memory test. Thirty-two 6-7 and 8-9-year- old children explored a laboratory-constructed funhouse, guided by instructions to study the layout or the route, and then were asked to describe the funhouse, with encouragement to sketch the space as they talked. Older children's descriptions of the space contained information about the temporal and spatial contiguity of areas in the space, with performance resembling that reported for adults. Younger children who were oriented to the layout tended to list places without reference to spatial relations, but descriptions provided by younger children who were oriented through the space did not differ from older children. - From Child Development Abstracts.

Gee, J. (1990). Memory and myth: A pespective on narrative. In A. McCabe, & C. Peterson (Eds), *Developing narrative structure*. Hillsdale, NJ: Lawrence Erlbaum Associates. NARRATIVES LANGUAGE AND MEMORY:

Gelman, Susan A., & Byrnes, James P. (1991). *Perspectives on language and thought : interrelations in development*. New York, NY: Cambridge University Press. LANGUAGE AND COGNITION LANGUAGE AND COGNITIVE DEVELOPMENT CATEGORIZATION SOCIAL INTERACTION LEXICAL DEVELOPMENT SEMANTIC DEVELOPMENT:

A collection of papers on semantic and lexical development which describe how children acquire their knowledge of the world and the ability to talk about it.

Gelman, Susan A., & Coley, John D. (1991). Language and categorization: The acquisition of natural kind terms. In S. A. Gelman, & J. Byrnes (Eds), *Perspectives on language and thought*. New York, NY: Cambridge University Press. LANGUAGE AND COGNITION LANGUAGE AND COGNITIVE DEVELOPMENT CATEGORIZATION SEMANTIC MAPPING LEXICAL DEVELOPMENT:

Gelman, Susan A., Wilcox, Sharon A., & Clark, Eve V. (1989). Conceptual and lexical hierarchies in young children. *Cognitive Development*, 4, 309-326. CATEGORIZATION COMPOUNDS SEMANTIC ORGANIZATION:

As predicted, compound nouns were easier to learn than single nouns, especially at the subordinate level. Age of child and category level influenced the kinds of errors children made. The most common error was to treat hierarchically related words as labeling mutually exclusive subsets so that terms from different levels contrasted at the same level. Both factors, linguistic form and conceptual level, influenced children's learning of new lexical hierarchies. - From Child Development Abstracts.

Gentile, Mary A., Boll, Thomas J., Stagno, Sergio, & Pass, Robert F. (1989). Intellectual ability of children after perinatal cytomegalovirus infection. *Developmental Medicine and Child Neurology*, 31, 782-786. AT-RISK CHILDREN LANGUAGE AND COGNITIVE DEVELOPMENT CONGENITAL DISORDERS:

The mental ability of 16 children who had not had congenital cytomegalovirus (CMV) infection, but acquired it before the age of six months, was compared with that of two other groups: one comprising 32 children who had CMV-excreting mothers but who were not infected themselves, the other comprising 18 healthy controls. Serial audiological, ophthalmological and psychometric examinations were performed on preschool and elementary school-aged children. Although the children with acquired CMV infection had lower mean arithmetic scores, the results suggest that healthy term infants who acquire early CMV infection are not at increased risk of intellectual impairment.- From Child Development Abstracts.

Gentner, Dedre, & Rattermann, MaryJo. (1991). Language and the career of similarity. In S. A. Gelman, & J. Byrnes (Eds), *Perspectives on language and thought*. New York, NY: Cambridge University Press. LANGUAGE AND COGNITION LANGUAGE AND COGNITIVE DEVELOPMENT RELATIONAL TERMS:

Gereben, Ferencné. (1972). Sprachperzeptorische Untersuchungen im Kreise an motorischen Aphasie leidenden Kinder. (Speech perception research in children suffering from motoric aphasia.). In *Papers in interdisciplinary speech research*. Budapest: Akademiai Kiado. APHASIAS MOTOR DISORDERS HUNGARIAN LANGUAGE AND MOTOR DEVELOPMENT: GERMAN

Gereben, Ferencné. (1978). Súlyos beszédhibák vizsgálata es terápiája (Diagnosis and treatment of severe speech disorders). *Magyar Fonetikai Füzetek*, 1, 35-42. INTERVENTION PROGRAMS CLASSIFICATION OF DISORDERS HUNGARIAN: HUNGARIAN

Gereben, Ferencné. (1979). Fruherfassung und Fruhbehandlung der Sprachbehinderten in Ungarn. (The early recognition and treatment of language delay in Hungary.). *Der Sprachheilpädagoge (Wien)*, 4, INTERVENTION PROGRAMS HUNGARIAN: GERMAN

Gereben, Ferencné. (1979). Individualisierte Gruppentherapie mit Spaltkindern. (Individualised group therapy for cleft palate children.). In *Sprachbehinderung und Gruppenaktivitaten Jugendund Volk*. Munchen/Wien: INTERVENTION PROGRAMS HUNGARIAN CLEFT PALATE: GERMAN

Gereben, Ferencné. (1988). Ajak es szájpadhasadékos gyermekek korai fejlesztése (Early intervention in cleft palate children). In *Korai fejlesztés a logopediában.*. Budapest: INTERVENTION PROGRAMS CLEFT PALATE HUNGARIAN: HUNGARIAN

Gerebenné, Várbíró K. (1986). A beszédfejlodési elmaradás korai felismerése hatása a pszichikus fejlödésre (The influence of early diagnosis of speech retardation on psychic development). In *Tanulmányok a beszédjavitásköréből. 1.* Budapest: Gyógypedagógiai Továbbképzés Könyvtára -- OPI. CLASSIFICATION OF DISORDERS ASSESSMENT PROCEDURES HUNGARIAN: HUNGARIAN

Gerebenné, Várbíró K., & Kissné, Eva Haffner. (1987). Beszédfejlesztés a gyógypedagógiai óvodákban. (Speech development in logopedic nurseries.). *Gyógypedagógia*, 5(6), 131-136. LANGUAGE AND EDUCATION INTERVENTION PROGRAMS: HUNGARIAN

Gerhardt, Julie. (1989). Monologue as a speech genre. In K. Nelson (Ed.), *Narratives from the crib*. Cambridge, MA: Harvard University Press. CRIB SPEECH NARRATIVES ASPECT TENSE PRONOUNS-PERSONAL SEMANTIC FEATURES VERBS MORPHOLOGICAL DEVELOPMENT:

Gerhardt follows the development of verb morphology for a six week period beginning when the subject is 1:10:16. She discusses the development of aspect and tense, and the use of the pronouns 'I' and 'my'. She subscribes to the view that aspect and tense develop from earlier discourse functions in the child's speech.

Gerhardt, Julie. (1991). The meaning and use of the modals 'hafta, needta' and 'wanna' in children's speech. *Journal of Pragmatics*, 16(6) , 531-590. MODALS AUXILIARIES:

German, D. J., & Simon, E. (1991). Analysis of children's word-finding skills in discourse. *Journal of Speech and Hearing Research*, 34, 309-316. CHILDREN'S DISCOURSE:

Gerratt, Bruce R., Till, James A., Rosenbek, John C., Wertz, Robert T., & Boysen, Allen E. (1991). Department of Veterans Affairs Dysarthia Survey. In C. A. Moore, K. M. Yorkston, & D. R. Beukleman (Eds), *Dysarthria and Apraxia of Speech*. Baltimore, MD: Paul H. Brookes Publishing Co. DYSARTHRIA:

Gettinger, Maribeth, Elliott, Stephen N., & Kratochwill, Thomas R. (1992). *Preschool and early childhood treatment directions*. Hillsdale, NJ: Lawrence Erlbaum Associates. ASSESSMENT PROCERDURES INTERVENTION PROGRAMS DEVELOPMENTAL SCALES AT-RISK CHILDREN LANGUAGE AND EDUCATION HANDICAPPED CHILDREN:

A text aimed at school psychologists which deals with the devising and validation of preschool predictive tests and treatment programs.

Gibbs, R. W. (1991). Semantic analyzability in children's understanding of idioms. *Journal of Speech and Hearing Research*, 34, 613-620. FIGURATIVE LANGUAGE:

Gierut, Judith A. (1992). The conditions and course of clinically induced phonological change. *Journal of Speech and Hearing Research*, 35, 1049-1063. PHONOLOGICAL DISORDERS TREATMENT GENERALIZATION:

Gilger, Jeffrey W., Eliason, Michele J., & Richman, Lynn C. (1989). A comparison of cognitive and behavioral patterns in learning-disabled children: Subtype and sex differences. *Developmental Neuropsychology*, 5, 227-243. SEX DIFFERENCES:

Learning disabled (LD) females (n = 83) were matched with LD males by age and full scale IQ and compared on a battery of cognitive and behavioral tests. Similar factor and profile structures were found for male and female LD children. - From Child Development Abstracts.

Gillam, R., & Johnston, Judith R. (1985). The development of print awareness in language disordered preschoolers. *Journal of Speech and Hearing Research*, 28, 521-526. LITERACY LANGUAGE AND EDUCATION READING DISORDERS:

An examination of the ability of normal and language impaired children to read environmental print which shows that the impaired subjects have difficulties with this task once such non-linguistic cues as color and typeface have been neutralized.

Gillam, R., & Johnston, Judith R. (1992). Spoken and written language relationships in lanuage/learning impaired and normally achieving school-age children. *Journal of Speech and Hearing Research*, 35, 1303-1315. WRITTEN LANGUAGE NARRATIVES DISCOURSE ANALYSIS DISCOURSE COHERENCE DISCOURSE DISORDERS LANGUAGE PROCESSING:

An analysis of eight variables characterizing the semantic and syntactic features of both sentential and discourse levels in written and spoken narratives. Written texts were found to be more semantically coherent but had fewer surface markers showing intersentential relationships. It was felt that this form/content interaction reflected the different cognitive processing demands of the two modalities. No inter-group differences were noted for written-spoken relationships.

Gillis, Steven. (1982). On prelinguistic prerequisites for linguistic reference. In S. Daalder, & M. Gerritsen (Eds), *Linguistics in the Netherlands*. Amsterdam: North Holland. LANGUAGE PRECURSORS REFERENCE FIRST WORDS LEXICAL DEVELOPMENT:

The semantic and pragmatic prerequisites of first word use are discussed and illustrated with the results of a case study.SG

Gillis, Steven. (1983). Interactie zonder woorden: de ontogenese van de communicatieve intentie. (Interaction without words: the ontogenesis of communicative intentions.). In F. Daems, & L. Goossens (Eds), *Een spyeghel voor G. Jo Steembergen*. Leuven: Acco. INTENTIONALITY INTERSUBJECTIVITY DUTCH: DUTCH

The paper discusses the development of prelinguistic communicative intentions in the light of Searle's theory of intentionality.SG

Gillis, Steven. (1983). Van pretalige naar talige interactie: semantische en pragmatische aspecten van de eenwoordfase in de taalverving. (From prelinguistic to linguistic interaction: semantic and pragmatic aspects of the one-word stage in language acquisition.). *Antwerp Papers in Linguistics*, 30, SINGLE-WORD SPEECH PRELINGUISTICS DUTCH LEXICAL DEVELOPMENT: DUTCH

The monograph is an extensive review of the literature on the one- word stage. It focuses on pragmatic, cognitive-semantic and formal models of the one-word stage.SG

Gillis, Steven. (1985). De ontwikkeling van het intentional communicatief handelen. (The development of intentional communication.). *TTT*, 5, 299-335. DUTCH INTENTIONALITY: DUTCH

This paper reviews the literature on the development of intentional communicative vocal acts.SG

Gillis, Steven. (1985). The development of the concept of reference in its interactional context. *Studia Filolgiczne*, 21, 73-89. REFERENCE CONTEXT COMMUNICATIVE DEVELOPMENT INTERSUBJECTIVITY:

This paper discusses the development of a child's concept of referential communicative acts.SG

Gillis, Steven. (1985). Protowoorden in de taalverwerving. (Protowords in language acquisition.). *Onze Taal*, 54, 112-113. PROTOWORDS: DUTCH

A discussion of the notion of protowords as precursors of genuine words in language acquisition.SG

Gillis, Steven. (1985). Towards the first word. In M. Spoelders, F. van Besien, F. Lowenthat, & F. van Damme (Eds), *Language acquisition and learning: essays in developmental pragmatics*. Leuven: Acco. PRELINGUISTICS FIRST WORDS PROTOWORDS LEXICAL DEVELOPMENT:

This paper discusses one child's 'meaningful' vocal production preceding the acquisition of the first word.SG

Gillis, Steven. (1986). De ontwikkeling van het intentioneel communicatief vocaliseren: cognitieve en sociaal-interactionele aspecten. (The development of intentional communicative vocalizing: cognitive and social-interactional aspects.). *Antwerp Papers in Linguistics*, 42, BABBLING VOCALIZATIONS PROTOWORDS TRANSITIONAL PHASES: DUTCH

This paper is a detailed study of the development of intentional vocalizing in the transitional phase between babbling and first words.SG

Gillis, Steven. (1986). This child's nominal insight is actually a process: the plateau-stage and the vocabulary spurt in early lexical development. *Antwerp Papers in Linguistics*, 45, VOCABULARY SPURT SINGLE-WORD SPEECH INTENTIONALITY TRANSITIONAL PHASES LEXICAL DEVELOPMENT CONTINUITY/DISCONTINUITY:

A detailed analysis of one child's vocabulary development in the one-word stage. The analysis shows no qualitative discontinuities in the child's word-use neither in the transitional stage from preverbal to early verbal behavior, nor in the period around the 'vocabulary spurt.' The incremental developments in the child's verbal behavior are documented and analyzed on a microanalytical level.SG

Gillis, Steven. (1986). Transitional phenomena revisited: Insights into the nominal insight. In B. Lindblom, & R. Zetterstroem (Eds), *Precursors of early speech.*. New York, NY: Stockton press. VOCABULARY SPURT TRANSITIONAL PHASES LEXICAL DEVELOPMENT CONTINUITY/DISCONTINUITY:

A concise version of Antwerp Papers in Linguistics, #42, which discusses the development of vocabulary in the single-word stage and touches on the nominal insight theory (vocabulary spurt) and social interaction.SG

Gillis, Steven. (1987). Een schets van recente ontwikkelingen in het onderzoek van de taalverwerving. (A sketch of recent developments in the study of language acquisition.) *Handlingen XLI der Koninklijke Zuidnederlandse Maatschippij voor Taal - en letterkunde en Geschiedenis*, 93-116. OVERVIEW-THEORY: DUTCH

This paper reviews the main trends in the study of child language acquisition from the late sixties onward.SG

Gillis, Steven. (1987). Woorden en betekenissen in de vroege taalverwerving. Deel 1, 2;. *Audiopedagogica*, 3, 2-13. LEXICAL DEVELOPMENT TRANSITIONAL PHASES PROTOWORDS VOCABULARY SPURT CONTINUITY/DISCONTINUITY: DUTCH

These two papers discuss the major phenomena in early lexical development.SG

Gillis, Steven. (1987). Words and categories at the onset of language acquisition. *Belgian Journal of Linguistics*, 2, 37-53. LEXICAL DEVELOPMENT FIRST WORDS CATEGORIZATION SEMANTIC MAPPING REFERENCE:

In this paper, it is argued that although the product of the child's extension of his early words indicates that words are used for categories of things, an analysis of the process underlying children's word-use reveals another picture. During the one-word stage, the process guiding the extension of a word to distinct referents shifts from extension on the basis of mere identification to extension on the basis of the notion of class or category of objects.SG

Gillis, Steven, & de Schutter, G. (1986). Le long cheminement vers le premier emploi des mots. (The long road to the first use of words.). *Linguisticae Investigationes*, 10, 67-83. FIRST WORDS LEXICAL DEVELOPMENT VOCABULARY SPURT CONTINUITY/DISCONTINUITY: FRENCH

The incremental changes of a child's verbal behavior in the one-word stage are closely scrutinized. The main thesis is that on a pragmatic as well as on a semantic level there is no discontinuity as suggested by the 'Nominal Insight' proponents.SG

Gillis, Steven, & de Schutter, G. (1988). De lange weg naar het eerste woordgebruik. (The long way towards the first word usage.). *Psychologica Belgica*, 28 (2), 105-121. FIRST WORDS LEXICAL DEVELOPMENT VOCABULARY SPURT CONTINUITY/DISCONTINUITY: DUTCH

This paper reports an intensive longitudinal case study of the developmental milestones leading up to a child's first words.SG

Gillis, Steven, & de Schutter, G. (1988). Taalverwerving als een transactioneel proces. (Language acquisition as a transactional process.). *Pedagogisch Tijdschrift*, 13 (4), 250-262. PIAGETIAN THEORY LANGUAGE AND COGNITIVE DEVELOPMENT SOCIAL INTERACTION HYPOTHESIS: DUTCH

J. Bruner's theory of language acquisition as a transactional process is critically examined and its complimentarity with Piaget's more cognitive oriented theory is discussed.SG

Gillis, Steven, Koopmans-van Beinum, F. J., & van der Stelt, J. M. (1982). De verwerving een woordveld bij 5:5 tot 6-jarigen: een verkennend onderzoek. (The acquisition of a semantic field by 4:5 to 6-year-olds. An exploratory investigation.). *Antwerp Papers in Linguistics*, 28, LEXICAL DEVELOPMENT VERBS-LOCATIVE VERBS-CAUSATIVE: DUTCH

The monograph reports an investigation of 4:5 to 6-year-olds acquisition of positional verbs zitten ('sit'), staan ('stand'), liggen ('lie') and their causative companions zetten ('put') and leggen ('lay'). The children's use of the intrinsic properties of the experimental objects in understanding the verbs and their relationships are discussed.SG

Gillis, Steven, Koopmans-van Beinum, F. J., & van der Stelt, J. M. (1988). De prelinguale periode. (The prelinguistic period.). *Antwerp Papers in Linguistics;*, 55, PRELINGUISTICS SOCIAL INTERACTION BABBLING LANGUAGE PRECURSORS: DUTCH

This paper reviews the literature on relevant preverbal developments for language acquisition, viz. social-interactional development and the development of vocal production. The paper focuses on the relationships between these two phenomena. Six stages in the preverbal period are distinguished. Also available in an English text.SG

Gillis, Steven, Koopmans-van Beinum, F. J., & van der Stelt, J. M. (1988). The prelinguistic stage. In P. Jordens, & J. Lalleman (Eds), *Language Development*. Dordrect: Foris. SOCIAL INTERACTION BABBLING LANGUAGE PRECURSORS PRELINGUISTICS:

This paper is a short version of *Antwerp Papers in Linguistics*, #55. It reviews the literature on relevant preverbal developments for language acquisition, viz. social-interactional development and the development of vocal production. The paper focuses on the relationships between these two. Six stages in the preverbal period are distinguished.SG

Gillis, Steven, & Schaerlaekens, A. M. (1985). Pragmatic aspects of early lexical acquisition and development. *Journal of Pragmatics*, 9 (4), 427-432. LEXICAL DEVELOPMENT PRAGMATIC DEVELOPMENT ADULT-CHILD INTERACTION:

An introduction to this special issue of *Journal of Pragmatics* considers the recent interest in the pragmatic aspects of early lexical acquisition and development. Adult-child interactions are assessed as an important step in the child's communicative understanding. Brief outlines of the articles in this issue are provided. SG

Gillis, Steven, & Verlinden, A. (1988). Nouns and verbs in early lexical development. *Antwerp Papers in Linguistics*, 54, LEXICAL DEVELOPMENT WORD CLASS NOUNS VERBS INPUT FACTORS PARENTAL INPUT:

This paper is a more extensive report of the research reported in 'Nouns and verbs in the input.' (cf. ABLA Papers 12, q.v. in CHILDES/BIB). It also discusses the question of directionality: the same structural characteristics of the mother's language are investigated at several stages of the child's vocabulary development: from preverbal to a vocabulary level of 400 words.SG

Gleitman, Lila R. (1990). The structural sources of verb meanings. *Language Acquisition*, 1, 3-55. VERBS SEMANTIC DEVELOPMENT SEMANTICS AND SYNTAX CUES-SYNTACTIC LEXICAL DEVELOPMENT:

Gleitman reviews the present state of understanding regarding the acquisition of verb meaning and suggests that it is basically an inadequate explanation. She goes on to propose that syntactic cues play an important role in the acquisition of verb meanings.

Gleitman, Lila R., & Gleitman, Henry. (1992). A picture is worth a thousand words, but that's the problem: The role of syntax in vocabulary acquisition. *Current Directions in Psychological Science*, 1(1), 31-35. VERBS VOCABULARY DEVELOPMENT SEMANTIC MAPPING SEMANTICS AND SYNTAX LEXICAL DEVELOPMENT CUES-SYNTACTIC:

Ostentation and semantic mapping alone are insufficient explanations of the acquisition of verb meaning. Children also make use of syntactic cues in the acquisition of verb meaning.

Gluck, Mark A., & Rumelhart, David E. (Eds). (1990). *Neuroscience and connectionist theory.* Hillsdale, NJ: Lawrence Erlbaum Associates. CONNECTIONISM:

A collection of essays introducing neural network models of human and higher vertebrate cognitive functions.

Golden, R. M., & Rumelhart, David E. (1991). A distributed representation and model for story comprehension and recall. In K. Hammond, & D. Gentner (Eds), *Proceedings of the Thirteenth Annual Conference of the Cognitive Science Society.* Hillsdale, NJ: Lawrence Erlbaum Associates. CONNECTIONISM NARRATIVES TEXT/STORY GRAMMARS DISCOURSE COMPREHENSION:

Goldfield, Beverly A. (1990). Pointing, naming, and talk about objects: Referential behavior in children and mothers. *First Language*, 10, 231-242. OSTENTATION LABELING GESTURE JOINT REFERENCE PARENTAL INPUT PARENTAL SPEECH:

This study investigates the relationships of children's communicative pointing and maternal language to the child's acquisition of object labels. At 14 months there were no differences between the two groups in either pointing or maternal language.

Goldfield, Beverley A., & Reznick, J. Steven. (1990). Early lexical acquisition: Rate, content, and the vocabulary spurt. *Journal of Child Language*, 17, 171-183. INDIVIDUAL VARIATION LEXICAL DEVELOPMENT VOCABULARY SPURT CONTINUITY/DISCONTINUITY DEVELOPMENTAL RATE METHODOLOGY-DIARY/CASE STUDY METHODOLOGY-LONGITUDINAL STUDY:

A longitudinal study of 18 children's word use, kept in diaries by the children's mothers, showed that the terms 'vocabulary spurt' and 'naming explosion' were best applied to children whose acquisition style was referential, i.e. children who concentrated their efforts on learning the names of things.

Goldin-Meadow, Susan. (1976). Structure in a manual communication system, development without a conventional language model: Language without a helping hand. In H. A. Whitaker, & H. Whitaker (Eds), *Studies in neurolinguistics* (vol. 4,). New York, NY: Academic Press. SIGNING DEAF CHILDREN:

Goldin-Meadow, Susan, & Mylander, Carolyn. (1990). Beyond the input given: The child's role in the acquisition of language. *Language*, 66, 323-355. DEAF CHILDREN GESTURE INPUT FACTORS SIGNING ACQUISITION THEORIES:

> The child's creative contribution to the language acquisition process is potentially most apparent in situations where the linguistic input available to the child is degraded, providing the child with ample opportunity to elaborate upon the input. The children described in this paper are deaf, with hearing losses so severe that they cannot naturally acquire spoken language, and their hearing parents have chosen not to expose them to sign language. Despite their lack of usable linguistic input, these children develop gestural communication systems which share many structural properties with early linguistic systems of young children learning from established language models. This paper reviews our findings on the structural properties of the deaf children's gesture systems and evaluates those properties in the context of data gained from other approaches to the question of the young child's language making capacity. - From Language.

Goldstein, Howard, & Mousetis, Lori. (1989). Generalized language learning by children with severe mental retardation: effects of peers' expressive modeling. *Journal of Applied Behavior Analysis*, 22(2), 245-259. RETARDED CHILDREN MODELING INTERVENTION PROGRAMS TREATMENT GENERALIZATION:

> From Stockholm Bibliographies.

Golinkoff, Roberta M. (Ed.). (1983). *The transition from prelingistics to linguistic communication.* Hillsdale, NJ: Lawrence Erlbaum Associates. TRANSITIONAL PHASES PRELINGUISTICS:

Golinkoff, Roberta M., & Hirsh-Pasek, Kathy. (1990). Let the mute speak: What infants can tell us about language acquisition. *Merrill-Palmer Quarterly*, 36, 67-92. SEGMENTATION EARLY SYNTACTIC DEVELOPMENT SEMANTIC MAPPING ACQUISITION THEORIES:

The period of infancy, before the child produces speech, may yield many of the secrets of the process of language acquisition. Infants must segment the acoustic-phonetic stream, parse the world into categories relevant to language, and discover the syntax by which language maps concepts onto speech. Research in each of these areas is reviewed. It is argued that the systems which contribute to language acquisition work complementarily in the real world to contribute to language acquisition.-From Child Development Abstracts.

Gombèrt, Jean E. (1990). *Le développement métalinguistique. (Metalinguistic development.)*. Paris: P.U.F. METALINGUISTICS: FRENCH

Available in English translations from University of Chicago Press, and The Harvester Press (London).

Goncz, Lajos. (1970). A kétnyelvüség hatása az intelligencia fejlödésére. (The influence of bilingualism on the development of intelligence.). *A Hungarológiai Intézet Tudományos Közleményei*, 3, 123-125. BILINGUALISM AND COGNITIVE DEVELOPMENT HUNGARIAN-SERBOCROATIAN SERBOCROATIAN-HUNGARIAN: HUNGARIAN

This paper contains information about forthcoming long-term investigations on the relation between Hungarian-Serbocroatian bilingualism and intelligence. A short review of different views on the structure and factors of developing intelligence is given and some methodological problems in such investigations are discussed.LG

Goncz, Lajos. (1973). Dvojezicnost kao faktor u objektivizaciji nekih aspekata misljenja kod dece. (Bilingualism as a factor in objectivizing some aspects of thinking in children.). *Zbornik Instituta za pedagoska istrazivanja u Beogradu*, 6, 201-205.

BILINGUALISM-COGNITIVE DEVELOPMENT LANGUAGE AND COGNITION: SERBOCROATIAN

In this paper we have presented the results of investigations about the influence of bilingualism on the development of some aspects of thinking in children. The following presupposition has been checked: is the unbreakable link between the word and the name - a phenomenon which represents a relevant aspect of nominal realism - as present in bilingual children as it is in monolingual ones at the age of 7?, i.e. the pupils of the first class of primary school. The instrument we used in investigating this problem was a list of 16 pairs of words, selected so that the longer word referred to an object or animal smaller than the other one named by a monosyllable word. Bilingual children have shown statistically much better results: the t test was significant at the level $P<0.05$.LG

Goncz, Lajos. (1974). Hogyan mérjük a kétnyelvüség különbözö aspektusait. (The measurement of different aspects of bilingualism.). *Oktatás és nevelés*, 5, 47-52.
BILINGUALISM-ASSESSMENT PROCEDURES METHODOLOGY-DESIGN: HUNGARIAN

Several techniques for measuring aspects of degree and types of bilingualism (questionnaires, word-list remembering, continued associations, reaction time, Osgood's semantic differential, psychogalvanic reaction) and their theoretical background is described.LG

Goncz, Lajos. (1974). Prilog neobihejvioristickih teorija znacenja teoriji dvojezicnosti. (Contribution of neobehavioristic theories of meaning to theories of bilingualism.). *Pedagoska stvarnost*, 8, 425-429. BILINGUALISM-LINGUISTIC THEORY LANGUAGE AND BEHAVIORISM: SERBOCROATIAN

Ervin Osgood's theory of coordinate-compound bilingualism is discussed in the context of contemporary neobehavioristic theories of meaning.LG

Goncz, Lajos. (1975). Jedna provera teorije dvojezicnosti o koordiniranim i slozenim jezickim sistemima kod dvojezicnih osoba. (A verification of the theory of coordinate and compound language systems in bilinguals.). In *Zbornik radova sa 5. Kongresa psihologa Jugoslaviije, Skopje.* HUNGARIAN-SERBOCROATIAN SERBOCROATIAN-HUNGARIAN BILINGUALISM-SIMULTANEOUS BILINGUALISM-SEQUENTIAL BILINGUALISM-SEMANTIC DEVELOPMENT BILINGUALISM-LEXICAL DEVELOPMENT: SERBOCROATIAN

Two groups of Hungarian-Serbocroatian bilingual high school students were tested: a coordinate and a compound bilingual group. The members of the coordinate group acquired their bilingual ability in a linguistically separated context, the language background of the compound group was mixed. The connotative meanings for the same words in the two languages, measured with semantic differential, was more different for the coordinate group, but the associative meaning was equal for the same words in the two groups.LG

Goncz, Lajos. (1975). Psiholoski aspekti ucenja jezika sredine na predskolskom uzrastu. (Psychological aspects of second language acquisition in the preschool period.). *Pedagoska stvarnost*, 6, 341-350. L2/L1 ACQUISITION BILINGUALISM-EDUCATION BILINGUALISM-COGNITIVE DEVELOPMENT CRITICAL PERIOD: SERBOCROATIAN

In this paper a series of research studies on various psychological aspects of bilingualism is reviewed. In the first group of studies the difference in acquisition of the first and second language, in the second the optimal period for the acquisition of second language and in the third the influence of early bilingualism on personality development is discussed.LG

Goncz, Lajos. (1976). Dvojezicna sredina kao faktor usvajanja i razvoja govora. (Bilingual environment as a factor of language acquisition and language development.). In *Jezik u drustvenoj sredini, Zbornik radova sa konferencije 'Jezik i drustvo'.* Novi Sad, Yugoslavia: SERBOCROATIAN-HUNGARIAN HUNGARIAN-SERBOCROATIAN BILINGUALISM LANGUAGE AND EDUCATION: SERBOCROATIAN

Bilingualism as a factor in language acquisition is discussed from the standpoint of developmental and educational psychology.LG

Goncz, Lajos. (1976). Stepen dvojezicnosti i ucestalost upotrebe razlicitih vrsta reci u maternjem i nematernjem jeziku. (The degree of bilingualism and the frequency of use of different types of words in the first and second language.). *Pedagoska stvarnost*, 6, 310-319. HUNGARIAN-SERBOCROATIAN SERBOCROATIAN-HUNGARIAN BILINGUALISM-LINGUISTIC THEORY BILINGUALISM-LANGUAGE CONTACT:

A list of 70 words was presented, in both Hungarian and Serbocroatian, to two groups of 20 balanced and 20 dominant Hungarian-Serbocroatian bilingual 18 year old high school students. The frequency of free word association with different types of words was different in the first language for the two groups. The dominant bilinguals gave more associations with adjectives, the balanced group with verbs. Missing answers were more frequent in the balanced group. The possible theoretical explications of these results are also discussed. LG.

Goncz, Lajos. (1977). Istrazivanja dvojezicnosti u Kanadi. (Investigations of bilingualism in Canada.). *Godisnjak Saveza drustava za primenjenu lingvistiku Jugoslavije;*, 2, 9-28. BILINGUALISM-LANGUAGE CONTACT BILINGUALISM-SEQUENTIAL BILINGUALISM-SIMULTANEOUS BILINGUALISM-LANGUAGE DIFFERENTIATION CODE-SWITCHING L2 EDUCATION IMMERSION BILINGUALISM-COGNITIVE DEVELOPMENT BILINGUALISM-NEUROLINGUISTICS BILINGUALISM-PROBLEMS/EFFECTS: SERBOCROATIAN

A review of Canadian investigations of bilingualism. The first part of the paper deals with studies of the bilingual's linguistic performance: problems of measuring the degree of bilingualism, the compound-coordinate distinction, the ability of bilinguals to keep their languages apart, and with switching mechanisms). Several studies are concerned with methods of second language teaching and with research findings bearing on the evaluation of immersion program pupils. The paper also describes studies dealing with bilingualism and cognitive functioning. It ends with a brief review of the investigations of social-psychological and neurological and neurolinguistic aspects of bilingualism and second language learning in Canada.LG

Goncz, Lajos. (1977). Kontinuirane asocijacije kao tehnika za merenje jezicke ravnoteze odnosno jezicke dominacije kod dvojezicnih osoba. (Continued associations as a means for the measurement of bilingual balance or linguistic dominance in bilingual persons.). *Psihologija*, 3-4, 107-115. BILINGUALISM-LANGUAGE PREFERENCE: SERBOCROATIAN

Two groups Of 20 dominant and 20 balanced bilingual (Hungarian-Serbocroat), pupils of secondary schools, were formed on the basis of their answers to a questionnaire about the ways they acquired their languages. Each group was given continuous associations on 4 Hungarian words and their equivalents in Serbocroat. Lambert (1955) showed that there is a great difference in the number of associations on identical words in the two languages. Statistic analysis applied in this case made it possible to determine the degree of the bilingual state of each pupil (i.e. difference in the knowledge and command of the two languages) by means of continuous associations. The last part of this paper examines the validity of such 'global' indicators of difference and development between the two above mentioned languages. LG.

Goncz, Lajos. (1979). O mogucnostima uticaja rane dvojezicnosti na kognitivni razoj. (On the possible influence of early bilingualism on cognitive growth.). *Godisnjak Saveza drustava za primenjenu lingvistiku Jugoslavije*, 3, 161-167. BILINGUALISM AND COGNITIVE DEVELOPMENT: SERBOCROATIAN

This paper specifies the ways in which early bilingualism might influence cognitive growth. These differences might affect cognitive development in a detrimental or in a stimulative way. The interference between the different languages and the reduced time the bilingual child spends with each language might have negative effects. However, the more diversified experience, the possibility of code-switching and making use of two different perspectives, and the faster process of objectification in the bilingual child might affect the cognitive development in a stimulative way.LG

Goncz, Lajos. (1979). Uticaj rane dvojezicnosti na kognitivni razoj. (The influence of early bilingualism on cognitive development.). *Psihologija*, 3-4, 81-92. BILINGUALISM-COGNITIVE DEVELOPMENT: SERBOCROATIAN

A group of 22 monolingual and two groups of 25 and 22 bilingual children were compared in several indicators of language development and general intelligence. The differences in vocabulary in favor of the monolingual group were explained.LG

Goncz, Lajos. (1982). A korai kétnyelvüség hatása a beszédfejlödésre. (The influence of early bilingualism on language development.). *Hungarológiai Közlemények*, 51, 141-174. BILINGUALISM: HUNGARIAN

Goncz, Lajos. (1983). A kétnyelvüség definiciója és fajai. (Definitions and types of bilingualism.). *Híd*, 10, 1180-1191. BILINGUALISM-SEQUENTIAL BILINGUALISM-SIMULTANEOUS: HUNGARIAN

This paper contains a review of different definitions and types of bilingualism.LG

Goncz, Lajos. (1984). Egy új kétnyelvüségi tipológia felállításának kisérlete. (An attempt at the establishmlent of a new typology of bilingualism.). *Hungarológiai Közlemények*, 1, 729-755. BILINGUALISM: HUNGARIAN

Goncz, Lajos. (1984). Psiholoska ispitivanja madjarsko-srpskohrvatske dvojezicnosi u Vojvodini-rezultati desetogodisnjih istrazivanja. (Psychological investigations of Hngarian-Serbocroatian bilingualism in Vojvodina: The results of 10 years of research.). In A. Necak-Luk, & I. Strukelj (Eds), *Dvojezicnost-individualne in druzbene razseznosti*. Ljubljana: Drustvo za uporabno jezikoslovlje Slovenije. HUNGARIAN-SERBOCROATIAN SERBOCROATIAN-HUNGARIAN BILINGUALISM-LINGUISTIC THEORY BILINGUALISM-COGNITIVE DEVELOPMENT BILINGUALISM-MOTIVATION BILINGUALISM-ATTITUDES: SERBOCROATIAN

This paper contains the results of a series of research studies of Hungarian-Serbocroation bilingualism in Vojvodina. The investigation can be divided into three groups: (a) The first group contains fundamental studies in the field of experimental psycholinguistics. They discuss the problem of interaction between the two languages of the bilingual individual and the types of bilingualism. (b) In the second group there are studies which investigate the relation between early bilingualism and cognitive growth, that is the developmental psychological aspects of bilingualism. (c) The third group contains studies which are concerned with the relation of the motivational variables and abilities in the acquisition of the second language. They discuss the problems of bilingualism from the standpoint of educational psychology and applied psycholinguistics.LG

Goncz, Lajos. (1985). *A kétnyelvüség pszichológiája. A magyar-szerbhorvát kétnyelvüség lélektani vizsgálata. (The psychology of bilingualism. Psychological investigation of Hungarian-Serbocroatian bilingualism.).* Novi Sad: Forum. HUNGARIAN-SERBOCROATIAN SERBOCROATIAN-HUNGARIAN BILINGUALISM-LINGUISTIC THEORY BILINGUALISM-NEUROLINGUISTICS BILINGUALISM-LANGUAGE PROCESSING BILINGUALISM-EDUCATION L2 EDUCATION L2/L1 ACQUISITION BILINGUALISM-SOCIAL FACTORS: HUNGARIAN

This book contains the results of 15 years of research on psychological aspects of Hungarian-Serbocroatian bilingualism in Vojvodina. The phenomenon of bilingualism was investigated from the standpoint of developmental psychology, social psychology, experimental psycholinguistics and educational psychology.LG

Goncz, Lajos. (1985). Rezultati istrazivanja psiholoskih aspekata dvojezicnosti u Vojvodini. (The results of investigations on psychological aspects of bilingualism in Vojvodina.). *Psihologija*, 1-2, 79-92. HUNGARIAN-SERBOCROATIAN SERBOCROATIAN-HUNGARIAN BILINGUALISM-COGNITIVE DEVELOPMENT BILINGUALISM-SEQUENTIAL BILINGUALISM-MOTIVATION BILINGUALISM-SIMULTANEOUS INTERLANGUAGE: SERBOCROATIAN

The paper reviews the results of 10 years of research about the psychological aspects of Hungarian-Serbocroatian bilinguals in Vojvodini (Yugoslavia). All the conducted research can be classified in three groups: The first group contains research in experimental psycholinguistics dealing with the problems of interactions between the linguistic systems in a bilingual person. The results contribute to a further precision in the definition of the concept of bilingualism and enable us to determine the sorts and types of bilingualism. The second group consists of those projects attempting to unveil the relationship between the early learning of two languages and other developing mental functions. These, namely, approach the problem of bilingualism from the aspect of developmental psychology and developmental psycholinguistics. The third group of research projects deal with the problem of bilingualism from the point of view of educational psychology and applied psycholinguistics and aim at determining the role of abilities and motivation in the learning of a new second language.LG

Goncz, Lajos. (1985). Ucenje jezika drustvene sredine i fenomen dvojezicnosti: pedagoski aspekti. (The acquisition of second language and the phenomenon of bilingualism: educational aspects.). *Zbornik Instituta za pedagogiju, Filozofski fakultet, Novi Sad*, 3, 11-27. BILINGUALISM-EDUCATION L2 EDUCATION LANGUAGE AND EDUCATION: SERBOCROATIAN

Goncz, Lajos. (1986). A két nyelv közötti kölcsönhatások színmegnevezési (Stroop) helyzetben magyar-szerbhorvát kétnyelvüeknél. (Interaction between two languages in a Stroop color naming situation in Hungarian-Serbocroatian bilinguals.). *Magyar Pszichológiai Szemle*, 2, 45-55. STROOP INTERFERENCE HUNGARIAN-SERBOCROATIAN SERBOCROATIAN-HUNGARIAN BILINGUALISM AND COGNITIVE DEVELOPMENT BILINGUALISM-LEXICAL DEVELOPMENT: HUNGARIAN

We tried to find out if a bilingual is able to exclude one of his languages while using the other. The phenomenon was studied in 23 Serbocroatian bilinguals by the bilingual version of Stroop's color naming test. The results of the experiment suggest that the seemingly inactive decoding system of the other language remains active, thus not supporting the 'one-switch' bilingual model offered by Penfield and Roberts. The results seem to verify the 'two-switch' model of Macnamara. According to this model there is a neurological mechanism which brings the decoding process of L1 and the coding process of L2 into function at the same time. The inability to exclude the inactive language in the experimental situation does not mean that bilinguals are unable to do so. There are factors (type of bilingualism, the nature of distractor, the degree of linguistic set, etc.) which can decrease the interaction between the language systems.LG

Goncz, Lajos. (1987). Prilog ispitivanju motivacije za ucenje jezika drustvene sredine i stranih jezika. (A contribution to the study of motivation for learning the language of the social community and foreign languages.). *Zbornik Instituta za pedagogiju, Filozofski fakultet, Novi Sad*, 5, 33-43. SERBOCROATIAN-HUNGARIAN HUNGARIAN-SERBOCROATIAN BILINGUALISM-MOTIVATION BILINGUALISM-ATTITUDES BILINGUALISM-EDUCATION L2 EDUCATION: SERBOCROATIAN

72 students whose mother tongue is Hungarian and who had studied Serbocroatian as the language of the social community in elementary and secondary school, were asked, on the basis of voice, to evaluate the personality traits of Hungarian-Serbocroatian bilingual persons when speaking the two languages. The attitudes established in this manner, do not show a more important connection with the indicators of achievement in learning the language of the social community. There is better achievement in the case of those subjects who had a high level of motivation and were instructed by a teacher they favored. In the same subjects, achievement in learning a foreign (world) language is improved if the learner has an integrated orientation toward language learning, high motivation, a more positive attitude toward learning a foreign language, if the subject is taught by a professor he likes and if his parents have a positive attitude toward learning the foreign language. It would seem, in the case of our subjects, that the complex of motivational variables called integrative motive in

foreign research studies, and which is in high correlation with success in the acquisition of a second language, is more influential on achievement in a forign (world) language than on achievement in the acquisition of the language of the social community. This could probably be explained by the different status of Serbocroatian as the language of the social community in Yugoslav conditions, than that of the second language in similar studies carried out in the USA and Canada. LG

Goncz, Lajos. (1988). Kako postati i istati dvokulturan i dvojezican uz pomoc skole u migrantskoj situaciji. (How to become and remain bicultural and bilingual through education in a migrant situation.). *Primijenjena psihologija*, 1-2, 113-130. BILINGUALISM-CULTURAL FACTORS BILINGUALISM-EDUCATION L2 EDUCATION: SERBOCROATIAN

Scientific research has shown that schooling can help develop bicultural and bilingual qualities in a migrant situation. Both migrant pupils and pupils of the receiving country can develop these characteristics, although this goal is achieved by different means as the starting positions of these two groups differ. Different types of education are reviewed in this report which, by correlating methods and linguistic aims of education, demonstrates how individual forms of the teaching process, given the language that is utilized (monolingual or bilingual) can influence some aspects of development (especially language learning) and school achievement. Education of children of migrant parents in the Federal Republic of Germany and Sweden is briefly reviewed.LG

Goncz, Lajos. (1988). A research study on the relation between early bilingualism and cognitive development. *Psychologische Beitrage*, 30, 1-2, 75-91. BILINGUALISM-COGNITIVE DEVELOPMENT HUNGARIAN-SERBOCROATIAN SERBOCROATIAN-HUNGARIAN BILINGUALISM-ATTITUDES:

This paper contains the results of a research study conducted in Vojvodina (Yugoslavia) on the relation between early Hungarian-Serbocroatian bilingualism and cognitive development. The hypotheses on the possible relation between early bilingualism and cognition were subjected to empirical verification on the basis of results computed from monolingual and bilingual groups of 6 and 10 year old children (69 and 126). It was shown that the investigated type of bilingualism (promoted mainly through the maintenance or language shelter school programs and in integrative social circumstances where the children's first language and culture is not replaced by a second one) is associated negatively at the age of 6, with the volume of passive vocabulary in the first language, also with the quality to derive relations and correlatives and with the earlier appearance of the ability to separate the verbal indicator from the object indicated. At the age of 10 the difference of passive vocabulary disappear and there is a positive association with the ability to derive relations and correlatives and a negative one with the knowledge of structures in the first language.LG

Goncz, Lajos. (1989). Psychological studies of bilingualism in Vojvodina. In M. Radovanovic (Ed.), *Yugoslav General Linguistics*. Philadelphia, PA: John Benjamins. BILINGUALISM-COGNITIVE DEVELOPMENT CODE-SWITCHING HUNGARIAN-SERBOCROATIAN SERBOCROATIAN-HUNGARIAN BILINGUALISM-EDUCATION:

This paper presents a short survey of the results obtained from a series of studies carried out in Vojvodina on various psychological aspects of bilingualism. The studies were made on groups of pupils and students ranging in age from pre-school to university level, who spoke either Hungarian only or both Hungarian and Serbocroatian. The objectives of this research were to establish the laws determining the phenomenon of bilingualism and to provide us with a suitable means of testing certain hypotheses of more general importance in psychology, psycholinguistics and didactics (e.g. the hypotheses concerning the relation between language and thought, in connection with the problems of code-switching).LG

Goncz, Lajos. (1990). Az iskola szerepe a többnyelvü es többkulturájú szemelyiség kialakításában: megoldások és lehetöségek. (The role of school in development of multilingual and multicultural individuals: solutions and possibilities.). *Oktatás és nevelés*, 2-3, 5-20. BILINGUALISM-EDUCATION: HUNGARIAN

The role of school in developing multilingual and multicultural individuals using scientific results on developmental aspects of bilingualism is discussed. A review of bilingual educational programs is also given.LG

Goncz, Lajos, Kodzopeljic, Jasmina, & Majstorovic, Nebojsa. (1989). Ucenje stranog jezika na predskolskom uzrastu i spospbnost jezicke analize. (The acquisition of a foreign language at preschool age and the ability for linguistic analysis.). *Psihologija*, 2, 5-15. BILINGUALISM-METALINGUISTIC DEVELOPMENT MUTUAL EXCLUSIVITY BILINGUALISM-PHONOLOGICAL DEVELOPMENT BILINGUALISM-COGNITIVE DEVELOPMENT BILINGUALISM-LEXICAL DEVELOPMENT BILINGUALISM-EDUCATION FRENCH-SERBOCROATIAN SERBOCROATIAN-FRENCH SERBOCROATIAN-ENGLISH ENGLISH-SERBOCROATIAN:

This research examined whether the situation of institutionalized foreign language acquisition at preschool age had similar effects to those observed in noninstitutionalized simulataneous bilingualism. The achievements in different aspects of linguistic analysis (readiness to change the labels attached to objects, syllabic and phonetic segmentation of words, the exclusion of the first sound as well as the remaining sounds of the word, the presence of nominal realism) were compared between three groups of children from Novi Sad whose first language was Serbocroatian: one group of 18 attended a preschool institution where French was spoken, another group of 39 learned English in addition to the regular education in Serbo-Croatian and the third group of 26 had no experience whatsoever with learning foreign languages. The results demonstrated that, there was a small but noticable experimental effect which appeared to have an impact on syllabic segmentation until about the age of 6.5.LG

Goncz, Lajos, & Varga, E. (1985). Interakcina medju jezickim sistemima dvojezicnih osaba. (Interaction between language systems of bilingualism.). *Revija za psihologiju*, 1-2, 13-24. STROOP INTERFERENCE HUNGARIAN-SERBOCROATIAN HUNGARIAN-GERMAN SERBOCROATIAN-GERMAN GERMAN-HUNGARIAN GERMAN-SERBOCROATIAN SERBOCROATIAN-HUNGARIAN BILINGUALISM-LINGUISTIC THEORY BILINGUALISM-NEUROLINGUISTICS BILINGUALISM-LANGUAGE PROCESSING: SERBOCROATIAN

The aim of this investigation was to determine whether, and to what extent, the decoding system of one language remains active when the bilingual is actually encoding in his other language. To examine this problem 34 subjects were tested using an adaptation of the Stroop Color-World Test in its bilingual version which simultaneously activates the bilingual's encoding process in one language and decoding in the other. The results of 34 subjects are presented. Twenty-four adults were tested for Hungarian-Serbocroatian, Hungarian-German and Serbocroatian-German bilingualism and ten 14-year-old school children for Hungarian-Serbocroatian bilingualism. The results indicate that a bilingual is unable to shut out one of his languages if the other is in function. This does not support the single switch model of bilingual functioning proposed by Penfield and Roberts, who suggest that if one language is on, the other must be off. The results are more in line with McNamara's two switch model of bilingual functioning, and support his hypothesis that a type of neurological mechanism activates both languages when the bilingual person is required to react in one language and is, at the same time, verbally distracted by stimuli from the other language. We find that the amount of interference depends on the kind of distractor and on the type of bilingualism.LG

Gonsalves, R. J. (1990). The representation of word meaning. In M. Piatelli-Palmarini (Ed.), *Proceedings of the Twelfth Annual Conference of the Cognitive Science Society*. Hillsdale, NJ: Lawrence Erlbaum Associates. SEMANTIC DEVELOPMENT LEXICAL DEVELOPMENT REPRESENTATIONS-LEXICAL REPRESENTATIONS-SEMANTIC:

Goodluck, Helen. (1989). When grammar wins over sense: children's judgments of extraposed relatives. *Journal of Psycholinguistic Research*, 18(4), 389-416. RELATIVIZATION SEMANTICS AND SYNTAX GRAMMATICALITY:

Goodluck, Helen. (1991). *Language acquisition : a linguistic introduction*. Oxford, UK: Basil Blackwell. ACQUISITION THEORIES ACQUISITION AND LINGUISTIC THEORY:

Goodluck, Helen, & Behne, D. (1991). Development in control and extraction. In J. Weissenborn, H. Goodluck, & T. Roeper (Eds), *Theoretical issues in language acquisition: Continuity and change in development*. Hillsdale, NJ: Lawrence Erlbaum Associates. ACQUISITION THEORIES CONTINUITY/DISCONTINUITY:

Goodnow, Jacqueline. (1992). Beyond modules. In M. R. Gunnar, & M. Maratsos (Eds), *Modularity and constraints in language and cognition*. Hillsdale, NJ: Lawrence Erlbaum Associates. MODULARITY LANGUAGE AND COGNITION LANGUAGE AND COGNITIVE DEVELOPMENT CONSTRAINTS:

Goodwin, H. M. (1990). *He-said-she-said: Talk as social organization among black children*. Bloomington, IN: Indiana University Press. SEX DIFFERENCES NONSTANDARD DIALECTS BLACK ENGLISH:

An ethnographic study which uses conversation analysis to show how children use their conversations to construct social worlds. Special attention is given to gender differences in social organization.

Gopnik, Alison, & Choi, Soonja. (1990). Do linguistic differences lead to cognitive differences? A cross-linguistic study of semantic and cognitive development. *First Language*, 10, 199-215. SAPIR-WHORF HYPOTHESIS LANGUAGE AND COGNITION CROSSLINGUISTIC STUDY FRENCH KOREAN CONSTRAINTS-COGNITIVE CONSTRAINTS-SEMANTIC SEMANTIC DEVELOPMENT:

Semantic and cognitive development were studied in eight Korean and French-speaking children, and these results were compared with results for 12 English-speakers. There were close and specific relations between semantic and cognitive developments. Non-English speakers used very different forms from English-speakers to encode disappearance, success and failure. Both categorization and naming developed later in the Korean-speakers than in English-speakers and French-speakers.

Gopnik, Alison, & Meltzoff, Andrew N. (1992). Categorization and naming-basic-level sorting in 18-month-olds and its relation to language. *Child Development*, 63, 1091-1103. CATEGORIZATION LABELING LANGUAGE AND COGNITIVE DEVELOPMENT:

Gopnik, Myrna. (1990). Feature blindness: A case study. *Language Acquisition*, 1, 139-164. DEVELOPMENTAL DISORDERS SEMANTICS AND SYNTAX DYSPHASIA CONGENITAL DISORDERS MORPHOSYNTACTIC DEVELOPMENT MORPHOLOGICAL DISORDERS INFLECTION:

Gopnik examines developmental dysphasia and proposes that its underlying cause is a linguistic feature deficit, and not a perceptual or cognitive deficit. She bases her argument on the fact that in developmental dysphasia the impairment appears to be restricted to morphosyntax, whereas other parts of the linguistic system are unaffected.

Gopnik, Myrna. (1993). *The biological basis of language*. New York, NY: Oxford Univesity Press. BIOLOGICAL FOUNDATIONS MODULARITY LANGUAGE AND PERCEPTION:

Gore, Madhuri. (1982). Some aspects of syntactic development in Marathi speaking children aged 2 1/2-3 years: a descriptive study. *Jaiish*, 13, 154. MARATHI SYNTACTIC DEVELOPMENT:

Gorrell, Paul, Crain, Stephen, & Fodor, Janet D. (1989). Contextual information and temporal terms. *Journal of Child Language*, 16(3), 623-632. TEMPORAL TERMS CONTEXT:

Goswami, Usha C. (1991). Learning about spelling sequences-the role of onsets and rimes in analogies in reading. *Child Development*, 62, 1110-1123. LITERACY SYLLABLES:

Goswami, Usha C., & Bryant, Peter E. (1991). *Phonological skills and learning to read*. Hillsdale, NJ: Lawrence Erlbaum Associates. LITERACY READING DISORDERS:

This book integrates recent exciting research on the precursors of reading and early reading strategies adopted by children in the classroom. The authors stress the importance of phonological skills and how phonological knowledge about rhymes and other units of sound help children form letter sequences as they learn how to read. Two contrasting theories are presented in this volume-one suggesting children's phonological awareness is a result of the experience of learning to read, and the other suggesting phonological awareness precedes, and is a causal determinant of, reading. Supporting the latter theory, the authors suggest that children make analogies and inferences about letter sequences in order to read and write new words. Contents include: Preface. Phonological awareness and reading. How children read words. Spelling and phonological awareness. How children read and write new words. Comparisons with backward readers and spellers. Correlations and longitudinal predictions. Teaching children about sounds. Do children read (and fail to learn to read) in different ways from each other? Theories about learning to read.

Gosy, Mária. (1979). A /r/ hang kialakulása a gyermeknyelvben (The evolution of the sound /r/ in child language.). *Magyar Fonetikai Füzetek*, 4, 172-182. LIQUIDS HUNGARIAN: HUNGARIAN

Gosy, Mária. (1981). A beszédhang kialakulása a gyermeknyelvben. (Development of speech sounds in child language). *Magyar Fonetikai Füzetek*, 7, 67-97. PHONEMIC DEVELOPMENT HUNGARIAN: HUNGARIAN

Gosy, Mária. (1984). A beszédmegertés kezdetei. (The beginnings of speech perception.). *Nyelvtudományi Közlemények*, 86, 23-35. SPEECH PERCEPTION HUNGARIAN: HUNGARIAN

Gosy, Mária. (1984). A hallás és a beszéd megertés kapcsolatáról (Interaction of hearing and speech understanding). *Magyar Nyelvör*, 108, 319-324. COMPREHENSION HUNGARIAN DEAF CHILDREN: HUNGARIAN

Gosy, Mária. (1984). Hangtani és szótani vizsgálatok hároméves gyermekek nyelvében (Phonetic and lexical examinations in the language of 3-year-old children). *Nyelvtudományi Ertekezések*, 119, 88. PHONETIC DEVELOPMENT LEXICAL DEVELOPMENT HUNGARIAN: HUNGARIAN

Gosy, Mária. (1985). Beszédhibás gyermek beszédmegertésének vizsgálata (The examination of speech comprehension in children with language impairments). *Gyógypedagógiai Szemle*, 2, 93-100. COMPREHENSION DISORDERS SPEECH ERRORS: HUNGARIAN

Gosy, Mária. (1988). A new test for speech audiometry of children. In J. Hirschberg, & Z. Labas (Eds), *Proceedings of the 4th International Congress of Pediatric Oto-Rhino-Laryngology Eger, Hungary*.. Budapest: AUDIOMETRY ASSESSMENT PROCEDURES HUNGARIAN G-O-H SYSTEM:

Gosy, Mária. (1988). Synthesized speech for auditory screening of children according to the G-O-H system. In J. Hirschberg, & Z. Labas (Eds), *Proceedings of the 4th International Congress of Pediatric Oto-Rhino-Laryngology Eger, Hungary*. Budapest: ASSESSMENT PROCEDURES G-O-H SYSTEM HUNGARIAN AUDIOMETRY:

Gosy, Mária. (1989). Beszédészlelési és beszédmegértési teljesítmény GMP-tesztcsomag. (Results of the GMP test battery for speech perception and comprehension.). In *GMP test-package for judgment of children's speech perception and comprehension ability*.. Budapest: LANGUAGE TESTING ASSESSMENT PROCEDURES GMP TEST HUNGARIAN: HUNGARIAN

Gosy, Mária. (1989). Beszélö számítógép az olvasás zavar megelözésében és javításában (Speaking computer for prevention and correction of children's reading difficulties). *Informatika*, 34-44. COMPUTER ASSISTED THERAPY READING DISORDERS HUNGARIAN: HUNGARIAN

Gosy, Mária. (1989). Identification of synthesized Hungarian vowels with 2 vs. 5 formants (by children and adults). In *Proceedings of the Eurospeech Conference II*. Paris: ACOUSTIC PHONETICS HUNGARIAN VOWELS:

Gosy, Mária. (1989). Speech perception performance: Evidence for or against a hearing aid. In *Hungarian Papers in Phonetics*. Budapest. SPEECH PERCEPTION AUDIOLOGY HUNGARIAN:

Gosy, Mária. (1989). Vowel harmony in children's speech. In W. Veenker (Ed.), *Mitteilungen der Societas Uralo-Altaica, vol. 8.* Hamburg: VOWEL HARMONY HUNGARIAN VOWELS:

Gosy, Mária. (1990). Beszédészlelés és olvasási készség. (Speech perception and reading ability). *A Tanító*, 18(12), 13-18. LITERACY HUNGARIAN SPEECH PERCEPTION: HUNGARIAN

Gosy, Mária. (1990). Beszédészlelés és olvasási készség. (Speech perception and reading ability.). *A Tanító*, XVIII (12), 13-18. LITERACY SPEECH PERCEPTION READING DISORDERS: HUNGARIAN

Gosy, Mária. (1990). A beszédészlelés idözítési zavarainak következményei az olvasás elsajátítására. (Consequences of perceptual temporal disorders on reading acquisition). *Hungarian Papers in Phonetics*, 23, TEMPORAL RELATIONS READING DISORDERS HUNGARIAN: HUNGARIAN

Gosy, Mária. (1990). Modell az olvasástanításhoz. (Model for teaching reading). *Fejlesztö Pedagógia*, 2, 28-32. LITERACY HUNGARIAN: HUNGARIAN

Gosy, Mária. (1990). On the predictability of reading performance. *Hungarian Papers in Phonetics*, 22, 84-93. LITERACY HUNGARIAN:

Gosy, Mária, Kassai, Ilona, & Szende, Tamás. (1982). Criteria of speech research in the explanation of language acquisition processes. *Budapesti Akusztikai Kollokvium.*, 8, 211-216. METHODOLOGY HUNGARIAN: HUNGARIAN

Gosy, Mária, & Laczko, Mária. (1987). A beszédmegertési teljesitmény fejlödése óvodáskortól felnöttkorig. (The development of speech understanding from the age of 3 up to adulthood). *Magyar Nyelvör*, 111, 444-452. COMPREHENSION HUNGARIAN COMPLEX SENTENCES LEXICAL DEVELOPMENT: HUNGARIAN

The authors examine the development of word and sentence identification abilities with the participation of more that 300 children (ages 3, 5, 7, 10, and 14 years) and of adults. The results show the gradual changes on the one hand and the breaks in the development on the other. The authors' hypothesis has been confirmed: the decisions on the lower levels of the speech understanding mechanism are more crucial for little children than the higher levels.MG

Gosy, Mária, Olaszy, G., Hirschberg, Jenö, & Farkas, Zsolt. (1987). Phonetically based new method for audiometry: the G-O-H measuring system using synthetic speech. *Hungarian Papers in Phonetics*, 17, 84-102. G-O-H SYSTEM AUDIOMETRY HUNGARIAN ASSESSMENT PROCEDURES:

Gough, Philip B., Ehri, Linnea C., & Treiman, Rebecca. (1992). *Reading acquisition*. Hillsdale, NJ: Lawrence Erlbaum Associates. LITERACY READING DISORDERS:

Gow, M. L., & Ingham, R. J. (1992). Modifying electroglottograph-identified intervals of phonation - the effect on stuttering. *Journal of Speech and Hearing Research*, 35, 495-511. STUTTERING:

Grainger, J., & O'Regan, J. K. (1993). A psychophysical investigation of language priming effects in two English-French bilinguals. In A. M. B. de Groot, & C. Barry (Eds), *The multilingual community*. Hillsdale, NJ: Lawrence Erlbaum Associates. FRENCH-ENGLISH ENGLISH-FRENCH BILINGUALISM-LANGUAGE PREFERENCE:

Grant, Eileen, & Standing, Lionel. (1989). Effects of a rapid decoding training on reading speed and comprehension. *Perceptual and Motor Skills*, 69, 515-521. LITERACY:

Two groups of poor readers, age 12 to 15 years were trained in rapid decoding of words presented either individually or in context. Twenty good and 20 poor readers provided additional untrained control groups. It was predicted that training would produce benefits in comprehension, especially for the subjects trained with words in context. Analysis showed that both trained groups significantly increased their reading rates. Improved comprehension scores were noted among all four groups, due to a general practice effect. However, context-trained subjects did not differ from the subjects trained with individual words, on either speed or comprehension. - From Child Development Abstracts.

Grant, June. (1987). *The hearing impaired: Birth to six.* San Diego, CA: Singular Group. DEAF CHILDREN INTERVENTION PROGRAMS FOR PARENTS BILINGUALISM-LANGUAGE DISORDERS PRELINGUISTICS BABBLING BIMODALITY BILINGUALISM:

An account of language development in deaf children including chapters on parental input, bilingualism, creativity, and early education.

Grant, Julia, Broerse, Jack, & Elias, Gordon. (1989). An application of Palinscar and Brown's comprehension instruction paradigm to listening. *Contemporary Educational Psychology*, 14, 164-172. LANGUAGE AND EDUCATION METHODOLOGY-ANALYSIS:

Gravel, J. S., & Wallace, I. F. (1992). Listening and language at 4 years of age-effects of early otitis media. *Journal of Speech and Hearing Research*, 35, 588-595. OTITIS MEDIA:

Greene, Anthony C., Sapp, Gary L., & Chissom, Brad. (1990). Validation of the Stanford-Binet Intelligence Scale: Fourth edition with exceptional Black male students. *Psychology in the Schools*, 27, 35-41. ASSESSMENT PROCEDURES STANFORD-BINET SCALE:

Standard Age Scores on the Stanford-Binet Intelligence Scale: Fourth Edition (SBIV) and WISC-R IQs of 51 urban black males receiving special education services were compared. Correlations between all combinations of scales ranged from.61 to.89, median r =.72. SBIV Composite mean scores did not differ significantly from the mean WISC-R Full Scale, Verbal, and Performance IQs. Regression analysis of the three subgroups (BD, LD, and EMR) indicated that the SBIV possesses differential validity for each group. These data suggest that SBIV possesses utility for assessing the intelligence of black students classified as BD and EMR. However, the use of the scale with LD students is unsupported. - From Child Development Abstracts.

Greenfield, Patricia M., Nelson, K., & Saltzman, E. (1977). The Development of rulebound strategies for manipulating seriated cups: A parallel between action and grammar. In M. S. Barbieri (Ed.), *Gli inizi del linguaggio: aspetti cognitivi e comunicativi (The emergence of language: cognitive and communicative aspects).*. La Nuova, Italy: Firenze. ISOMORPHISMS LANGUAGE AND ACTION LANGUAGE AND COGNITIVE DEVELOPMENT SYNTACTIC DEVELOPMENT:

Greenfield, Patricia M., & Savage-Rumbaugh, E. Sue. (1991). Imitation. Grammatical development and the invention of protogrammar by an ape. In N. A. Krasnegor, et al. (Eds), *Biological and behavioral determinants of language development.* Hillsdale, NJ: Lawrence Erlbaum Associates. IMITATION SYNTACTIC DEVELOPMENT LANGUAGE AND OTHER PRIMATES:

Grégoire, M. N., Rondal, Jean A., & Perée, F. (1984). Aspects morphosyntaxiques et lexicaux du langage spontané d'enfants de 2 à 5 ans. (Morphosyntactic and lexical aspects of the spontaneous speech of 2-5-year-olds). *Enfance*, 1, 51-65. LEXICAL DEVELOPMENT MORPHOSYNTACTIC DEVELOPMENT: FRENCH

Greiner, J. R., & Fitzgerald, H. E. (1992). Bimanual handwriting reveals delayed interhemispheric integration in childhood stuttering. *Developmental Neuropsychology*, 8, 395-411. STUTTERING LANGUAGE AND HANDEDNESS LATERALIZATION:

Grimm, Hannelore, & Weinert, Sabine. (1989). Mütterliche Sprache und Sprachverarbeitung dysphasischer Kinder. (Maternal speech and language processing in dysphasic children.). *Heilpädagogische Forschung*, 15 (1), SYNTACTIC DISORDERS PARENTAL INPUT PARENTAL SPEECH-ATYPICAL CHILDREN LANGUAGE PROCESSING: GERMAN

Two groups of children with comparable levels of language development were examined in a longitudinal study: eight dysphasic children, ages 3:9 to 4:8 years and eight children, ages 2:6 and 3:0 years, who showed normal language development. Three main questions were investigated: (1) In which respects dysphasic children's syntactic development different from the development observed in the normal controls? (2) Can the language deficits of the dysphasic children be traced back to specific structural and interactional aspects of the language input? (3) Do the two groups of children differ in their language-processing strategies? The findings suggest that the dysphasic children's syntactic development is not only delayed but also deviant. No causal relationship to the input language could be established. Instead, the data suggest that the dysphasic children's deviant language structures are the result of the insufficient language processing strategies. A two stage theory of language development is proposed.HG/SW

Grimm, Hannelore, & Weinert, Sabine. (1990). Is the syntax development of dysphasic children deviant and why? New findings to an old question. *Journal of Speech and Hearing Research*, 33,
SYNTACTIC DEVELOPMENT SYNTACTIC STRUCTURES SYNTACTIC DISORDERS:

The present study addresses three main issues: first, it considers whether the syntax development is adequately described as being purely quantitative retardation or whether there are qualitative differences as well. Second, the suggestion put forward by Grimm (1987) that the syntactic deficits of dysphasic children result from deficient language processing strategies is further explored. Third, it asks whether the language deficits are related to specific structural and interactional aspects of the language input. We examined two groups of children with comparable levels of language development: 8 dysphasic children, ages 3:9 to 4:8 years, and 8 control children, ages 2:1 to 2:11 years, who showed normal language development. The empirical evidence suggested that the dysphasic children's syntax development was not only delayed but also deviant, and that the children's deviant syntax structures were the result of insufficient language processing and could not be traced back to structural characteristics of the sentences used by their mothers.HG/SW

Grimm, Hannelore, & Weinert, Sabine. (1990). Syntaktische Sprachkompetenz: ein einheitliches Konstrukt? (Syntactic development: a uniform contruct?). *Sprache und Kognition*, 9 (2),
SYNTACTIC DEVELOPMENT SYNTACTIC STRUCTURES: GERMAN

In order to assess syntactic competence in children it is necessary to investigate how they are able to use the same syntactic structures in different tasks. Participants in the study were 32 preschool children between the ages of five and six as well as 32 students. In order to determine the interrelation among the actual on-line usage, the reproductive, and the productive use of syntactic structures, an imitation test, a word recognition test, and a transformation task were applied. Individual differences within and between tasks are pointed out. It is suggested that the children are not able to use their syntactic knowledge in a general and consistent way.HG/SW

Grodzinsky, Josef. (1990). *Theoretical perspectives on language deficits*. Cambridge, MA: MIT/Batsford. APHASIAS ACQUIRED APHASIA:

The author reviews the history of research on acquired aphasias and demonstrates how the linguistic analysis of aphasias is beneficial to the fields of neuropsychology, and psycholinguistics, as well as to linguistics itself.

Gropen, Jess, Pinker, Steven, Hollander, Michelle, & Goldbery, Richard. (1991). Syntax and semantics in the acquisition of locative verbs. *Journal of Child Language*, 18, 115-151. SEMANTICS AND SYNTAX VERBS-LOCATIVE CUES-SEMANTIC CUES-SYNTACTIC:

Two experiments were performed on the ability of children and adults to understand and produce locative verbs. The results confirm that children tend to make syntactic errors with sentences containing fill and empty, encoding the content argument as direct object. As predicted, children also misinterpreted the meanings of fill and empty as requiring not only that the container be brought into a full or empty state, but also that the content move in some specific manner (by pouring, or by dumping).

Grundy, Kim. (1989). *Linguistics in clinical practice.* San Diego, CA: Singular Group. CLINICAL LINGUISTICS DEVELOPMENTAL DISORDERS APHASIAS PROSODY DISFLUENCIES PHONOLOGICAL DISORDERS ASSESSMENT PROCEDURES:

Grunwell, Pamela. (1992). Assessment of child phonology in the clinical context. In C. A. Ferguson, L. Menn, & C. Stoel-Gammon (Eds), *Phonological development: Models, research, implications.* Monkton, MD: York Press. ASSESSMENT PROCEDURES PHONOLOGICAL DISORDERS ARTICULATION:

Gunnar, Megan R., & Maratsos, Michael P. (Eds) (1992). *Modularity and constraints in language and cognition.* Hillsdale, NJ: Lawrence Erlbaum Associates. MODULARITY LANGUAGE AND COGNITIVE DEVELOPMENT CONSTRAINTS:

> Papers presented at the 25th Minnesota Symposium on Child Psychology, held Oct. 25-27, 1990, at the University of Minnesota, which examine the roles of modularity and domain-specificity in higher cognitive functions.

Gunnar, Megan R., & Nelson, Charles A. (1991). *Developmental behavioral neuroscience.* Hillsdale, NJ: Lawrence Erlbaum Associates. NEUROLINGUISTICS LANGUAGE AND MOTOR DEVELOPMENT LANGUAGE AND AFFECT LANGUAGE AND COGNITIVE DEVELOPMENT:

> This volume provides an introduction to current research on the relation between brain development and the development of cognitive, linguistic, motor, and emotional behavior. At least two audiences will benefit from this book: psychologists interested in brain development and neuroscientists interested in behavioral development. Although each chapter is content-oriented, the volume as a whole provides a well integrated summary of the latest findings from developmental behavioral neuroscience.

Gupta, Anthea Fraser. (1985). Know what ho? Questions from a three year old Singaporean. In P. Fletcher, & M. Garman (Eds), *Child Language Seminar Papers 1985.* Reading, UK: Reading University. QUESTIONS PIDGINS/CREOLES:

The structure of interrogatives in a child acquiring Singapore Colloquial English as a dominant native language is outlined, together with a description of the child's acquisition of English.AFG

Gupta, Anthea Fraser. (1989). Singapore Colloquial English and Standard English. *Singapore Journal of Education*, 10 (2), 33-37. NONSTANDARD DIALECTS BIDIALECTISM LANGUAGE AND EDUCATION PIDGINS/CREOLES:

Based in part on a longitudinal study of the acquisition of Singapore Colloquial English as a native language, this paper outlines the differences between Standard English and the Singapore Colloquial English and suggests the appropriate places for each in the educational system.AFG

Gupta, Anthea Fraser. (1991). Acquisition of diglossia in Singapore English. In A. Kwan-Terry (Ed.), *Child Language and Development in Singapore and Malaysia;*. Singapore: Singapore University Press. BIDIALECTISM PIDGINS/CREOLES NONSTANDARD DIALECTS:

Singapore English is best seen as diglossic. The H-variety is Standard English and the L-variety is Singapore Colloquial English. Criterial features of each variety are explained, and the development of diglossia in four children from two Singapore Colloquial English-speaking families is outlined.AFG

Gupta, Anthea Fraser. (1991). Contact features of Singapore Colloquial English. In H. Kwok, & K. Bolton (Eds), *Sociolinguistics Today: International Perspectives*. London: Routledge. NONSTANDARD DIALECTS PIDGINS/CREOLES INTERLANGUAGE:

Singapore Colloquial English is a contact variety which can be analyzed using the terms of creolistics. An examination of the nominalizer 'one' and of the structure of interrogatives shows the various sources for structures in SCE. In the case of 'one' the substrate and the superstrate are both of importance: a marked structure emerges out of the formal overlap of pronoun and nominalizer. In the case of polar interrogatives, the superstrate contributes the formal features, while the substrate reinforces a pattern of distribution. There is a little or no formal influence from the substrate.AFG

Gupta, Anthea Fraser, & Yin, Ameline Lee Su. (1990). Gender representation in English language textbooks used in Singapore Primary Schools. *Language in Education*. LANGUAGE AND GENDER ROLES LANGUAGE AND EDUCATION SEX DIFFERENCES:

Two basal reader series used in the Singapore primary schools were analyzed for discrepancies in the treatment of male and female characters. Imbalances were found in the female:male ratio, in the amount of speech given to characters, and in role-representation. In both series, the importance of male characters becomes greater as the level of reader rises. The implications of this discrepancy are of some concern for Singapore's education system, where textbooks have long been seen as a major means of socialization.AFG

Gupta, P., & MacWhinney, Brian. (1992). Integrating category acquisition with inflectional marking: A model of the German nominal system. In *Proceedings of the Fourteenth Annual Conference of the Cognitive Science Society*. Hillsdale, NJ: Lawrence Erlbaum Associates. GERMAN INFLECTION NOUNS MORPHOSYNTACTIC DEVELOPMENT:

Gupta, P. Das, & Bryant, Peter E. (1989). Young children's causal inferences. *Child Development*, 60, 1138-1146. IMPLICATURE CAUSALITY:

The task was to work out what had caused the change to an object that started out as odd in 1 way and ended as odd in 2 ways. Three-year-olds often selected the instrument that could have caused the initial state and not the one that would produce the change. Four-year-olds hardly ever made this mistake. Three- year-olds made the correct choice when the change was from a canonical to a noncanonical state (cup-wet cup) but not with the reverse. - From Child Development Abstracts.

Guralnick, Michael J., & Paul-Brown, Diane. (1989). Peer-related communicative competence of preschool children: developmental and adoptive characteristics. *Journal of Speech and Hearing Research*, 32(4), 930-943. COMMUNICATIVE COMPETENCE:

Gustafson, G. E., & Green, J. A. (1991). Developmental coordination of cry sounds with visual regard and gestures. *Infant Behavior and Development*, 14, 51-57. CRYING GESTURE INTERSUBJECTIVITY:

Gutierrez-Clellen, V. F., & Iglesias, A. (1992). Causal coherence in the oral narratives of Spanish-speaking children. *Journal of Speech and Hearing Research*, 35, 363-372. DISCOURSE COHERENCE SPANISH NARRATIVES CAUSALITY:

Gutmann, Arlyne J., & Rondal, Jean A. (1979). Verbal operants in mother's speech to non-retarded and Down's syndrome children matched for linguistic level. *American Journal of Mental Deficiency*, 83, 446-452. DOWN SYNDROME PARENTAL SPEECH-STYLE:

Gyurke, James, Siegal, Linda S., Burns, William J., Spiker, Donna, & Lipsitt, Lewis P. (1991). The Bayley Scales of Infant Development: Issues of prediction and outcome revisited. In C. Rovee-Collier, & L. P. Lipsitt (Eds), *Advances in infancy research*. Norwood, NJ: Ablex. BAYLEY SCALES DEVELOPMENTAL SCALES:

H

Habermann, Gustáv M. (1980). *A müvelödési hátrány ényhítése szemelyiségfejlesztö programokkal: a pedagógiai eljárások hatekónysága a váltózónkénti adatok tükrében. (Alleviating cultural handicaps by programs of personality development: effectiveness of procedures as confiremd by univariate anlayses.).* Budapest: Hungarian Academy of Sciences, Research Group of Educational Sciences. LANGUAGE AND EDUCATION L2 EDUCATION: HUNGARIAN

Habermann, Gustáv M. (1980). A neveléspszichológia és a nyelvtudomány közeledésének új szakasza. (A new phase in the 'rapprochement' of educational psychology and linguistic science.). *Pedagógiai Szemle,* 30 (10), 885-897. HUNGARIAN LANGUAGE AND EDUCATION L2 EDUCATION: HUNGARIAN

Habermann, Gustáv M. (1981). A szemantikai és pragmatikai elöfeltévések kérdése a human információfeldolgozásban. (The problem of semantic and pragmatic suppositions in human information processing.). In I. Barkoczi (Ed.), *Magyar Pszichológiai Társaság V. Országos Tudományos Konferenciája.* Budapest: MPT. HUNGARIAN IMPLICATURE: HUNGARIAN

Habermann, Gustáv M. (1985). Megszabják-e szociális tényezök az elöfeltévéses és implikativ jelentésviszonyok megértéset? (Do social factors determine comprehension of presuppositional and implicative relations of meaning?). In C. Pléh, & J. Nagy (Eds), *Magyar Pszichológiai Társaság.* Budapest: MPT. IMPLICATURE LANGUAGE AND SOCIAL CLASS EDUCABILITY HUNGARIAN: HUNGARIAN

Habermann, Gustáv M. (1986). Az interpropozicionális viszonyok megértésének környezetfüggése a gimnáziumi és szakközépiskolai tanulóknál. (Environmental dependence of the comprehensoin of inter-propositional relations in grammar school and SVSS students.). *Neveléselmelet és Iskolakutatás*, 5 (4), 83-150. HUNGARIAN EDUCABILITY LANGUAGE AND EDUCATION: HUNGARIAN

Habermann, Gustáv M. (1987). Magasabb szintü strukturák a komplementum-felvevö predikátumokat tartalmazó mondatok megértési képességei körében. (Higher structures in the ability patterning of the comprehension of sentences involving complement governing predicates.). In I. Barkoczi (Ed.), *Magyar Pszichológiai Társaság VIII*. Budapest: Országos Pedagógiai Intézet. COMPLEMENTS HUNGARIAN COMPREHENSION COMPLEX SENTENCES: HUNGARIAN

Habermann, Gustáv M. (1988). Diachronic analysis of sentence comprehension abilities in a four-cycle multivariate study of efficiency. In M. Kalmar, & S. Jackson (Eds), *Third European Conference on Developmental Psychology*. Budapest: ISSBD/MPT. COMPLEX SENTENCES COMPREHENSION HUNGARIAN:

Habermann, Gustáv M. (1988). *The processing of inter-propositional relations in Hungarian sentences with complement governing predicates*. Budapest: National Institute of Education. COMPLEMENTS HUNGARIAN COMPREHENSION COMPLEX SENTENCES:

Habermann, Gustáv M. (1990). A propozicionális inferenciák problemája a mondatmegértésben. (The problem of propositional inferences in sentence comprehension.). *Pszichológia*, 10, IMPLICATURE HUNGARIAN COMPREHENSION: HUNGARIAN

Habermann, Gustáv M., & Klein, Stephanie. (1981). *Müvelödési hátrány releváns tanulói szemelyiség összetevök faktorstrukturája 5/6 osztályos általános iskolások körében. (Factor structure of personality constituents relevant to cultural handicaps in 5th and 6th grade elementary school pupils.)*. Budapest: Magyar Tudományos Pedagógiai Kutató Csoport. HUNGARIAN LANGUAGE AND EDUCATION EDUCABILITY: HUNGARIAN

Hadley, P. A., & Rice, Mabel L. (1991). Conversational responsiveness of speech-impaired and language-impaired preschoolers. *Journal of Speech and Hearing Research*, 34, 1308-1317. CONVERSATIONAL SKILLS CONVERSATIONAL DISORDERS:

Hagtvet, Bente, & Vedeler, Liv. (1983). Reynell-Zinkin testen: en utviklingsskala for synshemmede ssmabarn. (Reynell-Zinkin Scales-a developmental scale for blind preschool children). *Nordisk Tidsskrift for Specialpedagogikk*, 1, 40-48. BLIND CHILDREN ASSESSMENT PROCEDURES NORWEGIAN REYNELL-ZINKIN SCALES: NORWEGIAN

The Reynell-Zinkin Scales have been translated to Norwegian and tried out on 12 children aged 2 years 8 months to 6 years 7 months. The scales seem to be useful in clinical work. Weaknesses in the scales are discussed.

Haight, W., & Miller, P. J. (1992). The development of everyday pretend play-a longitudinal study of mother's participation. *Merrill-Palmer Quarterly* , 38, 331-349. LANGUAGE AND PLAY PARENTAL INPUT:

Haith, Marshall M. (1990). Progress in the understanding of sensory and perceptual processes in early infancy. *Merrill-Palmer Quarterly*, 36, 1-26. INFANT PERCEPTION:

This review focuses on infant sensation and perception. It is shown that progress has been dramatic in this area. Several activities seem especially promising: The exploration of the relations between brain development and perceptual development, the use of more dynamic and realistic perceptual settings, the study of the relations between perception and action, and new attempts to unify concepts and theory between the fields of infant perception and of older child and adult perception. - From Child Development Abstracts.

Hall, D. G. (1991). Acquiring proper nouns for familiar and unfamiliar animate objects-2-year-olds' word-learning biases. *Child Development*, 62, 1142-1154. NOUNS-PROPER VOCABULARY DEVELOPMENT LEXICAL DEVELOPMENT:

Hall, James W. (1991). *Handbook of auditory evoked responses*. San Diego, CA: Singular Publishing Group. NEONATES ATYPICAL DEVELOPMENT LANGUAGE DISORDERS AUDIOMETRY:

Overview of auditory evoked responses: past, present, and future. Anatomy and physiology. Effect of non-pathologic subject characteristics. Effect of stimulus factors. Effect of acquisition factors. Waveform analysis. Calibration, standards, and normative data. Test: protocols and procedures. Measurement problems and solutions. Basic audiometry. Peripheral auditory assessment. Neurodiagnosis: central nervous system. Newborn auditory screening. Intraoperative monitoring. Intensive care unit monitoring. Non-auditory evoked responses. Case reports: adults, children.

Halliday, Michael A. K., Gibbons, John, & Nicholas, Howard. (Eds) (1990). *Learning, keeping and using language*. Amsterdam, The Netherlands: John Benjamins. BILINGUALISM L2 ACQUISITION SOCIOLINGUISTIC FACTORS PARENTAL INPUT L2 EDUCATION:

Two volumes of selected papers from the proceedings of the Eighth World Congress of Applied Linguistics, Sydney, 1987. Volume 1 is concerned with language learning in monolingual and bilingual settings, and volume 2 is concerend with the use and maintenance of language in these settings.

Halperin, Jeffrey M., Healey, Jane M., Zeitchik, Ellen, Ludman, Wendy L., & Weinstein, Lissa. (1989). Development aspects of linguistic and mnestic abilities in normal children. *Journal of Clinical and Experimental Neuropsychology* , 11, 518-528. ASSESSMENT PROCEDURES LANGUAGE AND COGNITIVE DEVELOPMENT PEABODY PICTURE VOCABULARY TEST BOSTON NAMING TEST WECHSLER SCALES:

Peabody PVT-Revised, Boston Naming, (BNT), Paired Associate Learning of the Wechsler Memory Scale (PAL), and verbal fluency tests were administered to 241 normal children aged 6-12 years. Three factors emerged: factor 1 contained loadings from two semantic fluency measures (animals and food), factor 2 contained the PPVT-R and the BNT, and factor 3 contained two PAL measures.

Halpern, Diane F. (1991). *Sex differences in cognitive abilities.* Hillsdale, NJ: Lawrence Erlbaum Associates. SEX DIFFERENCES COGNITIVE DEVELOPMENT:

A comprehensive look at the how, why, and when, sex differences occur, and the extent of sex differences in cognitive development.

Hamayan, Else V., & Damico, Jack S. (1991). *Limiting bias in the assessment of bilingual students.* San Diego, CA: Singular Group. BILINGUALISM-ASSESSMENT PROCEDURES L2 ASSESSMENT PROCEDURES METHODOLOGY-RESPONSE BIAS ASSESSMENT PROCEDURES:

Contents deal with the reduction of bias in the assessment of Limited English Proficiency Students.

Hammen, Vicki L., Yorkston, Kathryn M., & Dowden, Patricia. (1991). Index of contextual intelligibility: Impact of semantic context in dysathria. In C. A. Moore, K. M. Yorkston, & D. R. Beukleman (Eds), *Dysathria and apraxia of speech.* Baltimore, MD: Paul H. Brookes Publishing Co. DYSARTHRIA CONTEXT INTELLIGIBILITY:

Hammond, Jennifer. (1990). Oral and written language in the educational context. In M. A. K. Halliday, J. Gibbons, & H. Nicholas (Eds), *Learning, keeping and using language* . Amsterdam, The Netherlands: John Benjamins. LANGUAGE AND EDUCATION WRITTEN LANGUAGE:

Selected paper from the proceedings of the Eighth World Congress of Applied Linguistics, Sydney, 1987.

Hannley, Maureen. (1986). *Basic principles of auditory assessment.* San Diego, CA: Singular Publishing CGroup. AUDIOLOGY AUDIOMETRY:

Calibration of test equipment. Preliminary principles. Principles and measurements of acoustic impedance. Clinical applications of acoustic immittance. Pure tone audiometry. Principles of masking. The audiogram. Sources of variance in pure tone audiometry. Speech audiometry. Interpretation. Putting it all together.

Hanson, Marci J. (1987). *Teaching the infant with Down Syndrome: a guide for parents and professionals*. San Diego, CA: Singular Publishing Group. LANGUAGE AND EDUCATION DOWN SYNDROME INTERVENTION PROGRAMS FOR PARENTS:

Experiences of parents of infants with Down Syndrome. Medical perspectives on Down Syndrome. Progress of infants with Down Syndrome taught by their parents. Interacting and teaching. Breaking behavior into small steps. Observing and recording the child's progress. Developmental milestones. Teaching activities: gross motor, cognitive, and fine motor, communication and social self help. After infancy. References. Glossary. Appendix I: types of Down Syndrome. Appendix II: medical concerns associated with Down Syndrome. Appendix III: child development resources. Appendix IV: parent and professional resources. Appendix V: child profiles. Baby's record.

Hardyck, C. (1976). A model of individual differences in hemispheric functioning. In H. A. Whitaker, & H. Whitaker (Eds), *Studies in neurolinguistics*, vol. 4. New York, NY: Academic Press. LATERALIZATION INDIVIDUAL VARIATION:

Harkness, S. (1990). A cultural model for the acquisition of language: Implications for the innateness debate. *Developmental Psychobiology*, 23(7), NATIVISM:

Harley, Birgit, et al. (1990). *The Development of second language proficiency*. New York, NY: Cambridge University Press. BILINGUALISM L2 ACQUISITION L2 EDUCATION L2 READING PROFICIENCY:

Papers prepared for a symposium held at the Ontario Institute for Studies in Education, November 1987.

Harris, John. (1990). *Early language development: implications for clinical and educational practice*. London, UK: Routledge. LANGUAGE AND EDUCATION INTERVENTION PROGRAMS:

Harris, Margaret. (1993). *Language experience and early language development: From input to uptake*. Hillsdale, NJ: Lawrence Erlbaum Associates. ENVIRONMENTAL INFLUENCES AT-RISK CHILDREN INPUT FACTORS SOCIAL INTERACTION ADULT-CHILD INTERACTION PARENTAL SPEECH PARENTAL INPUT:

Harris's point of view is that the linguistic and social environment in which the child acquires language must be an important factor in language development, otherwise there would be no point in undertaking intervention programs for children with language problems.

Harris, Margaret, & Barrett, Martyn D. (1989). Children's first words and their relation to maternal speech. In *Proceedings of the Child Language Seminar, 1989.*. Hatfield, UK: Hatfield Polytechnic. FIRST WORDS LEXICAL DEVELOPMENT INPUT FACTORS PARENTAL INPUT REPRESENTATIONS-LEXICAL:

Reports some preliminary findings from a longitudinal observational study of four mother-child dyads, in which it was found that the children's early words exhibited the full range of developmental changes predicted by Barrett's 1986 model of early lexical development. The mothers' uses of these same words bore no clear relationship to these developmental changes, suggesting that these changes were endogenously rather than environmentally driven. MDB.

Harris, Margaret, Clibbens, John, Chasin, Joan, & Tibbits, Ruth. (1989). The social context of early sign language development. *First Language*, 9, 81-97. SIGNING ADULT-CHILD INTERACTION PARENTAL INPUT:

An analysis of the relationship between mother's signing, the child's pattern of attention, and the nonverbal context of the signing revealed that a high proportion of signs were seen by the children and that, by 20 months of age, the majority of signs also had a nonverbal context which was salient for the child. There were general similarities in the pattern of strategies employed by the mothers to relate their signs to the nonverbal context but there were also interesting differences. - From Child Development Abstracts.

Harris, Paul L., Macrae, A. J., & Bassett, E. M. (1978). Disambiguation by young children. In R. N. Campbell & P. T. Smith. (Eds). *Recent advances in the psychology of language.* New York, NY: Plenumn. AMBIGUITY:

Harris, Sandra L., Handleman, Jan S., & Burton, Jean L. (1990). The Stanford Binet profiles of young children with autism. *Special Services in the Schools*, 6, 135-143. AUTISM:

Autistic children were assessed with the Stanford Binet Intelligence Scale. Inspection of the pattern of their responses yielded a distinctive profile with the subscale of Absurdities being consistently the lowest and Pattern Analysis the highest subtest.

Harris, Sandra L., Handleman, Jan S., Gordon, R., & Kristoff, B., et al. (1991). Changes in cognitive and language functioning of preschool children with autism. *Journal of Autism and Developmental Disorders*, 21, 281-290. AUTISM LANGUAGE AND COGNITIVE DEVELOPMENT:

Hart, Betty. (1991). Input frequency and children's first words. *First Language*, 11, 289-300. FIRST WORDS ENVIRONMENTAL INFLUENCES INPUT FACTORS:

Examination of free play sessions recorded at one-month intervals suggests that children's first words reflect the frequency of their use by adults in the child's environment. From Child Development Abstracts.

Haryu, Estuko. (1989). What facilitates learning to read characters by children?. *Japanese Journal of Educational Psychology*, 37, 264-269. LITERACY LITERACY READING DISORDERS JAPANESE: JAPANESE

The relative difficulty in learning to read Kanji and Hiragana by children was investigated. The result shows that the difficulty in learning characters depends not so much on their visual complexity as on the meaningfulness of their pronunciation. - From Child Development Abstracts..

Haryu, Etsuko. (1991). A developmental study of children's use of mutual exclusivity and context to interpret novel words. *Japanese Journal of Educational Psychology*, 39, 11-20. MUTUAL EXCLUSIVITY: JAPANESE

By the age of 5:0 children will accept the contextual information present when novel labels are applied to familiar objects. Prior to that age there is a tendency to reject the contextual information and rely upon mutual exclusivity to determine the correct label for the object. From Child Development Abstracts.

Hasan, Ruqaiya, & Cloran, Carmel. (1990). A sociolinguistic study of everyday talk between mothers and children. In M. A. K. Halliday, J. Gibbons, & H. Nicholas (Eds), *Learning, keeping and using language* . Amsterdam, The Netherlands: John Benjamins. ADULT-CHILD INTERACTION PARENTAL INPUT SOCIAL INTERACTION:

Selected paper from the proceedings of the Eighth World Congress of Applied Linguistics, Sydney, 1987.

Hastings, P. M., Lytinen, S. L., & Lindsay, R. K. (1991). Learning words: computers and kids. In K. Hammond, & D. Gentner (Eds), *Proceedings of the Thirteenth Annual Conference of the Cognitive Science Society*. Hillsdale, NJ: Lawrence Erlbaum Associates. LEXICAL DEVELOPMENT:

Hatzichristou, C., & Hopf, D. (1992). School performance and adjustment of Greek remigrant students in the schools of their home country. *Applied Psycholinguistics*, 13, 279-294. TRANSFER INTERFERENCE BILINGUALISM-EDUCATION LANGUAGE AND EDUCATION:

Hausendorf, Heiko, & Quasthoff, Uta M. (1989). Ein Modell zur Beschreibung von Erzählerwerb bei Kindern. (A model of the descriptions of children's narrative development.). In K. Ehlich, & K. Wagner (Eds), *Erzählerwerb*. Bern: NARRATIVES TEXT/STORY GRAMMARS: GERMAN

Hausendorf, Heiko, & Quasthoff, Uta M. (1992). Patterns of adult-child interaction as a mechanism of discourse acquisition.

Journal of Pragmatics., 17(3), 241-250. ADULT-CHILD INTERACTION DISCOURSE STRUCTURE:

Hauser, Marc D., & Marler, Peter. (1992). Do and should studies of animal communication affect interpretations of child phonological development? In C. A. Ferguson, L. Menn, & C. Stoel-Gammon (Eds), *Phonological development: Models, research, implications.* Monkton, MD: York Press. PHONOLOGICAL DEVELOPMENT ACQUISITON THEORIES-PHONOLOGY:

Hawkins, J. A. (1988). *Explaining language universals.* Oxford: Blackwell. ACQUISITION AND LINGUISTIC THEORY LANGUAGE UNIVERSALS:

Hawkins, J. A. (1988). Papers in Universal Grammar: Generative and typological approaches. *Lingua*, 74 (2/3), PARAMETER SETTING ACQUISITION AND LINGUISTIC THEORY:

Special edition.

Hay, D. F., Stimson, C. A., & Castle, J. (1991). A meeting of minds in infancy: Imitation and desire. In D. Frye, & C. Moore (Eds), *Children's theories of mind.* Hillsdale, NJ: Lawrence Erlbaum Associates. THEORY OF MIND IMITATION:

Healy, Alice F., Kosslyn, Stephen M., & Shiffrin, Richard M. (1992). *From learning processes to cognitive processes: Essays in honor of William K. Estes.* Hillsdale, NJ: Lawrence Erlbaum Associates. LANGUAGE PROCESSING LANGUAGE AND COGNITION CONNECTIONISM COGNITIVE DEVELOPMENT LANGUAGE AND BEHAVIORISM LANGUAGE AND EDUCATION:

A two volue set written in honor of Estes. Volume 1 features essays on mathematical and theoretical issues, and volume 2 deals with theoretical and experimental issues.

Hedderson, John. (1987). *SPSSx made simple.* Belmont, CA: Wadsworth. SPSS METHODOLOGY-ANALYSIS:

An introductory guide to using mainframe SPSSx (*Statistical Package for the Social Sciences*) which requires no previous knowledge and which introduces the programs in a concise, easy to understand and nonthreatening manner.

Hegde, M. N. (1985). *Treatment procedures in communicative disorders*. San Diego, CA: Singular Group. INTERVENTION PROGRAMS TREATMENT GENERALIZATION:

Introductory level text.

Hegde, M. N. (1987). *Clinical research in communicative disorders*. San Diego, CA: Singular Group. METHODOLOGY-DESIGN LANGUAGE DISORDERS:

Introductory level text.

Hegde, M. N. (1991). *Introduction to communicative disorders*. San Diego, CA: Singular Group. ARTICULATION DISORDERS DISFLUENCIES CLEFT PALATE CEREBRAL DISORDERS AUDIOLOGY:

Introductory level text.

Heitman, Robert J., & Gilley, William F. (1989). Effects of blocked versus random practice by mentally retarded subjects on learning a novel skill. *Perceptual and Motor Skills*, 69, 443-447. RETARDED CHILDREN:

Analysis showed no significant differences among practice conditions which provided 10 minutes of experience prior to test. - From Child Development Abstracts.

Helm-Estabrooks, Nancy, & Albert, Martin L. (1991). *Manual of aphasia therapy*. San Diego, CA: Singular Group. APHASIAS NEUROLINGUISTICS INTERVENTION PROGRAMS:

Neuroanatomy and neuropathology of language, process approaches to evaluation and treatment of aphasias, visual action therapy, involuntary utterances, melodic intonation therapy, perseveration, Wernicke's aphasia, drug therapy for aphasia, psychological, legal and social aspects of aphasia.

Hemphill, L., Picardi, N., & Tager-Flusberg, Helen. (1991). Narrative as an index of communicative competence in mildly mentally retarded children. *Applied Psycholinguistics*, 12, 263-279. RETARDED CHILDREN NARRATIVES COMMUNICATIVE COMPETENCE:

Hendershott, JoAnn L., Searight, H. Russell, Hatfield, Jimmy L., & Rogers, Billy. (1990). Correlations between the Stanford-Binet, Fourth Edition and the Kaufman Assessment Battery for Children for a preschool sample. *Perceptual and Motor Skills*, 71, 819-825. ASSESSMENT PROCEDURES KAUFMAN ASSESSMENT BATTERY FOR CHILDREN:

The Stanford-Binet IV and the Kaufman Assessment Battery for Children were administered to 36 preschool children to estimate the association of scores. No significant mean difference was obtained between the two composite scores. Correlations between conceptually similar factors were higher than those between dissimilar factors.

Henderson, Bruce B. (1991). Describing parent-child interaction during exploration: Situation definitions and negotiations. *Genetic, Social, and General Psychology Monographs*, 117, 79-89. ADULT-CHILD INTERACTION PARENTAL SPEECH:

Children aged 3:0-6:0 were videotaped exploring novel objects with both parents. When mismatches occurred, participants negotiations of definitions were coded, and questions were coded for complexity, function, and appropriateness of response. Definitions matched between the participants 80% of the time. - From Child Development Abstracts

Henderson, Donald, & Hendershott, A. (1991). ASL and the family system. *American Annals of the Deaf*, 136, 325-329. SIGNING-ASL DEAF CHILDREN:

Hendricks, H., Hickmann, Maya, & Liang, J. (1989). Diskurskohasion im Erstspracherwerb: Eine sprachvergleichende Untersuchung. (Discourse cohesion in first language acquisition -- A crosslinguistic study.). *Zeitschrift für Literaturwissenschaft und Linguistik*, 73, 53-74. DISCOURSE COHERENCE CROSSLINGUISTIC STUDY-DISCOURSE: GERMAN

Henly, Elizabeth, & Sheldon, Amy. (1986). Duration and context effects on the perception of English /r/ and /l/: A comparison of Cantonese and Japanese speakers. *Language Learning*, 36(4), 505-521. LIQUIDS L2 PHONOLOGY INTERLANGUAGE-PHONOLOGY JAPANESE-ENGLISH CANTONESE-ENGLISH CHINESE-ENGLISH ENGLISH-CANTONESE ENGLISH-JAPANESE ENGLISH-CHINESE:

Herman, Louis M., Pack, A. A., & Morrel-Samuels, P. (1993). Representational and conceptual skills of dolphins. In L. M. Herman, H. L. Roitblat, & P. E. Nachtigall (Eds), *Language and communication: Comparative perspectives*. Hillsdale, NJ: Lawrence Erlbaum Associates. ANIMAL COMMUNICATIONS:

Hernandorena, C. L. M., & Lamprecht, Regina R. (1988). Implicacoes da teoria da fonologia natural e da teoria dos tracos distintivos na fonologia clinica. (Implications of Natural Phonology and of Distinctive Feature Theory for clinical phonology.). *Letras de Hoje*, 23 (4), 57-79. PHONOLOGICAL DISORDERS PORTUGUESE: PORTUGUESE

> Discussion of the pros and cons of both Stampe's Natural Phonology and Distinctive Feature theory-as proposed by Chomsky & Halle and Ladefoged-applied to clinical phonology.RRL

Herrmann, D. J., Chaffin, R. J. S., Conti, Gina, Peters, D. A., & Robbins, P. (1979). Comprehension of antonymy and the generality of categorization models. *Journal of Experimental Psychology: Human Learning and Memory*, 5, 585-597. ANTONYMS CATEGORIZATION MUTUAL EXCLUSIVITY:

Herrmann, D. J., Frisina, R. D., & Conti, Gina. (1978). Categorization and familiarity in recognition involving a well-memorized list. *Journal of Experimental Psychology: Human Learning and Memory*, 4, 428-440. CATEGORIZATION:

Hess, Carla W., & Haug, Holly T. (1989). The reliability of type-token ratios for the oral language of school age children. *Journal of Speech and Hearing Research*, 32, 536-540. METHODOLOGY-ANALYSIS:

Alternate forms reliability of four type-token ratios (TTRs) of oral language samples were studied. The four TTRs included the basic type-token ratio, the corrected type-token ratio, the root type-token ratio, and the bilogarithmic type-token ratio. Within each TTR measure, there were no significant differences among the means for samples of the same size, but all means for a given sample differed significantly from the means of all other sample sizes. - From Child Development Abstracts.

Hess, L., & Johnston, Judith R. (1988). Acquisition of back channel responses to adequate messages. *Discourse Processes*, 11, 319-336. CONVERSATIONAL SKILLS PRAGMATIC DEVELOPMENT TOPIC MAINTENANCE TOPIC COLLABORATION COMMUNICATIVE COMPETENCE:

An examination of the acquisition of the communicative feedback responses used by listeners to let the speaker know that they are being understood, e.g. such minimal encouragers as nods, eye contacts, etc.JRJ

Hickey, Tina. (1989). Insealbhu na Gaeilge. (The acquisition of Irish). *Teangeolas*, 26, 19-24. IRISH: IRISH

The language of a child aged 1:4 to 2:1 acquiring Irish as a first language is described.TH

Hickey, Tina. (1990). The acquisition of Irish: a study of word order development. *Journal of Child Language*, 17 (1), WORD ORDER IRISH:

The claims of the 'naturalness agrument' regarding word order acquisition are reviewed in the light of data from three children acquiring Irish, a strict VSO language. Overall the children adhered to the positional restrictions on main verbs, which are sentence-initial, and verbal nouns and verbal adjectives, which occur post-subject. Their production of subject- initial utterances was higher than that found in input to them, and this resulted mainly from their elision of the verb 'to be' as auxiliary and main verb when it was given information.TH

Hickey, Tina. (1990). ILARSP: a grammatical profile of Irish. *Clinical Linguistics and Phonetics*, 4 (4), 363-376. IRISH ASSESSMENT PROCEDURES LARSP:

The adaptation to Irish of LARSP (the Language Assessment, Remediation and Screening Procedure) is described. The use of this method to profile acquisition in this language is discussed, and its applications are examined. This adaptation is based on longitudinal data from four children. The problems of comprehensiveness and representativeness in adapting the profile are discussed and the solutions arrived at are illustrated with examples of each utterance type at clause, phrase and word level for each stage.TH

Hickey, Tina. (1991). Mean length of utterance and the acquisition of Irish. *Journal of Child Language*, 18, 553-569. IRISH MEAN LENGTH OF UTTERANCE:

Hickman, Maya. (1991). Review of 'The acquisition of narratives' by M. Bamberg. *Language*, 67(1), 150-155. BOOK REVIEW NARRATIVES GERMAN:

Hickmann, Maya. (1990). The Development of discourse cohesion: Some functional and crosslinguistic issues. In G. Pierraut-Le Bonniec, & M. Dolitsky (Eds), *From basic language to discourse bases*. Amsterdam: John Benjamins. DISCOURSE COHERENCE CROSSLINGUISTIC STUDY-DISCOURSE:

Hickmann, Maya. (1990). Le discours rapporte: Aspects métapragmatiques du langage et de son développement. (Discourse production: metapragmatic aspects of language and its development). *Bulletin de Psychologie*, 25, METALINGUISTICS PRAGMATIC DEVELOPMENT COMMUNICATIVE COMPETENCE DISCOURSE DEVELOPMENT: FRENCH

Hickmann, Maya. (1992). The boundaries of reported speech. Some developmental aspects. In J. Lucy (Ed.), *Reflexive language: Reported speech and metapragmatics*.. Cambridge: Cambridge University Press. METALINGUISTICS PRAGMATIC DEVELOPMENT:

Hickmann, Maya, & Liang, J. (1990). Clause structure variation in Chinese narrative discourse: A developmental analysis. *Linguistics*, 28(6), 1167-1200. CHINESE NARRATIVES SYNTACTIC STRUCTURES:

Hicks, Deborah. (1990). Kinds of narratives: Genre skills among first graders from two communities. In A. McCabe, & C. Peterson (Eds), *Developing narrative structure.* Hillsdale, NJ: Lawrence Erlbaum Associates. NARRATIVES DISCOURSE FUNCTIONS:

Hicks, Deborah. (1990). Narrative skills and genre knowledge: Ways of telling in the primary grades. *Applied Psycholinguistics*, 11, 83-104. TEXT/STORY GRAMMARS NARRATIVES:

Children watched a silent movie and were then asked to produce a simultaneous three-minute commentary accompanying a film clip, a report of the story as a news item following the film, and a retelling of the story as a narrative after the end of the film. Analysis of the results showed that primary school children had still to develop their genre knowledge.

Higginson, Roy. (1988). The ISU/CHILDES database: A bibliographic addition to CHILDES. *Journal of Child Language*, 15(1), 175-177. BIBLIOGRAPHY CHILDES:

Describes the database/bibliography, the formats that it is available in, and its relationship to the CHILDES database.

Higginson, Roy. (1989). The CHILDES/BIB database. *Child Language, Teaching and Therapy*, 5(3), 335-342. BIBLIOGRAPHY CHILDES:

Describes the application of the database and bibliography in clinical settings.

Higginson, Roy. (1990). An update on the CHILDES/BIB (formerly ISU/CHILDES) database. *Journal of Child Language,*, 17, 473-479. BIBLIOGRAPHY CHILDES:

Announces the change of name and describes the changes that have taken place in the bibliography since its original release in 1988.

Higginson, Roy, & MacWhinney, Brian. (1991). *CHILDES/BIB: An annotated bibliography of child language and language disorders.* Hillsdale, NJ: Lawrence Erlbaum Associates. CHILDES BIBLIOGRAPHY:

Detailing more than one hundred years of research including the most current developments, CHILDES/BIB serves as a quick reference to literature on child language and language disorders. The coverage includes not only the field of language acquisition, but also bilingualism, second language acquisition, language and cognition, and atypical popluations. Available in both electronic and printed versions, the database contains more than 7,500 references to various journal articles and books.

Higginson, Roy, & MacWhinney, Brian. (1993). *CHILDES/BIB: An annotated bibliography of child language and language disorders - 1993 Supplement.* Hillsdale, NJ: Lawrence Erlbaum Associates. CHILDES BIBLIOGRAPHY:

The 1993 supplement to the earlier bibliography which adds a further 3,000 references to the original work. Many of the new references were added as a result of the highly successful response to the call for the submission of personal bibliographies which was sent to non-North-American members of the International Association for the Study of Child Language after the Fifth Child Language Congress (Budapest, 1990). As a result, the bibliography now presents a more comprehensive picture of the worldwide research conducted in the field since 1970. The bibliography is also available as a fully searchable electronic database.

Hilke, D. D. (1991). Infant vocalizations and changes in experience. In D. J. Napoli, & J. A. Kegl (Eds), *Bridges between psychology and linguistics: A Swarthmore Festschrift for Lila Gleitman.*. Hillsdale, NJ: Lawrence Erlbaum Associates. VOCALIZATIONS:

Hill, B. P., & Singer, L. T. (1990). Speech and language development after infant tracheostomy . *Journal of Speech and Hearing Disorders*, 55, 15-20. TRAUMATIC DISORDERS ATYPICAL DEVELOPMENT ARTICULATION DISORDERS:

Hirschberg, Jenö. (1978). A gyermek beszédfejlödésének orvosi vonatkozásai (Medical aspects of speech development). *Magyar Fonetikai Füzetek*, 1, 37-42. LANGUAGE DISORDERS HUNGARIAN: HUNGARIAN

Hirschberg, Jenö. (1988). Szajpad-elegtelenség (Cleft-palate). *Medicina.* CLEFT PALATE HUNGARIAN: HUNGARIAN

Hirschberg, Jenö, Gosy, Mária, Pataki, A., Pinter, E., & Nagy, László, et al. (1986). Test de la comprehensibilidad del habla (Test for evaluation of speech of children having speech defect). *Logopedia, Foniatria y Audilogia*, 3, 144-153. ASSESSMENT PROCEDURES HUNGARIAN: SPANISH

Hirschberg, Jenö, & Szende, Tamás. (1976). Acoustic cues for voice quality features. In *6th Acoustic Conference, Budapest 1976.*. Budapest: Az Optikai, Akusztikai es Filmtechnikai Egyesulet publication. ACOUSTIC PHONETICS HUNGARIAN:

Hirschberg, Jenö, & Szende, Tamás. (1976). Die rolle der akustischen Analyse in der Diagnostikpathologisch veranderter Sauglingsstimmen. (The role of acoustic analysis in the analysis of infant's sucking noises). In *Proc. 16th International Congr. Logopedics and Phoniatrics. Interlaken, 1974.*. Basel: ACOUSTIC PHONETICS VOCALIZATIONS HUNGARIAN: GERMAN

Hirschberg, Jenö, & Szende, Tamás. (1982). *Pathological cry, stridor and cough in infants.* Budapest. CRYING LANGUAGE DISORDERS HUNGARIAN:

Hirschberg, Jenö, & Szende, Tamás. (1985). *Pathologische Schreistimme, Stridor und Hustenton im Saulingsalter. (Pathological cry, stridor, and cough in infants.).* Budapest: Akademiai Kiado/ G. Fischer Verlag. CRYING LANGUAGE DISORDERS HUNGARIAN: GERMAN

Hirschfeld, Lawrence A. (1989). Discovering linguistic differences: Domain specificity and the young child's awareness of multiple languages. *Human Development*, 32, 223-236. METALINGUISTICS:

The child's rich and specific categorical skills have been the focus of considerable empirical research. Recent work supports the claim that even preschoolers acquire domain-specific and structured knowledge about natural kinds, on the one hand, and certain types of social and moral judgments on the other. The present paper considers the young child's recognition of multiple languages in light of these findings on domain specificity. We argue that the realization that more than one language exists is predicated on the emergence of metasocial as well as metalinguistic awareness. - From Child Development Abstracts.

Hirsh-Pasek, Kathy, & Golinkoff, Roberta M. (1991). Language comprehension: a new look at some old themes. In N. A. Krasnegor, et al. (Eds), *Biological and behavioral determinants of language development*. Hillsdale, NJ: Lawrence Erlbaum Associates. COMPREHENSION:

Hitch, Graham J., Halliday, M. Sebastian, Schaafstal, Alma M., & Heffernan, Thomas M. (1991). Speech, 'inner speech,' and the development of short-term memory: Effects of picture-labeling on recall. *Experimental Child Psychology*, 51, 220-234. INNER SPEECH LANGUAGE AND MEMORY:

Three experiments explored the effect of overt speech on children's use of 'inner speech' in short-term memory. Word length and phonemic similarity had greater effects in the older children and when pictures were labeled at presentation. There were no significant differences with respect to overall performance or effects of word length and phonemic similarity.

Hobbs, Margaret, & Bacharach, Verne R. (1990). Children's understanding of big buildings and big cars. *Child Study Journal*, 20, 1-18. DIMENSIONAL ADJECTIVES SPATIAL TERMS:

Children 3 and 5 were shown pairs of buildings and pairs of cars and judged which stimulus was the big one. All children used a height rule when interpreting big. 5-year-olds were more consistent in use of this rule.

Hobson, R. Peter. (1993). *Autism and the development of the mind.* Hillsdale, NJ: Lawrence Erlbaum Associates. AUTISM THEORY OF MIND INTERSUBJECTIVITY SELF-CONCEPT:

Hobson contends that autism is the result of the inability to differentiate between the self and the world in the early stages of development, and believes that an examination of the syndrome can throw light on normal child development.

Hodson, Barbara W., & Paden, Elaine P. (1991). *Targeting intelligible speech: A phonological approach to remediation, 2nd Ed.* San Diego, CA: Singular Group. PHONOLOGICAL DISORDERS INTERVENTION PROGRAMS INTELLIGIBILITY:

Procedures for the assessment, analysis and remediation of phonological disorders.

Hoff-Ginsberg, Erika. (1990). Maternal speech and the child's development of syntax: A further look. *Journal of Child Language*, 17, 85-99. PARENTAL INPUT PARENTAL SPEECH-SYNTAX FINE TUNING HYPOTHESIS:

The results suggest that maternal speech supports the child's development of syntax through linguistic interaction and exemplification of syntactic structures.

Hoff-Ginsberg, Erika, & Krueger, W. M. (1991). Older siblings as conversational partners. *Merrill-Palmer Quarterly*, 37, 465-482. SIBLING EFFECTS:

Hoffer, Pamela Corbett, & Bliss, Lynn S. (1990). Maternal verbal responsiveness with language-impaired, stage-matched, and age-matched normal children. *Journal of Applied Developmental Pshchology*, 11, 305-319. PARENTAL SPEECH-ATYPICAL CHILDREN LANGUAGE DISORDERS AT-RISK CHILDREN ADULT-CHILD INTERACTION:

The interactions between mothers and their children were coded using Schacter's (1979) analysis. Mothers of LI children were generally less responsive to their children's utterances than mothers in the control groups. Mothers of LI children also ignored and changed the topic of their children's utterances.

Hoffman, Charlotte. (1991). *An introduction to bilingualism.* London, UK: Longmans. BILINGUALISM-PROBLEMS/EFFECTS:

A discussion of the individual and societal effects of bilingualism.

Hoffman, Paul R., Schuckers, Gordon H., & Daniloff, Raymond G. (1989). *Children's phonetic disorders: Theory and treatment.* San Diego, CA: Singular Group. PHONOLOGICAL DISORDERS INTERVENTION PROGRAMS PHONOLOGICAL PROCESSES LANGUAGE PROCESSING:

Includes chapters on phonetic processing and acquisition, phonetic disorders and their assessment and treatment.

Holder, M. D., Herman, Louis M., & Kucsaj, Stan A., II. (1993). A bottle-nosed dolphin's responses to anomalous sequences expressed within an artificial. In L. M. Herman, H. L. Roitblat, & P. E. Nachtigall (Eds), *Language and communication: Comparative perspectives.* Hillsdale, NJ: Lawrence Erlbaum Associates. ANIMAL COMMUNICATIONS:

Holdgrafer, Gary E. (1991). Quantity of communicative behavior in children from birth to 30 months. *Perceptual and Motor Skills*, 72, 803-806. SEX DIFFERENCES INTENTIONALITY:

An examination of the free play behavior of 68 children revealed that girls produce more communicative output than boys, and that verbal children are significantly more productive than preverbal children. From Child Development Abstracts.

Holdgrafer, Gary E., & Dunst, Carl J. (1990). Use of low structured observation for assessing communicative intents in children. *First Language*, 10, 243-253. INTENTIONALITY ADULT-CHILD INTERACTION PARENTAL SPEECH-STYLE:

Thirty-six children were observed while playing with their mothers. Their communicative behaviors were recorded according to intent and level. Rejects occurred significantly less often than either comments or requests, which did not differ significantly, across age groups at nonverbal and verbal-contextual levels.

Holdgrafer, Gary E., Kysela, Gerard M., & McCarthy, Catherine. (1989). Joint action intervention and child language skills: A research note. *First Language*, 9, 299-305. JOINT REFERENCE INTERVENTION PROGRAMS LANGUAGE AND ACTION:

The impact of joint action-based early language intervention on the vocabulary development and socio- communicative word usage of four developmentally delayed children was investigated. Results from pre- and post-intervention language samples revealed increases in vocabulary size, especially for object words, for all children. Improvements in mother-child interaction were generally consistent with the goals of intervention. - From Child Development Abstracts.

Holender, D. (1990). Comment: writing systems and the modularity of language. In I. G. Mattingly, & M. Studdert-Kennedy (Eds), *Modularity and the motor theory of speech perception*. Hillsdale, NJ: Lawrence Erlbaum Associates. LITERACY WRITTEN LANGUAGE:

Holland, Audrey L. (1984). *Language disorders in children*. San Diego, CA: Singular Group. DEVELOPMENTAL DISORDERS CONGENITAL DISORDERS:

Holobow, N. E., Genesee, Fred, & Lambert, Wallace E. (1991). The effectiveness of a foreign language immersion program for children from different ethnic and social class backgrounds. *Applied Psycholinguistics* , 12, 179-198. IMMERSION LANGUAGE AND SOCIAL CLASS L2 EDUCATION LANGUAGE AND EDUCATION:

Honig, Alice S., & Park, Kyung-Ja. (1989). Family factors associated with language competence among toddlers in French, North African, and African families in France. *Early Child Development and Care*, 50, 31-49. CROSSCULTURAL STUDY FRENCH ARABIC CROSSLINGUISTIC STUDY-PARENTAL SPEECH:

Hoosain, Rumjahn. (1991). Cerebral lateralization of bilingual functions after handedness switch in childhood. *Journal of Genetic Psychology*, 152, 263-268. LANGUAGE AND HANDEDNESS LATERALIZATION BILINGUALISM-NEUROLINGUISTICS CHINESE-ENGLISH ENGLISH-CHINESE:

Adult bilingual speakers of Chinese/English who had been forced to switch dominant hands in childhood to the right-hand showed a weaker left-hemisphere dominance for word perception than natural right-hand dominant speakers. Their eprformance was similar to that of left-hand dominant speakers who had not been forced to switch hands. From Child Development Abstracts.

Hopkins, W. D., & Morris, R. D. (1993). Hemispheric priming as a technique in the study of lateralized cognition processes in chimpanzees: Some recent findings. In Herman, L. M., Roitblat, H. L. & Nachtigal, P. E. (Eds). *Language and communication: Comparative perspectives*. Hillsdale, NJ: Lawrence Erlbaum Associates. ANIMAL COMMUNICATIONS LANGUAGE AND OTHER PRIMATES LATERALIZATION:

Hornstein, Norbert. (1990). *As time goes by: Tense and universal grammar*. Cambridge, MA: MIT/Batsford. TENSE SEQUENCING CONNECTIVES-CONDITIONAL CONNECTIVES-ADVERBIAL CONNECTIVES-TEMPORAL:

This book adds to the acquisition literature by proposing a theory of natural language tense that is responsive to acquisition theory's question 'How do children construct complex grammars from the rude fragments available to them?'. Hornstein focusses on this logical problem and highlights the role of syntax in semantics. Topics covered include: adverbial modification, temporal adjunction, conditionals, and tense sequencing.

Hort, Barbara E., & Taylor, Marjorie. (1990). A sex difference in the salience of cues for inductive reference. *British Journal of Developmental Psychology*, 8, 39-50. SEX DIFFERENCES IMPLICATURE:

The present study of inductive inference tested the possibility that sex differences are due to the way the properties are described rather than the biological-non- biological difference in the items. The results indicate that the content of the items (biological versus non-biological) is irrelevant, sex differences in patterns of correct inference are a function of the way the items are described (actions/states versus consequences). Boys made significantly more correct inferences than chance for items whose properties were described as actions or states, while girls made significantly more correct inferences than chance for items whose properties were described as consequences. - From Child Development Abstracts.

Horton, M., & Markman, Ellen M. (1980). Developmental differences in the acquisition of basic and superordinate categories. *Child Development*, 51, 708-719. CATEGORIZATION INDIVIDUAL VARIATION SUPERORDINATION:

Hoshi, Miwako, Kunyama, Yoko, Hasumi, Motoko, & Hikasa, Mako. (1989). Developmental scale for symbolic function in manipulative play. *Japanese Journal of Educational Psychology*, 36, 345-351. LANGUAGE AND PLAY DEVELOPMENTAL SCALES SYMBOL DEVELOPMENT: JAPANESE

A developmental scale for symbolic functions in early childhood is proposed with Level 0 (no symbolization), Level 1 (symbolization of action), Level 2 (symbolization of object and action), and Level 3 (symbolization of action, object and agent). Five children ranging in age from 9 to 28 months old were observed once a month for 17 months in the play setting with toys and everyday objects provided. The above hypothetical stages were verified except in level 3 since the behaviors expected from the scale did not occur in the same age range.-From Child Development Abstracts.

Houdebine, A. M. (1983). *Aspects de la langage orale des enfants a l'entrée au Cours Préparatoire. (The oral language of preschoolers.).* Besancon, France: NRP/CRDP. LANGUAGE AND EDUCATION ACQUISITION THEORIES-OVERVIEW: FRENCH

Hovdhaugen, Even, & Simonsen, Hanne G. (1988). On the acquisition of the t-and k-languages by Samoan children. *Papers from the Tenth Scandinavian Conference of Linguistics*, 2, 1-15. SAMOAN NONSTANDARD DIALECTS BIDIALECTISM:

The article discusses how Samoan children acquire the two different sociolects of their language, illustrated with material from two children from Western Samoa (2.9 and 6.2).

Howarth, L., & Conti-Ramsden, Gina. (1987). Sing a song please: musical contexts and language learning. *European Journal of Speech Needs Education*, 2, 143-160. LANGUAGE AND MUSIC PARENTAL INPUT ADULT-CHILD INTERACTION:

Howe, Christine J. (1993). *Language learning: A special case for developmental psychology*. Hillsdale, NJ: Lawrence Erlbaum Associates. NATIVISM PARENTAL SPEECH ENVIRONMENTAL INFLUENCES CONTEXT QUESTIONS LEXICAL DEVELOPMENT SYNTACTIC DEVELOPMENT LITTLE LINGUIST THEORY:

This book challenges the notion that language development could not take place as quickly and as efficiently as it does if it did not rely upon innate grammatical principles. It presents a psychologically driven theory which can account for the development of language without having to rely upon innate linguistic knowledge.

Howe, N. (1991). Sibling-directed internal state language, perspective taking, and affective behavior. *Child Development*, 62, 1503-1512. PERSPECTIVE TAKING SOCIAL SPEECH:

Howell, Janet, & Dean, Elizabeth. (1991). *Treating phonological disorders in children: Metaphon-theory to practice*. San Diego, CA: Singular Group. PHONOLOGICAL DISORDERS METALINGUISTICS INTERVENTION PROGRAMS METAPHON THERAPY:

An overview of phonological disorders and metalinguistic awareness, followed by a description of Metaphon therapy and its efficacy.

Howell, Karen Kuehn, Harrison, Terry E., Stanford, Lisa D., Zahn, Bradley H., & Bracken, Bruce A. (1990). An empirical evaluation of three preschool language curricula. *Psychology in the Schools*, 27, 296-302. LANGUAGE AND EDUCATION INTERVENTION PROGRAMS:

The purpose of this study is to evaluate empirically the efficacy of three commercially produced preschool language curricula: the Boehm Resource Guide, the Bracken Concept Development Program, the Peabody Language Development Kit-Revised. Results of a 24-week experimental intervention with 76 preschool children indicated that there were no significant pretest-posttest gains on a dependent measure of basic concept acquisition among any of the three intervention groups or the control groups.

Howlin, Patricia, & Rutter, Michael. (1989). Mothers' speech to autistic children: a preliminary causal analysis. *Journal of Child Psychology and Psychiatry*, 30(6), 819-843. AUTISM PARENTAL SPEECH-ATYPICAL CHILDREN:

From Stockholm Bibliographies.

Hoyle, Susan M. (1991). Children's competence in the specialized register of sportscasting. *Journal of Child Language*, 18, 435-450. REGISTER COMMUNICATIVE COMPETENCE:

4 subjects spontaneous and elicited productions of sports commentary speech was compared with adult formal-register speech. Subjects commentary was characterized by incomplete syntactic structures, frequent passives, and heavy use of simple present tense. From Child Development Abstracts.

Hsia, S. (1992). Developmental knowledge of interword and intraword boundaries-evidence from American and Mandarin Chinese speaking beginning readers. *Applied Psycholinguistics*, 13, 341-372. MANDARIN CHINESE WORD BOUNDARIES LEXICAL DEVELOPMENT MORPHOLOGICAL DEVELOPMENT LITERACY:

Hsu, Jennifer R., & Cairns, Helen S. (1990). Interpreting PRO: From strategy to structure. In E. H. Bendix (Ed.), *The uses of linguistics*. New York, NY: New York Academy of Sciences. PARAMETER SETTING PRONOUNS SYNTACTIC DEVELOPMENT:

Hsu, Jennifer R., Cairns, Helen S., Eisenberg, Sarita, & Schlisselberg, Gloria. (1989). Control and coreference in early child language. *Journal of Child Language*, 16(3), 599-622. REFERENCE PRONOUNS SYNTACTIC DEVELOPMENT PARAMETER SETTING:

> Results replicate earlier studies and show five stages in the development of PRO. A significant relationship was observed between forward PRO and the presence of overt pronouns.

Hsu, Jennifer R., Cairns, Helen S., Eisenberg, Sarita, & Schlisselberg, Gloria. (1991). When do children avoid backwards coreference? *Journal of Child Language*, 18, 339-353. ANAPHORA:

> Young children's avoidance of backwards coreference was examined for the age range 3:1-8:0. Children and adults were asked to act out sentences containing pronominal anaphora. Results indicated a childhood preference for internal coreference even if it involved violating the syntactic structure. From Child Development Abstracts.

Hu, Q. (1993). Common features of mothers' vocabulary. In J. L. Sokolov, & C. E. Snow (Eds), *Handbook of research inlanguage development using CHILDES*. Hillsdale, NJ: Lawrence Erlbaum Associates. PARENTAL SPEECH-VOCABULARY METHODOLOGY-DESIGN METHODOLOGY-COMPUTERS CHILDES:

Hudson, J. A., & Shapiro, L. R. (1990). From knowing to telling: The development of children's scripts, stories and personal narratives. In A. McCabe, & C. Peterson (Eds), *Developing narrative structure*.

Hillsdale, NJ: Lawrence Erlbaum Associates. NARRATIVES EVENTS/SCRIPTS:

Hudson, J. A., & Slackman, E. A. (1990). Children's use of scripts in inferential text processing.. *Discourse Processes*, 13, 375-385. LITERACY EVENTS/SCRIPTS TEXT/STORY GRAMMARS:

Hudson, P. (1990). What's in a word? Levels of representation and word recognition. In D. A. Balota, G. B. Flores d'Arcais, & K. Rayner (Eds), *Comprehension processes in reading*. Hillsdale, NJ: Lawrence Erlbaum Associates. REPRESENTATIONS-LEXICAL:

Hudson, Thom, Detmer, Emily., & Brown, J. D. (1992). *A framework for testing cross-cultural pragmatics*. Honolulu, HI: University of Hawaii Press. L2 PRAGMATICS INTERLANGUAGE-PRAGMATICS L2 EDUCATION ASSESSMENT PROCEDURES:

Huebner, Thom, & Ferguson, Charles A. (Eds) (1991). *Crosscurrents in second language acquisition and linguistic theories*. Philadelphia, PA: John Benjamins. L2 ACQUISITION L2 ACQUISITION THEORIES L2 SYNTAX L2 PHONOLOGY SOCIOLINGUISTIC FACTORS L2 LINGUISTIC THEORY:

> A selection of revised and updated papers from a conference held at Stanford University in 1987 during the Linguistic Institute. The papers show that theory contributes to application (the usual current), but that application can make equal returns to theory (thus, crosscurrents). Moreover, the contributors show that, although there is a strong tendency in the field of linguistics to see 'theorists' working within formal models of syntax. SLA research can contribute to linguistic theory more broadly defined to include various functional as well as formal models of syntax, theories of phonology, variationist theories of sociolinguistics, etc.

Hughes, Diana L., & Carpenter, Robert L. (1989). Short-term syntax learning and generalization effects. *Child Language Teaching and Therapy*, 5, 202-220. TREATMENT GENERALIZATION SYNTACTIC DISORDERS:

Two language theory procedures, a structured, repetitive drill approach and a story-based question and answer approach were used to teach is and are to four language impaired children aged 4:4 to 6:3, over a four-week period. Effectiveness was measured by three methods: within-therapy data, structured probe data, and at-home spontaneous probe data. While levels of correct productions were high in therapy, production on spontaneous probes remained low. Structured probe performance varied, but was generally substantially higher than spontaneous probe performance. Results indicate that syntax learning depends on how such learning is measured. - From Child Development Abstracts.

Huiskens, L., Coppen, P. A., & Jagtman, M. (1991). Developing a tool for the description of language acquisition. *Linguistics*, 29(3), 451-479. METHODOLOGY:

Hulme, Charles, & MacKenzie, Susie. (1992). *Working memory and severe learning difficulties*. Hillsdale, NJ: Lawrence Erlbaum Associates. LANGUAGE AND MEMORY LITERACY LANGUAGE AND EDUCATION INTERVENTION PROGRAMS:

The impact of memory deficits on learning and development has far reaching consequences for LANGUAGE and reading. This book discusses the state of knowledge on memory deficits and proposes an intervention program.

Hulstijn, J. H., & Bossers, B. (1993). Individual differences in L2 proficiency as function of L1 proficiency. In A. M. B. de Groot, & C. Barry (Eds), *The multilingual community*. Hillsdale, NJ: Lawrence Erlbaum Associates. L2/L1 ACQUISITION INDIVIDUAL VARIATION:

Hunt, E. (1993). A proposal for computer modeling of animal linguistic comprehension. In L. M. Herman, H. L. Roitblat, & P. E. Nachtigall (Eds), *Language and communication: Comparative perspectives*. Hillsdale, NJ: Lawrence Erlbaum Associates. COMPUTER SIMULATIONS ANIMAL COMMUNICATIONS:

Hupet, Michael, & Tilmant, Brigitte. (1989). How to make young children produce cleft sentences. *Journal of Child Language*, 16(2), 251-261. CLEFTS:

Hurford, James R. (1987). *Language and number: the emergence of a cognitive system*. Oxford, UK: Basil Blackwell. NUMERALS LANGUAGE AND COGNITIVE DEVELOPMENT:

A theoretical discussion of the acquisition of numeral systems. (Reprinted 1990).

Hurford, James R. (1989). Biological evolution of the Saussurean sign as a component of the language acquisition device. *Lingua*, 77(2), 187-222. LANGUAGE ACQUISITION DEVICE BIOLOGICAL FOUNDATIONS:

Hurford, James R. (1990). Nativist and functional explanations in language acquisition. In I. Roca (Ed.), *Logical issues in language acquisition*. Dordrecht, The Netherlands: Foris Publications. NATIVISM ACQUISITION THEORIES:

Hurford, James R. (1991). The evolution of the critical period for language acquisition. *Cognition*, 40, 159-201. CRITICAL PERIOD:

Hurford, James R. (1992). An approach to the phylogeny of the language faculty. In J. A. Hawkins, & M. Gell-Mann (Eds), *The Evolution of Human Languages*. New York, NY: Addison Wesley. PHYLOGENETIC ORIGINS:

Huszár, Csilla. (1988). A logopédiai óvodában folyó anyanyelvinevelés (Mother tongue education in logopedic nurseries). *Gyosze XVI*, 3, 210-214. INTERVENTION PROGRAMS HUNGARIAN: HUNGARIAN

Huttenlocher, Janellen, & Higgins, E. T. (1978). Issues in the study of symbolic development. In W. E. Collins (Ed.), *Minnesota symposia on child psychology*. Hillsdale, NJ: Lawrence Erlbaum Associates. SYMBOL DEVELOPMENT:

Hyams, Nina. (1991). A reanalysis of null subjects in child language. In J. Weissenborn, H. Goodluck, & T. Roeper (Eds), *Theoretical Issues in Language Acquisition-Continuity and Change in Development*. Hillsdale, NJ: Lawrence Erlbaum Associates. PARAMETER SETTING NULL SUBJECTS SYNTACTIC DEVELOPMENT:

Hyams, Nina. (1992). Morphosyntactic development in Italian and its relevance to parameter-setting models-comment. *Journal of Child Language* , 19 , 695-709. ITALIAN MORPHOLOGICAL DEVELOPMENT MORPHOSYNTACTIC DEVELOPMENT PARAMETER SETTING:

Hyams, Nina, & Sigurjonsdottir, Sigridur. (1990). The development of 'long-distance anaphora': A crosslinguistic comparison with special reference to Icelandic. *Language Acquisition*, 1, 57-93. ANAPHORA PRONOUNS PARAMETER SETTING ICELANDIC CROSSLINGUISTIC STUDY-SYNTAX:

The authors examine the binding of pronominal anaphora over long syntactic distances. They review previous works which suggest that binding is a parameterized system and go on to use Icelandic to exemplify their theory.

Hyltenstam, Kenneth, & Obler, Loraine K. (1989). *Bilingualism across the lifespan*. New York, NY: Cambridge University Press. BILINGUALISM-LANGUAGE PROCESSING BILINGUALISM-CULTURAL FACTORS BILINGUALISM-SOCIAL FACTORS BILINGUALISM-COGNITIVE DEVELOPMENT BILINGUALISM-NEUROLINGUISTICS BILINGUALISM-LANGUAGE DIFFERENTIATION BILINGUALISM-LANGUAGE LOSS BILINGUALISM-LANGUAGE DISORDERS:

In this broad overview of current theoretical and empirical approaches to the study of bilingualism, the contributors examine the dynamics of bilingual language processing over time from the perspective of neurolinguistics, psycholinguistics, and sociolinguistics. This multidisciplinary approach is fundamental to an understanding of how the bilingual's two (or more) language systems interact with each other and with other higher cognitive systems, neurological substates, and social systems. Contributors examine the nature of bilingualism during various phases of the life cycle and in various health/pathology conditions. Topics range from code separation in the young bilingual child, across various types of language pathologies in adult bilinguals, to language choice problems in dementia.

I

Idiazabal, Itziar. (1984). Conciencia bilingüe del niño bilingüe (Bilingual conscience of the bilingual child.). In M. Siguan (Ed.), *Adquisición precoz de una segunda lengua*. Barcelona, Spain: Universidad de Barcelona. BILINGUALISM-COGNITIVE DEVELOPMENT LANGUAGE AND MORALITY: SPANISH

Idiazabal, Itziar, & Bronckart, J. P. (1984). La compréhension des énonces transitives en Basque. (The comprehension of transitive sentences in Basque.). *Journal de Psychologie Normal et Pathologique.*, 79(4), 357-388. BASQUE VERBS-TRANSITIVE: FRENCH

Idiazabal, Itziar, & Bronckart, J. P. (1986). Las estrategias de comprensión de los enunciados transitivos en vasco (Strategies of comprehension of transitive sentences in Basque). In M. Siguan (Ed.), *Estudios de Psicolingüistica*. Madrid: Piramide. BASQUE VERBS-TRANSITIVE COMPREHENSION: SPANISH

Imedadze, N. V. (1972). *Psychological research (Vol. 2)*. Tbilisi: Metsniereba Publishing House. LANGUAGE AND COGNITION SAPIR-WHORF HYPOTHESIS: RUSSIAN

The result of experimental research have shown that the 2 groups of school-age children belonging to various language communities (other variables equal) group the physical objects differently. That proves the possibility of linguistic differences (e.g. lexical segmentation in Georgian and Russian languages) on the nonverbal behavior.

Imedadze, N. V. (1975). The acquisition of second language grammatic by child. *Mazne (Messenger) Georgian Academy of Science*, 3, 25-35. GEORGIAN L2 SYNTAX OPERATING PRINCIPLES APPROACH INTERFERENCE L2 ACQUISITION STRATEGIES:

The acquisition of a second language by Georgian children is analyzed in terms of Slobin's operating principles. In the research it is shown that the definite modifications of these principles are due to native language interference.

Imedadze, N. V. (1979). Bessoznatelnoje v strategii ovladenija jazikom. (The Unconscious in the strategy of language acquisition.). In *The unconcious: nature, functions, methods of study*. Tbilisi, Georgia: Metsniereba Publishing House. ACQUISITION THEORIES-SOVIET SYNTACTIC DEVELOPMENT L2/L1 ACQUISITION BILINGUALISM-SOVIET RESEARCH: RUSSIAN

An analysis of the process of language acquisition reveals the paradoxal fact that the child derives a system of grammar rules from an unordered verbal input; the rules being actually absent in the child's consciouness. Language set is proposed as an explanatory concept. It constitutes the basis of heuristic intuitive activity, the specific content of which can be described in terms of strategy of 'operative principles of verbal input processing.' Evidence on an experimental teaching of a second language involving 6-7 year old children permits the differentiation of the child's spontaneous speech into: a) those due to native language interference and b) those of heuristic nature, pointing to a partial preservation of a strategy analogous to that used by the child in learning its mother tongue.

Imedadze, N. V. (1979). *Experimental-psychological study of second language acquisition and mastery*. Tbilisi: Metsniereba Publishing House. L2 EDUCATION L2 ACQUISITION STRATEGIES LANGUAGE AND COGNITION: RUSSIAN GEORGIAN

Monograph concern the psychological regularities of the process of second language acquisition and mastering (in pre-school, school children and students). Two groups of problems are analyzed in the study: the first is connected with the qualitative peculiarities of the forms of second language acquisition: the second, with the functioning of the formed second language system, typology and models of bilingualism, the interaction of native and second language systems.

Imedadze, N. V. (1984). Description of a program of experimental teaching of Russian language in Soviet Georgian elementary schools. *Contemporary Educational Psychology*, 9 (3), 269-274. BILINGUALISM-SEQUENTIAL L2 EDUCATION RUSSIAN-GEORGIAN GEORGIAN-RUSSIAN:

The study involved the observation of 6 and 7 year old Georgian school children learning a second language by experimental teaching techniques-under the conditions of 'non-learning behavior.' The results of experimental learning proved the effectiveness of the psychological principles used.

Imedadze, N. V. (1988). *Ontogenesis of metalinguistic function and bilingualism*. Moscow: Materials of Ix Symp. for Psycholinguistics. METALINGUISTICS BILINGUALISM-METALINGUISTIC DEVELOPMENT: RUSSIAN

The development of metalinguistic ability in monolingual and bilingual children (4-5 years) has been experimentally studied. The preference lies in bilingual children in some aspects of methalinguistic ability.

Imedadze, N. V., & Tuite, K. (1992). The acquisition of Georgian. In D. I. Slobin (Ed.), *The crosslinguistic study of language acquisition (Vol. 3)*. Hillsdale, NJ: Lawrence Erlbaum Associates. GEORGIAN:

Indefrey, P. (1990). Henning Wode: Einfuhrung in die Psycholinguistik. Rezension. (Henning Wode: Introduction to psycholinguistics - a review.). *Linguistische Berichte.*, 125, OVERVIEW-PSYCHOLINGUISTICS BOOK REVIEW: GERMAN

Ingham, R. (1992). The optional subject phenomenon in young children's English-a case study. *Journal of Child Language*, 19, 133-151. SYNTACTIC STRUCTURES GRAMMATICAL RELATIONS NULL SUBJECTS PARAMETER SETTING:

Ingham, R. J. (1990). On the valid role of reliability in identifying what is stuttering - comment. *Journal of Speech and Hearing Disorders*, 55, 394-397. STUTTERING:

Ingram, David. (1989). *First language acquisition: method, description, and explanation*. New York, NY: Cambridge University Press. OVERVIEW-SYNTAX OVERVIEW-GENERAL OVERVIEW-PHONOLOGY OVERVIEW-SEMANTICS MORPHOLOGICAL DEVELOPMENT LEXICAL DEVELOPMENT METHODOLOGY:

A closely analyzed exposition of how children acquire language that explores the receptive and productive abilities of children in all core areas of language-phonology, morphology, syntax, and semantics. Readers will acquire the fundamental knowledge and skill not only to interpret primary literature, but to approach their own research with sophistication. While the descriptive facts that are currently available on the first language acquisition are central to the book, its emphasis on methodology and explanation distinguishes this text from others. The various ways in which research is conducted is discussed in detail, as well as the strengths and weaknesses of different approaches, leading to new perspectives on key theoretical issues.

Ingram, David. (1990). *Phonological disability in children*. San Diego, CA: Singular Group. PHONOLOGICAL DISORDERS INTERVENTION PROGRAMS METHODOLOGY-DESIGN METHODOLOGY-ANALYSIS PHONOLOGICAL DEVELOPMENT:

Descriptions of phonological acquisition and the methodology for phonological data collection and anaylsis, deviant phonological development, and recent developments and issues in remediation.

Ingram, David. (1991). An historical observation on why mama and papa. *Journal of Child Language*, 18, 711-713. PHONOLOGICAL DEVELOPMENT:

Ingram, David. (1992). Early phonological acquisition: A crosslinguistic perspective. In C. A. Ferguson, L. Menn, & C. Stoel-Gammon (EdS), *Phonological development: Models, research, implications*. Monkton, MD: York Press. CROSSLINGUISTIC STUDY-PHONOLOGY:

Inhelder, Bärbel, & Karmiloff-Smith, Annette. (1978). Thought and language. In B. Preisseisen, D. Goldstein, & M. Appel (Eds), *Topics in Cognitive Development, Vol. 2*. New York, NY: Plenum Press. LANGUAGE AND COGNITIVE DEVELOPMENT:

Inhelder, Bärbel, Lezine, I., Sinclair, Hermina, & Stambak, Mira. (1972). Les débuts de la fonction semiotique. Modèles animaux du comportement humain. (The origins of semiotic functions. Animal models of human behavior.). *Colloque international du CNRS*, 198, 133-144. SEMIOTIC FUNCTIONS PIAGETIAN THEORY: FRENCH

Inhelder, Bärbel, Lezine, I., Sinclair, Hermina, & Stambak, Mira. (1972). Les débuts de la fonction symbolique. (The origins of symbolic function.). *Archives de Psychologie*, 41, 187-243. SYMBOL DEVELOPMENT PIAGETIAN THEORY: FRENCH

Itakura, S., & Matsuzawa, T. (1993). Acquisiton of personal pronouns by a chimpanzee. In Herman, L. M., Roitblat, H. L. & Nachtigal, P. E. (Eds). *Language and communication: Comparative perspectives*. Hillsdale, NJ: Lawrence Erlbaum Associates. PRONOUNS-PERSONAL LANGUAGE AND OTHER PRIMATES:

Ito, Ryoko, Kondo, Kiyomi, Kihara, Kumiko, Matsuda, Keiko, & Kojima, Mami. (1991). The effect of mother-child affective interaction on self-other cognition and communicative activity: Mother-child play in a group therapy for children with pervasive developmental disorders. *Reports of the Research Institute for the Education of Exceptional Children*, 40. AUTISM LANGUAGE AND PLAY ADULT-CHILD INTERACTION:

> Mother-child play was investigated in a group consisting of seven autistic children and their mothers. Results indicate that autistic children are better able to communicate with their mothers after they have had an empathic relationship with them. From Child Development Abstracts.

Ittyerah, Miriam, & Samparapungavan, Ala. (1989). The performance of congenitally blind children in cognitive developmental tasks. *British Journal of Developmental Psychology*, 7, 129-139. BLIND CHILDREN:

> The study compare the performance of a group of congenitally blind children and two groups of sighted children, one of which was blindfolded and the other, visually informed. Results indicate that cognitive development in the blind is not identical to that in the sighted groups. The differences in performance between groups are content or task specific and do not take the form of a global deficit across all developmental tasks. - From Child Development Abstracts..

J

Jackson, Catherine A. (1989). Language acquisition in two modalities: the role of nonlinguistic cues in linguistic mastery. *Sign Language Studies*, 62, 1-22. SIGNING BIMODALITY DEAF CHILDREN:

From Stockholm Bibliographies.

Jacobs, P. (1991). Making sense of lexical acquisition. In U. Zernik (Ed.), *Lexical acquisition: Exploiting on-line resources to build a lexicon*. Hillsdale, NJ : Lawrence Erlbaum Associates. LEXICAL DEVELOPMENT:

Jacobson, John T. (1985). *The auditory brainstem response.* San Diego, CA: Singular Publishing Group. TRAUMATIC DISORDERS AUDIOMETRY CONGENITAL DISORDERS ATYPICAL DEVELOPMENT AUDIOLOGY:

An overview of the auditory brainstem response. Neural generators of the auditory brainstem response. Instrumentation and signal processing. Stimulus calibration in ABR measurements. Normative aspects of the ABR. Interpretation: problems and pitfalls. Conductive hearing loss and the ABR. The effect of cochlear lesions on the ABR. Frequency specificity in evoked potential audiometry. ABR in eighth nerve and low brainstem lesions. ABR in upper brainstem lesions. Physiological responses in multiple sclerosis and other demyelinating diseases. The ABR in intraoperative monitoring. Monitoring neurologic status of comotose patients in the intensive care unit. Neurologic applications of the auditory brainstem response to the pediatric age group. Infant assessment: developmental and age-related considerations.

Identification of congenital hearing loss with the auditory brainstem response. Auditory brainstem response measures with multiply handicapped children and adults. Auditory brainstem response hearing aid applications. Auditory brainstem response testing strategies. Special case studies. Author index. Subject index.

Jacobson, John T., & Northern, Jerry L. (1991). *Diagnostic audiology*. San Diego, CA: Singular Publishing Group. AUDIOLOGY:

Overview of auditory diagnosis. Special auditory tests: a historical perspective. Audiologic instrumentation. Otologic evaluation. Otoneurologic diseases and associated audiologic profiles. Immittance measures in auditory disorders. Strategies for optimizing the detection of neuropathology from the auditory brainstem response. Diagnosis of middle ear pathology and evaluation of convective hearing loss. Evaluation and diagnosis of cochlear disorders. Acoustic neuroma: diagnosis and management. Central auditory disorders. Assessment of infants for hearing impairments. Balance disorders (the dizzy patient). Auditory test strategy. Index.

Jaeger, J. J. (1992). Not by the chair of my hinny hin hin - some general properties of slips of the tongue in young children. *Journal of Child Language*, 19, 335-366. SPEECH ERRORS:

James, Sharon L. (1990). *Normal language acquisition*. Boston, MA: College-Hill/Little, Brown. ACQUISITION THEORIES-OVERVIEW:

Jansonius-Schultheiss, Kino. (1981). Verbal apraxia in children and adults. *Logopedie en Foniatrie*, 53 (9), 408-426. APRAXIA:

Study in verbal dyspraxia and apraxia in relation to speech and linguistic factors. Description of method of assessment, differential diagnosis as well as method of treatment of young apractic children and adults by speech pathologists.KJS

Jansonius-Schultheiss, Kino. (1983). Readings in child phonology. *Logopedie en Foniatrie*, 55 (10), 340-342. OVERVIEW-PHONOLOGY ARTICULATION DISORDERS PHONOLOGICAL DEVELOPMENT:

The importance of child phonology in the treatment of articulation in young speech disturbed children.KJS

Jansonius-Schultheiss, Kino. (1985). Is there a relation between eating and learning to speak? In *Proceedings 9, Institute of Phonetic Sciences*. Amsterdam: University of Amsterdam. LANGUAGE AND MOTOR DEVELOPMENT:

Overview of the literature concerning the relation between mouth function (development) and speech development.KJS

Jansonius-Schultheiss, Kino. (1986). Dysphasia in children (in Dutch). *Logopedie en Foniatrie*, 58, 192-107. DEVELOPMENTAL DISORDERS READING DISORDERS: DUTCH

Overview of the literature on (developmental) dysphasia, assessment and suggestions for treatment also related to reading problems.KJS

Jansonius-Schultheiss, Kino. (1986). Mouth movements and mouth behaviours: a dialogue between dentists and speech pathologists. *Nederlands Tandartsenblad*, 41, 50-54. LANGUAGE AND MOTOR DEVELOPMENT ARTICULATION: DUTCH

Descriptions of the relations between oral functions and speech as well as suggestions for cooperation between dentists (engaged in regular as well as special dental care) and speech pathologists.KJS

Jansonius-Schultheiss, Kino. (1987). Not in touch: a communication disorder in development. In *Proceedings 11, Institute of Phonetic Sciences*. Amsterdam: University of Amsterdam. BABBLING CLEFT PALATE VOCALIZATIONS METHODOLOGY-LONGITUDINAL STUDY AT-RISK CHILDREN INTERSUBJECTIVITY ADULT-CHILD INTERACTION:

Longitudinal study on mother-infant communicative interaction in a mother-child pair (cleft palate baby 0:2-2:0

year) in which the verbal communication slowly is extinguished in the second year of life.KJS

Jansonius-Schultheiss, Kino. (1988). Mother-infant interaction in two-year-old cleft palate children (in Dutch). In P. Janssen (Ed.), *Afscheidssymposium Prof. Dr. P. H. Damste*. Utrecht: Afd. Foniatrie, AZU. INTERSUBJECTIVITY ADULT-CHILD INTERACTION CLEFT PALATE TURN TAKING IMITATION PARENTAL INPUT INPUT FACTORS: DUTCH

Mother-infant communications in two year old cleft palate children. Verbal interactions (turn-taking aspects as well as data on mother-child speech imitations) are related to parental opinions concerning child rearing practices.KJS

Jansonius-Schultheiss, Kino. (1989). The communicative development of two children with a cleft lip and palate (in Dutch). *Logopedie en Foniatrie*, 61, 348-352. CLEFT PALATE ADULT-CHILD INTERACTION INTERSUBJECTIVITY PARENTAL INPUT: DUTCH

Comparison of the speech development in interaction of two cleft lip and palate boys (0:2-2:0 year) with the maternal communicative pattern. Emphasis is given upon the amount of longitudinally described moments of communicative interactions in both of the children and the value of it for the speech development.KJS

Jansonius-Schultheiss, Kino. (1989). In dialogue: the development of communication of a mother and her cleft lip and palate baby during the first two years of life. In E. Beyaert, H. Bour, & W. v. Praag (Eds), *Effectonderzoek van Fysiotherapie en Logopedie*. Utrecht: CLEFT PALATE TURN TAKING ADULT-CHILD INTERACTION INTERSUBJECTIVITY GESTURE: DUTCH

Precursors of speech production delay in a two year old cleft palate boy: frequency of sound production, turn-taking aspects, communicative exchanges in the visual, mimic, handmovement mode of mother and child investigated.KJS

Jansonius-Schultheiss, Kino. (1989). Oral perception and communicative interaction in speech development: feeding a cleft lip and palate infant. In O. Kriens (Ed.), *What is a cleft lip and palate?*. Stuttgart, Germany: Georg Thieme Verlag. ADULT-CHILD INTERACTION LANGUAGE AND MOTOR DEVELOPMENT CLEFT PALATE BABBLING:

Relation between onset of milestones in speech movements in mother- child interaction in the process of feeding (i.e. oral stimulation) in the first year of life: overview of monthly analyzed speech productions of a cleft lip and palate baby (month 4 until 11) in the light of pre-child speech (speech facilitating) as well as post-child speech (speech reinforcement maternal communicative patterns).KJS

Jansonius-Schultheiss, Kino, Comijs, H., & Leyenaar, B. (1990). Developments in the treatment of cleft lip and palate. *Logopedie en Foniatrie*, 62 (9), 262-267. CLEFT PALATE INTERVENTION PROGRAMS:

Overview of relevant topics in medical intervention as well as speech and linguistic treatment of cleft lip and palate children. Critical evaluation of research data as presented at the 6th International Congress on Cleft Palate and Craniofacial Anomalies (June 1989, Jerusalem, Israel).KJS

Jansonius-Schultheiss, Kino, & Stam, C. (1985). Dysphasia in children. *Van Horen Zeggen*, 3, 79-85. DEVELOPMENTAL DISORDERS:

Discussion on developmental dysphasia.

Jansonius-Schultheiss, Kino, van Copenolle, L., & Beyaert, E. (1987). *Deviant mouth habits and speech: introduction, assessment and treatment*. Leuven, The Netherlands: Acco. LANGUAGE AND MOTOR DEVELOPMENT: DUTCH

Description as well as assessment of milestones in mouth development, mouth functions and noxious mouth habits, related to feeding and speech (development) as well as feeding and speech (developmental) problems.KJS

Jansonius-Schultheiss, Kino, & van der Stelt, J. M. (1990). Book for parents: questions about the development of your baby (in Dutch). In *Report nr 113, Instituut voor Fonetische Wetenschappen*. Amsterdam: Universiteit van Amsterdam. METHODOLOGY INTERVENTION PROGRAMS FOR PARENTS: DUTCH

Questionaires about daily routines, illnesses, psycho-motor and social development, infant temperament, speech productions, feeding and oral behaviors and child rearing practices.KJS

Jansonius-Schultheiss, Kino, & van der Stelt, J. M. (1990). Overview of literature belonging to the study on the influence of an oral plate upon the speech development and interaction in the first years of life of babies with a cleft lip and palate (in Dutch). In *Report nr 111, Instituut voor Fonetische Wetenschappen*. Amsterdam: Universiteit van Amsterdam. CLEFT PALATE: DUTCH

Jansonius-Schultheiss, Kino, van der Stelt, J. M., & Koopmans-van Beinum, F. J. (1986). Relation between mouth functioning and the onset of babbling (in Dutch). *Logopedie en Foniatrie*, 58, 238-241. BABBLING LANGUAGE AND MOTOR DEVELOPMENT: DUTCH

Data on the onset of babbling in relation to specific oral movements.KJS

Jarovinskij, Alexandr. (1977). K voprosu o razvitii kommunikativnoj kompetencii dvujazichnogo rebenka (On the question of the bilingual child's communicative competence development). In J. Linhart (Ed.), *Proceedings of the 3rd Prague Conference on Psychology of Human Learning and Development*. Prague: BILINGUALISM-COMMUNICATIVE COMPETENCE: SERBOCROATIAN

Jarovinskij, Alexandr. (1979). On the lexical competence of bilingual children of kindergarten age groups. *International Journal of Psycholinguistics*, 6 (15), 43-57. HUNGARIAN-RUSSIAN RUSSIAN-HUNGARIAN BILINGUALISM-LANGUAGE PREFERENCE:

16 children (10 female, 6 male) of intellectually mixed family background living in Budapest, with Russian mothers and Hungarian fathers were investigated. Two groups, A and B, with average age of 4:2 and 6:1 years, were formed. The social

background of families were reconstructed from data gained via questionnaires in both languages. A dominance coefficient for passive lexis was defined with a Hungarian version of the Peabody Picture Vocabulary Test and its Russian equivalent. The picture set of the same test was applied to gain dominant coefficients for active word use. Average results in both groups show that Hungarian dominates both passive and active vocabulary, while this effect seems to be stronger in Group A. Objective (birth order, the frequency of returning to a Russian language area) as well as subjective (motivational base in parents familial attitudes towards mastering the Russian language) were factors influencing the level of interlingual dominance in lexis brought about different patterns in Group A as compared to Group B.AJ

Jarovinskij, Alexandr. (1979). Vocabulary and syntax of bilingual children at preschool age. *Hungarológiai Közlemények*, 39 (40), 15-36. HUNGARIAN-RUSSIAN RUSSIAN-HUNGARIAN INTERFERENCE BILINGUALISM-SYNTACTIC DEVELOPMENT BILINGUALISM-VOCABULARY DEVELOPMENT TRANSFER: HUNGARIAN

The author studied the lexical and syntactic competence of Hungarian-Russian bilingual children in the preschool age. 18 children (10 girls and 8 boys) coming from 15 mixed families and attending Hungarian kindergartens participated in the experiment. In group A, consisting of 9 children, the mean age was 4:2, in group B (9 children)-6:1. All the children had Russian speaking mothers and Hungarian speaking fathers. Other children, group B, were in a more advantageous position regarding the acquisition of the Russian language. Average results in both groups showed that Hungarian dominates both passive and active vocabulary, while this effect was stronger in Group A. A qualitative analysis of word use - in case of PPVT - unambiguously proved that semantization of words in the less dominant language was insufficient in bilingual children. In balanced bilingualism a tendency has been revealed - in the case of describing pictures that correlated with the cognitive development of children. In older children there was a shift from dialogue-like description towards connected discourse. At the same time, the dominance of the environmental language (Hungarian) has an influence on picture description: more word types and tokens are used in Hungarian, as well as more complex sentences. A qualitative analysis of grammatical errors helped to reveal bilingual children's language acquisition strategies. There were two types of 'good' errors, connected to the acquisition strategies of Hungarian and Russian, and two other types, connected to transfer strategies. Syntactical models of Hungarian interfere more frequently in the Russian speech of children.AJ

Jarovinskij, Alexandr. (1980). Data on the vocabulary of bilingual nursery school-aged children. *Magyar Pszichológiai Szemle*, 4, 380-401. BILINGUALISM-MOTIVATION BILINGUALISM-LANGUAGE PREFERENCE: HUNGARIAN

An examination of the bilingual competence of the vocabulary of Hungarian-Russian bilingual children. 16 children-10 girls and 6 boys-took part in the survey. The children came from 14 intellectual families where the mother's language is Russian and that of the father is Hungarian. The families have lived in different parts of Budapest for six years on the average. The children we examined were divided into 2 groups according to their age: the age of children in group A was 4:2 months on the average and that of group B was 6:1 months. The data gained showed that in both groups the passive vocabulary and word usage dominates in Hungarian language but this dominance is somewhat stronger in group A. The objective factors influencing the vocabulary-dominance (sibling rank and the frequency of staying in Russian language area) and the subjective factors (the motivational base of the parents' family attitude toward learning the Russian language) formed differently in the two groups. The qualitative analysis of the answers (the so-called associative answers, the wrong answers with similar sounds, and the functional descriptions instead of naming) show that the semantization of words is insufficient in the less dominant language in case of bilingual children.AJ

Jarovinskij, Alexandr. (1983). Pszichológiai szempontok a gyermekkori kétnyelvüség megitelésében (Psychological aspects of childhood bilingualism). *Nyelvpedagógiai írások*, 4, 122-141. BILINGUALISM-PROBLEMS/EFFECTS BILINGUALISM-COGNITIVE DEVELOPMENT: HUNGARIAN

Jarovinskij, Alexandr. (1984). Faktori sredi vlijajucshie na bilingval'nuju kompetenciju dvujazichnih doshkol'nikov (Factors of environment influencing on the bilingual competence of preschool children). In M. Kodim, & I. Slamenik (Eds), *Proceedings of the 4th Prague International Conference*. Prague: Academia. BILINGUALISM-MOTIVATION BILINGUALISM-ATTITUDES BILINGUALISM-PROBLEMS/EFFECTS BILINGUALISM-COGNITIVE DEVELOPMENT BILINGUALISM-EDUCATION: SERBOCROATIAN

Jarovinskij, Alexandr. (1984). Picture description of bilingual children at preschool age. *Acta Linguistica Academiae Scientiarum Hungaricae*, 34(1-2), 95-106. CHILDREN'S DESCRIPTIONS BILINGUALISM-PRESCHOOLERS HUNGARIAN:

Jarovinskij, Alexandr. (1985). Magyar-orosz kétnyelvü óvodások képleírása (Picture description of Hungarian-Russian bilingual nursery school children). In J. Kádár (Ed.), *Beszéd és kommunikáció az óvodás- és kisiskoláskorban*. Budapest: Akadémiai Kiadó. HUNGARIAN-RUSSIAN RUSSSIAN-HUNGARIAN BILINGUALISM-EDUCATION: HUNGARIAN

Speech and communication in kindergarten and early school age.AJ

Jarovinskij, Alexandr. (1986). A gyermekkori termeszetés kétnyelvüség pszichológiai, pszicholingvisztikai kutatása (Psychological, psycholinguistic studies of natural childhood bilingualism). In K. Klaudy, & Z. Lengyel (Ed.), *Az idegen nyelvi nevelés-oktatás nehány iránya és lehetösége*. Budapest: BILINGUALISM-SEQUENTIAL L2 EDUCATION: HUNGARIAN

Some directions and possibilities in foreign language teaching and learning.AJ

Jarovinskij, Alexandr, & Fabricius, Ildikó. (1978). Kommunikatív folyamatok strategiája kétnyelvü gyermeknél. (The strategy of communicative processes in a bilingual child.). *Magyar*

Pszichológiai Szemle, 1, 72-80. BILINGUALISM-COMMUNICATIVE COMPETENCE: HUNGARIAN

Jarovinskij, Alexandr, & Fabricius, Ildiko. (1988). On communicative competence of a bilingual child. *Acta Linguistico Academiae Scientiarum Hungaricae*, 38, 2-13. BILINGUALISM-PRAGMATIC DEVELOPMENT CODE-SWITCHING BILINGUALISM-COMMUNICATIVE COMPETENCE:

Observations and experiences covering two years permit specific conclusions to be drawn on the basis of the material: (1) the two language systems show an approximate balance all along the period reported (age 1:8 to 2:1): (2) a dominance of the situative events cause the use of the inappropriate code by the child. He will fail to break the limit of a language system, associated with a situation earlier experienced as embedded in a communicative process: (3) in face to face interactions (two persons only), no confusion of the two language systems is observed in the given period of life. The child tries to remain within the confines of one language system at any rate by appealing to all verbal and non-verbal means available to him: (4) an early but clear-cut discrimination is proposed to evolve on the basis of emotional relations 'via different languages.' (v) A phenomenon of early- childhood 'interpreting' grows out of (the use of) equivalent, setting-specific linguistic schemes and pre-abstractional, situative translations: (5) monologues serve both for practicing of functions and for a social form of imaginary dialogue. In the case reported, they display a stratified structure with no confusions of signs from the two languages within one unit: (6) deficiency of communicative competence is recorded, in our case, concerning Russian language. The child is unable to generalize the communicative use of a language acquired exclusively through interaction with one person. Early acquisition of two languages is ultimately tied to specific situations and personal relations.AJ

Jensen, Arthur R. (1989). The relationship between learning and intelligence. *Learning and Individual Differences*, 1, 37-62. INDIVIDUAL VARIATION:

It is argued that observed correlations between individual differences in learning and intelligence can best be understood from the viewpoint of information processing theory, in particular, in terms of individual differences in the speed of operation of the various components of the information processing system. - From Child Development Abstracts.

Jensen, R. A. (1991). Family characteristics of autistic children - a further report. *Journal of Autism and Developmental Disorders*, 21, 557-558. AUTISM PARENTAL INPUT INPUT FACTORS AT-RISK CHILDREN ADULT-CHILD INTERACTION SOCIAL INTERACTION:

Jepson, Jil. (1989). The acquisition of categories in Chinese. *Lingua*, 78(2/3), 193-216. CHINESE CATEGORIZATION:

From Stockholm Bibliographies.

Jerger, James. (1984). *Pediatric audiology: current trends*. San Diego, CA: Singular Publishing Group. AUDIOLOGY AUDIOMETRY LANGUAGE AND EDUCATION DEAF CHILDREN:

Behavioral audiometry. Immittance audiometry. Speech audiometry. Electrophysiologic audiometry. Wearable amplification: a litany of persisting problems. Amplification in the educational setting. Habilitation of the hearing-impaired. Legislative issues in the habilitation of the hearing impaired.

Jerger, Susan, & Jerger, James. (1981). *Auditory disorders:a manual for clinical evaluation*. San Diego, CA: Singular Publishing Group. AUDIOLOGY CLASSIFICATION OF DISORDERS:

Acoustic schwannoma. Cerebrovascular disorders. Cholesteatoma. Collapsing ear canal. Diabetes mellitus. Discontinuity of the ossicular chain. Facial nerve disorders. Functional hearing disorders. Glomus jugulare tumors. Hereditary familial sensorineural hearing loss. Herpes. Zoster oticus. Intracranial tumors affecting the central auditory system. Malleus fixation. Meniere's disease. Multiple sclerosis. Noise-induced hearing loss. Otitis media. Otosclerosis. Ototoxicity. Paget's disease. Presbyacusis. Sudden (idiopathic) sensorineural hearing loss. Syphilis. Trauma. Glossary of selected test procedures. Glossary of terms and abbreviations.

Jeyifous, S. W. (1992). Developmental changes in the representation of word meaning-cross-cultural findings. *British Journal of Developmental Psychology*, 10, 285-299. CROSSLINGUISTIC STUDY-SEMANTICS REPRESENTATIONS-SEMANTIC:

Jirsa, P. E. (1992). The clinical utility of the P3-AERP in children with auditory processing disorders. *Journal of Speech and Hearing Research*, 35, 903-912. AUDITORY DISORDERS DEAF CHILDREN:

Jisa, Harriet. (1987). Sentence connectors in French children's monologue performance. *Journal of Pragmatics*, 11, 607-621. FRENCH CONNECTIVES DISCOURSE COHERENCE:

Sentence connectors play a principle role in the construction of texts. Learning to use sentence connectors, then, is an important step in the acquisition of skills necessary for the production of oral monologues. This work describes six monolingual French speaking children's (ages 3:2 to 4:10) uses of high frequency oral discourse connectors in nursery school situated narrative performance. The results show that part of the developmental process involves enlarging the set of connectors in the developing lexicon. In addition it is shown that children fine-tune the use of early acquired connectors in part by replacing existing functions with semantically more appropriate connectors. Finally, it is shown that an important factor in learning the appropriate conditions controlling high frequency connectors is learning when not to use them.HJ

Jisa, Harriet. (1989). The process of language replacement. In *Actes du Symposium AILA/CILA: Minorisation linguistique et interaction*. Commission Interuniversitaire Suiss de Linguistique Appliquee. BILINGUALISM-SIMULTANEOUS BILINGUALISM-LANGUAGE PREFERENCE:

Young children's simultaneous acquisition of two languages offers an excellent field for the exploration of a number of issues in language development. This paper underlines the importance of studies of childhood bilingualism for theories of language acquisition in general. Specifically, it discusses two bilingual children's replacement of the productively dominant language, French, by their non-dominant language, English.HJ

Jisa, Harriet. (1990). Le rôle des réformulations dans l'acquisition des langues: observation de la zone proximale du développement. (The role of clarification requests in the acquisiiton of language.). In *Actes du Colloque du Groupe de Recheche sur l'Acquisition des Langues*. Aix-en-Provence: Presses Universitaires. ADULT-CHILD INTERACTION CLARIFICATION REQUESTS: FRENCH

Learning to communicate is not necessarily equivalent to acquiring a language. Social interaction is, of course, the context in which the process of language acquisition can be observed, but one may ask what is the relationship between learning to communicate and learning linguistic forms. This article attempts to show how one can investigate the exact relation between conversation and acquisition through the study of clarification sequences in adult-child interaction.HJ

Jisa, Harriet, & Cosnier, Jacques. (1987). L'évolution de la fonction communicative. (The evolution of linguistic competence). *Pédiatrie*, 42, 509-517. INTENTIONALITY ADULT-CHILD INTERACTION INTERSUBJECTIVITY: FRENCH

This presentation in recent developments in child language research attempts to show that communicative competence is not built solely upon purely linguistic linguistic foundations. The development of communicative competence cannot be considered to begin with the first words. There is a growing body of evidence showing that functional communication appears long before the child's first uses of meaning-bearing sound sequences based on the adult language. Adult-child interaction, both during prelinguistic and early linguistic stages, provides an essential framework upon which verbal communication is based. The acquisition of what can be considered pragmatic competence, necessary for all communication, begins from birth.HJ

Jisa, Harriet, & Mariotte, Daniel. (1990). L'explication dans l'interaction enfant-enfant: co-construction de la cognition sociale. (The explanation in children's social speech with each other.). In *Les cahiers d'acquisition et pathologie du langage: Le jeune enfant et l'explication*. Paris, France: Presses Universitaires, Universite Rene Descartes. CHILDREN'S EXPLANATIONS SOCIAL INTERACTION SOCIAL SPEECH LANGUAGE SOCIALIZATION: FRENCH

Given situationally appropriate explanations is a pervasive activity in everyday life. The ability to engage in such an activity emerges gradually over time and over contexts. This study attempts to contribute to our understanding of the structures and functions of children's explanations in the contexts in which they emerge and develop. It argues that the evolution observed in children's performance should take into account developments in the child's understanding and representation of everyday life and conversation. It also argues that child-child interaction offers an excellent arena for the observation of how social cognition is co-constructed in what can be considered a dominant vehicle of socialization, everyday conversation.HJ

Joanette, Y., & Brownell, H.M. (1990). *Discourse ability and brain damage*. New York, NY: Springer-Verlag. TRAUMATIC DISORDERS DISCOURSE DISORDERS DEVELOPMENTAL DISORDERS:

The papers in this collection look at the historical and theoretical background of discourse analysis, and text analysis. It then turns to an examination of the impairments in discourse function suffered by adults and children who have suffered traumatic brain damage, and in congenital aphasias.

Joanette, Y., Goulet, P., & Hannequin, D. (1990). *Right hemisphere and verbal communication*. New York, NY: Springer-Verlag. LATERALIZATION COMMISUROTOMY TRAUMATIC DISORDERS PROSODY WRITTEN LANGUAGE PRAGMATIC DISORDERS LEXICAL DEVELOPMENT:

This books looks at the role of the right (nondominant language) hemisphere in verbal communication. It reviews previous work in the areas of commisurotomy and brain trauma, as well as experimental work with normal subjects. The final chapters discuss the nondominant hemisphere's role in lexical-semantics, written language, prosody, and pragmatics.

Johnson, Donna M. (1991). *Approaches to research in second language learning*. New York, NY: Longman. L2 RESEARCH DESIGN METHODOLOGY-DESIGN METHODOLOGY-ANALYSIS:

Johnson, Janice, Fabian, Veronica, & Pascual-Leone, Juan. (1989). Quantitative hardware stages that constrain language development. *Human Development*, 32(5), 245-271. CONSTRAINTS-BIOLOGICAL CONSTRAINTS-COGNITIVE:

From Stockholm Bibliographies.

Johnson, Janice, & Pascual-Lenoe, Juan. (1989). If you had my brain, where would I be? Children's understanding of the brain and identity. *Journal of Experimental Child Psychology*, 48, 1-31. FIGURATIVE LANGUAGE DEIXIS-PERSONAL PRONOUNS-PERSONAL:

Processing score increased with age in a predictable way. Growth in a mental attention resource accounted for much of the developmental variance in metaphor interpretation.

Johnson, J. M., Watkins, R. V., & Rice, Mabel L. (1992). Bimodal bilingual language development in a hearing child of deaf parents. *Applied Psycholinguistics*, 13, 31-52. BIMODALITY DEAF PARENTS:

Johnson, M. J. (1992). What's basic in a student-centered reading, writing, and thinking approach-one teachers perspective. *Volta Review*, 94 , 389-394. LITERACY WRITTEN LANGUAGE LANGUAGE AND EDUCATION:

Johnston, Judith R. (1981). Cognition and language in the preschool years. *Topics in Language Disorders*, 2(1), CAUSALITY SPATIAL TERMS TEMPORAL TERMS SYMBOL DEVELOPMENT LANGUAGE AND COGNITIVE DEVELOPMENT:

A special issue of *Topics in Language Disorders* edited by Judith Johnson concerning the relationship between language and cognition. The papers' topics include: symbol development, causality, space, number, time, and social aspects of language and cognition.

Johnston, Judith R. (1981). On location: Thinking and talking about space. *Topics in Language Disorders*, 2, 17-32. LOCATIVES SPATIAL TERMS NONLINGUISTIC STRATEGIES LANGUAGE AND COGNITIVE DEVELOPMENT:

A description of the relationship between the development of nonverbal spatial concepts and the acquisition of locatives.JRJ

Johnston, Judith R. (1982). Interpreting the Leiter IQ: Performance profiles of young normal and language disordered children. *Journal of Speech and Hearing Research*, 25, 291-296. ASSESSMENT PROCEDURES LEITER INTELLIGENCE TEST CONCEPT DEVELOPMENT DEVELOPMENTAL SCALES:

Demonstrates that this non-verbal intelligence test reflects only a very narrow range of intellectual abilities which helps to explain how it is possible to have a normal performance IQ and still be delayed in concept development and reasoning ability. JRJ.

Johnston, Judith R. (1982). Narratives: A new look at communication problems in older language disordered children. *Language, Speech and Hearing Services in Schools*, 13, 65-75. NARRATIVES TEXT/STORY GRAMMARS EVENTS/SCRIPTS DISCOURSE COHERENCE RECASTS METHODLOGY-DESIGN:

An analysis of a language impaired child's (eight-years-old) story telling which demonstrates that in a recasting situation the story being retold may not be the one that the original story teller meant to be shared. Stories are analyzed from the perspectives of Story Grammar, Script, Cohesion, and Communicative Effectiveness. JRJ.

Johnston, Judith R. (1983). What is language intervention? The role of theory. In J. Miller, D. Schiefelbusch, & D. Yoder (Ed.), *Contemporary issues in language intervention*. Rockville, MD: American Speech-Language-Hearing Association. INTERVENTION PROGRAMS ACQUISITION AND LINGUISTIC THEORY:

Argues that language intervention cannot be defined without reference to particular theories of language, learning, and impairment and contends that clinical work must be grounded in some implicit theory. JRJ.

Johnston, Judith R. (1985). The discourse symtpoms of developmental disorders. In T. V. Dijk (Ed.), *Handbook of discourse analysis*. San Diego, CA: Academic Press. DISCOURSE DISORDERS PRAGMATIC DISORDERS:

A critical review of the literature on atypical development which argues that the classification "pragmatic disorder" has yet to be justified. JRJ

Johnston, Judith R. (1985). Fit, focus, and functionality: An essay on early language intervention. *Child Language Teaching and Therapy*, 1, 125-134. INTERVENTION PROGRAMS METHODOLOGY-DESIGN:

Presents a set of general intervention principles and a theory that explains why they should lead to programs which accelerate language learning. JRJ.

Johnston, Judith R. (1988). Specific language disorders in the child. In N. Lass, L. McReynolds, J.Northern, & D. Yoder (EdS), *Handbook of speech-language-pathology and audiology*. Philadelphia, PA: B. C. Decker. SPECIFIC LANGUAGE IMPAIRMENT:

A comprehensive review of the literature on the cognitive, perceptual, and linguistic abilities of SLI children.JRJ

Johnston, Judith R. (1990). A second look at neo-nativism. *Journal of Speech Language Pathology and Audiology*, 14, 41-45. INTERVENTION PROGRAMS PARAMETER SETTING ACQUISITION AND LINGUISTIC THEORY NATIVISM:

A critique of Connell's attempt to apply Government Binding Theory and Universal Grammar frameworks to language intervention. JRJ.

Johnston, Judith R. (1991). The continuing relevance of cause. *Language, Speech, Hearing Services in Schools*, 22, 75-79. LANGUAGE AND COGNITION METHODOLOGY:

This article supports the view that even though psychological studies of language impaired children may not reveal the etiology of developmental disorders, they are useful as a means of examining the relationship between language and thought and can reveal knowledge about the mechanisms of language acquisition and language learning.JRJ

Johnston, Judith R. (1991). Questions about cognition in children with specific language impairment. In J. Miller (Ed.), *Research on child language disorders: A decade of progress*. Austin, TX: Pro-Ed. LANGUAGE DISORDERS LANGUAGE AND COGNITION LANGUAGE PROCESSING:

Identifies two areas for further study: symbolic function and cognitive processing.JRJ

Johnston, Judith R. (1992). Cognition and language impaired chldren. In P. Fletcher, & D. Hall (Eds), *Specific speech and language disorders in children*. London: Whurr. LANGUAGE DISORDERS DEVELOPMENTAL DISORDERS LANGUAGE AND COGNITION:

Review of work on nonverbal cognition and specific language impairment that stresses the likelihood that language impairment influences reasoning abilities and questions the value of "capacity limitation" as a useful explanantory construct. JRJ.

Johnston, Judith R. (1993). Definition and diagnosis of language development disorders. In G. Blanken, J.Dittman, H. Grimm, J. Marshall, & C. Wallesch (Ed.), *Linguistic disorders and pathologies: An international handbook*. Berlin: De Gruyter. DEVELOPMENTAL DISORDERS CLASSIFICATION OF DISORDERS:

A criticism of the "medical model" approach to describing and treating developmental language disorders. Reviews a selection of findings which describe developmental disorders in terms of general theories of normal language development. JRJ.

Johnston, Judith R. (1993). Specific language impairment, cognition, and the biological basis of language. In M. Gopnik (Ed.), *The biological basis of language*. New York, NY: Oxford University Press. BIOLOGICAL FOUNDATIONS MODULARITY ATTENTION LANGUAGE AND PERCEPTION SPECIFIC LANGUAGE IMPAIRMENT LANGUAGE AND COGNITION:

A review of the work on nonverbal cognition and its relationship to language learning.JRJ

Johnston, Judith R., Ammon, M., & Kahmi, Alan G. (1988). Language development chart. *Topics in Language Disorders*, 8, 42-53. MORPHOLOGICAL DEVELOPMENT EARLY SYNTACTIC DEVELOPMENT LEXICAL DEVELOPMENT FIRST WORDS DEVELOPMENTAL SCALES:

A two page summary of the major developments in the acquisition of English syntax, morphology, and the lexicon during the period from 2:0 to 3:0 years.JRJ

Johnston, Judith R., Blathchley, M., & Streit, G. Olness. (1990). Miniature language system learning in proficient and nonproficient learners. *Journal of Speech and Hearing Research*, 33, 335-343. MINIATURE LINGUISTIC SYSTEMS LANGUAGE AND PERCEPTION ATTENTION:

A within-child comparison of the relative difficulty of learning two miniature languages with differing grammars. The results indicate the role of perceptual salience in language learning, and reveal unusual patterns of attention (resource allocation) in poor learners. JRJ.

Johnston, Judith R., & Bowman, S. (1990). Garden Picture Vocabulary Tests: Relationships between performance in expression and reception. *International Journal of Clinical Neuropsychology*, 12,

103-106. ASSESSMENT PROCEDURES GARDEN PICTURE VOCABULARY TESTS TRAUMATIC DISORDERS VOCABULARY DEVELOPMENT:

Demonstrates that there is a disparity between the Expressive and Receptive Scales on this test which make it unacceptable as a means of assessing the relative strengths of language production and comprehension unless the subject of the test has suffered a neurological trauma. In the case of such a trauma, the Expressive Scale scores are depressed by the neuro-motor damage.JRJ

Johnston, Judith R., Miller, Jonathan F., Tallal, Paula, & Curtiss, Susan R. (1993). Conversations with language impaired children. *Journal of Speech and Hearing Research*. METHODOLOGY-DESIGN CHILDREN'S RESPONSES ATYPICAL DEVELOPMENT:

Looks at the effects of using a structured interview elicitation format to obtain language sample data. In particular the relationship between number of adult questions and the degree of ellipsis (and MLU) in chldren's speech. Compares normal and language impaired preschoolers. JRJ.

Johnston, Judith R., & Ramstad, V. (1983). Cognitive development in pre-adolescent language impaired children. *British Journal of Disorders of Communication*, 18, 49-55. LANGUAGE AND COGNITIVE DEVELOPMENT SPECIFIC LANGUAGE IMPAIRMENT CONCEPT DEVELOPMENT MODULARITY:

Demonstrates that older language impaired children are conceptually delayed and counters the whole notion of a "specific" language impairment. JRJ.

Jones, Charles. (1991). Comments on Goodluck and Behne. In J. Weissenborn, H. Goodluck, & T. Roeper (Eds), *Theoretical Issues in Language Acquisition-Continuity and Change in Development*. Hillsdale, NJ: Lawrence Erlbaum Associates. ACQUISITION THEORIES:

Jones, N. K. (1991). Development of morphophonemic segments in children's mental representations of words. *Applied Psycholinguistics*, 12, 217-239. REPRESENTATIONS-PHONOLOGICAL:

Jonkman, I., Licht, R., Bakker, D. J., & van den Broek-Sandmann, T. M. (1992). Shifting of attention in subtyped dyslexic children-an event-related potential study. *Developmental Neuropsychology*, 8, 243-259. DYSLEXIA READING DISORDERS:

Jordan, F. M., Murdoch, Bruce E., & Buttsworth, D. L. (1991). Closed-head-injured children's performance on narrative tasks. *Journal of Speech and Hearing Research*, 34, 572-582. TRAUMATIC DISORDERS NARRATIVES DISCOURSE DISORDERS:

Jordens, Peter. (1988). The acquisition of verb categories and word order in Dutch and German: Evidence from first and second language acquisition. In J. Pankhurst, M. S. Smith, & P. van Buren (Eds), *Learnability and Second Languages.* Dordrecht: Foris. GERMAN DUTCH GERMAN-DUTCH DUTCH-GERMAN L2 WORD ORDER WORD ORDER VERBS:

Jordens, Peter. (1988). The acquisition of word order in Dutch and German as L1 and L2. *Second Language Research.*, 4, 41-65. DUTCH-GERMAN GERMAN-DUTCH L2 WORD ORDER WORD ORDER GERMAN DUTCH:

Jordens, Peter. (1988). The aquisition of word order in L2 Dutch and German. In P. Jordens, & J. Lalleman (Eds), *Language development.* Dordrecht: Foris. L2 WORD ORDER DUTCH-GERMAN GERMAN-DUTCH WORD ORDER DUTCH GERMAN:

Jordens, Peter. (1988). Tweede-taalverwerving en universele grammatica. Taalverwerving en taalonderzoek. *Toegepaste Taalwetenschap in Artikelen*, 30, 31-47. DUTCH PARAMETER SETTING: DUTCH

Jordens, Peter. (1989). Case errors in German as a foreign language. Kinds and causes. In R. Freudenstein (Ed.), *Error in foreign languages. Analysis and treatment..* Marburg: Informationszentrum für Fremdsprachenforschung. CASE GERMAN L2 MORPHOSYNTAX:

Jordens, Peter. (1989). Talen kun je lernen. Tussen taaltheorie en praktij. In *Rede uitgesproken bij de aanvaarding van het ambt van gewoon hoogleraar in de Toegepaste Taalwetenschap aan de Vrije Universiteit to Amsterdam op donderdag 18 mei 1989*. Dordrecht: Foris. DUTCH: DUTCH

Jordens, Peter. (1990). The acquisition of verb placement in Dutch and German. *Linguistics*, 28(6), DUTCH GERMAN WORD ORDER SYNTACTIC STRUCTURES:

Jordens, Peter. (1990). Linguistics and second language acquisition. In T. Bongaerts (Ed.), *Balance and perspective. 25 years of Dutch applied linguistics. Toegepaste Taalwetenschap in Artikelen,* 36. L2 ACQUISITION L2 LINGUISTIC THEORY: DUTCH

Jordens, Peter, de Bot, K., & Trapman, H. (1989). Linguistic aspects of regression in German case marking. *Studies in Second Language Acquisition.*, 11, 179-204. L2 MORPHOSYNTAX CASE GERMAN UNLEARNING:

Jordens, Peter, & Lalleman, J. (1988). *Language development*. Dordrecht: Foris. OVERVIEW-GENERAL:

Jorm, A. F. (1991). The validity of word age-of-acquisition ratings-a longitudinal study of a child's word knowledge. *British Journal of Developmental Psychology*, 9, 437-444. VOCABULARY DEVELOPMENT:

Joshi, R. Malatesha. (1991). *Written language disorders*. Hingham, MA: Kluwer Academic Press. WRITTEN LANGUAGE AGRAPHIA BILINGUALISM-LANGUAGE DISORDERS:

A collection of papers dealing with the loss of spelling and writing abilities by both monolingual and bilingual speakers.

Juhász, Agnés. (1986). A beszéd és nyelvi fejlödés elmaradása mint vezetötünet. (Speech and language retardation as a critical symptom). *Gyógypedagógiai Szemle*, 4, LANGUAGE DISORDERS HUNGARIAN: HUNGARIAN

Juhász, Agnés, & Bittera, E. (1989). Examination of speech and language-from speech-therapist's point of view. *Hungarian Papers in Phonetics*, 21, 182-184. CLASSIFICATION OF DISORDERS HUNGARIAN:

Jung, Jack H. (1989). *Genetic syndromes in communication disorders.* San Diego, CA: Singular Group. CONGENITAL DISORDERS:

Topics include: principles of medical genetics, chromosomal syndromes, autosomal dominant and recessive diseases, X-linked diseases, polygenic-multifactorial syndromes, sporadic and environmental syndromes, and a glossary of medical terms.

Jusczyk, Peter W. (1992). Developing phonological categories from the speech signal. In C. A. Ferguson, L. Menn, & C. Stoel-Gammon (Eds), *Phonological development: Models, research, implications.* Monkton, MD: York Press. SPEECH PERCEPTION PHONEMIC DEVELOPMENT PHONOLOGICAL DEVELOPMENT:

Jusczyk, Peter W., Bertoncini, Josiane, Bijeljac-Babac, Ranka, Kennedy, Lori J., & Mehler, Jacques. (1990). The role of attention in speech perception by young infants. *Cognitive Development*, 5, 265-286. ATTENTION INFANT PERCEPTION NEONATES SPEECH PERCEPTION:

The present study explored how attentional focus affects the perceptions of speech in 4-day-old and 2-month-old infants. Attentional focus was manipulated by changing the composition of a set of syllables to which infants were habituated. Both 4-day-olds and 2-month-olds were able to detect the addition of a new syllable to the set. Two-month-olds, but not the 4-day- olds, were able to detect the addition of a new syllable that was similar to one of the familiarization set members.

K

Kagan, Aura, & Saling, Michael M. (1992). *An introduction to Luria's aphasiology*. Baltimore, MD: Paul H. Brookes. APHASIOLOGY ASSESSMENT PROCEDURES CLASSIFICATION OF DISORDERS LURIA-NEBRASKA NEUROPSYCHOLOGICAL BATTERY:

Explanation of the theoretical underpinning of Luria's work, classification and assessment of disorders, exemplification by case study, explains the Luria Neuropsychological Investigation and Luria-Nebraska Neuropsychological Battery instruments.

Kail, Michéle, & Weissenborn, Jürgen. (1991). Connectives: Developmental issues. In G. Pierraut-Le Bonniec, & M. Dolitsky (Ed.), *Language bases-Discourse bases: Some aspects of contemporary French psycholinguistics research*. Amsterdam, The Netherlands: John Benjamins. CONNECTIVES DISCOURSE COHERENCE FRENCH:

Kaler, Sandra R., & Kopp, Claire B. (1990). Compliance and comprehension in very young toddlers. *Child Development*, 61, 1997-2003. CHILDREN'S RESPONSES DISCOURSE COMPREHENSION ADULT-CHILD INTERACTION COMPREHENSION INTERSUBJECTIVITY:

Requests, using preselected words, were made to children in a naturalistic and pleasant play situation in a quasi-laboratory setting. Findings indicated significant shifts across age, with the most striking change occurring between 14-16 and 17-18 months. Comprehension influences compliance.

Kamhi, Alan G., Gentry, B., Mauer, D., & Gholson, B. (1990). Analogical learning and transfer in language-impaired children. *Journal of Speech and Hearing Disorders*, 55, 140-148. LANGUAGE AND COGNITION LANGUAGE AND COGNITIVE DEVELOPMENT LANGUAGE DISORDERS:

Kamhi, Alan G., & Johnston, Judith R. (1982). Towards an understanding of reatrded children's linguistic deficiencies. *Journal of Speech and Hearing Research*, 25, 435-445. RETARDED CHILDREN PRAGMATIC DISORDERS SPECIFIC LANGUAGE IMPAIRMENT LANGUAGE AND COGNITIVE DEVELOPMENT:

A comparison of the language devlopment of normal, language impaired, and mentally retarded children. The retarded children did not show the same kind of specific domain related deficiencies as the language impaired children, but they did show some pragmatic limitations. JRJ.

Kamhi, Alan G., & Johnston, Judith R. (1992). Semantic assessment: Determining propositional complexity. *Best Practices in Schools: Speech Language Pathology*, 2, 99-107. METHODOLOGY-ANALYSIS DISCOURSE ANALYSIS:

The authors set out a methodology for examining the propositional content of linguistic texts.JRJ

Kamps, D., Walker, D., Maher, J., & Rotholz, D. (1992). Academic and environmental effects of small group arrangements in classrooms for students with autism and other developmental disabilities. *Journal of Autism and Developmental Disorders*, 22, 277-293. LANGUAGE AND EDUCATION AUTISM DEVELOPMENTAL DISORDERS:

Karanth, P. (1989). Pronominal reversal in autism-a note. *NIMHANS Journal*, 7 (2), 181-184. AUTISM PRONOUNS-PERSONAL DEIXIS-PERSONAL SELF-CONCEPT:

The more recent past has witnessed a move from seeing autism as a condition involving social and emotional withdrawal to a view of autism as a disorder of development involving severe cognitive deficits. Autism is now considered as much a cognitive and linguistic disorder as it is a social and behavioural syndrome. The three major factors/disorders are now clearly implicated in autism, social abnormalities, cognitive dificits and language disorders. The question arises as to how these are inter-related: are they merely co-existent or are they causally related and if they are causally related which is the more basic-the social abnormality, the cognitive deficit or language disorder. The author in this paper has shared her clinical experience with children who have had language disorders, both autistic and nonautistic. This paper will limit itself to the phenomenon of pronominal reversal in autistic and other childhood disorders as against that of its acquisition and use in normals. Those who have worked with autistic children know that this description of the cognitive abilities of the one or two year old normal child is hardly matched by much older autistic children. The author reports that there is a need to look for the underlying cause of both the social and linguistic aberrances shown by the autistic child, including phenomena such as pronominal reversal.

Karmiloff-Smith, Annette. (1977). Développement cognitif et l'acquisition de la plurifonctionalité des déterminants. (Cognitive development and the acquisition of plurifunctionality of determinants.). In F. Bresson, et al. (Eds), *Genèse de la parole.* Paris: Presses Universitaires de France. PLURIFUNCTIONALITY LANGUAGE AND COGNITIVE DEVELOPMENT: FRENCH

Karmiloff-Smith, Annette. (1978). Adult simultaneous interpretation: a functional analysis of linguistic categories and a comparison with child development. In D. Gerver, & W. Sinaiko (Eds), *Language, interpretation and communication.* London: Plenum Press. CATEGORIZATION L2/L1 ACQUISITION:

Karmiloff-Smith, Annette. (1978). The interplay between syntax, semantics and phonology in language acquisition processes. In R. N. Campbell, & P. T. Smith (Eds), *Recent advances in the psychology of language.* London: Plenum Press. SEMANTICS AND SYNTAX MORPHOSYNTACTIC DEVELOPMENT:

Karmiloff-Smith, Annette. (1979). Language development after five. In P. Fletcher, & M. Garman (Eds), *Studies in language acquisition*. Cambridge: Cambridge University Press. LATER SYNTACTIC DEVELOPMENT:

Karmiloff-Smith, Annette. (1980). Psychological processes underlying pronominalization and non-pronominalization in children's connected discourse. In J. Kreiman, & E. Ojedo (Eds), *Papers from the parasession on pronouns and anaphora*. Chicago, IL: Chicago Linguistics Society. ANAPHORA PRONOUNS:

Karmiloff-Smith, Annette. (1981). L'importanza del linguagiio come ambito problematico per se nello sviluppo. (The importance of language as a problem space per se in child development.). In O. Andreani (Ed.), *Aspetti Biosocial dell Sviluppo*. Milano: Franco Angeli. LANGUAGE AND COGNITIVE DEVELOPMENT MODULARITY: ITALIAN

Karmiloff-Smith, Annette. (1983). A note on the concept of metaprocedural processes in linguistic and non-linguistic cognitive development. *Archives de Psychologie*, 51, 35-40. LANGUAGE AND COGNITIVE DEVELOPMENT METALINGUISTICS:

Karmiloff-Smith, Annette. (1985). A constructivist approach to modelling linguistic and cognitive development. *Archives de Psychologie*, 53, 113-126. LANGUAGE AND COGNITIVE DEVELOPMENT:

Karmiloff-Smith, Annette. (1985). Language and cognitive processes from a developmental perspective;. *Language and Cognitive Processes*, 1 (1), 60-85. LANGUAGE AND COGNITIVE DEVELOPMENT:

Karmiloff-Smith, Annette. (1986). Does metalinguistic awareness have any function in language acquisition processes? In *Proceedings of the Annual Child Language Forum*. Durham, UK: Durham University Publications. METALINGUISTICS:

Karmiloff-Smith, Annette. (1986). Some fundamental aspects of language acquisition after five. In P. Fletcher, & M. Garman (Eds). *Studies in language acquisition, 2nd Ed.* Cambridge: Cambridge University Press. LATER SYNTACTIC DEVELOPMENT:

Karmiloff-Smith, Annette. (1986). Stage/structure versus phase/process in modelling linguistic and cognitive development. In I. Levine (Ed.), *Stage and structure: Reopening the debate.* New York, NY: Ablex. LANGUAGE AND COGNITIVE DEVELOPMENT:

Karmiloff-Smith, Annette. (1987). Some recent issues in the study of language acquisition. In J. Lyons, R. Coates, M. Deuchar, & G. Gazdar (Eds), *New horizons in linguistics, 2.* Harmondsworth, UK: Penguin Books. ACQUISITION THEORIES LANGUAGE AND COGNITIVE DEVELOPMENT:

Karmiloff-Smith, Annette. (1988). A model of representational change in L1 and its implications for L2 learning. *Polyglot*, 9, L2/L1 ACQUISITION REPRESENTATIONS:

Karmiloff-Smith, Annette. (1988). A model of representational change in language acquisition. In *Proceedings of the Conference on the Basque Language.* Vasco: Servicio Central de Publicaciones del Gobierno. L2/L1 ACQUISITION LANGUAGE AND COGNITIVE DEVELOPMENT REPRESENTATIONS:

Karmiloff-Smith, Annette. (1990). Innate constraints and developmental change. In S. Carey, & R. Gelman (Eds), *Epigenesis of the mind: Essays in biology and knowledge;.* Hillsdale, NJ: Erlbaum. NATIVISM CONSTRAINTS-COGNITIVE:

Karmiloff-Smith, Annette. (1991). Piaget and Chomsky on language acquisition: divorce or marriage?;. *First Language*, 6, NATIVISM PIAGETIAN THEORY LANGUAGE AND COGNITIVE DEVELOPMENT:

Karmiloff-Smith, Annette. (1992). *Beyond modularity: a developmental perspective on cognitive science.* Cambridge, Mass.: MIT Press/Bradford Books. MODULARITY COGNITIVE DEVELOPMENT LANGUAGE AND COGNITIVE DEVELOPMENT:

Karniol, Rachel. (1990). Second language acquisition via immersion in daycare. *Journal of Child Language*, 17, 147-170. IMMERSION BILINGUALISM-PRESCHOOLERS ENGLISH-HEBREW HEBREW-ENGLISH METALINGUISTICS LANGUAGE PRECURSORS BOOTSTRAPPING TRANSFER L2 SEMANTICS:

A report of a program of second language acquisition via immersion by children aged 1:0-3:0. Following a period of silence there was a rapid onset of L2 production and many references to language itself. 8 types of language awareness were identified and it appeared that some of them were necessary precursors of L2 acquisition. Children appear to rely upon contingencies between speech and subsequent behavior to bootstrap the semantics of the second language.

Kasari, Connie, Mundy, Peter, Yirmiya, Nurit, & Sigman, Marian D. (1990). Affect and attention in children with Down syndrome. *American Journal on Mental Retardation*, 95, 55-67. ATTENTION DOWN SYNDROME LANGUAGE AND AFFECT:

The affective responsiveness and attention regulation with communication and language skills of children with Down syndrome was examined. Results both replicate and extend previous research on the attentional and affective characteristics of children with Down syndrome.

Kassai, Ilona. (1979). Az intonáció szerepe a gyermeknyelvben. (The role of intonation in child language.). *Magyar Fonetikai Füzetek*, 3, 80-83. INTONATION HUNGARIAN: HUNGARIAN

Kassai, Ilona. (1979). Gyermeknyelvi dallamminták. (Melodic patterns in child language.). *Magyar Fonetikai Füzetek*, 4, 147-171. PROSODY INTONATION HUNGARIAN BABBLING: HUNGARIAN

A description of melody, fundamental frequency and intonational intensity during the single word period.IK

Kassai, Ilona. (1981). A hangsúly kialakulása a gyermeknyelvben. (The emergence of stress in the child.). *Magyar Fonetikai Füzetek*, 7, 156-174. STRESS PROSODY: HUNGARIAN

Kassai, Ilona. (1981). Távhasonulás a gyermeknyelvben. (Consonant harmony in child language.). *Nyelvtudományi Közlemények*, 83, 160-167. HARMONY PHONOLOGICAL DEVELOPMENT CONSONANTS CONSTRAINTS-PHONOLOGICAL: HUNGARIAN

Author contends that consonant harmony should be considered as a syntagmatically motivated processing constraint.IK

Kassai, Ilona. (1983). A fonéma realitása a korai gyermeknyelvben. (Phonemic reality in early child language.). *Magyar Nyelvör*, 107, 420-423. PHONEMIC DEVELOPMENT LITERACY: HUNGARIAN

Author observes that children who have been in speech therapy perform better in learning to read than children who have not been in therapy and concludes that the phoneme has no psychological reality for children younger than 6:0.IK

Kassai, Ilona. (1987). A Bliss-nyelv nyelvtana. (Bliss-syntax for Hungarian.). In I. Kassai, & Z. Kálmán (Ed.), *Bliss-jelképszótár*. Budapest: HUNGARIAN BLISS SYMBOLS: HUNGARIAN

This paper gives the guidelines of building up sentences and longer messages by using blissymbols.IK

Kassai, Ilona. (1987). On the tonosyntax of a Hungarian child's early questions. *Magyar Fonetikai Füzetek*, 17, 102-115. INTONATION QUESTIONS HUNGARIAN: HUNGARIAN

The interaction of intonation and syntax in the development of questions from age 1:0 to 3:0.IK

Kassai, Ilona. (1988). Prosodic development of a Hungarian child: The one word stage. *Magyar Fonetikai Füzetek*, 19, 72-81. SINGLE-WORD SPEECH PROSODY HUNGARIAN: HUNGARIAN

Kassai, Ilona. (1990). Phonetic issues. In C. Pléh (Ed.), *Hungarian Child Language Research: 1970-1990*. Budapest: HUNGARIAN PHONOLOGICAL DEVELOPMENT:

This is an account of the fairly varied research on the phonetic aspects of the Hungarian child language during the last 20 years.IK

Kassai, Ilona, & Kovács, Emöke. (1978). Cluttering as a type of communication disorder. *Acta Linguistica Scientiarum Hungaricae*, 28, 115-119. COMMUNICATION DISORDERS CLUTTERING:

Examples of secondary school students cluttering in a variety of speech styles ranging from nonsense poetry to spontaneous speech.IK

Kastein, S. (1966). *The birth of language: The case history of a non-verbal child.* Springfield, IL: Thomas. ATYPICAL DEVELOPMENT:

Katz, W. F., Kripke, C., & Tallal, Paula. (1991). Anticipatory coarticulation in the speech of adults and young children-acoustic, perceptual, and video data. *Journal of Speech and Hearing Research*, 34, 1222-1232. COARTICULATION SPEECH PRODUCTION ARTICULATION:

Kavanagh, James F. (1991). *The Language continuum : from infancy to literacy.* Parkton, MD: York Press. LITERACY OVERVIEW-GENERAL:

Kay, Janice, Lesser, Ruth, & Coltheart, Max. (1990). *PALPA-Psycholinguistic assessments of language processing in aphasia.* Hove, UK: Lawrence Erlbaum Associates. APHASIAS PALPA ASSESSMENT PROCEDURES:

Approximately 60 tests which evaluate many aspects of the components of language structure. Package includes comprehensive guidelines for clinical use and test selection and all support materials.

Kaye, K. (1976). Infant's effects upon the mother's teaching strategies. In J. C. Glidewell (Ed.), *The social context of learning and development.* New York, NY : Gardner Press. FINE TUNING HYPOTHESIS SOCIAL INTERACTION HYPOTHESIS ADULT-CHILD INTERACTION PARENTAL SPEECH:

Kazman, R. (1991). Why do children say 'Me do it?'. In K. Hammond, & D. Gentner (Eds), *Proceedings of the Thirteenth Annual Conference of the Cognitive Science Society.* Hillsdale, NJ: Lawrence Erlbaum Associates. PRONOUNS-PERSONAL:

Keatley, C., & de Gelder, B. (1993). The bilingual primed lexical decision task: Cross-language priming disappears with speeded responses. In A. M. B. de Groot, & C. Barry (Eds), *The multilingual community*. Hillsdale, NJ: Lawrence Erlbaum Associates. BILINGUALISM-LEXICAL DEVELOPMENT:

Keil, Frank C. (1991). Theories, concepts, and the acquisition of word meaning. In S. A. Gelman, & J. Byrnes (Eds), *Perspectives on language and thought*. New York, NY: Cambridge University Press. SEMANTIC DEVELOPMENT LANGUAGE AND COGNITION LANGUAGE AND COGNITIVE DEVELOPMENT SEMANTIC MAPPING ACQUISITION THEORIES-SEMANTICS LEXICAL DEVELOPMENT CONCEPT DEVELOPMENT:

Keil, Frank C. (1992). The origins of an autonomous biology. In M. R. Gunnar, & M. Maratsos (EdS), *Modularity and constraints in language and cognition*. Hillsdale, NJ: Lawrence Erlbaum Associates. CONSTRAINTS-BIOLOGICAL:

Kemler-Nelson, Deborah G. (1990). When experimental findings conflict with every day observations. *Child Development*, 61, 606-610. CATEGORIZATION METHODOLOGY-DESIGN:

A discussion of the controversy concerning the effects of laboratory investigations of categorization and the fact that children appear to acquire real world categories more easily than laboratory categories.

Kemple, K., Speranza, H., & Hazen, N. (1992). Cohesive discourse and peer acceptance-longitudinal relations in the preschool years. *Merrill-Palmer Quarterly*, 38, 364-381. DISCOURSE COHERENCE SOCIOLINGUISTIC FACTORS SOCIAL SPEECH COMMUNICATIVE COMPETENCE:

Kennedy, M. D., Sheridan, M. K., Radlinski, S. H., & Beeghly, Marjorie. (1991). Play-language relationships in young children with developmental delays-implications for assessment. *Journal of Speech and Hearing Research*, 34, 112-122. LANGUAGE AND PLAY ASSESSMENT PROCEDURES SOCIAL SPEECH:

Kenny, Thomas, Gaes, Gerald, Saylor, William, Grossman, Linda, Kappelman, Murray, Chernoff, Robin, Toler, Susan, & Majer, Lani. (1990). The Pediatric Early Elementary Examination: Sensitivity and specificity. *Journal of Pediatric Psychology*, 15, 21-26. ASSESSMENT PROCEDURES LANGUAGE AND EDUCATION PEDIATRIC EARLY ELEMENTARY EXAMINATION:

The sensitivity and specificity of the Pediatric Early Elementary Examination (PEEX), a test designed to identify children at risk for learning problems was evaluated. The findings indicate that the PEEX correctly identified only 64.3% of children receiving special education services. The test has a high rate of false positives while still failing to identify 6-7.5% of the children receiving special education services.

Kent, Raymond D. (1991). *Intelligibility in speech disorders: theory, measurement and management*. Amsterdam, The Netherlands: John Benjamins. LANGUAGE DISORDERS INTELLIGIBILITY ARTICULATION INTERVENTION PROGRAMS:

Disorders that impair intelligibility are among the most serious disorders of communication. The papers in this volume, written by authors experienced in intelligibility issues in speech pathology and related fields, describe the basic dimensions by which speech intelligibility can and must be understood. The dimensions are auditory perceptual, linguistic, accoustic and physiologic. These, in turn, are applied to the fundamental problems of definition and theory, measurement and clinical management. Only relatively recently has there been significant progress in formal intelligibility assessment and few, if any books have been published on intelligibility concerns in speech pathology. It is hoped that this book represents the topic of intelligibility in a way that will encourage further invention in research and clinical efforts relating to this essential aspect of speech and language performance. - From promotional materials

Kent, Raymond D. (1991). *Reference manual for communicative sciences and disorders: Speech and language*. San Diego, CA: Singular. REFERENCE MANUAL PHONETICS PHONOLOGY ARTICULATION LANGUAGE DISORDERS PHONOLOGICAL DEVELOPMENT:

Human Development. Phonetics and Phonology. Speech and Related Functions. Respiration. Phonation. Articulalion, Upper Airway. Language. Related Psychological Data. Pharmacology. Commercial Sources. List of Professional/Scholarly Societies.

Kent, Raymond D. (1992). The biology of phonological development. In C. A. Ferguson, L. Menn, & C. Stoel-Gammon (Eds), *Phonological development: Models, research, implications*. Monkton, MD: York Press. LANGUAGE AND MOTOR DEVELOPMENT BIOLOGICAL FOUNDATIONS PHONOLOGICAL DEVELOPMENT ARTICULATION:

Kerek, Andrew. (1976). Phonological rules in the language of Hungarian children. In F. Ingemann (Ed.), *1975 Mid-America Linguistic Conference Papers*. Lawrence, Kansas.: University of Kansas, Dept. of Linguistics,. RULES-PHONOLOGICAL HUNGARIAN:

Kerkhoven, J. (1989). Intentional communication in the second half of the first year of life. *Report, Instituut voor Fonetische Wetenschappen, University of Amsterdam*, 107, DUTCH INTENTIONALITY COMMUNICATIVE DEVELOPMENT INTERSUBJECTIVITY:

Kessell, F. S. (1970). The role of syntax in children's comprehension from 6-12. *Monographs of the Society for Research in Child Development, #139*. Chicago, IL: University of Chicagoi Press. SEMANTICS AND SYNTAX COMPREHENSION LATER SYNTACTIC DEVELOPMENT:

Kessen, W., & Nelson, K. (1978). What the child brings to language. In B. Z. Preissen, D. Goldstein, & M. H. Appel (EdS), *Topics in cognitive development* (vol. 2,). New York, NY: Plenum. ACQUISITION THEORIES NATIVISM:

Kiger, Derrick M. (1989). Effects of music information load on a reading comprehension task. *Perceptual and Motor Skills*, 69, 531-534. LITERACY:

27 male and 27 female high school students read a passage of literature in the presence of silence, low information load, or high information load music. Comprehension was best in the first music condition, worst in the last condition. - From Child Development Abstracts.

Kilborn, K. (1989). Sentence processing in a second language: The timing of transfer. *Language and Speech.*, 32, 1-23. L2 LANGUAGE PROCESSING L2 SYNTAX TRANSFER:

Kilborn, K., & Ito, Takehiko. (1989). Sentence processing strategies in adult bilinguals: Mechanisms of second language acquisition. In B. MacWhinney, & E. Bates (Eds), *The crosslinguistic study of sentence processing*. Cambridge: Cambridge University Press. BILINGUALISM-LANGUAGE PROCESSING LANGUAGE PROCESSING:

Kim, Young-Joo. (1989). Theoretical implications of complements structure acquisition in Korean. *Journal of Child Language*, 16(3), 573-598. KOREAN COMPLEMENTS:

Kim, Y. T., & Lombardino, Linda J. (1991). The efficacy of script contexts in language comprehension intervention with children who have mental retardation. *Journal of Speech and Hearing Research*, 34, 845-857. RETARDED CHILDREN COMPREHENSION DISORDERS EVENTS/SCRIPTS:

King, Cynthia M., & Quigley, Stephen P. (1985). *Reading and deafness*. San Diego, CA: Singular. LITERACY DEAF CHILDREN ASSESSMENT PROCEDURES LANGUAGE AND COGNITIVE DEVELOPMENT READING DISORDERS LANGUAGE AND EDUCATION:

Cognition, Language, and Reading. Reading in Hearing Children. Reading in Deaf Children. Current Practices in Reading Instruction with deaf Children. Reading Materials I: Research. Reading Materials II: Description, Selection, and Use. Reading Assessment. Reading and Other Language-Variant Populations.

Kinnear, Paul R., & Gray, Colin. (1993). *SPSS/PC+ made simple.* Hillsdale, NJ: Lawrence Erlbaum Associates. SPSS METHODOLOGY-ANALYSIS METHODOLOGY-COMPUTERS:

A guide to the PC version of SPSS (*Statistical package for the social sciences*). The first five chapters cover an introducton to SPSS, the preparation of data commands, and the exploration of the data. The remaining ten chapters each deal with a particular test or procedure. The book is aimed at both newcomers and experienced users of the system.

Kirchner, Diane M. (1991). Reciprocal book reading: A discourse-based intervention strategy for the child with atypical language development. In T. M. Gallagher, & N. Rees (Eds), *Pragmatics of language: Clinical practice issues.*. San Diego, CA: Singular Group. INTERVENTION PROGRAMS PRAGMATIC DISORDERS SOCIAL INTERACTION ADULT CHILD INTERACTION INTERVENTION PROGRAMS FOR PARENTS:

A discussion of reciprocal reading routines and their impact on the development of language.

Kitterle, Frederick L. (Ed.). (1991). *Cerebral laterality: theory and research. The Toledo Symposium, vol.*. Hillsdale, NJ: Lawrence Erlbaum Associates. LATERALIZATION LANGUAGE AND HANDEDNESS COMPUTER SIMULATIONS:

The authors of these papers support the view that there are functional differences between the cerebral hemispheres. Research is reported which draws upon normal and clinical human populations as well as other primates. The book describes hemispheric interaction, hemispheric asymmetries, the relationship between handedness and lateralization, lateralization in other primates, and computational models of hemispheric activity.

Klausmeier, H. J., Ghatala, E. S., & Frayer, D. A. (1974). *Conceptual learning and development: A cognitive view.* New York, NY: Academic Press. CONCEPT DEVELOPMENT CATEGORIZATION SEMANTIC ORGANIZATION:

Klecan-Aker, Joan, & Blondeau, Rebecca. (1990). An examination of the written stories of hearing-impaired school-age children. *Volta Review*, 92, 275-282. DEAF CHILDREN WRITTEN LANGUAGE DISCOURSE COHERENCE NARRATIVES:

The purpose of the present investigation was to examine the written stories of school-age hearing-impaired children. Results indicated T-unit lengths within normal limits, and limited use of cohesive devices. The developmental level exhibited by most subjects was the truer narrative.

Klee, Thomas, Membrino, Irene, & May, Susan. (1991). Feasability of real-time transcription in the clinical setting. *Child Language, Teaching, and Therapy*, 7, 27-40. ASSESSMENT PROCEDURES METHODOLOGY-TRANSCRIPTION:

90% of the information captured by post-session audiotape transcription of children's language was captured by real-time transcription, and there was no significant reduction of intelligibility or MLU between the two methods. From Child Development Abstracts.

Klein, Harriet B., Lederer, S. H., & Cortese, E. E. (1991). Children's knowledge of auditory articulatory correspondences - phonologic and metaphonologic. *Journal of Speech and Hearing Research*, 34, 559-564. METALINGUISTICS ARTICULATION SPEECH PERCEPTION:

Klein, Wolfgang. (1989). Introspection into what? Review of C. Faerch and G. Kasper (1987) 'Introspection in second language research'. *Contemporary Psychology*, 34, 1119-1120. BOOK REVIEW L2 ACQUISITION L2 RESEARCH DESIGN:

Klein, Wolfgang. (1989). Kindersprache. La variation linguistique. *La sociolinguistique - En pays de langue allemande.*, 19, 101-124. METHODOLOGY ACQUISITION THEORIES OVERVIEW-GENERAL NONSTANDARD DIALECTS SOCIOCULTURAL FACTORS GERMAN: FRENCH

Klein, Wolfgang. (1989). *L'acquisition de langue étrangère. (Foreign language acquisition.).* Paris: Colin. BILINGUALISM L2 ACQUISITION: FRENCH GERMAN

French translation of Zweitspracherwerb: Eine Einfuhrung, 2nd Ed. 1987. Frankfurt am Main: Athenaum.

Klein, Wolfgang. (1989). Sprechen lernen - das Selbstverstandichste von der Welt. Einleitung. (Language learning - The most obvious thing in the world. Introduction). In W. Klein (Ed.), *Kindersprachen*. Lili: Zeitschrift fur Literaturwissenschaft und Linguistik. LANGUAGE AND COGNITION THEORY OF MIND SAPIR-WHORF HYPOTHESIS CONCEPT DEVELOPMENT SEMANTIC MAPPING: GERMAN

Klein, Wolfgang. (1990). A theory of language acquisition is not so easy. In Kleinschmidt (Ed.), *Studies in second language acquisition*. Amherst, MA: University of Massachusetts Press. L2 ACQUISITION THEORY:

Klein, Wolfgang. (1991). Prolegomena to a theory of language acquisition and implications for theoretical linguistics. In T. Huebner, & C. Ferguson (Eds), *Cross-currents in second language acquistion*. Amsterdam: John Benjamins. ACQUISITION THEORIES ACQUISITION AND LINGUISTIC THEORY:

Klein, Wolfgang, & Perdue, Clive. (1989). The learner's problem of arranging words. In B. MacWhinney, & E. Bates (Eds), *The crosslinguistic study of sentence processing*. Cambridge: Cambridge University Press. SYNTACTIC DEVELOPMENT LANGUAGE PROCESSING COMPLEX SENTENCES:

Klein, Wolfgang, Perdue, Clive, & Carrol, Mary, et al. (1992). *Utterance structure : developing grammars again*. Philadelphia, PA: John Benjamins. BILINGUALISM-SYNTACTIC DEVELOPMENT L2 SYNTAX:

Kleppe, S. A., Katayama, K. M., Shipley, K. G., & Foushee, D. R. (1990). The speech and language characteristics of children with Prader-Willi syndrome. *Journal of Speech and Hearing Disorders*, 55, 300-309. PRADER-WILLI SYNDROME LANGUAGE DISORDERS:

Klima, Edward S. (1990). Comment: Linguistic awareness and metalinguistic control. In I. G. Mattingly, & M. Studdert-Kennedy (Eds), *Modularity and the motor theory of speech perception*. Hillsdale, NJ: Lawrence Erlbaum Associates. METALINGUISTICS:

Klin, A. (1991). Young autistic children's listening preferences in regard to speech-a possible characterization of the symptom of social withdrawal. *Journal of Autism and Developmental Disorders*, 21, 29-42. AUTISM SOCIAL INTERACTION SPEECH PERCEPTION:

Klinge, Swantje. (1990). Prepositions in bilingual language acquisition. In M. J. Meisel (Ed.), *Two first languages - Early grammatical development in bilingual children*. Dordrecht: Foris. PREPOSITIONS BILINGUALISM-PREPOSITIONS BILINGUALISM-SIMULTANEOUS BILINGUALISM-SYNTACTIC DEVELOPMENT:

Kluwin, Thomas N., & Gaustad, Martha Gonter. (1991). Predicting family communication choices. *American Annals of the Deaf*, 136, 28-34. DEAF CHILDREN MODALITY PARENTAL INPUT:

> Results suggest that the mother takes the lead in determining the family's choice of a mode of communication. The single largest influence on the mother's mode of communication was the child's degree of hearing loss, followed by the child's mode of preschool education and the mother's level of education.

Kluwin, Thomas N., & Kelly, A. B. (1991). The effectiveness of dialogue journal writing in improving the writing skills of young deaf writers. *American Annals of the Deaf*, 136, 284-291. DEAF CHILDREN WRITTEN LANGUAGE LANGUAGE AND EDUCATION:

Kobayashi, R., Murata, T., & Yoshinaga, K. (1992). A follow-up study of 201 children with autism in Kyushu and Yamaguchi areas, Japan. *Journal of Autism and Developmental Disorders*, 22, 395-411. AUTISM CROSSLINGUISTIC STUDY-DISORDERS:

Koegel, R. L., Koegel, L. K., & Surratt, A. (1992). Language intervention and disruptive behavior in preschool children with autism. *Journal of Autism and Developmental Disorders*, 22, 141-153. AUTISM INTERVENTION PROGRAMS:

Koenig, Oliver. (1989). Hemispheric asymmetry in the analysis of Stroop stimuli: A developmental approach. *Developmental Neuropsychology*, 5, 245-260. STROOP INTERFERENCE LATERALIZATION:

> Errors and vocal reaction times of 108 righthanded 7 to 15 year old males were measured with Stroop color-word stimuli

for reading, naming, and interference. Results showed a right-visual-field advantage invariant with age in the reading condition and a left-visual-field advantage invariant with age in the naming condition. Only in the interference condition were there age-related differences in the pattern of visual asymmetry. Perhaps differences in visual asymmetries result from changes in subsets of cognitive components used to carry out different cognitive strategies. - From Child Development Abstracts.

Kohn, Amy S., & Landau, Barbara. (1990). A partial solution to the homonym problem: Parents' linguistic input to young children. *Journal of Psycholinguistic Research*, 19, 71-89. PARENTAL INPUT HOMONYMY:

Parents described homonyms by using explicit statements of category inclusion, subordinate forms (compounds, e.g., kiwi-bird), and specific forms that flagged the unusual homonym relationship. Parents especially provided distinctive alternative forms for homonym pairs (e.g., uceskate vs. skatefish) suggesting that they were attempting to preserve the unique form-meaning relationship violated by homonyms.

Kohn, B. (1991). On right-hemisphere comprehension of language, misrepresentations, and omissions-a reply to Bishop (1988) . *Developmental Neuropsychology*, 7, 115-119. LATERALIZATION:

Kohn, Caroline, & Müller, Natascha. (1990). Neuere Arbeitsergebnisse in der Bilingualismusforschung. (New essays in bilingual research.). *Deutschunterricht*, 5, 49-59. BILINGUALISM-OVERVIEW: GERMAN

Kohn, Kurt. (1990). *Dimensionen lernersprachlicher Performanz: Theoretische und empirische Untersuchungen zum Zweitsprachenerwerb. (Dimensions of language learning performance: Theoretical and empirical investigations of second language acquisition.).* Tübingen, Germany: Gunther Narr. L2 ACQUISITION INTERLANGUAGE L2 EDUCATION L2 COMMUNICATIVE COMPETENCE TRANSFER: GERMAN

Kohnstamm, G. A., & Schaerlaekens, A. M. (1981). *Nieuwe streeflijst woordenschat voor zesjarigen, gebaseerd op onderzoek in Nederland en Belgie. (Vocabulary list for six year old children: a renewed edition, based on a study in Belgium and the Netherlands.)*. Lisse, Holland: Swets & Zeitlinger. VOCABULARY DEVELOPMENT DEVELOPMENTAL SCALES ASSESSMENT PROCEDURES DUTCH: DUTCH

Konopczynski, Gabrielle. (1975). Perception (par des français et des étrangèrs) des structures intonatives d'enfants français: Analyse d'un test perceptuel. (Perception of French children's intonation patterns by native and non-native speakers). *Travaux du Department de Linguistique de Bésançon*, 3, 128-135. PROSODY INTONATION: FRENCH

Konopczynski, Gabrielle. (1976). Étude experimentale de quelques structures prosodiques employées par les enfants français entre 7 et 22 mois. (Experimental study of some prosodic structures used by French children aged 7 to 22 months.). *Travaux de l'Institut de Phonétique de Strasbourg*, 7, 171-205. PROSODY INTONATION: FRENCH

Konopczynski, Gabrielle. (1977). Acquisition du langage chez l'enfant de 0-2 ans: aperçu sur la réception et l'émission au niveau phonique. (Acquisition of language by children aged 0-2 years: thoughts on the perception and production of new sounds.). *Bulletin d'Audiophonologie*, 8(2), 50-70. SPEECH PERCEPTION SPEECH PRODUCTION PHONEMIC DEVELOPMENT PHONOLOGICAL DEVELOPMENT: FRENCH

Konopczynski, Gabrielle. (1977). Études sur l'intonation d'enfants français (6 mois-3 ans). (Studies of intonation in French children (0:6-3:0).). *Bulletin d'Audiophonologie*, 8(2), 95-112. INTONATION FRENCH: FRENCH

Konopczynski, Gabrielle. (1979). Le statut de la prosodie dans les recherches sur l'acquisition du langage: réflexions sur les corpus. (The state of prosody in acquisition research: reflections on the literature.). *Studia Phonetica*, 17, 49-60. FRENCH PROSODY: FRENCH

Konopczynski, Gabrielle. (1985). Acquisition de systèmes vocaliques sur différencies. L'example des régions de l'Est (Bésançon-Nancy). (The acquisition of regional dialects. The example of the Eastern regions-Bésançon-Nancy.). In A. M. Houdebine (Ed.), *La phonologie de l'enfant français de six ans, varietés régionales.*. Hamburg, Germany: Buske. NONSTANDARD DIALECTS VARIATION PHONOLOGICAL DEVELOPMENT: FRENCH

Konopczynski, Gabrielle. (1985). Acquisition du langage: la periode charnière et la structuration mélodique. (The acquisition of language: the babbling period and its melodic structure.). *Bulletin d'Audiophonologie*, NS1(2), 63-92. BABBLING PROSODY: FRENCH

Konopczynski, Gabrielle. (1986). Le bébé prélinguistique et le rhythme: prérequis pour l'acquisition du langage. (The prelinguistic child and rhythm: precursors of language acquisition.). *Bulletin d'Audiophonologie*, NS2(4), 279-306. PROSODY LANGUAGE PRECURSORS PRELINGUISTICS: FRENCH

Konopczynski, Gabrielle. (1988). *Prosodie du langage enfantin: une biliographie thématique. (Infant prosody: A thematic bibliography.)*. Hamburg, Germany: Buske. PROSODY BIBLIOGRAPHY: FRENCH

Compiler's note: The author has granted permission for this bibliography to be included in the next volume of CHILDES/BIB.

Konopczynski, Gabrielle. (1990). L'enfant et la construction de sa voix entre 0 et 1 an. (The child's construction of speech during the first year.). *Glossa*, 21, 12-23. PROSODY BABBLING: FRENCH

Konopczynski, Gabrielle. (1990). L'enfant et la construction de sa voix entre 0 et 2 ans. (The child and the construction of speech between birth and two years.). In N. Zavialoff (Ed.), *La lecture 1: De la neurobiologie a la pédagogie*. Paris, France: Editions l'Harmattan. ACQUISITION THEORIES-OVERVIEW: FRENCH

Konopczynski, Gabrielle. (1990). *Le langage émergent: caracteristiques rhythmiques. (Emerging language: characteristic rhythms.)*. Hamburg, Germany: Buske. PROSODY INTONATION: FRENCH

Konopczynski, Gabrielle. (1990). Le langage émergent: comment la mélodie dévient intonation. (Emerging language; How melody effects intonation.). In A. Zavialoff (Ed.), *La lecture, tome 1: De la neurobiologie a la pédagogie*. Editions l'Harmattan. INTONATION PROSODY: FRENCH

Konopczynski, Gabrielle. (1990). Travaux sur la prosodie du langage enfantin. (Works on infant prosody.). *Glossa*, 21, 38-40. PROSODY INTONATION BIBLIOGRAPHY: FRENCH

Konopczynski, Gabrielle. (1991). *Le langage émergent: Caracteristiques vocales et melodiques. (Emerging language: vocal and melodic characteristics.)*. Hamburg, Germany: Buske. PROSODY INTONATION: FRENCH

Konopczynski, Gabrielle, & Vinter, Shirley. (1989). L'analyse de la prosodie enfantine: son intérêt pour un bilan de prélangage. (The analysis of infant prosody: its interest for a prelinguistic check sheet.). *Bulletin d'Audiophonologie*, NS3(4), 261-290. PROSODY ASSESSMENT PROCEDURES METHODOLOGY-ANALYSIS: FRENCH

Konopczynski, Gabrielle, & Vinter, Shirley. (1989). La voix de l'enfant entendant et du déficient auditif profond a la periode charnière. (Hearing and profoundly deaf children's vocalizations during the babbling period.). *Acoustique*, 2, 265-277. LANGUAGE SOCIALIZATION BABBLING DEAF CHILDREN ADULT-CHILD INTERACTION PROSODY INTERSUBJECTIVITY VOCALIZATIONS PHONETIC GESTURES: FRENCH

Studies on the voice of babies are very seldom, and the babbling stage has been particulary ignored. So, 2 groups of babies, one with normal, and one with abnormal hearing were studied. 12 hearing and 12 profoundly deaf subjects were recorded regularly between 8 and 24 months in two different situations: playing alone and interacting with an adult. It has been demonstrated in earlier studies, that in the playing alone situation, the hearing child uses pure gibberish utterances, whereas in interacting he uses Proto-Language. Each of these categories has its own syllabic, temporal and melodic structure. It is demonstrated here, that the child also uses a special kind of voice in each situation. For instance, the hearing child has quite a different attitude when playing alone, or interacting with an adult: in the first case, he practices exploratory voice activities, utilizing a very wide range, from low creaking to extremely high squealing: on the other hand, when interacting, he places his voice in the medium zone. On the contraty, the deaf child does not babble when alone and has no exploratory activities. He only produces sounds when he is interacting, and the range is reduced. But for both groups the usual Fo is quite stable, and lower than generally supposed. Thus it can be concluded that there is not only an evolution in the voice, but there is also a building up of the voice with the building up of language and socialization.GK

Konopczynski, Gabrielle, & Vinter, Shirley. (1989). La voix de l'enfant entendant et du déficient profond à la periode charniére. (The voice of the hearing and profoundly deficient child in the babbling phase.). *Acoustique*, 2, 265-492. DEAF CHILDREN BABBLING VOCALIZATIONS: FRENCH

Konstantareas, M. Mary, Homatidis, Soula, & Busch, Julie. (1990). Cognitive communication, and social differences between autistic boys and girls. *Journal of Applied Developmental Psychology*, 11, 411-424. SEX DIFFERENCES AUTISM:

This study confirmed a preliminary investigation which demonstrated that girls are more severely affected by autism than boys.

Konstantareas, M. Mary, Zadjeman, Helena, Homatidis, Soula, & McCabe, Ann E. (1988). Maternal speech to verbal and high functioning versus nonverbal and low functioning autistic children. *Journal of Autism and Developmental Disorders*, 18, 647-656. AUTISM PARENTAL INPUT:

There were significant differences between the speech of the mothers of the two groups of children. The verbal, high functioning children's mothers asked more questions and provided much more linguistic input and reinforcement for their children than the other mothers. The mothers of the nonverbal, low functioning group had shorter MLUs, were much more directive and tended to reinforce motor rather than linguistic behavior.

Konya, Aniko. (1990). A jelentés szóbeli hangsúlyozása. (Linguistic emphasis of meaning.). *Pszichológia*, 10, 121-141. LEXICAL DEVELOPMENT HUNGARIAN SEMANTIC MAPPING: HUNGARIAN

Koopmans-van Beinum, F. J. (1987). Cleft lip/palate. In C. Reynolds, & L. Mann (Eds), *Encyclopedia of special education, vol. 1.* New York, NY: J. Wiley & Sons. CLEFT PALATE:

Koopmans-van Beinum, F. J. (1987). Early capacities for speech communication. *Proceedings of the Institute of Phonetic Sciences, University of Amsterdam*, 11, PRELINGUISTICS LANGUAGE PRECURSORS:

Koopmans-van Beinum, F. J., Jansonius-Schultheiss, Kino, & van der Stelt, J. M. (1990). The influence of an oral plate upon the speech development and interaction in the first two years of life of cleft palate babies. *Report,Instituut voor Fonetische Wetenschappen, Universiteit van Amsterdam*, 110, CLEFT PALATE ADULT-CHILD INTERACTION INTERSUBJECTIVITY: DUTCH

Longitudinal research with monthly video-recordings of mother- infant interaction in a naturalistic (home-) situation. Time-series (micro-) analysis of verbal and non-verbal communicative development: medical intervention and treatment aspects, psycho-social, psycho-linguistic and educational (child-rearing) aspects. Twelve cleft lip- and/or palate babies and 6 normal children in interaction with their mothers are studied.KvB

Koopmans-van Beinum, F. J., & van der Stelt, J. M. (1979). Early stages in infant speech development. In *Proceedings 5, Institute of Phonetic Sciences.* Amsterdam: University of Amsterdam. BABBLING VOCALIZATIONS LANGUAGE AND MOTOR DEVELOPMENT:

Defines three speech motor milestones in the early development of sound production.KvB

Koopmans-van Beinum, F. J., & van der Stelt, J. M. (1981). The development of speech motor aspects in the first year of life. *Logopedie en Foniatrie*, 53, 320-328. BABBLING:

The onset of babbling in 50 normal children related to sex, place in the family, generational age, sleeping position, thumbsucking, feeding methods, and SES.KvB

Koopmans-van Beinum, F. J., & van der Stelt, J. M. (1988). Baby-babbling: from birth cry to dialogue (in Dutch).. In M. Vandenbroecke (Ed.), *Ter Sprake*. Dordrecht: Foris Publications. BABBLING INDIVIDUAL VARIATION: DUTCH

Speech development described for the general public. Maternal verbal behaviour in relation to the babbling milestone: precursors for 'expressive' and 'referential' children?KvB

Koopmans-van Beinum, F. J., van der Stelt, J. M., & Jansonius-Schultheiss, Kino. (1984). Speech development and interaction in the first years of life of normal and cleft palate babies. In *Proceedings 8, Institute of Phonetic Sciences*. Amsterdam: University of Amsterdam. CLEFT PALATE ADULT-CHILD INTERACTION INTERSUBJECTIVITY:

Outline of the study on speech development and interaction in normal and cleft palate babies.KJS

Koopmans-van Beinum, F. J., van der Stelt, J. M., & Jansonius-Schultheiss, Kino. (1988). The development of speech communication in normal and cleft-palate babies: state of the art of a project. *Proceedings of the Institute of Phonetic Sciences, University of Amsterdam*, 12, CLEFT PALATE SOCIAL INTERACTION:

Koppitz, Elizabeth M. (1975). *The Bender Gestalt Test for young children, 2 vols.* Boston, MA: Allyn & Bacon. ASSESSMENT PROCEDURES BENDER GESTALT TEST DEVELOPMENTAL SCALES ATYPICAL DEVELOPMENT:

Covers the interpretation of Bender Gestalt test results for children age 5-10 years. All aspects of the test are considered:

its reliability, its relationship to cultural factors and IQ, its use as a diagnostic tool, and as a developmental scale for emotionally disturbed children.

Kovács, Emöke. (1970). Beszédhiba és az olvasás kapcsolata (Interrelation of speech disorders and reading.). *Ovodái Nevelés*, 23, 197-199. LITERACY READING DISORDERS LANGUAGE DISORDERS: HUNGARIAN

Kovács, Emöke. (1970). A peszeség. Az orrhangzós beszéd. (Sigmatism and rhinophonia.). In E. Kovács (Ed.), *Logopédiai jegyzet I*. Budapest: ARTICULATION DISORDERS: HUNGARIAN

Kovács, Emöke. (1990). Methodische Schritte zur Dyslexie-Prävention. (Methodological steps in dyslexia - prevention.). In W. Bachmann, & Z. Mesterhazy (Ed.), *Trende und Perspektiven der ungarisschen Heilpädagogik*. Geissen, Germany: Justus Liebig Universität. DYSLEXIA INTERVENTION PROGRAMS READING DISORDERS: GERMAN

Kovács, Emöke, Ligeti, Róbert, & Palotás, Gábor. (1979). Nehány újabb szempont a gyerekkori dyslexia osztályozásában. (Some new criteria for the classification of childhood dyslexia.). In E. Kovács (Ed.), *Szemelvények a dyslexia köréböl*. Budapest: DYSLEXIA HUNGARIAN READING DISORDERS: HUNGARIAN

Kovács, Emöke, & Meixner, Ildikó. (1979). Az olvasáserettség megállapítása óvodáskorban. (Assessing reading ability in preschoolers.). In E. Kovács (Ed.), *Szemelvények a dyslexia köréböl*. READING DISORDERS LITERACY HUNGARIAN: HUNGARIAN

Kovács, Z. Fehérné. (1987). A gyermek dysphoniások tünetcsoportjának terápiájáról (On the therapy of childhood dysphonic symptoms). *A Gyógypedagógiai Tanárképzö Föiskola Tudományos Közleményei.*, 10, 383-386. INTERVENTION PROGRAMS HUNGARIAN PHONOLOGICAL DISORDERS: HUNGARIAN

Kraft, Barbara. (1986). Die Analyse mündlicher Kommunikation von Kindern unter dem Aspekt des Interaktions-bzw. Kommunikations-typs-Nutzen und Probleme. (Am Beispiel des Kommunikationstyps GEMEINSAM PLANEN). (The analysis of children's oral communication under the aspects of interactions and respective communication types -- usage and problems.). *Linguistische Studien/Zentralinstitut für Sprachwissenschaft, Reibe A*, 149, 68-83. GERMAN DISCOURSE ANALYSIS DISCOURSE FUNCTIONS: GERMAN

Kraft, Barbara. (1989). Methodologische Aspekte der linguistischen Analyse von Gesprächen aus der Perspektive eines tätigkeitsorientiert Forschungsansatzes. (Methodological aspects of the linguistic analysis of conversation from the persepctive of an activity oriented research position.). *Zeitschrift für Phonetik, Sprachwissenschaft, und Kommunikationsforschung*, 42, 168-177. GERMAN CONVERSATION DISCOURSE ANALYSIS LANGUAGE FUNCTIONS METHODOLOGY-ANALYSIS: GERMAN

Kraft, Barbara. (1990). Aspekte sprachlich-kommunikativen Handelns der Erzieherin im Kindergarten. (Aspects of language transactions of kindergarten teachers.). *Linguistische Studien/Zentralinstitut für Sprachwissenschaft, Reibe A*, 204, 71-123. GERMAN LANGUAGE AND EDUCATION LANGUAGE FUNCTIONS COMMUNICATIVE FUNCTIONS: GERMAN

Kraft, Barbara. (1991). Beobachtungen zum Erwerb kooperationsorganisierender Sprechandlungen bei drei- und sechsjährigen Kindern. (Observations on the development of the cooperative organization of language by 3-to-6 year old children.). In K. Wagner (Ed.), *Sprechhandlungserwerb*. Bern: Peter Lang. GERMAN TURN TAKING CONVERSATIONAL COMPETENCE: GERMAN

Kraft, Barbara, & Meng, Katharina. (1984). Methodische Probleme der Analyse und Sequenzierung mündlicher Kommunikation. (Methodological problems of the analysis and sequencing of oral communication.). *Linguistische Studien/Zentralinstitut für Sprachwissenschaft, Reibe A*, 118, 94-134. METHODOLOGY-ANALYSIS METHODOLOGY-TRANSCRIPTION: GERMAN

Kraft, Barbara, & Vollhardt, Constanze. (1990). Widersprechen bei Fünfjährigen. (Contradictions by five-year- olds.). In K. Wagner (Ed.), *Sprechhandlungserwerb*. Bern: Peter Lang. GERMAN CHILDREN'S DISCOURSE CHILDREN'S RESPONSES: GERMAN

Kramer, Thayer L., Bukowski, William M., & Garvey, Catherine. (1989). The influence of the dyadic context on the conversational and linguistic behavior of its members. *Merrill-Palmer Quarterly*, 35, 327-341. SOCIAL SPEECH CHILDREN'S DISCOURSE TOPIC COLLABORATION:

Triads of mixed-sex, same-age, and previously acquainted children (aged 34 to 67 months) were observed in a laboratory playroom. The results indicate that although there was considerable consistency in the linguistic output of dyads within a 15 min interaction, there was no consistency across the dyads that shared a common member. - From Child Development Abstracts.

Krashen, Stephen D. (1989). *Language acquisition and language education: Extensions and applications*. Englewood Cliffs, NJ: Prentice-Hall. LANGUAGE AND EDUCATION ACQUISITION THEORIES L2 ACQUISITION THEORIES:

Krasnegor, Norman A., Rumbaugh, Duane M., Schiefelbusch, Richard L., & Studdert-Kennedy, Michael (Ed.). (1991). *Biological and behavioral determinants of language development*. Hillsdale, NJ: Lawrence Erlbaum Associates. ACQUISITION THEORIES BIOLOGICAL FOUNDATIONS LANGUAGE DISORDERS LANGUAGE AND OTHER PRIMATES:

Inspired by a conference sponsored by the Human Learning and Behavior Branch of the National Institute of Child Health and Human Development, this book is devoted to an examination of the biobehavioral bases of language acquisition. What sets this book apart from others is its emphasis on the development of language within the dual contexts of evolution and ontogeny. Major themes revolve around the questions of how language came to be the dominant form of human communication and how language emerges in humans during the period spanning infancy through adulthood. Of interest to developmental psychologists, psycholinguists, and neurospychologists, this volume will also be of value to researchers and clinicians working with retarded children and the learning disabled since the theoretical discussions and empirical findings presented bear directly on the diagnosis and treatment of children with impaired language capacity. Biological and hehavioral Determinants of Language Development may also be used as a text in medical and graduate level courses that focus upon pediatric psychology, behavioral medicine, child development, and pediatrics.

Kratochwill, Thomas R., & Levin, Joel R. (Ed.). (1992). *Single-case research design and analysis: New directions for psychology and education.* Hillsdale, NJ: Lawrence Erlbaum Associates. METHODOLOGY-DIARY/CASE STUDY METHODOLOGY-DESIGN METHODOLOGY-ANALYSIS:

A collection of seven case studies which are offered as examples of well-organized single subject research studies. Topics covered include: time series experiments, nonparametric statistics for single case studies, and single case design and analysis techniques.

Kricos, Patricia, Lesner, Sharon, & Lazarus, Gloria. (1990). Influence of visual information on speech assessment with hearing-impaired children. *Volta Review*, 92, 213-222. DEAF CHILDREN ASSESSMENT PROCEDURES:

The influence of visual information on speech assessment with hearing-impaired children was studied. Three hearing-impaired children were studied and evaluated using Ling's Phonetic Level Speech Evaluation procedure, as well as 12 three-syllable sentences developed by McGarr. Administration of these tests was videotaped for judgement in two conditions: audio-only, and audio-video. Judgement of speech accuracy was influenced by availability of visual information.

Krovetz, R. (1991). Lexical acquisition and information retrieval. In U. Zernik (Ed.), *Lexical acquisition - Exploiting on-line resources to build a lexicon*. Hillsdale, NJ : Lawrence Erlbaum Associates. LEXICAL DEVELOPMENT:

Kucsaj, Stan A., II, & Kirkpatrick, V. M. (1993). Similarities and differences in human and animal language research: Toward a comparative psychology of language. In L. M. Herman, H. L. Roitblat, & P. E. Nachtigall (Eds), *Language and communication: Comparative perspectives*. Hillsdale, NJ: Lawrence Erlbaum Associates. LANGUAGE AND OTHER PRIMATES METHODOLOGY ANIMAL COMMUNICATIONS:

Kuehn, David P., Lemme, Margaret L., & Baumyartner, John M. (1989). *Neural Bases of Speech, Hearing and Language*. San Diego, CA: Singular. NEUROLINGUISTICS AUDIOLOGY:

Studying the Nervous System: Communication Science Perspective. Basic Neuroanatomy. Basic Neurophysiology. Develomental Neuroanatomy an Neurophysiology. Neuroanatomy of Speech. Neurophysiology of Speech. Nueroanatomy of Hearing. Neurophysiology of Hearing. Neural Correlates of Language Function. Neurolinguistics.

Kurita, H., Kita, M., & Miyake, Y. (1992). A comparative study of development and symptoms among disintegrative psychosis and infantile autism with and without speech loss. *Journal of Autism and Developmental Disorders*, 22 , 175-188. PSYCHOPATHOLOGICAL CHILDREN AUTISM:

Kuure, Olli, & Kuure, L. (1990). Svenskan hos hogstadieelever i finska klasser i Sverige. (Swedish among Finnish junior high school pupils in Sweden.). In G. Tingbjorn (Ed.), *Andra symposiet om svenska som andrasprak i Goteborg 1989*. Stockholm: Skriptor. SWEDISH-FINNISH FINNISH-SWEDISH BILINGUALISM: SWEDISH

Kuure, Olli, & Siponen, K. (1990). Om tvasprakighetstypologier. (On the typologies of bilingualism.). In K. Herberts (Ed.), *Sjatte nordiska tvasprakighetskonferensen*. University Abo Akademi. BILINGUALISM: SWEDISH

Kwan-Terry, Anna. (1983). A longitudinal study of the simultaneous acquistion of English and Chinese in a pre-school child in Singapore. In F. Eppert (Ed.), *Transfer and translation in language learning and teaching*. Singapore: RELC. BILINGUALISM-SIMULTANEOUS ENGLISH-CHINESE CHINESE-ENGLISH:

Kwan-Terry, Anna. (1986). The acquisition of word-order in English and Chinese interrogative sentences: A Singapore case study. *RELC Journal*, June, 14-39. L2 WORD ORDER QUESTIONS BILINGUALISM-SIMULTANEOUS ENGLISH-CHINESE CHINESE-ENGLISH:

Kwan-Terry, Anna. (1988). Interlingual processes: A child's development in the use of the English BE+ING structure and its Cantonese equivalent. In V. Bickley (Ed.), *Language in education in a bilingual and multi-lingual setting*. Hong Kong: Institute of Languages in Education. CHINESE-ENGLISH ENGLISH-CHINESE INTERLANGUAGE-MORPHOLOGY BILINGUALISM-MORPHOLOGICAL DEVELOPMENT:

Kwan-Terry, Anna. (1990). The role of transfer in simultaneous language acquisition. In M. A. K. Halliday, J. Gibbons, & H. Nicholas (EdS), *Learning, keeping and using language* . Amsterdam, The Netherlands: John Benjamins. TRANSFER BILINGUALISM-SIMULTANEOUS:

Selected paper from the proceedings of the Eighth World Congress of Applied Linguistics, Sydney, 1987.

Kwan-Terry, Anna. (1990). The use of pragmatic particles in bilingual acquistion. In T. Le, T. Do, & J. Hepburn (Eds), *Proceedings of the International Coinference on Language Teaching and Learning: Theory into Practice*. Tasmania: Department of Adult Learning and Postgraduate Studies, School of Education. BILINGUALISM-PRAGMATIC DEVELOPMENT BILINGUALISM-MORPHOLOGICAL DEVELOPMENT BILINGUALISM-SYNTACTIC DEVELOPMENT PARTICLES:

Kwan-Terry, Anna. (1991). *Child language development in Singapore and Malaysia*. Singapore : Singapore University Press. LANGUAGE AND COGNITION CROSSLINGUISTIC STUDY CROSSCULTURAL STUDY TAMIL CHINESE MALAY:

Kwiatkowski, Joan, & Shriberg, Lawrence D. (1992). Intelligibility assessment in developmental phonological disorders-accuracy of caregiver gloss. *Journal of Speech and Hearing Research*, 35, 1095-1104. PHONOLOGICAL DISORDERS INTELLIGIBILITY:

L

Labarca, Angela, Bailey, Leslie M., & Di Pietro, Roberto J. (1990). *Issues in L2 : theory as practice, practice as theory*. Norwood, NJ: Ablex Pub. Corp. L2 EDUCATION L2 ACQUISITION L2 TEACHING:

Proceedings of the 7th Delaware Symposium on Language Studies, October 1985, the University of Delaware.

Labelle, Mary. (1990). Predication, WH-movement, and the development of relative clauses. *Language Acquisition*, 1, 95-119. QUESTIONS-WH RELATIVIZATION FRENCH CROSSLINGUISTIC STUDY-SYNTAX:

Labelle examines the development of WH-movement in relative clauses in French and contrasts it with the development of the same process in English and concludes that although the two adult languages are syntactically similar, they differ in how the development of this process proceeds. In English, children appear to acquire WH-movement in relative clauses at an early age, but in French the same structure is present but the underlying movement strategy does not appear to be present before about the age of 6.0 years.

Laczko, Mária. (1988). An experiment on the relation between speech understanding and dyslexia. *Hungarian Papers in Phonetics*, 19, 82-92. DYSLEXIA READING DISORDERS:

The paper deals with the problem of dyslexia since the number of children having difficulties in understanding what they read, or giving expression to what they think is on the increase. On the basis of the author's own experiments it is claimed that deficiencies in the hearing and/or of the speech perception process that are responsible for reading defects.ML

Laczko, Mária. (1989). Speech understanding and dyslexia: experimental evidence. *Hungarian Papers in Phonetics*, 21, 184-187. DYSLEXIA READING DISORDERS LANGUAGE AND EDUCATION:

The term dyslexia is used to cover reading and writing disturbances of different origin, extent and types. The paper presents the author's experimental data concerning the reading comprehension of children and supports the hypothesis that serious difficulties of speech comprehension tend to underlie the children's poor school performance and actual reading defects.ML

Lafontaine, D., Arguelles, M., Boulanger, M., Counet, S., Denis, C., Miermans, M. C., Sarantou, P., Stafilas, E., Seron, Xavier, Moreau, M. L., Richelle, M., & Rondal, Jean A. (1981). Bilingualisme et scolarité: une enquête sociolinguistique sur les enfants espagnols des écoles primaires liègeoises. (Bilingualism and education: A sociolinguistic investigation of Spanish children in primary schools in Liège.). *Psychologica Belgica*, 21, 41-63. BILINGUALISM-EDUCATION FRENCH-SPANISH SPANISH-FRENCH L2 EDUCATION: FRENCH

Lahey, Margaret. (1989). *Disorders of communication - The science of intervention*. San Diego, CA: Singular. COMMUNICATION DISORDERS INTERVENTION PROGRAMS CLASSIFICATION OF DISORDERS PHONOLOGICAL DISORDERS MOTOR DISORDERS ARTICULATION DISORDERS CLEFT PALATE APHASIAS APRAXIA DYSARTHRIA:

Philosophy in Intervention. Aspects of the Anatomy and Physiology of Speech. The Classification of Communicative Disorders. The Epidemiology of Communication Disorders. The Profession at Work. Language Disorders in Children. Childhood Phonological Disorders. Childhood Articulatory Disorders of Neurogenic Origin. Childhood Voice Disorders. Childhood Stuttering. Cleft Palate and Other Craniofacial Anomalies in Children. Aphasia: Theory-Based Intervention. Assessment of Dysarthria: The Critical Prerequisite to Treatment. Apraxia of Speech. Voice Disorders in Adults. Adult

Stuttering. Surgical Rehabilitation in Adults. Conclusion: Developing the Science of Intervention.

Lahey, Margaret. (1992). Linguistic and cultural diversity: further problems for determining who shall be called language disordered. *Journal of Speech and Hearing Research*, 35, 638-639. ASSESSMENT PROCEDURES CROSSCULTURAL STUDY CULTURAL FACTORS LANGUAGE DISORDERS:

Lahey, Margaret, Liebergott, J. W., Chesnick, M., & Menyuk, Paula, et al. (1992). Variability in children's use of grammatical morphemes. *Applied Psycholinguistics*, 13, 373-398. INDIVIDUAL VARIATION MORPHOSYNTACTIC DEVELOPMENT:

Lam, A. S. L., Perfetti, Charles A., & Bell, L. (1991). Automatic phonetic transfer in bidialectal reading. *Applied Psycholinguistics*, 12, 299-311. LITERACY BIDIALECTISM TRANSFER:

Lambert, J. L., & Rondal, Jean A. (1978). *Le mongolisme. (Down syndrome.)*. Bruxelles: Mardaga. DOWN SYNDROME: FRENCH

Lambert, J. L., & Rondal, Jean A. (1980). Note tecnique. À propos d'un indice de développement syntaxique chez les arrières mentaux. (Technical note: About an index of syntactic development by the mentally retarded.). *Le Langage et l'Homme*, 43, 43-44. ASSESSMENT PROCEDURES SYNTACTIC DISORDERS RETARDED CHILDREN: FRENCH

Lambert, J. L., & Rondal, Jean A. (1981). Performance verbale et capacités communicatives chez les handicapes mentaux adultes. (Verbal performance and communicative capacity of mentally handicapped adults.). In J. A. Rondal, J. Lambert, & H. Chipman (Eds), *Psycholinguistique et handicap mental: recherches récentes et perspectives*. Bruxelles: Mardaga. LANGUAGE AND COGNITION RETARDED CHILDREN: FRENCH

Lambert, J. L., & Rondal, Jean A. (1983). The language of Down's syndrome adults. In *Proceedings de la Conference on Down's Syndrome*. Madrid, Spain: Instituto Internacional Para La Investigacion Y Asesoramiento Sobre La Deficiencia Mental. DOWN SYNDROME:

Lambert, J. L., Rondal, Jean A., & Seron, Xavier. (1982). L'intervention langagière: problèmes et perspectives. (Language intervention: problems and perspectives.). In J. Rondal, & X. Seron (Ed.), *Troubles du langage: Diagnostic et rééducation*. Bruxelles: Mardaga. INTERVENTION PROGRAMS: FRENCH

Lambert, J. L., Rondal, Jean A., & Sohier, C. (1980). Analyse des troubles articulatoires chez des enfants arrières mentaux mongoliens et non-mongoliens. (Analysis of the articulatory troubles of retarded infants with and without Down syndrome). *Bulletin d'Audiophonologie*, 10, 13-20. RETARDED CHILDREN DOWN SYNDROME ARTICULATION DISORDERS: FRENCH

Lambert, Wallace E., et al. (Eds). (1981). *Faces and facets of bilingualism.* Washington, DC: Center for Applied Linguistics. BILINGUALISM:

Lamp, Robert E., & Krohn, Emily J. (1990). Stability of the Stanford-Binet Fourth Edition and K-ABC for young black and white children from low income families. *Journal of Psychoeducational Assessment*, 8, 139-149. LANGUAGE AND SOCIAL CLASS ASSESSMENT PROCEDURES STANFORD-BINET SCALE KAUFMAN ASSESSMENT BATTERY FOR CHILDREN CROSSCULTURAL STUDY SOCIOLINGUISTIC FACTORS:

The results for children aged 4:0-6:0 were highly stable across tests, and there were no significant differences between the cultural groups.

Lamprecht, Regina R. (1985). O periodo dos enunciados de uma palavra na linguagem da crianca-abordagens atuais. (The one-word utterance period in child language-contemporary approaches.). *Letras de Hoje*, 18, 33-45. PORTUGUESE SINGLE-WORD SPEECH: PORTUGUESE

Presentation and discussion of Greenfield & Smith's (1976) semantic relations, Dore's (1979) pragmatic relations, and Freire's (1980) pragmatic- semantic relations (based on Skarakis & Prutting, 1977).RRL

Lamprecht, Regina R. (1990). Aquisicao da linguagem pela crianca apos os 5 anos de idade. (Language acquisition in children over 5 years of age.). In M. Tasca (Ed.), *Desenvolvendo a lingua falada e escrita*. Porto Alegre: Sagra. PORTUGUESE LATER SYNTACTIC DEVELOPMENT LANGUAGE AND EDUCATION : PORTUGUESE

Analogical to the work of C. Chomsky and A. Karmiloff-Smith, this article discusses syntactic and pragmatic aspects of Brazilian Portuguese which may still represent some kind of difficulty to children over 5. The relevance of these developmental facts for teachers is discussed.RRL

Landau, Barbara. (1993). Language learning in blind children. In H. Tager-Flusberg (Ed.), *Constraints on language acquisition: Studies of atypical children*. Hillsdale, NJ: Lawrence Erlbaum Associates. ATYPICAL DEVELOPMENT BLIND CHILDREN:

Landau, Barbara, & Stecker, Deanna S. (1990). Objects and places: Geometric and syntactic representations in early lexical learning. *Cognitive Development*, 5, 287-312. PREPOSITIONS NOUNS CUES-SYNTACTIC REPRESENTATIONS-SYNTACTIC:

Three experiments investigated differences in the geometric properties of objects and places underlying children's knowledge of count nouns and prepositions. Both children and adults could use the syntactic contexts to make appropriate semantic inferences, assuming that the noun referred to the object itself and the preposition to the object's location.

Landis, L. (1990). Otitis media in early childhood and its relationship to later phonological development - comment. *Journal of Speech and Hearing Disorders*, 55, 172-172. OTITIS MEDIA ATYPICAL DEVELOPMENT PHONOLOGICAL DEVELOPMENT PHONOLOGICAL DISORDERS:

Landolfi, L., Barbieri, Maria S., & Brandimonte, A. (1990). Imparare a spiegare, gli effetti del linguaggio materno sul bambino. (Learning how to explain: Effects of mother's language on the child.). *Eta Evolutiva*. CHILDREN'S EXPLANATIONS PARENTAL INPUT VYGOTSKYAN THEORY ADULT-CHILD INTERACTION: ITALIAN

Within a neo-Vygotskian framework, explanations are a basic device for development and socialization. This paper describes a study of mother-child interaction designed to analyze the contents and strategies of the mother's explanations, and their effects on the child. The aim was to test whether the children incorporate maternal explanations, and to explain how they do so. 9 mother-child pairs, with children at three age levels (30, 45 and 60 months), were videotaped reading a booklet in two successive sessions at 20-day intervals. Each session was loosely organized into four stages, in such a way as to permit checkingof the child's baseline and of her/his learning after the mother's explanations. The results of the first analyses show important differences between the first and second sessions as regards the quantity and content of the language produced by the child, and there were also few differences related to age.MSB

Landry, Susan H., & Loveland, Katherine A. (1989). The effect of social context on the functional communication skills of autistic children. *Developmental Disorders*, 19, 283-299. AUTISM CONTEXT:

Autistic children's attention-directed behavior differed most from that of the other groups in spontaneous interaction and they did not produce more attention-directing behavior when a high degree of adult direction was provided.

Lange, Sven. (1976). *En preliminar grammatisk analys av spraket hos Freja fran 20 til 41 manaders alder. ((A preliminary grammatical analysis of the language of Freja from 20 to 41 months of age).* Stockholm: University of Stockholm. SWEDISH EARLY SYNTACTIC DEVELOPMENT: SWEDISH

Companion publications under the same title were issued in 1974 and 1975. SL.

Lange, Sven. (1976). *Prepositionerna i ett barns spontana tal. En langdsnittsstudie. ((Prepositions in a child's spontaneous speech. A longitudinal study.).* Stockholm: University of Stockholm. PREPOSITIONS SWEDISH METHODOLOGY-LONGITUDINAL STUDY: SWEDISH

Lange, Sven, & Larsson, Kenneth. (1977). Studier i det tidiga barnsprakets grammatik. (Studies in early child grammar.). In *Project Child Language Syntax, PM No. 11*. Stolkholm: Department of Scandinavian Languages. SWEDISH SYNTACTIC DEVELOPMENT: SWEDISH

Langevin, C., & Rondal, Jean A. (1980). Le nouveau programme de français au primaire au Quebec (The new French program in the primary school in Quebec.). *L'École Belge*, K3, 136-140. LANGUAGE AND EDUCATION FRENCH BILINGUALISM-EDUCATION: FRENCH

Langley, M. Beth, & Lombardino, Linda J. (1991). *Neurodevelopmental strategies for managing communication disorders in children with severe motor dysfunction*. San Diego, CA: Singular. INTERVENTION PROGRAMS COMMUNICATION DISORDERS MOTOR DISORDERS ASSESSMENT PROCEDURES:

> Introduction to the Neurodevelopmental Approach for Assesslng and Treating Communication Disorders in Neurologically Impaired Children. Respiratory Components of Communication: Assessment and Treatment. Prespeech Development, Assessment, and Treatment Strategies. Alternative Feeding Methods. Nutritional Assessment. Sensory Preparation of the Oral Motor Area: Organization for Function. Augmenting Communication in Children with severe cognitive, Sensory, and Motor Dysfunction: Issues and Strategies. Assessment: A Multidimensional Process. Facilitation of Learning. Teaming: Integrated services within a Neurodevelopmental Framework.

Lankamp, R. F. (1989). *A study on the effect of terminology on language two reading comprehension: Should specialist terms in medical texts be avoided?*. Amsterdam:Rodopi. L2 READING PROFICIENCY L2 JARGON:

Lanza, E. (1992). Can bilingual 2-year-olds code-switch. *Journal of Child Language*, 19, 633-658. CODE-SWITCHING:

Lapadat, Judith C. (1991). Pragmatic language skills of students with language and/or learning disabilities. *Journal of Learning Disabilities*, 24, 147-157. CONVERSATIONAL DISORDERS:

A meta-analytical review of 33 studies investigating the pragmatic language skills of 3- to 12-year-old students with language disorders, language-learning disabilities, or learning disabilities as compared with the pragmatic language skills of nondisabled peers was conducted. The students with language and/or learning disabilities demonstrated consistent and pervasive pragmatic deficits in conversation compared to nondisordered peers across settings, conversational partners, age groups, and types of pragmatic skills measured.

LaPointe, Leonard L. (1991). *Base-10 response form and revised manual*. San Diego, CA: Singular Group. ASSESSMENT PROCEDURES INTERVENTION PROGRAMS BASE-10 RESPONSE FORM:

A clinical assessment instrument which allows a graphic representation of the status of the child's language development to be made. The form can also be used to produce environments to stimulate the language of children with disorders.

Largo, Remo H., Graf, S., Kundu, S., Hunziker, U., & Molinari, L. (1990). Predicting developmental outcome at school age from infant tests of normal, at-risk, and retarded infants. *Developmental Medicine and Child Neurology*, 32, 30-45. ASSESSMENT PROCEDURES RETARDED CHILDREN AT-RISK CHILDREN GRIFFITHS MENTAL DEVELOPMENT SCALES:

The performance of groups of 118 preterm, 119 term, and 78 retarded children was examined for predictive validity for verbal, performance, and locomotor development. The Griffiths Language and Performance Scales proved to be the best predictors of later intellectual functioning. The social score had a moderate predictive value, while the locomotor score was of little predictive value.

Larkin, Jill H., & Chabay, Ruth W. (1992). *Computer assisted instruction and intelligent tutoring systems*. Hillsdale, NJ: Lawrence Erlbaum Associates. C.A.L.L. COMPUTER ASSISTED THERAPY LANGUAGE AND EDUCATION L2 EDUCATION INTERVENTION PROGRAMS:

Although not specifically related to language issues, this book should be of interest to all those people who use computers in language therapy and teaching.

Larsen-Freeman, Diane. (1992). *Discourse analysis in second language research*. Rowely, MA: Newbury House. L2 DISCOURSE L2 EDUCATION L2 RESEARCH DESIGN:

Larsen-Freeman, Diane, & Long, Michael H. (1991). *An introduction to second language acquisition research*. New York, NY: Longman. L2 ACQUISITION L2 RESEARCH DESIGN:

Larsson, Kenneth. (1976). *En preliminar grammatisk analys av spraket hos Tor fran 20 til 43 mandaders alder. (A preliminary grammatical analysis of the language of Tor from 20 to 43 months of age.)*. Stockholm: University of Stockholm. EARLY SYNTACTIC DEVELOPMENT SWEDISH: SWEDISH

A companion publication under the same title was issued in 1975. KL.

Larsson, L., & Brodin, Jane. (1988). *Kommunikationshjalpmedel och anpassningar for forstandshandikappade. (Communication aids and adaptations for the mentally retarded.)*. Stockholm: Handikappinstitutet. RETARDED CHILDREN INTERVENTION PROGRAMS: SWEDISH

Communication is something difficult and complicated for all people with mental retardation and multiple handicaps. One of the problems is to find communication aids that can be used by individuals with mental retardation. In Sweden all technical handicap aids can be obtained free of charge if there is a need. The staff from the county councils who are responsible for the prescription of technical aids sometimes have difficulties finding the best help for each individual with mental retardation. The aim of this study has been to invent what communication aids are available on the Swedish market and to elaborate how these can be modified for mentally retarded. The study has resulted in a publication with photos of communication aids and different adaption.

Lass, N., McReynolds, L., Northern, Jerry L., & Yoder, D. (1988). *Handbook of speech-language-pathology and audiology*. Philadelphia, PA: B. C. Decker. LANGUAGE DISORDERS AUDIOLOGY ASSESSMENT PROCEDURES INTERVENTION PROGRAMS:

See also related volume published by W. D. Saunders (Philadelphia, PA) in 1982 under the title Speech, language, and hearing.

Laudanna, A., & Volterra, Virginia. (1991). Order of words, signs, and gestures - a first comparison. *Applied Psycholinguistics*, 12, 135-150. GESTURE SIGNING FIRST WORDS:

Laufer-Dvorkin, Batia. (1991). *Similar lexical forms in interlanguage.* Tubingen, Germany: Gunther Narr. TRANSFER INTERLANGUAGE L2 EDUCATION:

Le Rouzo, Marie-Louise. (1990). Le développement de la production vocale en rélation avec la parole entendue et le développement moteur. (The development of vocalizations with specific reference to shared speech and motor development.). *Glossa*, 21, 4-11. LANGUAGE AND MOTOR DEVELOPMENT VOCALIZATIONS BABBLING INTERSUBJECTIVITY: FRENCH

Leavell, C., & Lewandowski, L. (1990). Neurolinguistic deficits and the left hemisphere in the reading disabled. *Developmental Neuropsychology*, 6, 319-337. READING DISORDERS LATERALIZATION NEUROLINGUISTICS:

Lebrun, Yvan. (1990). *Mutism*. San Diego, CA: Singular. MUTE CHILDREN:

The Psychology of Silence. The Syndrome of Mutism: Introduction. The Syndrome of Mutism: Functional Mutism. The Syndrome of Mutism: Functional Mutism. The Syndrome of Muiism: Organic Mutism. Epilogue.

Lederberg, Amy R. (1991). Social interaction among deaf preschoolers-the effects of language ability and age . *American Annals of the Deaf*, 136, 53-59. DEAF CHILDREN SOCIAL INTERACTION SOCIAL SPEECH:

Lederberg, Amy R., & Mobley, Caryl E. (1990). The effect of hearing impairment on the quality of attachment and mother-toddler interaction. *Child Development*, 61, 1596-1604. DEAF CHILDREN ADULT-CHILD INTERACTION INTERSUBJECTIVITY:

> Hearing impaired and hearing toddlers together with their hearing mothers were observed in Ainsworth's Strange Situation and during free play. Security of attachment and ratings of maternal and toddler behavior during free play were remarkably similar for the hearing impaired and hearing dyads. Security of attachment was related to maternal and toddler behavior in a similar way for the hearing impaired and hearing toddlers.

Lee, C. D., & Gasser, M. (1992). Where do underlying representations come from? A connectionist approach to the acquisition of phonological rules. In J. Dinsmore (Ed.), *The symbolic and connectionist paradigms: Closing the gap* . Hillsdale, NJ: Lawrence Earlbaum Associates. REPRESENTATIONS-PHONOLOGICAL CONNECTIONISM RULES-PHONOLOGICAL:

Lee, C. J. (1990). Some hypotheses concerning the evolution of polysemous words. *Journal of Psycholinguistic Research*, 19, 211-219. POLYSEMY LEXICAL DEVELOPMENT:

Lee, Rene Friemoth, & Kamhi, Alan G. (1990). Metaphoric competence in children with learning disabilities. *Journal of Learning Disabilities*, 23, 476-482. FIGURATIVE LANGUAGE LANGUAGE DISORDERS PRAGMATIC DISORDERS:

> Metaphoric competence was examined in two groups of children with learning disabilities and one group of nondisabled peers. The group with a history of language impairment consistently performed more poorly on the metaphor tasks than the group without a history of language impairment, who, in turn, performed more poorly than the nondisabled children.

Lee, Thomas Hun-tak. (1991). Linearity as a scope principle for Chinese: the evidence from first language acquisition. In D. Napoli, & J. Kegl (Eds), *Bridges between psychology and linguistics: A Swarthmore Festschrift for Lila Gleitman*. Hillsdale, NJ: Lawrence Erlbaum Associates. CHINESE SYNTACTIC DEVELOPMENT:

Lee, Thomas Hun-tak, & Gradman, Harry L. (1990). A comparison of performance on Chinese and English dichotic listening tasks by bilingual native Mandarin speakers. In M. A. K. Halliday, & J. G. S. H. Nicholas (Eds), *Learning, keeping and using language*. Amsterdam, The Netherlands: John Benjamins. MANDARIN CHINESE-ENGLISH ENGLISH-CHINESE DICHOTIC LISTENING BILINGUALISM-NEUROLINGUISTICS:

Selected paper from the proceedings of the Eighth World Congress of Applied Linguistics, Sydney, 1987.

Lees, Janet, & Urwin, Shelagh. (1990). *Children with language disorders*. San Diego, CA: Singular. INTERVENTION PROGRAMS ASSESSMENT PROCEDURES LANGUAGE DISORDERS:

Written from a clinical point of view, this text examines what speech-language pathologists really do, working individually and in multidisciplinary teams, with language-impaired children. Presents a holistic view of the child the family, the environment, and progress with language. Includes case examples througout drawn from actual clinical practice.

Legerstee, Maria. (1990). Infants use multimodal information to imitate speech sounds. *Infant Behavior and Development*, 13, 343-354. MODALITY IMITATION INFANT PERCEPTION VOWELS:

The role of audition and vision in eliciting early imitation of speech sounds was examined in this study. Thirty infants were presented with the vowel sounds 'a' and 'u'. For one half of the infants, these sounds were paired with an adult who silently articulated the same vowel. For the other half, the adult articulated the opposite one. Only the infants who were exposed to matched auditory and visual information were observed to imitate the vowels.

Lehman, Mark E., & Sharf, Donald J. (1989). Perception/production relationships in the development of vowel duration cue to final consonant voicing. *Journal of Speech and Hearing Research*, 32(4), 803-815. VOWELS CONSONANTS-FINAL CUES-PHONOLOGICAL PRODUCTION/PERCEPTION:

Lehrer, Adrienne, & Kittay, Eva F. (1992). *Frames, fields, and contrasts: New essays in semantic and lexical organisation.* Hillsdale, NJ: Lawrence Erlbaum Associates. SEMANTIC ORGANISATION SEMANTIC RELATIONS LEXICAL DEVELOPMENT REPRESENTATIONS-LEXICAL REPRESENTATIONS-SEMANTIC:

A collection of essays dealing with semantic and lexical organisation, processing and representation.

Leith, William R., & Johnston, Robert G. (1986). *Handbook of voice therapy for the school clinician.* San Diego, CA: Singular Publishing Group. REFERENCE MANUAL ARTICULATION DISORDERS:

Lempert, Henrietta. (1989). Animacy constraints on preschool children's acquisition of syntax. *Child Development*, 60(1), 237-245. CONSTRAINTS-SYNTACTIC ANIMACY:

Lengyel, Zsolt. (1974). Razvoj sistema nominalne deklinacija u govoru dvogodisnjeg detata koje usvaja madarski kao materhji jezik (Acquisition of Noun System by Two-Year-Old Hungarian Children). In *Modeli u sintaksi decjeg gavora.*. Novi-Sad. HUNGARIAN CASE MORPHOSYNTACTIC DEVELOPMENT: SERBOCROATIAN

This study is an emperical investigation of the first case form in Hungarian noun systems.

Lengyel, Zsolt. (1976). Formation and development of the verb system in the language of a two year old child. In *Kolloquium uber Kindersprache.*. Tubingen: Narr. VERBS HUNGARIAN:

This study is a grammatical analysis of the very first verb form in Hungarian child language.

Lengyel, Zsolt. (1976). Magyar gyermeknyelvi kutatások a XIX. században (Hungarian Child Language Investigation in the 19th Century). *Magyar Nyelvor*, 81-90. OVERVIEW-GENERAL HUNGARIAN: HUNGARIAN

Lengyel, Zsolt. (1977). Developments of parts of speech in the Hungarian child language. *International Journal of Psycholinguistics*, 4, 50-64. WORD CLASS HUNGARIAN:

The early system of parts of speech in Hungarian child language is analyzed in this study.ZL

Lengyel, Zsolt. (1979). *A pszicho- es szociolingvisztika helye az anya- és idegennyelvek oktatásában (The place of psycholinguistics and sociolinguistics in mother tongue and Foreign Language Teaching).* Debrecen. LANGUAGE AND EDUCATION L2 EDUCATION BILINGUALISM-EDUCATION: HUNGARIAN

This book deals with language teaching questions and problems. It trys to show the way of applying the most important results of psycholinguistics and sociolinguistics in practical education (the process of understanding and generating of linguistic messages, the language register, the connections between social roles and verbal behavior, etc.).ZL

Lengyel, Zsolt. (1981). *A gyermeknyelv (Child language).* Budapest: Gondolat. OVERVIEW-GENERAL HUNGARIAN SOVIET RESEARCH CROSSLINGUISTIC STUDY: HUNGARIAN

This book shows the state of researches of child language of the 70's to Hungarian specialists. This work tries to treat at first the most important trends and tendencies of American works on child language, but there are also including some important results of Russian, German, and French literature.ZL

Lengyel, Zsolt. (1981). *Tanulmányok a nyelvelsajátítás köréből (Studies on language acquisition).* Budapest: Akadémiai. INTENTIONALITY HUNGARIAN SINGLE-WORD SPEECH EARLY SYNTACTIC DEVELOPMENT WORD ORDER: HUNGARIAN

In this work there are several studies with rich empirical data of the ontogenetic speech development of 2-6 year-old Hungarian children.ZL

Lengyel, Zsolt. (1982). Gyermenknyelvi kutatasok Magyarorszagon: 1975-80 (Child language research in Hungary: 1975-80). In *Hungarológiai Közlemények*. Novi Sad: HUNGARIAN OVERVIEW-GENERAL: HUNGARIAN

A review of books and articles about child language researches in Hungary. Researches involve subjects from psycho- and sociolinguistics to educational fields.ZL

Lengyel, Zsolt. (1985). *Nyelv-lélek-társadalom: Az anyanyelvi nevelés pszicho- és szociolingvsztikai vonatkozásai (Language-Mind-Society: Some questions of mother tongue teaching from psycho- and sociolinguistic points of view)*. Budapest: Tankönyvkiadó. LANGUAGE AND EDUCATION: HUNGARIAN

This book is a review of the most important and recent psycholinguistic and sociolinguistic tendencies and theses with their possible applications in mother tongue teaching.ZL

Lengyel, Zsolt. (1989). Metanyelv es nyelvtanulas (Acquisition of language and metalinguistic knowledge). *Magyar Nyelvor*, 3, 332-340. METALINGUISTICS WORD CLASS HUNGARIAN:

During the process of language acquistion children learn not only grammatical, semantic structures of their native language, but some metalinguistic rules too. In this article the 'first' meaning of such expressions (noun, singular, etc.) for children is analyzed.ZL

Leonard, Laurence B. (1989). Language learnability and specific language impairment in children. *Applied Psycholinguistics*, 10(2), 179-202. SPECIFIC LANGUAGE IMPAIRMENT LEARNABILITY :

Leonard, Laurence B. (1992). Models of phonological development and children with phonological disorders. In C. A. Ferguson, L. Menn, & C. Stoel-Gammon (Eds), *Phonological development: Models, research, implications*. Monkton, MD: York Press. PHONOLOGICAL DISORDERS PHONOLOGICAL DEVELOPMENT:

Leonard, Laurence B., Bortolini, Umberrta, Caselli, M. Cristina, & McGregor, Karla K. (1992). Morphological deficits in children with specific language impairment: The status of features in underlying grammar. *Language Acquisition*, 2, 151-179. SPECIFIC LANGUAGE IMPAIRMENT MORPHOLOGICAL DISORDERS CROSSLINGUISTIC ITALIAN STUDY-DISORDERS MORPHOSYNTACTIC DEVELOPMENT:

The authors conducted a crosslinguistic study of Italian and English children with SLI and concluded that there were no grounds to support the notion that the disorder is caused by the absence of morphosyntactic features in the underlying grammar.

Leonard, Laurence B., & Fey, Marc E. (1991). Facilitating grammatical development: The contribution of pragmatics. In T. M. Gallagher, & N. Rees (Eds), *Pragmatics of language: Clinical practice issues.*. San Diego, CA: Singular Group. SYNTACTIC DISORDERS INTERVENTION PROGRAMS:

An examination of the interaction between pragmatics and syntactic development, and how pragmatics can be used to enhance the syntactic development of children with syntactic disorders.

Leonard, Laurence B., & McGregor, Karla K. (1991). Unusual phonological patterns and their underlying representations: A case study. *Journal of Child Language*, 18, 261-271. PHONOLOGICAL PATTERNS REPRESENTATIONS-PHONOLOGICAL:

Leonard, Laurence B., McGregor, Karla K., & Allen, George D. (1992). Grammatical morphology and speech perception in children with specific language impairment. *Journal of Speech and Hearing Research*, 35, 1076-1085. MORPHOSYNTACTIC DEVELOPMENT SPEECH PERCEPTION SPECIFIC LANGUAGE IMPAIRMENT:

Leonard, Laurence B., Schwartz, Richard G., Allen, George D., Swanson, Lori A., & Froem-Loeb, Diane. (1989). Unusual phonological behavior and the avoidance of homonymy in children. *Journal of Speech and Hearing Research*, 32(3), 583-590. SELECTION/AVOIDANCE HOMONYMY:

Leong, Che Kan, & Randhawa, Bikkar S. (1989). *Understanding literacy and cognition*. New York, NY: Plenum. LITERACY LANGUAGE AND EDUCATION LANGUAGE AND COGNITION CROSSLINGUISTIC STUDY-LITERACY:

Topics include: literate thought, literacy and cognition metaphors, artificial intelligence and automated tutoring, Swedish work on 'text windows', and a comparative study of rural India.

Lesser, Ruth. (1989). *Linguistic investigations of aphasia, 2nd Ed.* San Diego, CA: Singular. APHASIAS SEMANTIC DISORDERS SYNTACTIC DISORDERS:

Glossary of Terms. Interpretations of Aphasia. Linguistics and Aphasia. Linguistic Dichotomies. Performances in Aphasia. Semantic Relationships: Associations, Fields and Features. Semantic Relationships: Categories, Complexes, and Retrieval. Investigations of Syntax. Investigations and Prosody. Psycholinguistic and Sociolinguistic Applications of Linguistics to Aphasia.

Levelt, Willem J. M., Mills, Anne, & Karmiloff-Smith, Annette. (1981). *Child language research in ESF countries*. Strasbourg: European Science Foundation Publications. OVERVIEW-THEORY:

Levin, Bonnie E. (1990). Organizational deficits in dyslexia: Possible frontal lobe dysfunction. *Developmental Neuropsychology*, 6, 95-110. DYSLEXIA NEUROLINGUISTICS:

The performance on a battery of cognitive tests of a group of 20 dyslexics was compared with the performance of a control group. The dyslexics appeared to have deficits in control and problem-solving strategies.

Levin, Iris, & Tolchinsky-Landsmann, Liliana. (1989). Becoming literate: referential and phonetic strategies in early reading and writing. *European Journal of Behavioral Development*, 12, 369-384. WRITTEN LANGUAGE LITERACY:

Levine, Daniel S. (1991). *Introduction to neural and cognitive modeling*. Hillsdale, NJ: Lawrence Erlbaum Associates. CONNECTIONISM COMPUTER SIMULATIONS:

An introduction to neural networks which integrates research from several disciplines. Contents include: the history of neural networks, network organizational principles, the development of cognitive functions, and some computer simulation exercises.

Levine, Gustav. (1990). *A guide to SPSS for analysis of variance*. Hillsdale, NJ: Lawrence Erlbaum Associates. SPSS METHODOLOGY-ANALYSIS METHODOLOGY-COMPUTERS:

This book contains copies of programs that can be used for the analysis of variance and related statistical tests using SPSS (*Statistical package for the social sciences*) software. First two chapters are a reference guide to the use of SPSS. The rest of the book contains the programs which include programs for: Omnibus F-tests, analysis of covariance, repeated measures analysis, multiple factors analysis, and trend analysis.

Levitt, Andrea G., & Utman, J. G. A. (1992). From babbling towards the sound systems of English and French - a longitudinal 2-case study. *Journal of Child Language*, 19, 19-49. CROSSLINGUISTIC STUDY-PHONOLOGY PROSODY FRENCH BABBLING PHONETIC INVENTORIES PHONEMIC DEVELOPMENT:

Levorato, Maria C. (1988). *Racconti, storie e narrazioni. I processi di comprensione dei testi. (Recounting, stories, and narratives: The processes of text comprehension)*. Bologna,Italy: Il Mulino. DISCOURSE ANALYSIS DISCOURSE COMPREHENSION TEXT/STORY GRAMMARS: ITALIAN

A monograph on text comprehension in children and adults.MCL

Levorato, Maria C., & Cacciari, Christina. (1992). Children's comprehension and production of idioms-the role of context and familiarity. *Journal of Child Language*, 19, 415-433. FIGURATIVE LANGUAGE CONTEXT:

Levorato, Maria C., & de Zuani, E. (1985). L'integrazione delle informazioni visive e verbali nel ricordo di storie nei bambinidieta prescolare e scolare. (The integration of visual and verbal information in the recall of stories by children.). *Giornale Italiano di Psicologia*, 12, 3O9-332. LANGUAGE AND MEMORY NARRATIVES CONGRUENCY-SEMANTIC: ITALIAN

An analysis of children's recalled accounts of stories presented together with vignettes.MCL

Levorato, Maria C., & Zammuner, V. L. (1984). Semantic discontinuities introduced by 'but' in children's discourse. *Ricerche di Psicologia*, 1, 90-113. CONNECTIVES-CONDITIONAL SEMANTIC DEVELOPMENT CONGRUENCY-SEMANTIC: ITALIAN

An analysis of the semantic functions of the adversative 'but' in children's discourse.MCL

Levorato, Maria C., & Zuani, E. De. (1987). Lo sviluppo dei processi diintegrazione di informazioni visive e verbali congruenti, incomplete e incongruenti. (The integration of visual and verbal information congruent, incongruent and incomplete.). *Giornale Italiano di Psicologia*, 14, 459-478. LANGUAGE AND MEMORY NARRATIVES CONGRUENCY-SEMANTIC: ITALIAN

Children were first presented with vignettes and sentences and then they were asked to recall them. The visual stimuli could be either congruent, incongruent or incomplete when compared with the verbal stimuli.MCL

Levy, Elena. (1989). Monologue as development of the text-forming function of language. In K. Nelson (Ed.), *Narratives from the crib*. Cambridge, MA: Harvard University Press. CRIB SPEECH NARRATIVES ANAPHORA PRONOUNS:

Levy examines the subject's presleep monologues and reports that contrary to the literature the child appears to have a grasp of anaphoric pronouns as early as 1:9. Heretofore, it has been reported that anaphoric reference is not intact until after 5:0 (Karmiloff-Smith, 1986).

Levy, E. T., & McNeill, David. (1992). Speech, gesture, and discourse. *Discourse Processes*, 15, 277-301. GESTURE DISCOURSE DEVELOPMENT:

Levy, Stine, Zoltak, Brenda, & Saelens, Tom. (1988). A comparison of obstetrical records of autistic and nonautistic referrals for psychoeducational evaluation. *Journal of Autism and Developmental Disorders*, 18, 573-581. AT-RISK CHILDREN AUTISM NEONATES:

The birth records of 59 autistic children and 28 nonautistic children matched for intellectual level were compared for abnormal presentation. The autistic group had a higher frequency of abnormal presentation than the control group.

Levy, Yonata, Amir, N., & Shalev, R. (1993). Morphology in a child with congenital left hemisphere brain lesion: Implications for normal acquisition. In H. Tager-Flusberg (Ed.), *Constraints on language acquisition: Studies of atypical children*. Hillsdale, NJ: Lawrence Erlbaum Associates. ATYPICAL DEVELOPMENT CONGENITAL DISORDERS MORPHOLOGICAL DEVELOPMENT LATERALIZATION:

Lewinsky, T. Z., Koenig, S., Otis-Wilborn, A., & Messenheimer-Young, T. (1992). Language and literacy in early childhood-camping, canoes, and adventure for profoundly hearing-impaired children. *Volta Review* , 94 , 359-364. LITERACY DEAF CHILDREN:

Lewis, B. A. (1990). Familial phonological disorders - 4 pedigrees. *Journal of Speech and Hearing Disorders*, 55, 160-170. PHONOLOGICAL DISORDERS HERITABILITY:

Lewis, B. A., & Freebairn, L. (1992). Residual effects of preschool phonology disorders in grade school, adolescence, and adulthood. *Journal of Speech and Hearing Research*, 35, 819-831. PHONOLOGICAL DISORDERS:

Lewis, B. A., & Thompson, L. A. (1992). A study of developmental speech and language disorders in twins. *Journal of Speech and Hearing Research*, 35, 1086-1094. MULTIPLE BIRTHS LANGUAGE DISORDERS SIBLING EFFECTS DEVELOPMENTAL DISORDERS:

Lewis, Vicky, & Boucher, Jill. (1991). Skill, content and generative strategies in autistic children's drawings. *British Journal of Developmental Psychology*, 9, 393-416. AUTISM:

Leybaert, J. (1992). Determinants of reading ability in deaf individuals: The roles of phonolgocal codes. In M. Marschark, & M. D. Clark (Ed.), *Psychological perspectives on deafness*. Hillsdale, NJ: Lawrence Erlbaum Associates. DEAF CHILDREN LITERACY LANGUAGE AND EDUCATION:

Li, Ping. (1988). Acquisition of spatial reference in Chinese. In P. Jordens, & J. Lalleman (EdS), *Language development in the Netherlands*. Dordrecht: Foris. CHINESE SPATIAL TERMS REFERENCE DEIXIS-SPATIAL:

Libby, Marion N., & Aries, Elizabeth. (1989). Gender differences in preschool children's narrative fantasy. *Psychology of Women Quarterly*, 13, 293-306. SEX DIFFERENCES NARRATIVES:

> Twenty-two female and 20 male 3- to 5-year-old children were presented with six story starts and were asked to finish the stories. Girls introduced significantly more friendly figures who offered assistance. Boys introduced significantly more aggressive behavior and attempts to master situations through the use of aggressive activity. Girls told significantly more stories about girls, boys tended to tell more stories about boys. The analysis of the fantasy narratives showed boys to be more concerned with coping with aggressive drives and channeling them into attempts at mastery, and girls with caretaking and responding to the needs of others. - From Child Development Abstracts.

Liberg, C. (1990). 'I am not guessing!' Children's early achievement of literacy. In G. Conti-Ramsden, & C. E. Snow (Eds), *Children's language*. Hillsdale, NJ: Lawrence Erlbaum Associates. LITERACY:

Lichtenstein, Robert, & Ireton, Harry. (1984). *Preschool screening: Identifying young children with developmental and emotional problems*. Boston, MA: Allyn & Bacon. ASSESSMENT PROCEDURES ATYPICAL DEVELOPMENT DEVELOPMENTAL SCALES:

This book covers early identification procedures, practical and technical factors of testing young children, and recommendations for future practice.

Lieberman, Philip, & Blumstein, Sheila E. (1988). *Speech physiology, speech perception, and acoustic phonetics*. New York, NY: Cambridge University Press. ACOUSTIC PHONETICS SPEECH PRODUCTION SPEECH PERCEPTION ARTICULATION BIOLOGICAL FOUNDATIONS NEUROLINGUISTICS-NEURAL SUBSTRATES COMPUTER SIMULATIONS:

An introductory textbook which covers the many aspects of speech production and perception including: acoustic phonetics, articulatory phonetics, biological and neurological substrates of speech, and the principles involved in making computer models of speech processes.

Lieven, Elena V. M., Pine, Julian M., & Barnes, H. D. (1992). Individual differences in early vocabulary development-redefining the referential-expressive distinction. *Journal of Child Language*, 19, 287-310. INDIVIDUAL VARIATION FIRST WORDS VOCABULARY DEVELOPMENT:

Lightfoot, David. (1991). *How to set parameters : arguments from language change*. Cambridge, MA: MIT Press. PARAMETER SETTING LANGUAGE CHANGE SYNTACTIC DEVELOPMENT:

Lillo-Martin, Diane C. (1991). Comments on Hyams and Weissenborn: on licensing and identification. In J. Weissenborn, H. Goodluck, & T. Roeper (Eds), *Theoretical issues in language acquisition - Continuity and change in development*. Hillsdale, NJ: Lawrence Erlbaum Associates. PARAMETER SETTING NULL SUBJECTS:

Lillo-Martin, Diane C. (1992). Deaf readers and Universal Grammar. In M. Marschark, & M. D. Clark (Eds), *Psychological perspectives on deafness*. Hillsdale, NJ: Lawrence Erlbaum Associates. DEAF CHILDREN SYNTACTIC DEVELOPMENT PARAMETER SETTING:

Lillo-Martin, Diane C., Hanson, V. L., & Smith, Suzanne T. (1992). Deaf readers comprehension of relative clause structures. *Applied Psycholinguistics*, 13, 13-30. LITERACY DEAF CHILDREN RELATIVIZATION:

Lindblom, Björn. (1991). The status of phonetic gestures. In I. G. Mattingly & M. Studdert-Kennedy. (Eds). *Modularity and the motor theory of speech perception*. Hillsdale, NJ: Lawrence Erlbaum Associates. PHONETIC GESTURES SPEECH PERCEPTION:

Lindblom, Björn. (1992). Phonological units as adaptive emergents of lexical development. In C. A. Ferguson, L. Menn, & C. Stoel-Gammon (Eds), *Phonological development: Models, research, implications*. Monkton, MD: York Press. LEXICAL DEVELOPMENT REPRESENTATIONS-PHONOLOGICAL:

Lindner, K., & Johnston, Judith R. (1992). Grammatical morphology in language impaired children acquiring English or German as their first language: A functional perspective. *Applied Psycholinguistics*, 13, 115-130. CROSSLINGUISTIC STUDY-MORPHOLOGY GERMAN LANGUAGE DISORDERS SEMANTIC RELATIONS:

An examination of the morphological development in German and English using children with language impairments as subjects. The German children appeared to have less difficulty with morphological acquisition and the authors speculate that this may be due to the greater importance of morphology as a means of expressing semantic relations in German than in English.JRJ

Ling, Daniel. (1984). *Early intervention for hearing impaired children: oral options*. San Diego, CA: Singular Publishing Group. DEAF CHILDREN INTERVENTION PROGRAMS:

Early oral intervention. An introduction. The Helen Neebe Speech and Hearing Center. An early auditory-oral intervention program. The McGill University Project. An acoupedic program. Comments and conclusions.

Lipsitt, Lewis P. (1990). Learning and memory in infants. *Merrill-Palmer Quarterly*, 36, 53-66. NEONATES:

Ample evidence demonstrates that newborn infants process information in every sensory modality and respond differentially to stimuli from birth. The human infant also exhibits the ability to learn and to engage in self-regulatory behavior. Such behavior can affect physiological processes. Hedonic mediation of approach-avoidance and learned behavior, as well as memory, are important factors in the interaction of the infant and the environment. - From Child Development Abstracts.

Lleo, Conxita. (1986). The evolution of syllabic structure as an example of interaction between universal restrictions and individual strategies in first language acquisition.. In M. Brame, H. Contreras, & F. Newmeyer (Eds), *A Festschrift for Sol Saporta.* Seattle: Noit Amrofer. SYLLABLES-STRUCTURE:

Lleo, Conxita. (1988). Adquisicio lexico-fonologica de dues llengues i homonimia: algunes hipotesis. (Lexico-phonological acquisition of two languages and homonymy: some hypotheses.). In *Miscellania Antoni M. Badia i Margarit 8.* Barcelona: Abadia de Montserrat. HOMONYMY CATALAN-SPANISH SPANISH-CATALAN BILINGUALISM-PHONOLOGICAL DEVELOPMENT BILINGUALISM-LEXICAL DEVELOPMENT: CATALAN

Lleo, Conxita. (1990). Homonymy and reduplication revisited: on the extended availability of two strategies in phonological acquisition. *Journal of Child Language*, 17, 267-278. REDUPLICATION HOMONYMY BABBLING:

Lleo, Conxita. (1991). Adquisición de la fonología de la lengua materna. In J. Liceras (Ed.), *La adquisición del lenguaje: Teoría y métodologia.* Madrid: Fundación Ortega y Gassett. PHONOLOGICAL DEVELOPMENT SPANISH: SPANISH

Lleo, Conxita. (1991). Adquisición de la fonología de las segundas lenguas. (Acquisition of second language phonology.). In J. Liceras (Ed.), *La adquisición del lenguaje: Teoría y métodologia*. Madrid: Fundación Ortega y Gasset. BILINGUALISM-PHONOLOGICAL DEVELOPMENT INTERLANGUAGE-PHONOLOGY: SPANISH

Lleo, Conxita. (1991). Cap a la recerca sistematica sobre l'adquisicio fonologica delcatala com a primera llengua en criatures multilingues. (Towards systematic research on the phonological acquisition of Catalan as a first language by multilingual children.). *Zeitschrift fur Katalanistik*, 4, 78-92. PHONOLOGICAL DEVELOPMENT CATALAN BILINGUALISM-PHONOLOGICAL DEVELOPMENT: CATALAN

Lleo, Conxita. (1991). One phonological system or two in early bilingual acquisition. *Multilingual Matters*, 9, INTERLANGUAGE-PHONOLOGY BILINGUALISM-PHONOLOGICAL DEVELOPMENT:

Lloyd, Lyle L., & Kaplan, Harriet. (1978). *Audiometric interpretation: a manual of basic audiometry*. San Diego, CA: Singular Publishing Group. AUDIOMETRY:

Overview. Reading the pure tone audiogram. Interpreting speech audiometry. Use of masking. Determining the educational and communicative significance of the hearing loss. Audiometric inconsistencies. Index.

Lloyd, P. (1991). Strategies used to communicate route directions by telephone: a comparison of the performance of 7-year-olds, 10-year-olds and adults. *Journal of Child Language*, 18, 171-189. COMMUNICATIVE COMPETENCE CHILDREN'S EXPLANANTIONS CHILDREN'S DESCRIPTIONS:

Lloyd, P. (1992). The role of clarification requests in children's communication of route directions by telephone. *Discourse Processes* , 15, 357-374. CHILDREN'S DESCRIPTIONS REQUESTS:

Lloyd, P., Boada, H., & Forns, M. (1992). New directions in referential communication research. *British Journal of Developmental Psychology*, 10, 385-403. REFERENTIAL COMMUNICATION:

Lock, Andrew. (1991). The role of social interaction in early language development. In N. A. Krasnegor, et al. (EdS), *Biological and behavioral determinants of language development.* Hillsdale, NJ: Lawrence Erlbaum Associates. SOCIAL INTERACTION HYPOTHESIS:

Locke, John L. (1990). Structure and stimulation in the ontogeny of spoken language. *Developmental Psychobiology*, 23(7), NATIVISM:

Locke, John L., & Mather, Patricia L. (1989). Genetic factors in the ontogeny of spoken language: Evidence from monozygotic and dizygotic twins. *Journal of Child Language*, 16, 553-559. HERITABILITY MULTIPLE BIRTHS NATIVISM ARTICULATION:

A reanalysis of the Mather and Black (1984) data revealed that there were significant differences between the articulations of mono- and dizygotic twins. The authors argue that this evidence weakens the claims for the genetic transmission of language.

Locke, John L., & Pearson, Dawn M. (1992). Vocal learning and the emergence of phonological capacity: A neurobiological approach. In C. A. Ferguson, L. Menn, & C. Stoel-Gammon (Eds), *Phonological development: Models, research, implications.* Monkton, MD: York Press. PHONOLOGICAL DEVELOPMENT:

Logan, Robert J. (1991). *The three dimensions of stuttering - neurology, behavior, and emotion.* San Diego, CA: Singular. STUTTERING:

Introduction. The Neurophysiological Bases of Emotion and Their Effects on Sensorimotor Speech. The Three-Dimensional Model of Stuttering. Clinical Implications of the Three-Dimensional Model.

Loke, Kit-Ken. (1990). A semantic analysis of young children's use of Mandarin shape classifiers. In A. Kwan-Terry (Ed.), *Child language development in Singapore and Malaysia.* Singapore: Singapore University Press. CLASSIFIERS MARKEDNESS MANDARIN CHINESE PARTICLES:

This paper is a reinterpretation of the data used by Loke and Harrison (1986), whose analysis of the appropriate and inappropriate use of shaped classifiers by the children is now rejected on the basis of it being an error analysis of children's use of the classifiers against the adults. It is proposed that a semantic analysis which reflects how the children themselves actually use the shape classifiers will reflect the semantic relationship the children perceive between the classifiers and the objects classified. This semantic relationship is described in terms of a set of binary semantic features, which captures the meanings assigned to the classifiers by the children. It is also suggested that the implicational order of acquisition of the shape classifiers based on their total frequencies of use be interpreted in terms of markedness and Denny's (1976) notion of extendedness.KKL

Loke, Kit-Ken, & Harrison, Godfrey. (1986). Young children's use of Chinese (Cantonese and Mandarin) sortal classifiers. In H. Kao, & R. Hoosain (Eds), *Linguistics, Psychology, and the Chinese Language*. Hong Kong: Centre of Asian Studies, University of Hong Kong. CANTONESE CHINESE MANDARIN CATEGORIZATION GENDER CLASSIFIERS:

A study of 40 Cantonese speaking children in Macau, aged 3-7 years, and a separate study of 21 Mandarin acquiring kindergarten children in Singapore, aged between 5:0 and 6:10, show that in a counting task, these children used the 'general classifier' goh (Cantonese) and ge (Mandarin) predominantly. The Mandarin data also shows the following appropriate use of shape classifiers: zhi for long and rigid objects, tiao for long and flexible objects, li for round objects, zhang and pian for flat objects. It is argued that this classification is necessarily based on the children's awareness of the shapes of the objects and their ability to match these shapes with the meanings of the classifiers. An examination of the order of acquisition for these shape classifiers in terms of their total frequency of use shows that the order is compatible with Clark's (1977) findings on the shape criteria used by young children in over-extension, i.e., rounds --> length --> flatness.KKL

Loke, Kit-Ken, & Harrison, Godfrey. (1988). Children's discovery of Mandarin shape classifiers. In *Revised Summaries and 24 Reprinted Abstracts by the Child Language Research Institute*. Lund, Sweden: Department of Linguistics, Lund University. CLASSIFIERS GENDER MANDARIN CHINESE:

> Based on data collected from 44 kindergarten children in an identification and counting task, two methods of analysis of children's use of Mandarin shape classifiers are presented. The first looks at the children's use of Mandarin shape classifiers for distinctive shape categories. The second establishes the children's discovered meanings for the shape classifiers by assigning semantic features to the shape classifiers on the basis of the shared attributes of the objects classified. Results are further interpreted in a wider cognitive context.KKL

Loke, Kit-Ken, & Low, Johna Mei-Yin. (1988). A proposed descriptive framework for the pragmatic meanings of the particle la in colloquial Singaporean English. In B. McCarthy (Ed.), *Asian Pacific Papers, Occasional Papers Number 10*. Sydney: Applied Linguistics Association of Australia. INTONATION TONE PARTICLES PIDGINS/CREOLES:

> It is argued that Kwan-Terry's (1978) basis of distinction of two forms of la, i.e., stress and duration, is problematic. This paper examines data collected from the speech of pre-school children, and presents the various discourse intonational patterns and pragmatic meanings of the particle la in Colloquial Singaporean English. It is argued that there are three variants of la based on pitch heights with pitch variations, on which duration and stress can be further superimposed. A tonal-intonational framework of la is thus proposed to capture its full range of subtle pragmatic meanings.KKL

Loosemore, R. P. W., Brown, G. D. A., & Watson, F. L. (1991). A connectionist model of alphabetic spelling development and developmental and acquired dysgraphia. In K. Hammond, & D. Gentner (Ed.), *Proceedings of the Thirteenth Annual Conference of the Cognitive Science Society*. Hillsdale, NJ: CONNECTIONISM AGRAPHIA LITERACY:

Lord, Catherine, Mulloy, Catherine, Wendelboe, Michael, & Schopler, Eric. (1991). Pre- and perinatal factors in high-functioning females and males with autism. *Journal of Autism and Developmental Disorders* , 21, 197-209. AUTISM:

High-functioning females and males of similar IQ were compared with 54 normally developing siblings. Both male and female autistic children had higher non-optimality scores than their siblings. Much of the difference was accounted for by first borns and fourth- or later borns in the autistic group. Estimated weeks of gestation greater than 42 occurred more often for autistic subjects than siblings, and autistic males tended to come from larger families than autistic females.

Lörik, József. (1982). Allami gondozott gyermekek fonémaállományának fejlettsége (Phoneme system of foster home children). *Gyógypedagóiai Szemle*, 100-112. PHONEMIC DEVELOPMENT SOCIOLINGUISTIC FACTORS FOSTERED CHILDREN HUNGARIAN: HUNGARIAN

Lörik, József. (1982). Qualitative und quantitative Mangel der verbalen Kommunikation in der Erziehungsheimen, und ihre Auswirkung auf die Sprachentwicklung. (The extent of the deficiencies of insitutionalized children's verbal communication, and its effect on language development.). In H. Aschenbrenner (Ed.), *Jugend und Volk*. Munchen/Wien: HUNGARIAN COMMUNICATIVE DISORDERS INSTITUTIONALIZED CHILDREN: GERMAN

Lörik, József. (1984). Adalékok a többváltozatü névszótövek gyermeki elsajátításához (Contributions to the study of the acquisition of nominal allomorphs). *Gyógypedagógiai Szemle*, 95-101. MORPHOPHONEMIC DEVELOPMENT HUNGARIAN: HUNGARIAN

Loveland, Katherine A., & Tunali, Belgin. (1991). Social scripts for conversational interactions in autism and Down syndrome. *Journal of Autism and Developmental Disorders*, 21, 177-186. AUTISM DOWN SYNDROME ADULT-CHILD INTERACTION:

Loveland, Katherine A., Tunali, Belgin, McEvoy, Robin E., & Kelley, Michelle L. (1989). Referential communication and response adequacy in autism and Down's syndrome. *Applied Psycholinguistics*, 10, 301-313. AUTISM DOWN SYNDROME REFERENTIAL DISORDERS REFERENTIAL COMMUNICATION:

Subjects, 13 with autism and 14 with Down's syndrome, matched on verbal mental age, learned a simple board game, and were asked to teach it to a listener who used varying levels of prompting to produce target information. Autistic subjects required specific prompting to produce target information, whereas most Down's subjects did not. - From Child Development Abstracts.

Lowenfeld, Margaret. (1991[1935]). *Play in childhood.* New York, NY: Cambridge University Press. LANGUAGE AND PLAY:

A re-issue of the 1935 classic work on play and human development.

Lowenthal, F., van Damme, F., & Cordeir, J. (Eds). (1982). *Language and language acquisition.* New York, NY: Plenum. ACQUISITION THEORIES ACQUISITION AND LINGUISTIC THEORY:

Lucariello, Joan. (1991). Canonicality and consciousness in child's narrative. In B. Britton, & A. Pellegrini (Eds), *Narrative Thought and Narrative Language.* Hillsdale, NJ : Lawrence Erlbaum Associates. NARRATIVES:

Lucariello, Joan, Kyratzis, A., & Nelson, Katherine. (1992). Taxonomic knowledge - what kind and when? *Child Development* , 63, 978-998. CATEGORIZATION:

Lucas, Ceil (Ed.). (1989). *Sign language research: Theoretical issues.* Washington, DC: Gallaudet University Press. SIGNING:

Luczynski, Jan. (1988). Review of L.F.M. Scinto's Written Language and Psychological Development. *Psychologia Wychowawcza.*, 31(3), 357-359. BOOK REVIEW LITERACY WRITTEN LANGUAGE:

Luczynski, Jan. (1989). Review of M. Nystrand's The Structure of Written Communication. Studies in Reciprocity Between Writers and Readers. *Psychologia Wychowawcza.*, 32(2), 207-211. BOOK REVIEW WRITTEN LANGUAGE LITERACY:

Luczynski, Jan. (1989). Text strategies and cognition: The organization of meaning in written text and the development of operational intelligence. In P. Boscolo (Ed.), *Writng: Trends in European research. Proceedings of the International Workshop on Writing.*. Padova, Italy: UPSEL Editore. POLISH WRITTEN LANGUAGE LITERACY LANGUAGE AND COGNITION TEXT/STORY GRAMMARS PIAGETIAN THEORY:

The study reported in this paper was designed to reveal whether any difference exists in strategies for functional composition of texts written by children on the concrete operational level and the formal operational level. The texts analyzed in the study were written in Polish by 20 subjects, 10 concrete operational and 10 low formal operational. The proceedure of text analysis, based on the functional sentence perspective developed by the Prague School, was adopted from an earlier study. The results obtained in the study suggest that a link exists between the growing ability to produce coherent and integrated narrative texts and the shift from concrete operational to low formal operational level. Furthermore, there is evidence that the situation of writing a text gives children an opportunity to elaborate their thought operations in a similar way to the situation in which action on objects is performed. This is reflected in parallels between the strategies of functional text compositions and the logical structure of thought operations. Conclusions, however, should be drawn carefully and with respect to external factors such as educational patterns.JL

Luczysnki, Jan. (1990). Inteligencja operacyjuna a rozwoj strategii komponowania tekstow pisanych (Operational intelligence and the development of strategies for written text composition). *Psychologia Wychowawcza.*, 33(3), 111-129. POLISH LITERACY WRITTEN LANGUAGE LANGUAGE AND COGNITION PIAGETIAN THEORY: POLISH

This article deals with the relationship between the learning of skills in writing narrative texts, and the development of operational intelligence. Following Vygotsky, Bruner, and Scinto, it was supposed that situations of writing narrative texts provide children with occasions for accumulating experience that is important in the development of formal-operational structures. Empirical investigations compared texts written by subjects on three levels of operational intelligence development: concrete-operational, formal-operational A, and formal-operational B. The procedure used for analysis of the meaning organization of text was based on the theory of functional sentence perspective (FSP). Results partially support the hypothesis, but show as well the possible interference of such social-cultural factors as ethnic language and pedagogical influence.JL

Ludlow, Christy L. (1991). Measures and designs for research in dysarthia. In C. A. Moore, K. M. Yorkston, & D. R. Beukleman (Eds), *Dysarthria and apraxia of speech*. Baltimore, MD: Paul Brookes. DYSARTHRIA METHODOLOGY-DESIGN:

Luelsdorff, Philip A. (1990). Orthographic complexity and orthographic acquisition. In M. A. K. Halliday, J. Gibbons, & H. Nicholas (Eds), *Learning, keeping and using language* . Amsterdam, The Netherlands: John Benjamins. WRITTEN LANGUAGE LITERACY:

Selected paper from the proceedings of the Eighth World Congress of Applied Linguistics, Sydney, 1987.

Luetkest-Ahlman, B. (1991). Following the rules - consistency in sign. *Journal of Speech and Hearing Research*, 34, 1293-1298. SIGNING:

Lund, Nancy J., & Duchan, Judith F. (1992). *Assessing children's language in naturalistic contexts, 3rd ed.* Englewood Cliffs, NJ: Prentice-Hall. ASSESSMENT PROCEDURES COMMUNICATIVE COMPETENCE:

First edition, 1983, second edition, 1988.

Luschei, Erich S. (1991). Development of objective standards of nonspeech oral strength and performance: an advocate's view. In C. A. Moore, K. M. Yorkston, & D. R. Beukleman (Eds), *Dysarthia and apraxia of speech*. Baltimore, MD: Paul H. Brookes. DYSARTHRIA APRAXIA:

Lust, Barbara, & Eisele, J. (1991). On the acquisition of syntax in Tamil - a comment on Garman (1974). *Journal of Child Language*, 18, 215-226. TAMIL SYNTACTIC DEVELOPMENT:

Lust, Barbara, & Mazuka, Reiko. (1989). Crosslinguistic studies of directionality in first language acquisition: the Japanese data-a response to O'Grady, Suzuki-Wei & Cho 1986. *Journal of Child Language*, 16(3), 665-684. JAPANESE SYNTACTIC DEVELOPMENT CROSSLINGUISTIC STUDY-SYNTAX:

Luterman, David M. (1987). *Deafness in the family*. San Diego, CA: Singular Publishing Group. DEAF CHILDREN INTERVENTION PROGRAMS FOR PARENTS:

Family in theory. Family in practice: the Wagners. Parents. Family in practice: the Murphys. Siblings. Family in practice: the Marshalls. Grandparents. Working with the deaf family. Index.

Luterman, David M. (1991). *Counseling the communicatively disordered and their families*. San Diego, CA: Singular Publishing Group. INTERVENTION PROGRAMS:

A discussion of individual, group, and family counselling techniques and practices and how they can used by speech/language clinicians in their dealings with clients.

Lynch, Michael P., Oller, D. Kimbrough, & Steffens, Michele. (1989). Development of speech-like vocalizations in a child with congenital absence of cochleas: The case of total deafness. *Applied Psycholinguistics*, 10, 315-333. DEAF CHILDREN VOCALIZATIONS:

Taped utterances of a 3-year-old child born without cochleas were examined. Initially, the subject's speech consisted almost exclusively of small numbers of sounds characteristic of early infancy. As the subject participated in extensive vocal stimulation activities and received intermittent exposure to tactile speech information, the subject made rapid improvement in the quality of his vocalizations. - From Child Development Abstracts.

Lysens, M. Th., & Rondal, Jean A. (1990). *Actes du Premier Congrès Européen sur le syndrome de Down. (Proceedings of the 1st European Congress on Down syndrome.).* Heusy-Verviers: APLM. DOWN SYNDROME: FRENCH

Lyytinen, Paula. (1978). The acquisition of Finnish Morphology in Early Childhood. *Jyvaskyla Studies in Education, Psychology and Social Research*, 37, FINNISH MORPHOSYNTACTIC DEVELOPMENT:

Lyytinen, Paula. (1982). The acquisition process of Finnish morphology in 2-7-year-old children. *Acta Psychologica Fennica*, 9, 112-125. FINNISH MORPHOLOGICAL DEVELOPMENT INFLECTION:

Lyytinen, Paula. (1983). Symbolic play and early language. In *Reports from the Department of Psychology*. Finland: University of Jyvaskyla. LANGUAGE AND PLAY:

Lyytinen, Paula. (1984). Rules in child language. In L. Pulkkinen, & P. Lyytinen (Eds), *Human action and personality. Essays in honor of Martti Takala*. Jyvaskyla, Finland: Jyvaskyla Studies in Education, Psychology and Social Research. RULES:

Lyytinen, Paula. (1987). Cognitive Skills and Finnish Language Inflection. *Scandinavian Journal of Psychology*, 28, 304-312. FINNISH MORPHOSYNTACTIC DEVELOPMENT INFLECTION:

Lyytinen, Paula. (1988). *Developmental changes in children's pretend play*. Jyvaskyla, Finland: Department of Psychology, University of Finland. LANGUAGE AND PLAY:

The development of pretend play was investigated in children 2-6 years of age (18 in each five age groups) by examining changes in action and language based expressions of pretending. Play behavior was assessed by using a selected set of Duplo Lego toys. The analyzed time of the videotaped play session was 8 minutes for each child. Interest focused on the occurence of decentration, decontextualization, and integration at different age levels. 2- year-olds differed significantly from 5-and 6-year-olds in the total number of play acts and action integrations. While the decentered play acts increased with age being the most common forms of action-based pretense in all age groups, substitution and invention showed no increasing occurrence with age. Single-acheme combinations were uncommon at all ages. Multischeme combinations showed a more regular incremental pattern with age. The proportion of the events and long episodes and their included action themes was highest among 6- year-olds. Significant age trends did not occur for language pretending. The results, however, indicated that the attribution of an independent agency emerged earlier in language than in action. The active other-directed utterances comprised the most frequently occurring category of linguistic pretense in all age groups. Similar trend in action was found only at the age of four.PL

Lyytinen, Paula. (1988). Morfologiatesti. Taivutusmuotojen hallinnan mittausmenetelma lapsille. (The Morphological Test: A measure of the mastery of children's inflectional forms). *University of Jyvaskyla, Finland. Reports from the Department of Psychology,* 298, FINNISH INFLECTION ASSESSMENT PROCEDURES: FINNISH

This test has been published by the Finnish Test Service Corporation.

Lyytinen, Paula. (1988). Suomen Kielen Taivutusmuotojen Hallinta 2-9 vuotiailla lapsilla. Katsaus psykologiseen tutimekseen. (The mastery of Finnish inflectional forms in 2 to 9 year olds. A review of psychological studies.). *University of Jyvaskyla, Finland. Reports from the Department of Psycology*, 297, FINNISH INFLECTION MORPHOSYNTACTIC DEVELOPMENT: FINNISH

Lyytinen, Paula. (1989). Effects of modelling on children's pretend play. *Scandinavian Journal of Psychology*, 30, 177-184. LANGUAGE AND PLAY MODELING:

The effects of modelling on pretend play were studied in children between 2.6 and 3.6 years of age by examining changes both in the action and language-based expressions of pretending. Three modelled scenes were demonstrated with the same realistic toys used by the child in the pre- modelling phase. The results gave support to the idea of the effectiveness of modelling. The effects of the modelled scenes were clearest among children whose pre-modelling play consisted of object-centered actions including few of pretending. The post-modelling play of this subgroup showed better quality of action and language categories and integration measures. Among the decentered players no significant action benefit could be achieved. This might have been an outcome of the contextual limits of the toy material and of the drop of play motivation caused by the model interruption. However, these children expressed verbal pretending revealing significant pre-post effects for inventive utterances.PL

Lyytinen, Paula. (1989). *The mastery of Finnish inflectional forms*. Jyvaskyla: Department of Psychology, University of Jyvaskyla. FINNISH INFLECTION MORPHOLOGICAL DISORDERS COMPARATIVES SUPERLATIVES NOUNS ADJECTIVES VERBS MORPHOSYNTACTIC DEVELOPMENT:

The production of Finnish inflectional forms was assessed using a Berko-type morphological test. Subjects were 2:6 to 9-year-old language normally developed children, pre-school age language-delayed and school-age dysphasic children. By analyzing children's correct and erroneous response patterns the attempt was to reveal developmental steps in acquisition of morphology. The results showed children at age of 2:6 and still at 3:6 had difficulties inflecting test words, whereas 4:6 and 5:6-year-olds had made progress in both verb and noun inflection and in use of adjectives. 6:6-year- olds still produced incorrect inflectional patterns in the superlative, substituting comparatives for them. 9-year-olds mastered all the suffixes included in the morphological test. The acquisition order and the mastery level of morphology of language-delayed and dysphasic children correspond to the achievements of 3:6 and 4:6-year-olds.PL

Lyytinen, Paula. (1990). Symbolinen leikki: apsen kehitystason arviointimetelmana. (Symbolic play in assessing the child's cognitive level.). *University of Jyvaskyla, Finland. Reports from the Department of Psychology*, 312, LANGUAGE AND PLAY: FINNISH

Lyytinen, Paula. (1991). Developmental trends in children's pretend play. *Child Care Health and Development*, 17, 9-25. LANGUAGE AND PLAY:

M

Macario, Jason F. (1991). Young children's use of color classification: Foods and canonically colored objects. *Cognitive Development*, 6, 17-46. CATEGORIZATION:

2-4 year olds reliably chose sticks of appropriate colors when prompted by category labels, and rejected inappropriately colored objects for the same categories. Color was more salient than shape for classifying food objects, and vice versa for play objects. From Child Development Abstracts.

Macken, Marlys A. (1992). Where's phonology? In C. A. Ferguson, L. Menn, & C. Stoel-Gammon (Eds), *Phonological development: Models, research, implications*. Monkton, MD: York Press. ACQUISITION AND LINGUISTIC THEORY PHONOLOGICAL DEVELOPMENT:

MacLean, Darla J., & Schuler, Maureen. (1989). Conceptual development in infancy: The understanding of containment. *Child Development*, 60, 1126-1137. CONCEPT DEVELOPMENT:

After being habituated to videotaped episodes of sand being poured into and out of a cylinder, infants saw a 'possible' event and then an 'impossible' event. Next, infants were involved in a game of dropping blocks into a cup. Fourteen-month-olds were contrasted with 20-month-olds. The latter but not the former demonstrate understanding of containment. Some infants were trained through playing with both cans and tubes in their home. They performed in both tests similarly to untrained 20-month-olds. - From Child Development Abstracts.

MacNeilage, Patricia F. (1991). The 'postural origins' theory of primate neurobiological asymmetrics. In N. A. Krasnegor et al. (Eds). *Biological and behavioral determinants of language development*. Hillsdale, NJ: Lawrence Erlbaum Associates. LATERALIZATION BIOLOGICAL FOUNDATIONS:

MacWhinney, Brian. (1972). Hungarian child language references. In D. I. Slobin (Eds), *Leopold's bibliography of child language*. Bloomington: Indiana University Press. BIBLIOGRAPHY HUNGARIAN:

MacWhinney, Brian. (1975). Pragmatic patterns in child syntax. *Papers and Reports on Child Language Development*, 10, 153-165. SYNTACTIC DEVELOPMENT PRAGMATIC DEVELOPMENT:

MacWhinney, Brian. (1978). Limitations on the use of rules in describing behavior. In J. Scandura, & C. Brainerd (Eds), *Structural/process models of complex human behavior*. Alphen aan den Rijn: Sijthoff and Noordhoff. RULES:

MacWhinney, Brian. (1980). Review of "Language acquisition: Studies in first language development" edited by P. Fletcher and M. Garman. *Contemporary Psychology*, 25, 718-719. BOOK REVIEW ACQUISITION THEORIES:

MacWhinney, Brian. (1983). Review of "Language Acquisition and Linguistic Theory" edited by S. Tavakolian. *Journal of Child Language*, 10, 667-672. BOOK REVIEW ACQUISITION AND LINGUISTIC THEORY:

MacWhinney, Brian. (1985). Grammatical devices for sharing points. In R. Schiefelbusch (Ed.), *Communicative competence: Acquisition and intervention*. Baltimore, MD: University Park Press. CUES-SYNTACTIC CUES-PRAGMATIC:

MacWhinney, Brian. (1985). Topic and perspective as cognitive functions: Commentary on "Topic as Starting Point for Syntax" by H. Lempert. *Monographs of the Society for Research in Child Development*, 24, 140-147. TOPIC-COMMENT SYNTACTIC DEVELOPMENT:

MacWhinney, Brian. (1987). Cues, competition, and learning. In J. Miller (Ed.), *Wisconsin Papers on Language Development*. Madison, WI: University of Wisconsin. COMPETITION MODEL CUES:

MacWhinney, Brian. (1989). Competition and lexical categorization. In R. Corrigan, F. Eckman, & M. Noonan. (Eds), *Linguistic categorization*. New York: Benjamins. COMPETITION MODEL LEXICAL DEVELOPMENT MUTUAL EXCLUSIVITY CATEGORIZATION SEMANTIC ORGANIZATION:

MacWhinney, Brian. (1989). Competition in language and thought. In J. Montangero (Ed.), *Language and cognition. Cahiers Jean Piaget 10*. Geneva: Fondation Archives Jean Piaget. COMPETITION MODEL LANGUAGE AND COGNITIVE DEVELOPMENT:

MacWhinney, Brian. (1989). Making words make sense: Commentary on "The Mutual Exclusivity Bias in children's word learning" by W. Merriman and L. Bowman. *Monographs of the Society for Research in Child Development*, 220, 124-129. MUTUAL EXCLUSIVITY LEXICAL DEVELOPMENT CATEGORIZATION:

MacWhinney, Brian. (1989). Review of "Category Acquisition" edited by Y. Levy, I. Schlesinger, & M. Braine. *Language and Speech*, 31, 383-386. BOOK REVIEW CATEGORIZATION:

MacWhinney, Brian. (1989). Review of "Connections and symbols" edited by S. Pinker and J. Mehler. *Applied Psycholinguistics*, 12, 26-28. BOOK REVIEW CONNECTIONISM:

MacWhinney, Brian. (1990). Connectionism as a framework for language acquisition theory. In J. Miller (Ed.), *Progress in research on child language disorders*. Austin, TX: Pro-Ed. CONNECTIONISM ACQUISITION THEORIES :

MacWhinney, Brian. (1990). Psycholinguistics and foreign language acquisition. In J. Tommola (Ed.), *AFinLA Yearbook 1990*. Turku: AFinLA. L2 EDUCATION L2 LINGUISTIC THEORY LANGUAGE AND EDUCATION:

MacWhinney, Brian. (1991). *The CHILDES project - Computational tools for analyzing talk*. Hillsdale, NJ: Lawrence Erlbaum Associates. CHILDES CHILD LANGUAGE CORPORA

METHODOLOGY-TRANSCRIPTION METHODOLOGY-ANALYSIS METHODOLOGY-COMPUTERS :

MinCHAT. File headers. Transcribing words. Transcribing morphemes on the main line. Utterences and tone roots. Prosody within words. Scoped symbols. Dependent tiers. UNIBETs and diacritics. PHONASCII. Error coding. Speech act codes. Morphological and syntactic coding. Examples of transcribed data. Tecniques for recording and transcription. Changes to CHAT symbol summary. Introduction to CLAN. Learning CLAN. DOS, Macintosh, and UNIX. The programs. CLAN Options. Word lists. Testing, bugs, and modifications. Database introduction. English data. Non English data. Narrative data. Data from books. Data on language impairments. Second language acquisition data. The organization of the CHILDES system. Future directions.

MacWhinney, Brian. (1991). The Competition Model and foreign language acquisition. In M. Swartz (Ed.), *Tutoring System for Foreign Language Acquisition*. Amsterdam: Kluwer. COMPETITION MODEL L2 EDUCATION L2 LINGUISTIC THEORY LANGUAGE AND EDUCATION:

MacWhinney, Brian. (1991). Reply to Woodward and Markman. *Developmental Review*, 11, 192-194. LEXICAL DEVELOPMENT MUTUAL EXCLUSIVITY CATEGORIZATION:

MacWhinney, Brian. (1991). Universals in language processing. In W. Bright (Ed.), *Oxford International Encyclopedia of Linguistics*. London: Oxford University Press. LANGUAGE PROCESSING LANGUAGE UNIVERSALS:

MacWhinney, Brian. (1992). *The CHILDES Database, 2nd Ed.* Dublin, OH: Discovery Systems. CHILDES CHILD LANGUAGE CORPORA METHODOLOGY-ANALYSIS METHODOLOGY-COMPUTERS

MacWhinney, Brian. (1992). Transfer and competition in second language learning. In R. Harris (Ed.), *Cognitive processing in bilinguals*. Amsterdam: Elsevier. BILINGUALISM TRANSFER COMPETITION MODEL L2 EDUCATION L2 LINGUISTIC THEORY:

MacWhinney, Brian. (1993). The dinosaurs and the ring. In R. Corrigan, S. Lima, & M. Noonan (Eds), *The reality of linguistic rules*. San Diego: Academic. RULES CUES CONNECTIONISM:

MacWhinney, Brian. (1993). Some updates and future directions in CHILDES. In J. L. Sokolov, & C. E. Snow (Eds), *Handbook of research in language development using CHILDES*. Hillsdale, NJ: Lawrence Erlbaum Associates. CHILD LANGUAGE CORPORA CHILDES METHODOLOGY-COMPUTERS METHODOLOGY-DESIGN METHODOLOGY-ANALYSIS:

MacWhinney, Brian, & Anderson, J. (1986). The acquisition of grammar. In I. Gopnik, & M. Gopnik (Eds), *From models to modules*. Norwood, N.J.: Ablex. SYNTACTIC DEVELOPMENT:

MacWhinney, Brian, & Bates, Elizabeth. (1978). Sentential devices for conveying givenness and newness: A cross-cultural developmental study. *Journal of Verbal Learning and Verbal Behavior*, 17, 539-558. GIVEN-NEW:

MacWhinney, Brian, & Bates, Elizabeth. (1990). *The cross-linguistic study of sentence processing*. New York, NY: Cambridge University Press. LANGUAGE PROCESSING CROSSLINGUISTIC STUDY-SYNTAX COMPETITION MODEL APHASIAS BILINGUALISM-LANGUAGE PROCESSING CONNECTIONISM SYNTACTIC DEVELOPMENT COMPLEX SENTENCES:

Languages differ in myriad ways, yet all share certain core features. How has nature devised the human mind and the child to cope with both this commonality and this diversity? Most psycholinguistists are interested in universal processes, but the vast majority of psycholinguistic studies are of English speakers. This study presents the results of psychologists working within the general framework of a processing model called the Competition Model, as they explore ways in which human beings in different cultures adapt to the tasks of learning and using language. Taking the view that natural languages are extremely important research variables, the contributors investigate bilingualism, aphasia, first language learning, comprehension, production, and PDP connectionist models of learning.

MacWhinney, Brian, Bates, Elizabeth, & Kliegl, R. (1984). Cue validity and sentence interpretation in English, German, and Italian. *Journal of Verbal Learning and Verbal Behavior*, 23, 127-150. CROSSLINGUISTIC STUDY-PRAGMATICS CUES-PRAGMATIC CUES-SYNTACTIC GERMAN ITALIAN COMPLEX SENTENCES:

MacWhinney, Brian, & Leinbach, Jared. (1991). Implementations are not conceptualizations: Revising the verb learning model. *Cognition*, 29, 121-157. VERBS CONNECTIONISM:

MacWhinney, Brian, Leinbach, Jared, Taraban, Roman M., & McDonald, Janet L. (1989). Language learning: Cues or rules? *Journal of Memory and Language*, 28(3), 255-277. RULES CUES COMPETITION MODEL CONNECTIONISM GERMAN CASE MORPHOSYNTACTIC DEVELOPMENT:

A description of an artifical neural network's learning of German case morphology which refutes the argument that artifical neural networks are incapable of learning behaviors as complex as language.

MacWhinney, Brian, & Snow, Catherine E. (1990). The Child Language Data Exchange System. *ICAME Journal*, 14, 3-25. CHILDES CHILD LANGUAGE CORPORA METHODOLOGY-COMPUTERS METHODOLOGY-ANALYSIS:

MacWhinney, Brian, & Snow, Catherine E. (1992). Tools for analyzing child language corpora. In A. Mackie, T. McAuley, & C. Simmons. (Eds), *For Henry Kucera: Studies in Slavic philology and computational linguistics*. Ann Arbor: Michigan Slavic Publications. CHILDES METHODOLOGY-ANALYSIS METHODOLOGY-COMPUTERS CHILD LANGUAGE CORPORA:

MacWhinney, Brian, & Snow, Catherine E. (1992). The wheat and the chaff - or four confusions regarding CHILDES. *Journal of Child Language*, 19, 459-471. CHILDES CHILD LANGUAGE CORPORA METHODOLOGY:

Maegiste, E. (1993). Second language learning in elementary and high school students. In A. M. B. de Groot, & C. Barry (Eds), *The multilingual community*. Hillsdale, NJ: Lawrence Erlbaum Associates. L2 EDUCATION BILINGUALISM-EDUCATION LANGUAGE AND EDUCATION:

Maestas, J., Moores, Y., & Rondal, Jean A. (1981). Le premier environnement linguistique des enfants née des parents sourds. (The early linguistic environment of children born to deaf parents.). *Enfance*, 4 (5), 245-252. PARENTAL INPUT DEAF PARENTS FRENCH: FRENCH

Magnusson, David, & Bergman, Lars R. (1990). *Data quality in longitudinal research*. New York, NY: Cambridge University Press. METHODOLOGY-LONGITUDINAL STUDY METHODOLOGY-ANALYSIS:

An examination of: the reliability and validity of longitudinal research data, subject attrition, sampling, aggregation, and confidentiality issues.

Magnusson, David, Rudinger, Georg, & Torestad, Bertil. (1991). *Problems and methods in longitudinal research : stability and change*. New York, NY: Cambridge University Press. METHODOLOGY-LONGITUDINAL STUDY:

An examination of the special problems and demands of longitudinal research.

Malatesta-Magai, Carol, & Dirval, Bruce. (1992). Language, affect, and social order. In M. R. Gunnar, & M. Maratsos (EdS), *Modularity and constraints in language and cognition*. Hillsdale, NJ: Lawrence Erlbaum Associates. CONSTRAINTS MODULARITY LANGUAGE AND AFFECT:

Malave-Lopez, Lilliam M., & Duquette, Georges. (1991). *Language, culture, and cognition : a collection of studies in first and second language acquisition*. Philadelphia, PA: Multilingual Matters. L2/L1 ACQUISITION L2 ACQUISITION BILINGUALISM LANGUAGE AND COGNITION LANGUAGE AND COGNITIVE DEVELOPMENT SAPIR-WHORF HYPOTHESIS SOCIOLINGUISTIC FACTORS:

Malone, D. Michael, & Stoneman, Zolinda. (1990). Cognitive play of mentally retarded preschoolers: Observations in the home and school. *American Journal on Mental Retardation*, 94, 475-487. RETARDED CHILDREN LANGUAGE AND PLAY:

A within-subjects design was used to examine the cognitive play of 12 mainstreamed mentally retarded preschool boys during group free-play at school and in an independent play situation at home. Children not only played more in the home condition, but this play was more sophisticated than that in the school condition. Increased differences between home and school performance were positively associated with communicative developmental age. - From Child Development Abstracts.

Maratsos, Michael P. (1990). Are actions to verbs as objects are to nouns? On the differential semantic bases of form, class, category. *Linguistics*, 28(6), 1351-1379. CONCEPT DEVELOPMENT SEMANTIC MAPPING SEMANTIC DEVELOPMENT LEXICAL DEVELOPMENT VERBS NOUNS CATEGORIZATION:

Maratsos, Michael P. (1991). How the acquisition of nouns may be different from that of verbs. In N. A. Krasnegor, et al. (Eds), *Biological and behavioral determinants of language development*. Hillsdale, NJ: Lawrence Erlbaum Associates. WORD CLASS NOUNS VERBS:

Maratsos, Michael P. (1992). Constraints, modules, and domain specificity : an introduction. In M. R. Gunnar, & M. Maratsos (Eds), *Modularity and constraints in language and cognition*. Hillsdale, NJ: Lawrence Erlbaum Associates. MODULARITY CONSTRAINTS:

Marchman, Virginia A., Bates, Elizabeth, Burkardt, Antionette, & Good, Amy B. (1991). Functional constraints of the acquisition of the passive: Toward a model of the competence to perform. *First Language*, 11, 65-92. PASSIVES:

In two experiments, children and adults described intransitive, prototypically transitive, and non-protypically transitive scenes presented in an animated film in response to a probe about one or several of the characters. The results suggest that young children do appear to have knowledge of the passive. However, the overall frequencey of passive usage increased across development.

Marchman, Virginia A., Miller, Ruth, & Bates, Elizabeth. (1991). Babble and first words in children with focal brain injury. *Applied Psycholinguistics*, 12, 1-22. GESTURE BABBLING FIRST WORDS TRAUMATIC DISORDERS:

Results indicate that all children were delayed in the number of gestures they were reported to produce, as well as in reported lexical production. Reported comprehension was also typically well below age level. However, age-appropriate comprehension was observed in one child througout the period sampled. Phonological analysis revealed both similarities and differences between the early vocalizations of the neurologically involved children and those of the control group.

Marchman, Virginia A., & Plunkett, Kim. (1989). Token frequency and phonological predictability in a pattern association network. Implications for child language acquisition. In *Proceedings of the Eleventh Annual Conference of the Cognitive Science Society.*. Hillsdale, NJ: Lawrence Erlbaum. CONNECTIONISM REPRESENTATIONS-PHONOLOGICAL LEXICAL DEVELOPMENT TENSE:

A description of an artificial neural network learning English past tense markers.

Marcotte, A. C., O'Brien, B., Holbdy, P., & Labarba, R. C. (1992). Cerebral lateralization for speech production in congenitally blind adolescents. *Developmental Neuropsychology*, 8, 29-39. BLIND CHILDREN LATERALIZATION:

Marcus, Gary F., et al. (1992). *Overregularization in language acquisition.* Chicago, IL: University of Chicago Press. OVERGENERALIZATION SEMANTIC DEVELOPMENT:

Commentary by Harald Clahsen. Includes bibliographical references.

Marcus, Gary F., Ullman, Michael, Pinker, Steven, Hollander, Michelle, Rosen, John T, & Xu, F. (1990). Overregularization. *MIT Center for Cognitive Science Occasional Paper*, 41. CONNECTIONISM TENSE RULES-MORPHOLOGICAL OVERGENERALIZATION-MORPHOSYNTACTIC:

> An analysis of 11,500 irregular past tense utterances made by 69 subjects reveals that overregularizations are rare which suggests that the previously proposed need for children to relearn syntactic rules which have been acquired erroneously is invalid. The report does confirm that there is a 'U' shaped developmental curve of irregular past tense morphemes but the authors believe that the rate of irregular past tense usage is low and that it extends well into the school years. The authors reject Rumelhart and McClelland's (1986) hypothesis that the increasing input of regular past tense forms has an impact on the previously learned past tense system which causes the overregularization of the past tense morpheme and maintain that the overrregularization error occurs as a result of the onset of 'obligatoriness' which requires the marking of past tense forms. The authors also maintain that there is a frequency effect involved in the use of irregular past tense forms and that there may be some form of protective barrier or filter which prevents the spread of past tense rules to irregular verbs. The authors believe that like adults, children obligatorily mark tense using one of two mechanisms: either memory for regulars, or a regular affixation rule. They propose that if the child retrieves an irregular past tense form it blocks the operation of the affixation rule, but because children's memory traces for irregular forms are not strong enough to guarantee perfect retrieval, they sometimes fail to retrieve an irregular form and the affixation rule operates in error to produce the overregularized form.

Markman, Ellen M. (1991). The whole object, taxonomic, and mutual exclusivity assumptions as initial constraints on word meanings. In S. A. Gelman, & J. Byrnes (EdS), *Perspectives on language and thought*. New York, NY: Cambridge University Press. LANGUAGE AND COGNITION LANGUAGE AND COGNITIVE DEVELOPMENT MUTUAL

EXCLUSIVITY SEMANTIC MAPPING LEXICAL DEVELOPMENT CATEGORIZATION CONCEPT DEVELOPMENT CONSTRAINTS-SEMANTIC:

Markman, Ellen M. (1992). Constraints on word learning : speculations about their nature, origins, and domain specificity. In M. R. Gunnar, & M. Maratsos (Eds), *Modularity and constraints in language and cognition*. Hillsdale, NJ: Lawrence Erlbaum Associates. LEXICAL DEVELOPMENT SEMANTIC MAPPING CONSTRAINTS-SEMANTIC MUTUAL EXCLUSIVITY:

Marks, Lawrence E., Hammeal, Robin J., & Bornstein, Marc H. (1987). *Perceiving similarity and comprehending metaphor*. Chicago, IL: University of Chicago Press. FIGURATIVE LANGUAGE DISCOURSE COMPREHENSION SEMANTIC DEVELOPMENT:

The author describe three experiments in which children are asked to match pitch to brightness, loudness to brightness, and pitch to size. They describe a theory to explain the comprehension of metaphors in speech.

Marler, Peter. (1990). Innate learning preferences: Signals for communication. *Developmental Psychobiology*, 23(7), NATIVISM:

Marschark, Marc. (1992). Origins,and interactions in social, cognitive, and language development in deaf children. In M. Marschark, & M. D. Clark (Eds), *Psychological perspectives on deafness*. Hillsdale, NJ: Lawrence Erlbaum Associates. DEAF CHILDREN LANGUAGE AND COGNITION LANGUAGE AND COGNITIVE DEVELOPMENT SOCIAL INTERACTION:

Marschark, Marc, & Clark, M. Diane. (1992). *Psychological perspectives on deafness*. Hillsdale, NJ: Lawrence Erlbaum Associates. DEAF CHILDREN LANGUAGE AND EDUCATION SIGNING:

Marschark, Marc, Everhart, V. S., & Dempsey, P. R. (1991). Nonliteral content in language productions of deaf, hearing, and native-signing hearing mothers. *Merrill-Palmer Quarterly*, 37, 305-323. SIGNING DEAF CHILDREN PARENTAL INPUT PARENTAL SPEECH FIGURATIVE LANGUAGE:

Marsh, R. W., Chen, May Jane, & Lei, Lau Lei. (1989). Piaget's theory of serial memory development: Some new evidence. *British Journal of Developmental Psychology*, 7, 363-369. PIAGETIAN THEORY SERIATION:

The results of the present study, contrary to Piaget & Inhelder's findings (1975), showed that serial memory is probably present at age 4 years.

Marslen-Wilson, William D. (Ed.). (1989). *Lexical representation and process*. Cambridge, MA: MIT/Batsford. LANGUAGE PROCESSING REPRESENTATIONS-LEXICAL CONNECTIONISM LEXICAL ACCESS:

Covers a wide variety of approaches from connectionism to symbolism and discusses the role of lexical representations in language processing. Topics covered include processing models, considerations of input factors, lexical structure, parsing, and interpretation.

Martin, Frederick N. (1987). *Hearing disorders in children: pediatric audiology*. San Diego, CA: Singular Group. DEAF CHILDREN AUDIOLOGY ATYPICAL DEVELOPMENT AUDIOMETRY INTERVENTION PROGRAMS FOR PARENTS LANGUAGE AND EDUCATION:

Causes and treatment of hearing loss in children. Some effects of early hearing impairment on English language development. The psychological world of the hearing impaired child and the family. Recognizing children with language disorders. Auditory brainstem response and middle ear assessment in children. Tests of hearing-the infant. Pure-tone tests with preschool children. Counseling parents of hearing impaired children. The educational management of hearing impaired children. Pediatric amplification. Identification audiometry. Audiology in the public school setting. Author index. Subject index.

Martin, J. (1991). Representing and acquiring metaphor-based polysemy. In U. Zernik (Ed.), *Lexical acquisition - Exploiting on-line resources to build a lexicon* . Hillsdale, NJ : Lawrence Erlbaum Associates. LEXICAL DEVELOPMENT FIGURATIVE LANGUAGE POLYSEMY:

Martin, J. D. (1990). Learning overlapping categories. In M. Piatelli-Palmarini (Ed.), *Proceedings of the Twelfth Annual Conference of the Cognitive Science Society*. Hillsdale, NJ: Lawrence Erlbaum Associates. CATEGORIZATION:

Martin, Michael. (1989). *Speech audiometry*. San Diego, CA: Singular Publishing Group. DEAF CHILDREN AUDIOLOGY ASSESSMENT PROCEDURES AUDIOMETRY CROSSLINGUISTIC STUDY:

> Basic properties. Towards a theory of speech audiometry tests. Speech tests in quiet and noise. Equipment for speech audiometry and its calibration. The German path to standardization in speech audiometry. Speech audiometry for differential diagnosis. The uses and misuses of speech audiometry in rehabilitiation. Speech tests of hearing for children. Speech perception tests for the profoundly deaf. Testing visual and auditory visual speech perception. Speech audiometry in the USA. The Scandinavian approach to speech audiometry. Speech audiometry in Australia. Speech tests in audiological assessment at the National Accoustic Laboratories. Non-European languages. Appendix: Equipment for speech audiometry: a draft standard. References. Index.

Martin, R. R., & Haroldson, S. K. (1992). Stuttering and speech naturalness-audio and audiovisual judgments. *Journal of Speech and Hearing Research*, 35, 521-528. STUTTERING:

Martins, Isabel Pavao, Castro-Caldas, Alexandre, van Dongen, Hugo R., & van Hout, Anne. (Eds) (1991). *Acquired aphasia in children*. Amsterdam, The Netherlands: Kluwer. ACQUIRED APHASIA DEVELOPMENTAL DISORDERS APHASIAS NEUROLINGUISTICS CEREBRAL DISORDERS TRAUMATIC DISORDERS:

Masataka, N. (1992). Early ontogeny of vocal behavior of Japanese infants in response to maternal speech. *Child Development*, 63, 1177-1185. PARENTAL INPUT SOCIAL INTERACTION ADULT-CHILD INTERACTION JAPANESE:

Masataka, N. (1992). Pitch characteristics of Japanese maternal speech to infants. *Journal of Child Language*, 19, 213-223. PARENTAL SPEECH-PROSODY JAPANESE:

Massaro, D. (1988). Some criticisms of connectionist models of human performance. *Journal of Memory and Language*, 27, 213-234. CONNECTIONISM:

Masterson, J. J., & Kamhi, Alan G. (1991). The effects of sampling conditions on sentence production in normal, reading-disabled, and language-learning-disabled children. *Journal of Speech and Hearing Research*, 34, 549-558. METHODOLOGY-DESIGN:

Masterson, J. J., & Kamhi, Alan G. (1992). Linguistic trade-offs in school-age children with and without language disorders. *Journal of Speech and Hearing Research*, 35, 1064-1075. LANGUAGE DISORDERS LANGUAGE PROCESSING:

Matthei, Edward H. (1989). Crossing boundaries: more evidence for phonological constraints on early multi-word utterances. *Journal of Child Language*, 16(1), 41-54. CONSTRAINTS-PHONOLOGICAL:

Mattingly, Ignatius G. (1990). Reading and the biological function of linguistic representations. In I. G. Mattingly, & M. Studdert-Kennedy (Eds), *Modularity and the motor theory of speech perception*. Hillsdale, NJ: Lawrence Erlbaum Associates. REPRESENTATIONS LITERACY:

Mattingly, Ignatius G., & Studdert-Kennedy, Michael. (1990). *Modularity and the motor theory of speech perception*. Hillsdale, NJ: Lawrence Erlbaum Associates. SPEECH PERCEPTION PHONETIC GESTURES MODULARITY ARTICULATION SIGNING LITERACY LANGUAGE AND MOTOR DEVELOPMENT:

A compilation of the proceedings of a conference held to honor Alvin M. Liberman for his outstanding contributions to research in speech perception, this volume deals with two closely related and controversial proposals for which Liberman and his collegues at Haskins Laboratories have argued forcefully over the past 15 years. The first is that articulatory gestures are the units not only of speech production but also of speech perception. The second is that speech production and perception are not cognitive processes, but rather functions of a special mechanism. This book explores the implications of these proposals not only for speech production and speech perception, but for the neurophysiology of language, language acquisition, higher-level linguistic processing, the visual perception of phonetic gestures, the production and perception of sign language, the reading process, and learning to read. The contributors to this volume include linguists, pscholinguists, speech scientists, neurophysiologists, and ethologists. Liberman himself responds in the final chapter.

Maxfield, T. L., & Plunkett, B. (Eds) (1991). *Papers on the acquisition of WH: Proceedings of the University of Massachusetts Roundtable.* Amherst: University of Massachusetts. SYNTACTIC DEVELOPMENT QUESTIONS-WH:

A special edition of *University of Massachusetts Occasional Papers.*

Maxon, A. B., & Welch, A. J. (1992). The role of language competence on comprehension of television messages by children with hearing impairment. *Volta Review* , 94, 315-326. TELEVISION AND LANGUAGE DEVELOPMENT DEAF CHILDREN:

Maxwell, Madeline M. (1989). A signing deaf child's use of speech. *Sign Language Studies*, 62, 23-42. BIMODALITY DEAF CHILDREN:

Mayer, S., & Musatti, T. (1992). Towards the use of symbol-play with objects and communication with adults and peers in the seconnd year. *Infant Behavior and Development*, 15, 1-13. LANGUAGE AND PLAY:

McAnally, Patricia L., Rose, Susan, & Quigley, Stephen P. (1987). *Language learning practices with deaf children.* San Diego, CA: Singular Publishing Group. DEAF CHILDREN INTERVENTION PROGRAMS LANGUAGE AND EDUCATION SIGNING-ASL:

Normal language development. Language development in prelinguistically deaf children. Historical overview of teaching methods and materials. Natural language approach: principles and practices. Structured and combined approaches to teaching languages. Using American sign language to teach English. Specialized aspects of language development. A brief synthesis.

McCabe, Allyssa. (1992). *Language games to play with your child : enhancing communication from infancy through late childhood, (revised ed.).* New York, NY: Insight Books. LITERACY LANGUAGE AND PLAY LANGUAGE AND EDUCATION INTERVENTION PROGRAMS FOR PARENTS:

McCabe, Allyssa, & Peterson, Carole. (1990). *Developing narrative structure.* Hillsdale, NJ: Lawrence Erlbaum Associates. NARRATIVES LANGUAGE AND MEMORY EVENTS/SCRIPTS CONNECTIVES:

McCabe, Ann E. (1989). Differential language learning styles in young children: The importance of context. *Developmental Review*, 9, 1-20. INDIVIDUAL VARIATION CONTEXT:

Style differences, it is argued, do not reflect more or less attempts on the part of the child to master the language system but rather functional variations which result from differences in status on contextual characteristics. - From Child Development Abstracts.

McCartney, Kathleen, Robeson, W. W., Jordan, E., & Mouradian, V. (1991). Mother's language with first and second born children. In K. Pillemer, & K. McCartney (EdS), *Parent-child relations throughout life.* Hillsdale, NJ: Lawrence Erlbaum Associates. PARENTAL SPEECH:

McCauley, R. J., & Demetras, M. J. (1990). The identification of language impairment in the selection of specifically language-impaired subjects. *Journal of Speech and Hearing Disorders*, 55, 468-475. ASSESSMENT PROCEDURES SPECIFIC LANGUAGE IMPAIRMENT:

McCormick, Barry. (1988). *Pediatric audiology: 0-5 years.* San Diego, CA: Singular Publishing Group. NEONATES AUDIOLOGY AUDIOMETRY DEAF CHILDREN:

Epidemiological basis for screening hearing. Otological considerations in the first five years of life. Neonatal hearing screening tests. Behavioral hearing tests 6 months to 5 years. Visual reinforcement audiometry. Pure tone audiometry. Electric response audiometry. Oto-acoustic emissions. Acoustic measurement of auditory function. Hearing aid systems. Hearing aid selection and evaluation for pre-school children. Earmoulds.

McCune, Lorraine. (1992). First words: A dynamic systems view. In C. A. Ferguson, L. Menn, & C. Stoel-Gammon (Eds), *Phonological development: Models, research, implications*. Monkton, MD: York Press. FIRST WORDS LEXICAL DEVELOPMENT:

McDaniel, Dana, & Cairns, Helen S. (1990). The child as informant - Eliciting linguistic intuitions from young children. *Journal of Psycholinguistic Research*, 19, 331-344. METHODOLOGY-DESIGN:

McDaniel, Dana, Cairns, Helen S., & Hsu, Jennifer R. (1990). Binding principles in the grammars of young children. *Language Acquisition*, 1, 121-139. SYNTACTIC DEVELOPMENT NOUNS-PROPER PRONOUNS ANAPHORA:

The authors examine the binding phenomena in the grammars of children ranging from 3:9 to 5:4 and attempt to extend and explain the current literature and some of its contradictions. Among other arguments, they pay close attention to the coreferencing of proper nouns and pronouns.

McDaniel, Dana, Cairns, Helen S., & Hsu, Jennifer R. (1991). Control principles in the grammars of young children. *Language Acquisition*, 1, 297-335. LANGUAGE AND ACTION COMPLEMENTS ADVERBS SYNTACTIC STRUCTURES:

The authors report two experiments investigating control principles in chilren's grammars. In the first experiment, twenty children acted out and gave grammaticality judgments on sentences containing complements and adverbial clauses. In the second, the development of these structures was followed in fourteen subjects from 4:1 to 4:10. The results indicated that children fell into several grammatical types which included: those who applied PRO reference arbitrarily, and those who had a coreference requirement for adverbial clauses which caused pronouns to behave like PRO in some constructions.

McFarlane, Stephen C., Fujiki, Martin, & Brinton, Bonnie. (1988). *Coping with communicative handicaps: resources for the practicing clinician*. San Diego, CA: Singular Publishing Group. INTERVENTION PROGRAMS FOR PARENTS INTERVENTION PROGRAMS LANGUAGE AND EDUCATION:

Counseling parents of communicatively handicapped children. Working with parents in the diagnostic setting. Working with parents of children with language disorders. Working with parents of children with voice and fluency disorders. Coping with the reluctant client. Teaming with the classroom teacher. Working with the medical-dental community. Speech pathology: views from medicine and dentistry. Author index. Subject index.

McGhee-Bidlack, Betty. (1991). The development of noun definitions: A metalinguistic analysis. *Journal of Child Language*, 18, 417-434. LEXICAL DEVELOPMENT SEMANTIC MAPPING NOUNS:

There are significant differences in the manner in which concrete and abstract noun definitions are defined. Only adults were able to define abstract nouns by class and characteristic response. From Child Development Abstracts.

McGregor, Karla K., & Schwartz, Richard G. (1992). Converging evidence for underlying phonological representation in a child who misarticulates. *Journal of Speech and Hearing Research*, 35, 596-603. REPRESENTATIONS-PHONOLOGICAL:

McGrother, C. W., & Marshall, B. (1990). Recent trends in incidence, morbidity and survival in Down's syndrome. *Journal of Mental Deficiency Research*, 34, 49-57. DOWN SYNDROME:

The number of young adults with Down's syndrome is currently increasing due to improvements in survival and a period of increased incident numbers in the 1960's. Deaths from infection have shown the largest decline.

McGuiness, Diane, Olson, Amy, & Chapman, Julia. (1990). Sex differences in incidental recall for words and pictures. *Learning and Individual Differences*, 2, 263-285. SEX DIFFERENCES LANGUAGE AND MEMORY:

A series of experiments was carried out to investigate sex differences in incidental recall trials for words and pictures following an irrelevant task which was either meaningful or meaningless. A strong female advantage was observed. Younger children and older males had better recall for pictures than words, whereas older children and older females had better recall for words. All subjects showed an increase in net recall over trials (hypermnesia) for words and pictures rated in a meaningful way.

McKee, Cecile. (1992). A comparison of pronouns and anaphors in Italian and English acquisition. *Language Acquisition*, 2, 21-54. ANAPHORA PRONOUNS ITALIAN CROSSLINGUISTIC STUDY-SYNTAX:

McKee examines the development of binding for pronouns and anaphors in Italian and English. The results indicate that Italian children abide by binding conditions A and B, but that English children's understanding of pronominal binding lags behind their understanding of anaphors and R-expressions. McKee interprets this to be a negation of the notions that the development of binding involves maturational or pragmatic constraints. In order to explain the differences between the acquisition of the two languages, she proposes a lexical misclassification solution, and a solution based upon children's early hypotheses about government.

McKellar, Gordon B. (1990). The language of neurolinguistics; principles and perspectives in the application of linguistic theory to the neuropsychology of language. In M. A. K. Halliday, J. Gibbons, & H. Nicholas (Eds), *Learning, keeping and using language* . Amsterdam, The Netherlands: John Benjamins. NEUROLINGUISTICS:

Selected paper from the proceedings of the Eighth World Congress of Applied Linguistics, Sydney, 1987.

McKeown, M. G. (1991). Learning word meanings from definitions: problems and potential. In P. Schwanenflugel (Ed.), *The psychology of word meanings*. Hillsdale, NJ: Lawrence Erlbaum Associates. SEMANTIC DEVELOPMENT SEMANTIC MAPPING LEXICAL DEVELOPMENT:

McLane, Joan Brooks, & McNamee, Gillian Dowley. (1990). *Early literacy*. Cambridge, MA: Harvard University Press. LITERACY:

McLean, James E., & Snyder-McLean, Lee K. (1991). Communicative intent and its realizations among persons with severe intellectual deficits. In N. A. Krasnegor, et al. (Eds), *Biological and behavioral determinants of language development*. Hillsdale, NJ: Lawrence Erlbaum Associates. RETARDED CHILDREN INTENTIONALITY :

McNeil, Malcom R., Rosenbek, John C., & Aronson, Arnold E. (1984). *The dysarthrias: physiology, acoustics, perception, management*. San Diego, CA: Singular Publishing Group. DYSARTHRIA ARTICULATION DISORDERS INTERVENTION PROGRAMS:

A neurobiologic view. Respiratory kinematics in speakers with motor neuron disease. Physiological analyses of Parkinsonian tremors in the orofacial sustem. Articulatory characteristics of Parkinsonian dysarthria: segmental and phase-level timing, spirantization, and glottal- supraglottal coordination. Assessment of stress patterning. Relationships between perceptual ratings and accoustical measures of hypokinetic speech. Relationships between articulation rate, intelligibility, and naturalness in spastic and ataxic speakers. Role of feedback, reinforcement, and compliance on training and transfer in biofeedback-based rehabilitation of motor speech disorders. Efficacy of modified palatal lifts for improving resonance.

McNeill, David. (1966). The capacity for language acquisition. *Volta Review*, 852, 5-21. LANGUAGE ACQUISITION DEVICE ACQUISITION THEORIES:

McNeill, David. (1992). The spectrum from gesture to sign. In M. Marschark, & M. D. Clark (Eds), *Psychological perspectives on deafness*. Hillsdale, NJ: Lawrence Erlbaum Associates. DEAF CHILDREN GESTURE SIGNING:

McPherson, Leslie M. (1991). A little goes a long way: Evidence for a perceptual basis of learning for the noun categories count and mass. *Journal of Child Language*, 18, 315-338. NOUNS-COUNT/MASS LEXICAL DEVELOPMENT:

Despite the presence of incongruent syntactic cues, children with a mean age of 2:10 systematically chose count/mass characteristics based upon the physical properties (object or substance) of the stimulus. From Child Development Abstracts.

McReynolds, Leija V., & Kerns, Kevin P. (1983). *Single-subject experimental designs in communicative disorders*. San Diego, CA: Singular Publishing Group. METHODOLOGY-DESIGN:

Preliminaries to single-subject experiments. Withdrawal and reversal designs. Multiple-baseline designs. Criteria for evaluationg data for treatment effectiveness. Reliability and observational codes. Beyond the basic designs. Reflections. References. Author index. Subject index.

McShane, John. (1991). *Cognitive development*. Cambridge, MA: Basil Blackwell. OVERVIEW-COGNITIVE DEVELOPMENT PIAGETIAN THEORY LANGUAGE AND COGNITIVE DEVELOPMENT NEOPIAGETIAN THEORY:

Integrates Piagetian theory into later developments in the field and focusses on mechanisms of developmental change, and what actually develops. Covers perception, memory, number, quantity, inferential reasoning, concepts, language, reading, and related theoretical issues.

McTear, Michael, & Conti-Ramsden, Gina. (1989). Assessment of pragmatic skills. In K. Grundy (Ed.), *Linguistics in clinical practice*. London: Taylor & Francis. ASSESSMENT PROCEDURES PRAGMATIC DISORDERS PRAGMATIC DEVELOPMENT:

McTear, Michael, & Conti-Ramsden, Gina. (1991). *Pragmatic disability in children*. London: Whurr Publishers. PRAGMATIC DISORDERS:

Meggyes, Klara S. (1972). The synchrony of different developmental stages in the language of a two year old child. In K. Ohnesorg (Ed.), *Colloquium Paedolinguisticum (Proceedings of the First International Symposium of Paedolinguistics held in Brno, October 14-16, 1970)*.. The Hague: Mouton. DEVELOPMENTAL UNIVERSALS HUNGARIAN:

Meggyes, Klara S. (1973). Az ösztönös es a naív szófejtések kérdéséhez (To the topic of instinctive and naive etymology). In E. Abaffy, F. Nagy, & E. Zelliger (Ed.), *Adalékok a magyar nyelv életrajzához*.. Budapest: HUNGARIAN NATIVISM: HUNGARIAN

Meggyes, Klara S. (1974). A késöi gyermeknyelv kutatásának funkciója a jelentéstanban. (Semantics and the research of late child language). In S. Imre, I. Szathmari, & L. Szuts (Eds), *Jelentéstan és stilisztika*.. Budapest: SEMANTIC DEVELOPMENT: HUNGARIAN

Meggyes, Klara S. (1977). A szó elsajátítása a nyelvelsajátítás folyamatában (Word acquisition and language acquisition). *Nyelvtudományi Közlemények*, 79, 238-244. LEXICAL DEVELOPMENT HUNGARIAN: HUNGARIAN

Meggyes, Klara S. (1979). Fiktív szövegkörnyezet és szituáció a gyermeki mondatmegértésben (Invented context and situation in sentence understanding of children). *Nyelvtudományi Közlemények*, 81, 153-160. CONTEXT DISCOURSE COMPREHENSION COMPREHENSION HUNGARIAN: HUNGARIAN

Meggyes, Klara S. (1980). Az ige idöváltás szerepe a magyar gyermek nyelvi szövegek egyik tipúsában (The role of shifting the verbal tense in one type of text produced by children). *Nyelvtudományi Közlemények*, 82, 237-250. TENSE HUNGARIAN: HUNGARIAN

Meggyes, Klara S. (1980). Jegyzetek a képi ábrázolás gyermeki verbálizálásáról (Notes on how children describe pictures). In K. Radics, & J. László (Eds), *Dialógus és interakció*. Budapest: CHILDREN'S DESCRIPTIONS HUNGARIAN: HUNGARIAN

Meggyes, Klara S. (1981). Kép, szöveg és idö a hatéves óvodások képleírásában (Picture, text and time in picture descriptions by six-year-old preschoolers). In M. Losonczy (Ed.), *Ovodai anyanyelvi nevelés továbbfejlesztése*. Kecskemét: CHILDREN'S DESCRIPTIONS HUNGARIAN: HUNGARIAN

Meggyes, Klara S. (1981). A mondat- és szövegalkotás nehány sajátosságai hatévesgyermekek képleírásában (Some features of sentence and text processing in picture descriptions of six-year-old preschoolers.). *Pszichológia*, 1, 541-551. CHILDREN'S DESCRIPTIONS HUNGARIAN: HUNGARIAN

Meggyes, Klara S. (1985). A gyermeki szókincs jelentésbeli oldalának vizsgálatárol. (On investigating the semantic aspect of children's vocabulary). *Magyar Nyelvör*, 109, 149-152. VOCABULARY DEVELOPMENT SEMANTIC DEVELOPMENT HUNGARIAN: HUNGARIAN

Meggyes, Klara S. (1985). A hatéves óvoda gyermek szófelhasználása összefüggö beszédben. (Word usage of six-year-old preschool children in continuous discourse.). In J. S. Kadar (Ed.), *Beszéd és kommunikáció az óvodás és kisiskoláskorban*. Budapest: Akadémiai Kiadó. CHILDREN'S DISCOURSE HUNGARIAN: HUNGARIAN

Meggyes, Klara S. (1988). Falusi es városi óvodások elbeszélö-leíró szövegeinek különbsége. (Differences in the narratives of preschool children living in urban and rural settings.). In J. Kiss, & L. Szuts (Eds), *A magyar nyelv retegzödése.*. Budapest: NARRATIVES SOCIOLINGUISTIC FACTORS HUNGARIAN: HUNGARIAN

Mehler, Jacques, & Bertoncini, Josiane. (1979). Infants' perception of speech and other acoustic stimuli. In J. Morton, & J. C. Marshall (Eds), *Psycholinguistics 2: Structures and processes*. Cambridge, MA: MIT Press. INFANT PERCEPTION SPEECH PERCEPTION PRELINGUISTICS:

Mehler, Jacques, & de Boysson-Bardies, Bénédicte. (1971). Études sur le rappel de phrases. (Studies on the recall of sentences.). *L'Année Psychologique*, 71 (2), 548-579. LANGUAGE AND MEMORY COMPLEX SENTENCES: FRENCH

Mehmet, Yavas. (1991). *Phonological disorders in children: Theory, research and practice*. London, UK: Routledge. PHONOLOGICAL DISORDERS:

Meier, Richard P., & Newport, Elissa L. (1990). Out of the hands: On a possible sign advantage in language acquisition. *Language*, 66(1), 1-23. SIGNING SINGLE-WORD SPEECH TWO-WORD SPEECH MODALITY:

Recent research has examined the early stages of language development in signed and spoken language. In this paper we discuss claims that, in the timing of early language milestones, there is an advantage for the acquisition of signed language. In particular, we will review the evidence that the emergence of the first signs and of the first two-sign combinations is precocious in signing children as compared to the appearance of the first words and the first two-word strings in speaking children. We conclude that the evidence for early syntax in signing children is not at all compelling. Finally, we discuss the import of a short-lived sign advantage in early language acquisition, in terms of understanding maturational timing mechanisms more generally. Specifically, we address the question of whether or not a single timing mechanism underlies early milestones in the acquisition of both vocabulary and syntax. - From Language.

Meisel, Jürgen M. (1983). Language development and linguistic theory. Review of 'Derek Bickerton (1981), Roots of Language'. *Lingua*, 61, 231-257. BOOK REVIEW ACQUISITION AND LINGUISTIC THEORY:

Meisel, Jürgen M. (1985). Les phases initiales du développement de notions temporelles, aspectuelles et de modes d'action. Étude basée sur le langage d'enfants bilingues: français-allemends (First steps to notions of tense, aspect, and aktionsart, in bilingual children: French and German). *Lingua*, 66 (4), 321-374. GERMAN-FRENCH FRENCH-GERMAN BILINGUALISM-ASPECT BILINGUALISM-TENSE BILINGUALISM-VOICE BILINGUALISM-VERBS VERBS: FRENCH

Meisel, Jürgen M. (1989). Early differentiation of languages in bilingual children. In K. Hyltenstam, & L. Obler (Ed.), *Bilingualism across the life span: In health and in pathology*. Cambridge: Cambridge University Press. BILINGUALISM-LANGUAGE DIFFERENTIATION:

Meisel, Jürgen M. (1990). INFL-ection: subjects and subject-verb agreement. In M. J. Meisel (Ed.), *Two first languages: Early grammatical development in bilingual children*. Dordrecht: Foris. AGREEMENT BILINGUALISM-SYNTACTIC DEVELOPMENT BILINGUALISM-MORPHOLOGICAL DEVELOPMENT:

Meisel, Jürgen M. (1990). *Two first languages : early grammatical development in bilingual children*. Dordrecht, The Netherlands: Foris. FRENCH-GERMAN GERMAN-FRENCH BILINGUALISM-SYNTACTIC DEVELOPMENT:

Meisel, Jürgen M. (1992). *The acquisition of verb placement: Functional categories and V2 phenomena in language development*. Dordrecht, The Netherlands: Kluwer Academic. VERBS SYNTACTIC DEVELOPMENT CROSSLINGISTIC STUDY-SYNTAX SYNTACTIC STRUCTURES:

Meisel, Jürgen M. (1992). La adquisición simultanea de dos primeras lenguas. Discusión general e implicaciónes para el estudio del bilingüismo en euskadi. (The simultaneous acquisition of two first languages.). *Iberoamericana*, 33, 5-34. BILINGUALISM-SIMULTANEOUS: SPANISH

Meixner, Ildikó. (1986). A diszlexia felismeréséröl és pedagógiai vonatkozásairól. (Diagnosis and educational aspects of dyslexia). In A. Horanyi, O. Kasané, & V. Ormani (Ed.), *Pedagógusok és pszichológusok*. Budapest: Egyöttmüködés a szociálizációs zavarok megelözéséért. DYSLEXIA HUNGARIAN: HUNGARIAN

Melekian, Badrig A. (1990). Family characteristics of children with dyslexia. *Journal of Learning Disabilities*, 23, 386-391. DYSLEXIA LANGUAGE AND EDUCATION LANGUAGE AND SOCIAL CLASS AT-RISK CHILDREN SIBLING EFFECTS:

The present study was based on a retrospective review of children with severe dyslexia. The major findings were the low occupational status and educational level of parents and the predominance of high-ranking children in large sibships. Parental age was not found to be an important risk factor.

Melhuish, E. C., Lloyd, E., Martin, S., & Mooney, A. (1990). Type of children at 18 months-II. Relations with cognitive and language development. *Child Psychology and Psychiatry*, 31, 861-870. LANGUAGE AND COGNITIVE DEVELOPMENT LANGUAGE AND SOCIAL CLASS LANGUAGE AND EDUCATION PARENTAL INPUT:

The relationship between type of day care experience and cognitive and language development at 18 months of age was considered. There was a strong association between socio-economic characteristics and type of day care. The results for cognitive development indicate a relationship with mother's education but not with type of day care. For language development the results indicate that children who experience group care were less likely to show much production of different word combinations, but that this was related to the children's language environments.

Melo, Lelia E. (1989). Speech disorders and personal, familial, environmental antecedents. In *Anais de I Encontro Sobre Acquisicao Linguagem*, 205-220. Porto Allegre, Brazil. LANGUAGE DISORDERS SIBLING EFFECTS ENVIRONMENTAL INFLUENCES:

Meltzoff, Andrew N., & Moore, N. Keith. (1989). Imitation in new born infants: Exploring the range of gestures initiated and underlying mechanisms. *Developmental Psychology*, 25, 954-962. IMITATION GESTURE NEONATES:

Head movement and tongue-protrusion gestures were used. Imitation was not limited to the intervals during which the experimenter's movements were displayed. Newborn imitation is not constrained to a few privileged oral movements. - From Child Development Abstracts.

Menard, Scott. (1991). *Longitudinal research*. Newbury Park, CA: Sage Publications, Inc. METHODOLOGY-LONGITUDINAL STUDY METHODOLOGY-DESIGN:

Written in non-technical language, this practical volume covers the major issues involved in longitudinal research, including research design strategies, methods of data collection, and commonly encountered problems. In addition, it compares longitudinal and cross-sectional research in terms of consistency and accuracy of results.

Meng, Katharina. (1981). Untersuchungen zur sprachlichen Kommunikation (von kindern) - Ausgangsbegriffe und theoretische Fragen. (Examinations of children's communication-results and theoretical questions.). *Linguistische Studien/Zentralinstitut für Sprachwissenschaft, Reibe A*, 84, 1-39. CHILDREN'S DISCOURSE GERMAN: GERMAN

Meng, Katharina. (1985). Sequences for securing understanding in child communication. *Rassegna Italiana di Linguistica Applicata*, 17, 175-185. CHILDREN'S DISCOURSE CONVERSATIONAL COMPETENCE CONVERSATIONAL REPAIRS:

Meng, Katharina. (1985). Untersuchungen zur Ontogenese der sprachliche Kommunikation. (Examinations of the ontogenesis of communication.). *Zeitschrift für Phonetik, Sprachwissenschaft und Kommunikationsforschung*, 38, 45-57. GERMAN COMMUNICATIVE DEVELOPMENT: GERMAN

Meng, Katharina. (1986). Kommunikationslinguistische und Sprachpädagogische Überlegungen zu Rubensteins 'Psychologie der Rede' (Linguistics and language education: Reflections on Rubenstein's 'Psychology of Speech'.). *Linguistische Studien/Zentralinstitut für Sprachwissenschaft, Reibe A*, 139, 127-165. LANGUAGE AND EDUCATION: GERMAN

Meng, Katharina. (1986). Zur Rekonstruktion intuitiven Kommunikationswissens. (On the reconstruction of intuitive communicative knowledge.). *Linguistische Studien/Zentralinstitut für Sprachwissenschaft, Reibe A*, 149, 57-67. GERMAN COMMUNICATIVE COMPETENCE: GERMAN

Meng, Katharina. (1987). Narrating and listening in the kindergarten: first findings with 3- year-olds. In H. Geissner (Ed.), *On Narratives. Proceedings of the 10th International Colloquium on Speech Communication.* Frankfurt: NARRATIVES LANGUAGE AND EDUCATION:

Meng, Katharina. (1988). Erzählen und Zuhören im Alltag. Skizze eines Kommunikationstyps. (Narrating and listening in the "day care(?)"-Sketches of a communicative category.). *Linguistische Studien/Zentralinstitut für Sprachwissenschaft, Reibe A*, 181, 1-68. GERMAN NARRATIVES DISCOURSE FUNCTIONS DISCOURSE STRUCTURE TEXT/STORY GRAMMARS LANGUAGE AND EDUCATION: GERMAN

Meng, Katherina. (1988). Interacktion und Kommunikation bei Kindern: Entwicklungslininen im Vorschulalter. (Children's interaction and communication: Developmental lines in preschoolers.). In H. Pätzold, & K. Funke (Eds), *Zur psychischen Entwicklungg der Persönlichkeit im Kindes- und Jugendalter: Theoretische und methodologische Probleme und Ergebnisse etappenorientierter Forschungsstrategien.* Berlin, Germany: Auftrag der Gesellschaft für Psychologie der DDR. GERMAN COMMUNICATIVE DEVELOPMENT INTERSUBJECTIVITY SOCIAL INTERACTION: GERMAN

Meng, Katharina. (1988). Kommunikationslinguistik und Kommunikationerziehung. (The linguistics of communication and communication education.). In *Kann man Kommunikation lehren? Konzepte mündlicher Kommunikation und ihrer Vermittlung.* Frankfurt: Norbert Gutenberg. COMMUNICATIVE DEVELOPMENT LANGUAGE AND EDUCATION GERMAN: GERMAN

Meng, Katherina, & Kraft, Barbara. (1976). Kommunikationsmerkmale als Variable sprachdiagnostischer Situationen. (Characteristics of communication as variables in diagnostic situations.). *Zeitschrift für Psychologie*, 184, 191-202. GERMAN COMMUNICATIVE DEVELOPMENT COMMUNICATIVE DISORDERS INTERVENTION PROGRAMS ASSESSMENT PROCEDURES: GERMAN

Meng, Katharina, Kraft, Barbara, & Nitsche, Ulla. (1991). *Kommunikation im Kindergarten. Studien zur Aneignung der kommunikativen Kompetenz. (Communication on the kindergarten. Studies on the appropriateness of communicative competence.).* Berlin: Akademie-Verlag. GERMAN COMMUNICATIVE COMPETENCE: GERMAN

Meng, Katherina, & Kruse, Karen. (1984). Verständnissicherung: Allgemeine und ontogenese Aspekte eines Typs von Sequenzen kommunikativer Handlungen. (Comprehension: General and ontogentic aspects of types of sequences of communicative acts.). *Linguistische Studien/Zentralinstitut für Sprachwissenschaft, Reibe A*, 118, 1-65. COMPREHENSION COMMUNICATIVE DEVELOPMENT GERMAN: GERMAN

Meng, Katharina, & Nitsche, Ulla. (1989). Verständnissicherung im Gesprach. (Comprehension of language.). *Deutsch als Fremdsprache*, 3, 158-163. COMPREHENSION COMMUNICATIVE DEVELOPMENT: GERMAN

Meng, Katherina, & Quasthoff, Uta M. (1992). *Narrative development in a social context.* Hillsdale, NJ: Lawrence Erlbaum Associates. NARRATIVES:

A special issue of the *Journal of Narrative and Life History* (volume 2, part 3) containing papers originally presented at the Fifth International Child Language Congress (Budapest, 1990) based around the topic of narrative interaction.

Menn, Lise. (1992). Bulding our own models: developmental phonology comes of age. In C. A. Ferguson, L. Menn, & C. Stoel-Gammon (Eds), *Phonological development: Models, research, implications.* Monkton, MD: York Press. ACQUISITION THEORIES-PHONOLOGY ACQUISITION AND LINGUISTIC THEORY:

Menn, Lise, & Matthei, Edward H. (1992). The "two-lexicon" account of child phonology: Looking back, looking ahead. In C. A. Ferguson, L. Menn, & C. Stoel-Gammon (Ed.), *Phonological development: Models, research, implications.* Monkton, MD: York Press. REPRESENTATIONS-PHONOLOGICAL LEXICAL DEVELOPMENT PHONOLOGICAL DEVELOPMENT:

Mentis, Michelle, & Thompson, Sandra A. (1991). Discourse: A means for understanding normal and disordered language. In T. M. Gallagher, & N. Rees (Ed.), *Pragmatics of language: Clinical practice issues*. San Diego, CA: Singular Group. DISCOURSE ANALYSIS DISCOURSE DISORDERS:

Menyuk, Paula, Chesnick, M., Liebergott, J. W., & Korngold, B., et al. (1991). Predicting reading problems in at-risk children. *Journal of Speech and Hearing Research*, 34, 893-903. AT-RISK CHILDREN READING DISORDERS:

Menyuk, Paula, Liebergott, J. W., Schultz, M., & Chesnick, M., et al. (1991). Patterns of early lexical and cognitive development in premature and full-term infants. *Journal of Speech and Hearing Research*, 34, 88-94. LEXICAL DEVELOPMENT LANGUAGE AND COGNITIVE DEVELOPMENT:

Merriman, William E., & Schuster, J. M. (1991). Young children's disambiguation of object name reference. *Child Development*, 62, 1288-1301. LABELING AMBIGUITY MUTUAL EXCLUSIVITY CONCEPT DEVELOPMENT LEXICAL DEVELOPMENT SEMANTIC MAPPING:

Mervis, Carolyn B. (1991). Studying lexical development: The value of the diary method. In C. Rovee-Collier, & L. P. Lipsitt (Eds), *Advances in infancy research*. Norwood, NJ: Ablex. LEXICAL DEVELOPMENT METHODOLOGY-DIARY/CASE STUDY METHODOLOGY-DESIGN:

Metter, E. Jeffery, & Hanson, Wayne R. (1991). Dysarthria in progressive supranuclear palsy. In C. Moore, K. M. Yorkston, & D. R. Beukelman (Eds), *Dysarthria and apraxia of speech*. Baltimore, MD: Paul H. Brookes. DYSARTHRIA:

Metz, Dale E., Schiavetti, Nicholas, Sitler, Ronald W., & Samar, Vincent J. (1990). Speech production stability characteristics of hearing-impaired speakers. *Volta Review*, 92, 223-235. DEAF CHILDREN ARTICULATION DISORDERS ARTICULATION:

> The within-subject standard deviations on eight acoustic variables over repeated speech productions of hearing-impaired speakers was examined. The findings suggest that hearing-impaired speakers who exhibit low overall speech intelligibility may fall into two distinct groups: those who are

extremely consistent in their abherrant production patterns, and those who are extremely inconsistent in their error patterns.

Meyer-Schepers, Ursula. (1991). *Linguistik und Problematik des Schriftspracherwerbs: von der Sachlogik des Zusammenhangs von Laut- und Schriftsprache über die Logik der Aneignung von Schriftsprachkompetenz zur Diagnose und Therapie von Fehlersyndromen.* Frankfurt am Main, Germany: P. Lang. GERMAN WRITTEN LANGUAGE AGRAPHIA: GERMAN

Michaels, S. (1990). The dismantling of narrative. In A. McCabe, & C. Peterson (Eds), *Developing narrative structure.* Hillsdale, NJ: Lawrence Erlbaum Associates. NARRATIVES:

Mikeš, Melanie. (1982). Microsociolinguistics of Hungarian-Serbocroatian bilingualism. In R. L. Cooper (Ed.), *Language spread: Studies in diffusion and social change.* Bloomington, IN: Indiana University Press. HUNGARIAN-SERBOCROATIAN SERBOCROATIAN-HUNGARIAN BILINGUALISM-CULTURAL FACTORS BILINGUALISM-SOCIAL FACTORS:

Mikeš, Melanie. (1989). The early acquistion of German as a foreign language. *Grazer Linguistische Studien.*, 32, GERMAN L2 ACQUISITION:

Mikeš, Melanie. (1990). Some issues of lexical development in early bi- and trilinguals. In C. E. Snow, & G. Conti-Ramsden (Ed.), *Children's language.* Hillsdale, NJ: Lawrence Erlbaum Associates. BILINGUALISM-LEXICAL DEVELOPMENT:

Mikeš, Melania, & Dezsö, Lásló. (1972). Diachronic syntax and the ontogenesis of language. In *Proceedings of the Eleventh International Congress of Linguistics..* Bologna: ACQUISITION AND LINGUISTIC THEORY SYNTACTIC DEVELOPMENT:

Mikeš, Melanie, & Dezsö, Lásló. (1972). Sentence-programming span in child language. In K. Ohnesorg (Ed.), *Colloquium Paedolinguisticum..* The Hague, The Netherlands: Mouton. COMPLEX SENTENCES LANGUAGE AND MEMORY:

Mikeš, Melanie, & Gadler, H. (1986). Der Erwerb der Müttersprache beim einsprachigen und beim dreisprachigen Kind. (The acquisition of a native language by mono- and multilingual children.). *Gräzer Linguistische Studien*, 27, L2/L1 ACQUISITION BILINGUALISM-LANGUAGE DIFFERENTIATION BILINGUALISM-SIMULATANEOUS: GERMAN

Mikeš, Melanie, & Savič, Svenka. (1974). The expanding of the noun phrase in child language. *Journal of Child Language*, 1(1), SYNTACTIC STRUCTURES NOUNS:

Mikeš, Melania, Tallman, J., & Goncz, Lajos. (1971). Adalékok a szociálizáció fejlödéséhez kétnyelvü óvodás gyermekeknél. (A contribution to the problem of socialization among bilingual children in kindergartens.). *A Hungarológiai Intézet Tudományos Közleményei*, 8, 60-73. BILINGUALISM-SOCIAL FACTORS HUNGARIAN-SERBOCROATIAN SERBOCROATIAN-HUNGARIAN SOCIAL SPEECH: HUNGARIAN

The aim of our research work has been to show how the knowledge of a second language influences socialization in a kindergarten group consisting of 26 children, 16 boys and 10 girls, between 5 and 6 years of age. At the beginning of the examination period-the first half of October 1970-11 children were Hungarian-Serbocroatian bilinguals, 9 of them incipient bilinguals, and 6 of them Serbocroatian monolinguals. The degree of socialization has been measured by interactions, taking into account the frequency of contacts between or among children, the children involved in each contact and the occurrence of speech. Our first statement is concerned with the general comparison of the bilingual kindergarten with a monolingual kindergarten which has been treated as the control group. The major interactions are the initiated and sharing interactions in both kindergartens and in both periods of observation. This would indicate that the contact among the children was positive, more friendly than angry behavior, and that the children tended to play more collectively than individually. The bilingual children had the greatest number of interactions: almost half again as many as the children belonging to the group of incipient bilinguals, and almost twice as much as the monolingual children in fall, while this proportion changed somewhat in spring. As to the language use a clear tendency is seen from the results. Although all the children use more Serbocroatian than Hungarian, the bilinguals use less Serbocroatian than the incipient bilinguals. With regard to the occurrence of speech in interactions, bilinguals tended to use more speech than incipient bilinguals in fall, and both used more speech than monolinguals in fall and spring.LG

Mikeš, Melanie, & Vlahovič, P. (1970). Approche méthodologique aux recherches de l'apprentissage du langage par l'enfant. (Methodological approaches to research in language acquisition by children.). In *Actes du Dixième Congrès International des Linguistes.*. Bucarest: METHODOLOGY-DESIGN METHODOLOGY-ANALYSIS: FRENCH

Mikeš, Melanie, Vlahovič, P., & Dezsö, Láslő. (1972). Développement des constructions de complément d'objet et de lieu dans le langage des enfants sèrbocroates et hongrois. (The development of object complements and locatives (?) in the language of Serbocroatian and Hungarian children.). In K. Ohnesorg (Ed.), *Colloquium Paedolinguisticum*. The Hague, The netherlands: Mouton. SERBOCROATIAN HUNGARIAN COMPLEMENTS LOCATIVES: FRENCH

Miles, Elaine. (1989). *The Bangor dyslexia teaching system*. San Diego, CA: Singular Publishing Group. DYSLEXIA LANGUAGE AND EDUCATION INTERVENTION PROGRAMS:

This book describes the author's teaching system, perfected at the University College of North Wales (Bangor, Wales), for children who are dyslexic or have specific learning difficulties. The text is in two sections, the first covering elementary school ages, the second covering high school ages.

Miller, Joanne L., & Jusczyk, Peter W. (1989). Seeking the neurobiological bases of speech perception. *Cognition*, 33(1-2), 111-137. SPEECH PERCEPTION BIOLOGICAL FOUNDATIONS:

Miller, Jonathan F. (1991). *Research on child language disorders: A decade of progress*. San Diego, CA: Singular Publishing Group. LANGUAGE DISORDERS INTERVENTION PROGRAMS:

Introduction. Language development. Theory and models. Language disorders. Directions for future research: research resources. Intervention. Speech sound system. Language processes. Index.

Miller, Max, & Weissenborn, Jürgen. (1991). Sprachliche Sozialisation. (Speech socialization.). In K. Hurrelmann, & D. Ulich (Eds), *Handbuch der Sozialisationsforschung*. Munich: Psychologie Verlagsunion. LANGUAGE AND SOCIAL TRANSMISSION LANGUAGE SOCIALIZATION: GERMAN

Miller, P. J. (1993). Troubles in the garden and how they get resolved: A young child's transformation of his favorite story. In C. A. Nelson (Ed.), *Memory and affect in development*. Hillsdale, NJ: Lawrence Erlbaum Associates. LANGUAGE AND MEMORY NARRATIVES:

Milloy, Nancy, & Lesley, Summers. (1989). Six years on -- do claims still hold? Four children reassessed on a procedure to identify developmental articulatory dyspraxia. *Child Language Teaching and Therapy*, 5, 287-303. ASSESSMENT PROCEDURES MILLOY ASSESSMENT OF PRAXIS ARTICULATION ARTICULATION DISORDERS:

Children diagnosed after three administrations of the MAP at six monthly intervals continued to present the characteristics of dyspraxia, or showed the expected improvements predicted for immature articulatory praxis. - From Child Development Abstracts.

Milner, E. (1976). CNS maturation and language acquisition. In H. A. Whitaker, & H. Whitaker (Eds), *Studies in neurolinguistics*, vol. 1. New York, NY: Academic Press. LATERALIZATION NEUROLINGUISTICS CORTICAL STRUCTURES:

Milosky, Linda M. (1990). *World knowledge and language*. Rockville, MD: Aspen System Corporation. LANGUAGE AND COGNITION CONCEPT DEVELOPMENT SEMANTIC MAPPING CATEGORIZATION SAPIR-WHORF HYPOTHESIS:

Minami, Masahuko, & Kennedy, Bruce P. (1991). *Language issues in literacy and bilingual/multicultural education*. Cambridge, MA: Harvard Educational Review. BILINGUALISM-EDUCATION LITERACY L2 EDUCATION LANGUAGE AND EDUCATION:

A collection of essays previously published in The Review dealing with language and literacy covering areas such as: acquisition theory, syntactic acquisition, language acquisition and reading, language education, adult literacy, and bilingual education.

Mineo, B. A., & Goldstein, Howard. (1990). Generalized learning of receptive and expressive action-object responses by language-delayed preschoolers. *Journal of Speech and Hearing Disorders,* 55(4), 665-678. TREATMENT GENERALIZATION:

Mitchell, P., & Robinson, E. J. (1992). Children's understanding of the evidential connotation of 'know' in relation to overestimation of their own knowledge. *Journal of Child Language*, 19, 167-182. VERBS-MENTAL:

Mitchell, Peter, & Russell, James. (1991). Children's judgments of whether slightly and grossly discrepant objects were intended by a speaker. *British Journal of Developmental Psychology*, 9, 271-279. COMMUNICATIVE COMPETENCE CHILDREN'S DESCRIPTIONS:

5 and 9 year olds judged whether or not objects they found matched the descriptions for objects requested by speakers. Both age groups judged positively for grossly discrepant objects, but only 9 year olds showed a preference for judging positively when the discrepancy was slight. From Child Development Abstracts.

Mitchell, Pamela R., & Kent, Raymond D. (1990). Phonetic variation in multisyllable babbling. *Journal of Child Language*, 17, 247-265. BABBLING:

Phonetic variation in multisyllable babbling of infants was investigated. Eight infants were audio-taperecorded in their homes. The multisyllable vocalizations were categorized based on the presence or absence of phonetic variation, and the source of that variation. Multisyllables were produced with phonetic variation at or near the beginning of multisyllable babbling, which failed to support the existence of distinct stages of repetive or nonrepetitive babbling.

Mithun, Marianne. (1989). The acquisition of polysynthesis. *Journal of Child Language*, 16(2), 285-312. MOHAWK NATIVE AMERICAN LANGUAGES POLYSYNTHESIS MORPHOLOGICAL STRUCTURES:

Moerk, Ernst L. (1989). The LAD was a lady and the tasks were ill-defined. *Developmental Review*, 9, 21-57. ACQUISITION THEORIES INPUT FACTORS LANGUAGE ACQUISITION DEVICE:

The theoretical controversies and the factual evidence regarding causal factors and psychological processes in first language development are reconsidered. The informative value of the input is conceived as deriving from relationships between utterances, such as, corrections or closely spaced repetitions of identical syntactic forms. The incremental nature of language acquisition is emphasized and it is concluded that the processing demands faced by the child at each step are much less exorbitant than previously maintained. The tasks of the researcher are redefined in three domains: the conceptualization of cause-effect relationships, the delimitation of the significant input, and the explication of the psychological processes involved in the acquisition of language. - From Child Development Abstracts.

Moerk, Ernst L. (1991). *A first language taught and learned.* Baltimore, MD: Paul H. Brookes. TENSE INTERVENTION PROGRAMS PROGRESSIVES EARLY SYNTACTIC DEVELOPMENT SYNTACTIC STRUCTURES PREPOSITIONS:

A reanalysis of Roger Brown's transcripts of Eve and her mother which provides a detailed account of the acquisition of progressives, prepositional phrases, tense, and SOV structures. Presents a new teaching and learning model for intervention.

Moerk, Ernst L., & Vilaseca-Momplet, Rosa M. (1987). Time-binding in mother-child interactions: The morphemes for past and future. *Papers and Reports in Child Language Development*, 26, 80-87. TENSE:

Mogford, K., & Sadler, J. (1989). *Child language disability: Implications in an educational setting*. New York, NY: Multilingual Matters. LANGUAGE DISORDERS LANGUAGE AND EDUCATION:

Mohanon, K. P. (1992). Emergence of complexity in phonological development. In C. A. Ferguson, L. Menn, & C. Stoel-Gammon (Eds), *Phonological development: Models, research, implications*. Monkton, MD: York Press. PHONOLOGICAL DEVELOPMENT:

Mohr, János. (1978). A dadogók kezelésének tervezhetösége 'terápiásprogramban' (Plans in the therapeutic treatment of stuttering). *Magyar Fonetikai Füzetek*, 1, 117-120. STUTTERING HUNGARIAN: HUNGARIAN

Moilanen, Irma, Myhrman, Antero, & Kuure, Ollo. (1989). Linguistic problems of return migrant school children. In J. Niemi (Ed.), *Proceedings from the 11th Scandinavian Conference of Linguistics in Joensuu*. Finland: University of Joensuu. BILINGUALISM-PROBLEMS/EFFECTS SWEDISH-FINNISH FINNISH-SWEDISH:

> According to the present results, the use of language has very important consequences on returning emigrant children's school achievement and mental well being. The highest risk factor seems to be that of no clear linguistic identity, while the loyalty conflict, often described in the psychiatric literature, does not seem to be very common or could not be found using the present instruments. Cultural shock, indicated by the obligation to change the language of main communication, may have some consequences on the children's mood as reported by themselves, but a well-developed first language and the possibility to communicate with the mother in this language neutralize these feelings, apparently preventing the development of psychosomatic symptoms or behavioral disorders.OK

Moilanen, Irma, Myhrman, Antero, & Kuure, Olli. (1989). Tvasprakighet bland finska atervandarbarn. (Bilingualism among Finnish return migrant children.). In R. Soderbergh (Ed.), *Proceedings from the Second Scandinavian child language symposium*. Lund: Dept. of Linguistics, Lund University. BILINGUALISM-PROBLEMS/EFFECTS SWEDISH-FINNISH FINNISH-SWEDISH: SWEDISH

Children who had spoken both Finnish and Swedish with their mothers had more problems with reading and general psycholgical wellbeing than those who had spoken only Finnish with their mothers but used Swedish outside the home.

Molfese, Dennis L. (1989). Electrophysiological correlates of word meanings in 14 month old human infants.. *Developmental Neuropsychology*, 5, 79-103. METHODOLOGY-DESIGN LEXICAL DEVELOPMENT PHONETIC INVENTORIES SELECTION/AVOIDANCE:

In an initial study, auditory-evoked responses (AERs) to words that 14 month olds understood were reliably different from those infants did not appear to know. A second study showed that familiarity with the word sounds alone produced different AERs than novel speech-sound sequences, but these AER effects were different in both latency and electrode site from the differences shown in the first study. The findings suggest that AERs can be used to detect differences in word meanings in infants. - From Child Development Abstracts.

Molfese, Dennis L., Burger-Judisch, Lisa M., & Hans, Laura L. (1991). Consonant discrimination by newborn infants: Electrophysiological differences. *Developmental Neuropsychology*, 7, 177-195. NEONATES INFANT PERCEPTION SPEECH PERCEPTION SEX DIFFERENCES:

Evoked potential techniques were used to show that 38 neonates were capable of discriminating between /b/ and /g/. Significant performance differences were noted for males and females. - From Child Development Abstracts.

Molfese, Dennis L., & Molfese, Victoria J. (1976). VOT distinctions in infants; Learned or innate? In H. A. Whitaker, & H. Whitaker (Eds), *Studies in neurolinguistics*, vol. 4. New York, NY: Academic Press. VOICE-ONSET-TIME NATIVISM INFANT PERCEPTION SPEECH PERCEPTION:

Molfese, Dennis L., & Morse, Philip A. (1991). Developmental changes in non-human primate pattern of brain lateralization for the perception of speech cues: neuroelectrical correlates. In N. A. Krasnegor, et al. (Eds), *Biological and behavioral determinants of language development*. Hillsdale, NJ: Lawrence Erlbaum Associates. LANGUAGE AND OTHER PRIMATES LATERALIZATION SPEECH PERCEPTION:

Molfese, Dennis L., & Wetzel, W. F. (1992). Short-term and long-term auditory recognition memory in 14-month-old human infants-electrophysiological correlates. *Developmental Neuropsychology* , 8, 135-160. INFANT PERCEPTION SPEECH PERCEPTION LANGUAGE AND MEMORY:

Moll, Luis C. (1990). *Vygotsky and education*. New York, NY: Cambridge University Press. LANGUAGE AND EDUCATION VYGOTSKYAN THEORY:

More than any other theorist, the Soviet psychologist L.S. Vygotsky (1896-1934) viewed education as central to cognitive development. Vygotsky set out to develop a general approach to psychology that recognized the inseparability of the individual from the social: that addressed how thinking develops under particular social and historical conditions. He argued that higher or uniquely human psychological processes developed in children through enculturation into the practices of society: through the acquisition of society's technology, its signs and tools: through the process of education. As such, human pedagogy, in all its forms, is the defining characteristic of his approach, the central concept in his system. For Vygotsky, schools and other informal educational situations represented the best cultural laboratories to study thinking. He viewed schools as socially defined systems of activities, with special modes of discourse, and with major consequences for the development of thinking. This volume is devoted to analyzing educational implications and applications of Vygotsky's ideas as a means of bringing to light the relevance of Vygotskian concepts to education and the centrality of education to Vygotskian psychology.

Molnár, Ildikó. (1978). A hanghelyettesítések tipúsai a gyermeknyelvben 18-21 hónapos kor között (The types of sound-substitutions in child language between the ages of 18-21 months). *Magyar Fonetikai Füzetek*, 1, 22-52. PHONOLOGICAL SUBSTITUTIONS HUNGARIAN: HUNGARIAN

Montagh, Imre, Lörik, József, & Subosits, István. (1978). A laterális szigmatizmus akusztikai elemzése és terápiája (Acoustic features and therapy of lateral stigmatism). *Gyógypedagógia*, 4, ARTICULATION DISORDERS HUNGARIAN: HUNGARIAN

Montgomery, James W., Scudder, Rosalind R., & Moore, Christopher A. (1990). Language-impaired children's real-time comprehension of spoken language. *Applied Psycholinguistics*, 11, 273-290. CONTEXT COMPREHENSION DISORDERS:

The present investigation compared the real-time language processing abilities of language-impaired and normal children using a word-recognition reaction time paradigm. Results showed that the language-impaired and normal children used linguistic context to facilitate word recognition, but were slower to do so than their normally developing peers.

Moon, Christine, Bever, Thomas G., & Fifer, William P. (1992). Canonical and non-canonical syllable discrimination by 2-day-old infants. *Journal of Child Language*, 19, 1-17. NEONATES INFANT PERCEPTION SYLLABLES-STRUCTURE:

Moon, Christine, & Fifer, William P. (1990). Syllables as signals for 2-day-old infants. *Infant Behavior and Development*, 13, 377-390. NEONATES INFANT PERCEPTION SYLLABLES:

Neonates demonstrated two-stimulus auditory operant discrimination learning by altering nonnutritive sucking patterns during an 18-min session. Discriminative stimulus were two isolated, repeated syllables, and reinforcers were a recording of mothers' adult-directed speech and quiet. During the first 6 min, 16 of 20 subjects initiated bursts of sucking relatively more frequently during the syllable which signalled the availability of the recording of the mothers' voice versus quiet.

Moore, Chris, & Davidge, Jane. (1989). The development of mental terms: pragmatics or semantics? *Journal of Child Language*, 16, 633-641. VERBS-MENTAL:

An examination of the terms 'know, think, ' and 'sure'. Subjects were 60 children between the ages of 3:0 and 6:0. Improvement of usage of correct contrast between 'know-think' and 'sure-think' was age related with 'think' being treated as a less reliable index than 'know' and 'sure' by the age of 4:0 to 5:0. This indicates that expressing degrees of certainty is within the grasp of 4-5 year olds, but it is probably not based on the factive properties of the terms.

Moore, Chris, & Frye, Douglas. (1991). The acquisition and utility of theories of mind. In D. Frye, & C. Moore (Eds), *Children's theories of mind*. Hillsdale, NJ: Lawrence Erlbaum Associates. THEORY OF MIND:

Moore, Chris, & Furrow, David. (1991). The development of the language of belief: The expression of relative certainty. In D. Frye, & C. Moore (Eds), *Children's theories of mind*. Hillsdale, NJ: Lawrence Erlbaum Associates. THEORY OF MIND VERBS-MENTAL TRUTH VALUES:

Moore, Chris, Pure, Kiran, & Furrow, David. (1990). Children's understanding of the modal expression of speaker certainty and uncertainty and its relation to the development of a representational theory of mind. *Child Development*, 61, 722-730. MODALS VERBS-CONDITIONAL THEORY OF MIND VERBS-MENTAL:

A guessing game, object location task was used to examine children's (3:0-6:0) understanding of the modal verbs 'could, must, 'and 'might', and the modal adjuncts 'probably, possibly, ' and 'maybe'. At 3:0 children do not differentiate between any of the modals whereas 4 year olds and above were able to locate the object and use modal contrast. 4:0-6:0 were then tested to see how their understanding of mental and modal terms impacted on their theory of mind. Tasks assessing false beliefs, representational change, and appearance-reality distinctions were all intercorrelated.

Moore, Christopher A., Yorkston, Kathryn M., & Beukelman, David R. (Eds) (1991). *Dysarthria and apraxia of speech*. Baltimore, MD: Paul H. Brookes. MOTOR DISORDERS LANGUAGE DISORDERS APRAXIA DYSARTHRIA CLASSIFICATION OF DISORDERS:

Results of the Fifth Biennial Clinical Dysarthria Conference. The authors provide a description of the latest techniques and treatment processes for the treatment of motor speech disorders.

Moore, M. E., & Johnston, Judith R. (1993). Expressions of past time by normal and language impaired children. *Applied Psycholingistics*, 14, TENSE MORPHOSYNTACTIC DEVELOPMENT ADVERBS TEMPORAL TERMS DEIXIS-TEMPORAL:

An examination of the knowledge of past time adverbs and past tense morphemes in language impaired five-year-olds. An assymetry was found between the domains in developmental rate. JRJ.

Moore, M. E., Morreau, L., & Johnston, Judith R. (1991). A priority lexicon for hearing impaired children: Staff perceptions. *Journal of the American Deafness and Rehabilitation Association*, 24, 104-117. DEAF CHILDREN VOCABULARY DEVELOPMENT:

A comparative study which examined the set of words that teachers thought should be the initial set acquired by children with the data on vocabulary acquisiiton in the research literature.

Moore, S. E., & Perkins, W. H. (1990). Validity and reliability of judgements of authentic and simulated stuttering. *Journal of Speech and Hearing Disorders*, 55, 383-391. STUTTERING:

Moore, Vanessa, & Law, James. (1990). Coping ability of preschool children with delayed language development. *Developmental Medicine and Child Neurology*, 32, 249-257. LANGUAGE DELAY REYNELL DEVELOPMENTAL LANGUAGE SCALES GRIFFITHS MENTAL DEVELOPMENT SCALES:

> 92 children aged 2:6 with delayed language development were compared with 100 controls on a copying task from the Griffiths Scales, and on the comprehension and expressive Reynell Scales. The language delayed children scored lower on both scales than the controls.

Moore, William G., Josephson, Jean A., & Mauk, Gary W. (1991). Identification of children with hearing impairments: A baseline survey. *Volta Review*, 93, 187-196. DEAF CHILDREN ASSESSMENT PROCEDURES AT-RISK CHILDREN:

> An Oregon study of the patterns and ages of children with hearing impediments conducted prior to initiating a birth certificate screening program. From Child Development Abstracts.

Moravscik, Edith A. (1973). Reduplicative constructions. In J. H. Greenberg, C. A. Ferguson, & E. A. Moravscik (Eds), *Universals of human language*, vol. 3. Stanford, CA: Stanford University Press. REDUPLICATION BABBLING:

Morford, M., & Goldin-Meadow, Susan. (1992). Comprehension and production of gesture in combination with speech in one-word speakers. *Journal of Child Language*, 19, 559-580. GESTURE SINGLE-WORD SPEECH:

Morgan, James L. (1990). Input, innateness, and induction in language acquisition. *Developmental Psychobiology*, 23(7), NATIVISM:

Morgan, James L., & Travis, Lisa L. (1989). Limits on negative information in language input. *Journal of Child Language*, 16(3), 531-552. NEGATIVE EVIDENCE INPUT FACTORS:

Morgan, Sam B., Cutrer, Pamela S., Coplin, Jane W., & Rodrigue, James R. (1989). Do autistic children differ from retarded and normal children in Piagetian sensorimotor functioning? *Journal of Child Psychology and Psychiatry*, 30, 857-864. AUTISM PIAGETIAN THEORY:

Piagetian sensorimotor functioning of autistic, retarded, and normal children was assessed. The three groups showed no significant differences in overall performance or specific subtest performance contrary to previous reports of early sensorimotor deficits specific to autism. - From Child Development Abstracts.

Morisset, Colleen E., Barnard, Kathryn E., Greenberg, Mark T., Booth, Cathryn L., & Spieker, Susan J. (1990). Environmental influence on early language development: The context of social risk. *Development and Psychopathology*, 2, 127-149. LANGUAGE AND SOCIAL CLASS PARENTAL INPUT ADULT-CHILD INTERACTION SOCIAL INTERACTION LANGUAGE DISORDERS AT-RISK CHILDREN:

The impact of environmental risk on toddlers' cognitive and linguistic development was investigated in a longitudinal study of high-risk families. The risk factors examined were family social status, mothers' psychosocial functioning, and quality of dyadic involvement at 1 year of age. Data indicate that dyadic involvement was an important mediator in the relation between environmental risk and subsequent child competence.

Morra Pellegrino, Maria L., & Garibbo Giuganino, B. M. (1970). Confonto di alcuni indici psicolinguistici applicabili al linguaggio scritto e orale in eta evolutiva. (The development of oral and written language in children: comparison between two different psycholinguistic indexes.). *Rivista de Psicologia Sociale*, 17 (1), 1-11. WRITTEN LANGUAGE: ITALIAN

Morra Pellegrino, Maria L., & Scopesi, Alda. (1976). Linguaggio orale e scritto en eta evolutia: lo sviluppo sintattico del linguaggio descrittivo. (Oral and written language in children: syntactical development of descriptive language.). *Rassegna Italiana di*

Linguistica Applicata, 3 (1), 1-18. WRITTEN LANGUAGE SYNTACTIC STRUCTURES DISCOURSE STRUCTURE: ITALIAN

90 subjects divided into three age levels (8 to 9, 10 to 11, and 13 to 14 years) produced an oral and a written text each, in an experimental situation giving preference to the descriptive function. The syntactical structures of these texts were analyzed by calculating the incidence of various forms, expressly chosen and graded from the most rudimentary (enumeration, expanded enumeration, simple unexpanded sentences), to medium complex forms (simple expanded sentence, compound sentence) to more elaborate forms (complex sentence). The qualitative differences regarding the complexity introducers were also noted. The results show that the oral language presents a greater number of sentences compared with the written, at all age levels: less structured forms are more frequent in the oral than in the written. There is no great differentiation between oral and written forms at the 8 to 9 age level, whereas a greater differentiation is noted at the subsequent age level (10 to 11), becoming most evident at the highest age level (13 to 14).MMP/AS

Morra Pellegrino, Maria L., & Scopesi, Alda. (1978). Oral and written language: syntactical development of narrative language. *International Journal of Psycholinguistics*, 5 (1), 5-19. NARRATIVES WRITTEN LANGUAGE SYNTACTIC STRUCTURES DISCOURSE STRUCTURE:

Morra Pellegrino, Maria L., & Scopesi, Alda. (1979). Narrare e descrivere sono abilita linguistiche a sviluppo differenziato? (Is there any difference in the development of narrative vs. descriptive competence?). *Eta Evolutiva*, 4, 19-28. NARRATIVES COMMUNICATIVE COMPETENCE: ITALIAN

Morra Pellegrino, Maria L., & Scopesi, Alda. (1989). *Dal dialogo preverbale alla conversazione. Lo sviluppo in eta prescolare della comunicazione tra bambini e con l'adulto. (From preverbal dialogue to conversation. The development of communication among peers and with adults in preschoolers.).* Milano, Italy: Angeli. ADULT-CHILD INTERACTION CHILDREN'S DISCOURSE CHILDREN'S DIALOGUES SOCIAL INTERACTION SOCIAL SPEECH: ITALIAN

Morra Pellegrino, Maria L., & Scopesi, Alda. (1990). Structure and function of baby talk in a day-care center. *Journal of Child Language*, 17, 101-114. ITALIAN PARENTAL SPEECH-STYLE PARENTAL INPUT ADULT-CHILD INTERACTION LANGUAGE AND EDUCATION:

> The speech of five Italian teachers in a day- care center was examined for adjustments in style dependent upon the age of the children addressed, and the size of the group addressed.MMP/AS

Morra Pellegrino, Maria L., Scopesi, Alda, & D'Aniello, P. (1983). Scambi verbali tra coetanei nell'asilo nido. (Verbal interaction among peers in day care centers.). In T. Musatti, & S. Mantovani (Eds), *Adulti e bambini: educare e comunicare*. Bergamo, Italy: Juvenilia. SOCIAL INTERACTION LANGUAGE AND EDUCATION SOCIAL SPEECH: ITALIAN

Morra Pellegrino, Maria L., Scopesi, Alda, D'Aniello, P., & Zanobini, M. (1987). La comunicazione verbale in eta prescolare. Sviluppo delle comunicative e della competenza dialogica. (Verbal communication in preschool children. Developmental trends of communicative intentions and dialogs.). *Giornale Italiano di Psicolgia*, 14 (1), 47-72. SOCIAL INTERACTION SOCIAL SPEECH CHILDREN'S DIALOGUES CHILDREN'S DISCOURSE COMMUNICATIVE COMPETENCE LANGUAGE AND EDUCATION: ITALIAN

> Child-child and child-adult verbal exchanges are explored during free play sessions in day-care centers and kindergartens. Data are analyzed at two different levels. I level: We want to establish whether a change occurs from age two to five according to preferred addressee (peer/adult), communicative intentions (speech acts), adjustment to the partner. II level: The developmental trends of dialogue among peers are explored. Method: Groups of three children and an adult are observed in day-care centers and kindergartens. Each registration lasts 20 minutes: the adult interacts actively for 10 minutes, then only watches the children's play. Results. I level: preferred addressee changes with age: frequencies of communicative intentions addressed to adult and peers vary according to situation and age, the distribution in classes of

communicative intentions suggests a very early ability of the child to adjust to the partner. II level: a) also children in the first age level produce well structured dialogic sequences: b) strategies and contents of dialogues are different at each age level.MMP/AS

Morrel-Samuels, P., & Herman, L. M. (1993). Cognitive factors affecting comprehension of gesture language signs: A brief comparison of dolphins and humans. In L. M. Herman, H. L. Roitblat, & P. E. Nactigal. (Eds). *Language and communication: Comparative perspectives*. Hillsdale, NJ: Lawrence Erlbaum Associates. ANIMAL COMMUNICATIONS SIGNING:

Morris, David W. H. (1988). *A dictionary of speech therapy*. San Diego, CA: Singular Publishing Group. REFERENCE MANUAL INTERVENTION PROGRAMS LANGUAGE DISORDERS:

A well-received dictionary covering the terms used in speech pathology. Also describes therapy techniques, diagnostic tests, and contemporary theories on testing and therapy.

Morris, R. G. M. (1990). *Parallel distributed processing: Implications and psychology and neurobiology*. New York, NY: Oxford University Press. CONNECTIONISM COMPUTER SIMULATIONS:

In recent years there has been a substantial growth of interest in parallel distributed processing among experimental psychologists and neurobiologists. Many hope that developments in formal analysis of neural networks will provide a bridge between psychological accounts of cognitive function and those at the neural level. This volume examines the implications of these developments and their influence on experimental psychology and neurobiology.

Morrison, Judy A., & Shriberg, Lawrence D. (1992). Articulation testing versus conversational speech sampling. *Journal of Speech and Hearing Research*, 35, 259-273. ASSESSMENT PROCEDURES ARTICULATION:

Morrongiello, Barbara A. (1988). The development of auditory pattern perception skills. In C. Rovee-Collier, & L. P. Lipsitt (Ed.), *Advances in infancy research*. Norwood, NJ: Ablex. AUDITORY DEVELOPMENT:

Morrongiello, Barbara A., Fenwick, Kimberley D., & Chance, Graham. (1990). Sound localization acuity in very young infants: An observer-based testing procedure. *Developmental Psychology*, 26, 75-84. INFANT PERCEPTION:

Infants 8 to 28 weeks were tested to determine the smallest sound shift off midline and along the horizontal axis that could be reliably discriminated. Both sound-shift and no-shift trials were presented. The results indicated increasing localization acuity with age. - From Child Developmental Abstracts.

Morrongiello, Barbara A., & Rocca, Patrick T. (1990). Infants' localization of sounds within hemifields: Estimates of minimum audible angle. *Child Development*, 61, 1258-1270. INFANT PERCEPTION:

Infants, 6, 12, and 18 months of age were tested for minimum audible angle using a conditioned head-turn procedure with an equal number of no-change (control) trials and sound-shift (experimental) trials. A correct response resulted in a visual reinforcement. Localization acuity for sounds within hemifields was fairly poor and improved systematically with increasing age.

Mosconi, A. (1989). A psycho-rhetorical approach to explanations. In M. S. Barbieri (Ed.), *La speigazione nell'interazione sociale* . Torino, Italy: Loescher. CHILDREN'S EXPLANATIONS: ITALIAN

Assuming that explanation is a social act, whose aim is that of making the partner restructure his/her state of knowledge, the author shows how a different arrangement of the same quantity of information can make comprehension easier or harder for a potential partner.MSB

Moskowitz, A. I. (1973). The acquisition of phonology and syntax: A preliminary study. In K. J. J. Hintikka, & J. M. E. Moravscik (Eds), *Approaches to natural language: Proceedings of the 1970 Stanford Workshop on Grammar and Semantics*. Dordrecht, The Netherlands: Reidel. PHONOLOGICAL DEVELOPMENT SYNTACTIC DEVELOPMENT:

Most, T., & Frank, Y. (1991). The relationship between the perception and the production of intonation by hearing-impaired children. *Volta Review*, 93, 301-310. INTONATION DEAF CHILDREN:

Mount, Robin, Reznick, J. Steven, Kagan, Jerome, Hiatt, Susan, & Szpak, Mark. (1989). Direction of gaze and emergence of speech in the second year. *Brain and Language*, 36(3), 406-410. GAZE PRELINGUISTICS:

Mousset, Marie-Rose. (1990). L'évolution des productions vocales chez le jeune enfant porteur d'une fente palatine. (The evolution of vocalizations by young children with cleft palates.). *Glossa*, 21, 30-33. CLEFT PALATE VOCALIZATIONS BABBLING: FRENCH

Mozer, M. C. (1990). Discovering faithful 'Wickelfeature' representations in a connectionist network. In M. Piatelli-Palmarini (Ed.), *Proceedings of the Twelfth Annual Conference of the Cognitive Science Society*. Hillsdale, NJ: Lawrence Erlbaum Associates. CONNECTIONISM REPRESENTATIONS-PHONOLOGICAL:

Müller, Natascha. (1990). Developing two gender assignment systems simultaneously. In M. J. Meisel (Ed.), *Two first languages: Early grammatical development in bilingual children*. Dordrecht: Foris. GENDER BILINGUALISM-MORPHOLOGICAL DEVELOPMENT:

Müller, Natascha. (1990). Erwerb der Wortstellung bei bilingualen Kindern (Französisch- Deutsch). Zur Distribution von Finitheitsmerkmalen. (The development of word order in bilingual children - French/German.). *Linguistische Berichte*. GERMAN WORD ORDER BILINGUALISM-SYNTACTIC DEVELOPMENT: GERMAN

Murdoch, Bruce E. (1990). *Acquired neurological speech: Language disorders in childhood*. Hillsdale, NJ: Lawrence Erlbaum Associates. TRAUMATIC DISORDERS ACQUIRED DISORDERS:

An examination of the common and less common causes of traumatic speech/language disorders, including cerebral anoxia, metabolic and neural tube defects, radiation and infection induced damage, and convulsive disorders as well as the more common causes.

Murdoch, Bruce E. (1990). *Acquired speech and language disorders: A neuroanatomical and functional neurological approach*. Baltimore, MD: Paul H. Brookes. ACQUIRED APHASIA DEVELOPMENTAL DISORDERS NEUROLINGUISTICS-NEURAL SUBSTRATES:

Murphy, Walker D., Shea, Sandra L., & Aslin, Richard N. (1989). Identification of vowels in 'vowelless' syllables by 3-year-olds. *Perception and Psychophysics*, 46, 375-383. VOWELS SYLLABLES CONSONANTS-SYLLABIC:

The ability of 3-year-old to perceive the identity of vowels in full-vowel and silent center, consonant-vowel-consonant (CVC) syllables was investigated. The performance of individual children fell into two subgroups: those who performed like adults by maintaining correct vowel identification and those who identified the full-vowel syllables correctly but performed at chance. - From Child Development Abstracts.

Murray, Ann D., Johnson, Jeanne, & Peters, Jo. (1990). Fine-tuning of utterance length to preverbal infants: Effects on later language development. *Journal of Child Language*, 17, 511-525. FINE TUNING HYPOTHESIS PARENTAL INPUT PARENTAL SPEECH-STYLE SEX DIFFERENCES HOME SCALES INDIVIDUAL VARIATION:

The purpose of this study was to determine whether mothers simplify their speech during the second half of the first year of development when infants begin to comprehend words and use gestures to communicate intentionally, and whether individual differences in mothers' speech adjustments influence their infants' later language acquisition. Mothers who provided responsive and stimulating environments, as indicated by

HOME scores, also reduced their MLU over the age range studied. Mothers' MLU adjustments during the first year were more predictive than the HOME scale in forecasting receptive language development. In contrast, expressive language abilities were unrelated to the environmental variables measured but were predicted by child characteristics such as the infants' sex.

Musselman, Carol, & Churchill, Adele. (1991). Conversational control in mother-child dyads: auditory-oral versus total communication. *American Annals of the Deaf*, 136, 5-16. DEAF CHILDREN PARENTAL SPEECH-ATYPICAL CHILDREN PARENTAL SPEECH-STYLE:

The conversational control of hearing mothers who use auditory-oral communication (A/O) and those who use total communication (TC) was investigated. The mothers of both A/O and TC children were found to exert similarily high levels of conversational control. TC children exerted more control than the A/O children. For both the A/O and TC groups, maternal conversational style reflected the child's spoken language ability. Within the TC group, maternal style was related to the child's social development.

Musselwhite, Caroline R. (1986). *Apaptive play for special needs children: Strategies to enhance communication and learning*. San Diego, CA: Singular Publishing Group. LANGUAGE AND PLAY INTERVENTION PROGRAMS:

Main section headings: overview of adaptive play. Selecting, adapting, and making play materials. Adaptive play strategies for communicative goals. Developing support for adaptive play.

N

Nagy, József. (1978). A szófajokgyakorisági jellemzöi 8-10 éves tanulók nyelvhasználatában (Frequency characteristics of parts of speech in language use of 8-10 yr old students). *Magyar Nyelvor*, 186-204. METHODOLOGY-FREQUENCY COUNT WORD CLASS HUNGARIAN: HUNGARIAN

Naigles, Letitia. (1990). Children use syntax to learn verb meanings. *Journal of Child Language*, 17, 357-374. LEXICAL DEVELOPMENT VERBS BOOTSTRAPPING SEMANTICS AND SYNTAX CUES-SYNTACTIC:

> An experimental validation of Landau & Gleitman's (1985) syntactic bootstrapping procedure. Pairs of actions were presented simultaneously with a nonsense verb in one of two syntactic structures. The actions were subsequently separated, and the children were asked to select which action was the referent for the verb. The children's choice of referent was found to be a function of the syntactic structure in which the verb had been appeased.

Napoli, D., & Kegl, J. (Eds) (1991). *Bridges between psychology and linguistics: A Swarthmore Festschrift for Lila Gleitman*. Hillsdale, NJ: Lawrence Erlbaum Associates. DYSLEXIA LANGUAGE AND COGNITIVE DEVELOPMENT ACQUISITION AND LINGUISTIC THEORY :

> The papers in this book build a solid bridge between psychology and linguistics. It begins with a thorough examination of issues in developmental psychology, continues with questions on perception and cognition, studies the realm of psycholinguistics, and concludes with an exploration of theoretical linguistics.

Nation, James E., & Aram, Dorothy M. (1990). *Speech and language disorders*. San Diego, CA: Singular Group. CLASSIFICATION OF DISORDERS LANGUAGE DISORDERS:

Introductory text for undergraduate classes.

Neisser, Ulric. (1989). *Concepts and conceptual development*. New York, NY: Cambridge University Press. CONCEPT DEVELOPMENT LANGUAGE AND COGNITIVE DEVELOPMENT CATEGORIZATION:

Categories straddle the boundary between the mind and the world: they are socially developed mental representations, but they must fit the properties of real objects in the real environment if they are to be useful. This volume reflects the emerging consensus that a full understanding of categorization must take all these constraints into account. Everyday terms and categories depend not only on the implicit theories that people have about the world, but also on the objective properties of particular objects and the perceptible similarities among these objects. A new understanding of these multiple relationships is beginning to reshape the study of concepts and conceptual development.

Nelfelt, K., & Stromqvist, Sven. (1990). Semantiska aspekter pa horselskadade barns sprakutveckling-en projecktbeskrivning (Semantic Aspects of Language Development in the Hearing Impaired-A Project Description). Project Report Number One. *Gothenburg Papers in Theoretical Linguistics*, S15, DEAF CHILDREN LEXICAL DEVELOPMENT SEMANTIC DEVELOPMENT: SWEDISH

Nelson, E. M. M. (1992). Memory for metaphor by nonfluent bilinguals. *Journal of Psycholinguistic Research*, 21, 111-125. LANGUAGE AND MEMORY FIGURATIVE LANGUAGE BILINGUALISM:

Nelson, K. (1977). Structure and strategy in learning to talk. In M. S. Barbieri (Ed.), *Gli inizi del linguaggio: aspetti cognitivi e comunicativi (The emergence of language: cognitive and communicative aspects)*.. La Nuova, Italy: Firenze. ACQUISITION THEORIES SYNTACTIC DEVELOPMENT:

Nelson, K., Loncke, F., & Camarata, Stephen. (1992). Implications of research on deaf and hearing children's language learning. In M. Marschark, & M. D. Clark (Eds), *Psychological perspectives on deafness*. Hillsdale, NJ: Lawrence Erlbaum Associates. DEAF CHILDREN:

Nelson, Katherine. (1989). Monologue as representation of real-life experience. In K. Nelson (Ed.), *Narratives from the crib*. Cambridge, MA: Harvard University Press. CRIB SPEECH NARRATIVES LANGUAGE AND MEMORY EVENTS/SCRIPTS:

Nelson describes three themes in the subject's crib speech: accounts of recalled events, descriptions of expected events, and descriptions of routine events. Her writings are closely related to her other published works on children's events and scripts representation. She provides a corpus of twelve monologues as an appendix to this article.

Nelson, Katherine. (1989). Monologue as the linguistic construction of self in time. In K. Nelson (Ed.), *Narratives from the crib*. Cambridge, MA: Harvard University Press. CRIB SPEECH NARRATIVES:

Nelson draws together earlier chapters in the book and concludes that the linguistic structures and pragmatic functions of children's presleep monologues are radically different to the speech they exchange during interactions with adults in their environment.

Nelson, Katherine (Ed.). (1989). *Narratives from the crib*. Cambridge, MA: Harvard University Press. NARRATIVES CRIB SPEECH:

This book follows on from Wier and Kucsaj's works on crib speech and contains articles written by nine researchers. The book is divided into three sections which each contain three chapters: Part 1 --Constructing a world, Part 2 --Constructing a language, and Part 3 -- Constructing a self. The book is reviewed by J. S. Falk in Language 66(3), pages 558-562.

Nelson, Katherine. (1990). Language development in context. In E. H. Bendix (Ed.), *The uses of linguistics*. New York, NY: New York Academy of Sciences. OVERVIEW-GENERAL:

Nelson, Katherine. (1991). Concepts and meaning in language development. In N. A. Krasnegor, et al. (Eds), *Biological and behavioral determinants of language development*. Hillsdale, NJ: Lawrence Erlbaum Associates. LEXICAL DEVELOPMENT CONCEPT DEVELOPMENT SEMANTIC MAPPING:

Nelson, Katherine. (1991). The matter of time: Interdependences between language and thought in development. In S. A. Gelman, & J. Byrnes (Eds), *Perspectives on language and thought*. New York, NY: Cambridge University Press. LANGUAGE AND COGNITION LANGUAGE AND COGNITIVE DEVELOPMENT TEMPORAL TERMS:

Nelson, Katherine (1993). Events, narratives, memory: What develops? In C. A. Nelson (Ed.), *Memory and affect in development*. Hillsdale, NJ: Lawrence Erlbaum Associates. EVENTS/SCRIPTS NARRATIVES LANGUAGE AND MEMORY:

Nelson, Katherine, & Nelson, Agatha P. (1991). Category production in response to script and category cues by kindergarteners and second-grade children. *Journal of Applied Developmental Psychology*, 11, 431-446. CATEGORIZATION EVENTS/SCRIPTS:

> In condition one children produced items from three familiar categories following taxonomic category instructions, and in condition two after hearing two script contexts for each category. Second-graders and 5:0 year olds with school experience produced more items than 5:0 year olds without school experience, and second graders produced more items in the taxonomic condition. Kindergarteners produced more items in the script condition. From Child Development Abstracts.

Nelson, Keith E. (1991). On differentiated language learning models and differentiated interventions. In N. A. Krasnegor, et al. (Eds), *Biological and behavioral determinants of language development*. Hillsdale, NJ: Lawrence Erlbaum Associates. INTERVENTION PROGRAMS:

Nelson, L. K., & Bauer, Harold R. (1991). Speech and language production at age 2-evidence for tradeoffs between linguistic and phonetic processing. *Journal of Speech and Hearing Research*, 34, 879-892. LANGUAGE PROCESSING SPEECH PRODUCTION:

Netsell, Ronald. (1991). *A neurobiologic view of speech production and the dysarthrias, 2nd Ed.* San Diego, CA: Singular Group. SPEECH PRODUCTION DYSARTHRIA MOTOR DISORDERS NEUROLINGUISTICS:

Neumann, Klaus, & Charlton, Michael. (1990). *Spracherwerb und Mediengebrauch. (Language acquisition and use of the mass media.).* Tübingen, Germany: Gunther Narr. TELEVISION AND LANGUAGE DEVELOPMENT: GERMAN

Neumann, O. (1990). Lexical access: some comments on models and metaphors. In D. A. Balota, G. B. Flores d'Arcais, & K. Rayner (Eds), *Comprehension processes in reading.* Hillsdale, NJ: Lawrence Erlbaum Associates. LEXICAL ACCESS:

Neville, H. J. (1991). Whence the specialization of the language hemisphere? In I. G. Mattingly, & M. Studdert-Kennedy (Eds), *Modularity and the motor theory of speech perception.* Hillsdale, NJ: Lawrence Erlbaum Associates. LATERALIZATION:

Newman, Linda L., & Pratt, S. R. (1990). Adaptive self-stabilization in adult child interactions-temporal congruence with varied switch-pause durations. *Discourse Processes*, 13, 363-374. ADULT-CHILD INTERACTION INTERSUBJECTIVITY:

Newman, Linda L., & Smith, Anne B. (1989). Some effects of variations in response time latency on speech rate, interruptions, and fluency in children's speech. *Journal of Speech and Hearing Research*, 32(3), 635-644. SPEAKING RATE INPUT FACTORS:

Newport, Elissa L. (1991). Contrasting conceptions of the critical period for language. In S. Carey, & R. Gelman (Eds), *Epigenesis of mind: Essays on biology and cognition.*. Hillsdale, NJ: Lawrence Erlbaum Associates. CRITICAL PERIOD L2 AGE INFLUENCES:

Nicolas, C. (1987). Développement genétique de l'articulation (Development of phonotactics). *Rééducation orthophonique*, 25 (152), 363-370. FRENCH PHONOTACTICS: FRENCH

Nicolson, R. I., & Fawcett, A. J. (1990). Automaticity: A new framework for dyslexia research? *Cognition*, 35, 159-182. DYSLEXIA METHODOLOGY-DESIGN LANGUAGE AND MOTOR DEVELOPMENT:

A group of twenty-three 13 year old dyslexics ability to perform tests of motor balance was compared with a control group. On 19 out of 20 of the tests the dyslexics performed worse than the controls.

Nikolaus, Kurt, & Quasthoff, Uta M. (1982). What Makes a Good Story? In Flammer, & A. W. Kintsch (Ed.), *Discourse Processing.*. Amsterdam: NARRATIVES DISCOURSE STRUCTURE TEXT/STORY GRAMMARS:

Ninio, Anat. (1992). The relation of children's single word utterances to single word utterances in the input. *Journal of Child Language*, 19, 87-110. SINGLE-WORD SPEECH INPUT FACTORS:

Nippold, Marilyn A. (1988). *Later language development.* San Diego, CA: Singular Publishing Group. LITERACY WRITTEN LANGUAGE LATER SYNTACTIC DEVELOPMENT LANGUAGE SOCIALIZATION FIGURATIVE LANGUAGE LANGUAGE AND SOCIAL TRANSMISSION AMBIGUITY PRAGMATIC DEVELOPMENT:

The nature of literacy. The literacy lexicon. Spoken and written syntax. Reading and writing. Cognition. Verbal reasoning. Figurative language. Linguistic ambiguity. Language and socialization. Pragmatics. Subject index.

Nippold, Marilyn A. (1990). Concomitant speech and language disorders in stuttering children: A critique of the literature. *Journal of Speech and Hearing Disorders*, 55, 51-60. STUTTERING:

Nippold, Marilyn A. (1990). Concomitant speech and language disorders in stuttering children - a critique of the literature: reply. *Journal of Speech and Hearing Disorders*, 55, 803-804. STUTTERING:

Nitrouer, Susan, Studdert-Kennedy, Michael, & McGowan, Richard. (1989). The emergence of phonetic segments: evidence from the spectral structure of fricative-vowel syllables spoken by children and adults. *Journal of Speech and Hearing Research*, 32(1), 120-132. ACOUSTIC PHONETICS PHONEMIC DEVELOPMENT FRICATIVES VOWELS SYLLABLES PHONETIC INVENTORIES PHONOLOGICAL DEVELOPMENT:

Nitsche, Ulla. (1987). Untersuchungen zum Kommunikationstyp der Verständnissicherung bei Erwachsenen und Kindern. (Examinations of the communication strategies used for securing comprehension by adults and children.). *Linguistische Studien/Zentralinstitut für Sprachwissenschaft, Reibe A*, 158, 126-163. COMPREHENSION COMMUNICATIVE DEVELOPMENT GERMAN: GERMAN

Nitsche, Ulla. (1990). Zum Zustandekommen von Verstehensschwierigkeiten in Instruktionen und deren Bearbeitung durch ältere Vorschulkinder. (On the causes of difficulty understanding instructions and their treatment in older preschoolers.). *Linguistische Studien/Zentralinstitut für Sprachwissenschaft, Reibe A*, 204, 124-144. COMPREHENSION DISORDERS GERMAN INTERVENTION PROGRAMS LANGUAGE AND EDUCATION: GERMAN

Norris, D. (1990). Connectionism: A case for modularity. In D. A. Balota, G. B. Flores d'Arcais, & K. Rayner (Eds), *Comprehension processes in reading*. Hillsdale, NJ: Lawrence Erlbaum Associates. CONNECTIONISM MODULARITY:

Nozza, R. J., Miller, S. L., Rossman, R. N. F., & Bond, L. C. (1991). Reliability and validity of infant speech-sound discrimination-in-noise thresholds. *Journal of Speech and Hearing Research*, 34, 643-650. INFANT PERCEPTION AUDITORY DISCRIMINATION:

Nugent, J. Kevin, Lester, Barry M., & Brazelton, T. Berry (Eds). (1989). *Biology, culture and infant development*. Norwood, NJ: Ablex. CROSSCULTURAL STUDY SOCIAL INTERACTION NEONATES ADULT-CHILD INTERACTION INTERSUBJECTIVITY PARENTAL INPUT PARENTAL SPEECH NAVAJO NATIVE AMERICAN LANGUAGES:

The first volume in the series 'The cultural context of infancy'. Collection of papers covering: biosocial influences on the neonate, infants and parents in context, mother-infant interaction during the first year, and the crosscultural comparison of infant behaviors. Includes papers on several cultural groups including: Israeli, Efe, Puerto Rican, Portuguese, British, Malay, Navajo, and Hmong child rearing practices.

Nugent, J. Kevin, Lester, Barry M., & Brazelton, T. Berry (Eds). (1990). *Multicultural and interdisciplinary approaches to parent-infant relations, vol..* Norwood, NJ: Ablex. CROSSCULTURAL STUDY SOCIAL INTERACTION ADULT-CHILD INTERACTION NEONATES PARENTAL INPUT PARENTAL SPEECH INTERSUBJECTIVITY:

The second volume in the series 'The cultural context of infancy', covering: neonate behavior, mother-infant interaction in context, and cultural perspectives on high risk families. Examines German, Dutch, Kenyan, West Indian, Swedish, Danish, Mexican, Italian, Maghreb, Indonesian and Zulu parental interactions and neonatal behaviors.

O

O'Boyle, Michael W., & Hellige, Joseph B. (1989). Cerebral hemisphere asymmetry and individual differences in cognition. *Learning and Individual Differences*, 1, 7-35. LATERALIZATION INDIVIDUAL VARIATION:

> The authors identify several hemispheric dimensions on which individuals may differ, and investigate the possibility that underlying patterns of cerebral hemisphere asymmetry may be related to differences in cognitive abilities as reported for males and females, left- and righthanders, intellectually precocious and dyslexic individuals. - From Child Development Abstracts.

O'Connor, K. N., Roitblat, Herbert L., & Bever, Thomas G. (1993). Auditory sequence complexity and hemispheric assymetry of function in rats. In *Language and communication: Comparative perspectives*. Hillsdale, NJ: Lawrence Erlbaum Associates. ANIMAL COMMUNICATIONS:

O'Grady, William, Peters, Ann M., & Masterson, Deborah. (1989). The transition from optional to required subjects. *Journal of Child Language*, 16(3), 513-529. SUBJECTIVITY SYNTACTIC STRUCTURES:

Oakes, Lisa M., & Cohen, Leslie B. (1990). Infant perception of a causal event. *Cognitive Development*, 5, 193-207. CAUSALITY CONNECTIVES-CAUSAL:

Two examinations of 0:6 and 0:10 month-olds' perception of launching events revealed that 10 month olds, but not 6 month olds had some understanding of causality.

Ochs, Elinor, & Schieffelin, Bambi B. (Eds). (1979). *Developmental pragmatics.* New York, NY: Academic Press. PRAGMATIC DEVELOPMENT:

Odell, K., McNeil, Malcom R., Rosenbek, John C., & Hunter, L. (1991). Perceptual characteristics of vowel and prosody production in apraxic, aphasic, and dysarthric speakers. *Journal of Speech and Hearing Research*, 34, 67-80. APRAXIA APHASIAS DYSARTHRIA:

Oden, David L., Thompson, Roger K., & Premack, David. (1990). Infant chimpanzees spontaneously perceive both concrete and abstract same/different relations. *Child Development*, 61, 621-631. RELATIONAL TERMS LANGUAGE AND OTHER PRIMATES:

The results of a familiarization- novelty procedure suggest that four infant chimpanzees could perceive same/different relationships.

Odor, L. (1980). *Balázs beszélni tanul (Balázs learns to talk).* Budapest: Minerva. METHODOLOGY-DIARY/CASE STUDY HUNGARIAN: HUNGARIAN

Ogilvy, C. M., Boath, E. H., Cheyne, W. M., & Jahoda, G., et al. (1992). Staff-child interaction styles in multi-ethnic nursery schools. *British Journal of Developmental Psychology*, 10, 85-97. LANGUAGE AND EDUCATION ADULT-CHILD INTERACTION:

Ogura, Tamiko. (1991). A longitudinal study of the relationship between early language development and play development. *Journal of Child Language*, 18, 273-294. LANGUAGE AND PLAY JAPANESE:

In the development of four Japanese children, there were correspondences between the onset of six language landmarks and the onset of play subcategories. From Child Development Abstracts.

Oksaar, Els. (1989). Mehrsprachigkeit im Vorschulalter. (Bilingualism in preschoolers.). *Die Neueren Sprachen*, 88(4), 310-327. BILINGUALISM-PRESCHOOLERS: GERMAN

From Stockholm Bibliographies.

Oldenburg, Jane. (1990). Learning the language and learning through language in early childhood. In M. A. K. Halliday, J. Gibbons, & H. Nicholas (Eds), *Learning, keeping and using language* . Amsterdam, The Netherlands: John Benjamins. LANGUAGE AND SOCIAL TRANSMISSION LANGUAGE AND COGNITIVE DEVELOPMENT:

Olkiewicz, Eva. (1990). *Invandrarfamiljer i forandring : en studie over finska och jugoslaviska invandrarungdomar och deras foraldrar.* Stockholm, Sweden: Institute of International Education, University of Stockholm. L2 EDUCATION FINNISH-SWEDISH SWEDISH-FINNISH SERBOCROATIAN-SWEDISH SWEDISH-SERBOCROATIAN: SWEDISH

Oller, D. Kimbrough, & Lynch, Michael P. (1992). Infant vocalizations and innovations in infraphonology: toward a broader theory of development. In C. A. Ferguson, L. Menn, & C. Stoel-Gammon (Eds), *Phonological development: Models, research, implications.* Monkton, MD: York Press. VOCALIZATIONS BABBLING:

Olmstead, D. (1971). *Out of the mouth of babes.* The Hague, The Netherlands: Mouton. OVERVIEW-GENERAL:

Olson, David R. (1956). On conceptual strategies. In J. S. Bruner, et al. (Eds), *Studies in cognitive growth.* New York, NY: Wiley. CONCEPT DEVELOPMENT:

Olson, David R., & Torrance, Nancy. (1991). *Literacy and orality.* New York, NY: Cambridge University Press. LITERACY WRITTEN LANGUAGE:

In this study of the social and psychological implications of literacy, seventeen distinguished scholars provide a sustained and detailed examination of the relations between orality and literacy, the traditions based on them, the functions served by them, and the psychological and linguistic processes recruited and enhanced by them. By shedding the romantic view that literacy is the road to rationality and modernity, the volume provides a more functional view of literacy. The articles place new emphasis on the relationship between speaking and writing and highlight the different ways in which people exploit the particular resources of speech and writing for special purposes, such as building communities, creating records, and specializing genres, such as prose fiction, enhancing private study and meditation, and enhancing the specialization and organization of knowledge.

Olson, S. L., Bates, J. E., & Kaskie, B. (1992). Caregiver-infant interaction antecedents of children's school-age cognitive ability. *Merrill-Palmer Quarterly* , 38, 309-330. ADULT-CHILD INTERACTION LANGUAGE AND COGNITIVE DEVELOPMENT PARENTAL INPUT:

Onslow, M., Costa, L., & Rue, S. (1990). Direct early intervention with stuttering - some preliminary data. *Journal of Speech and Hearing Disorders*, 55, 405-416. STUTTERING INTERVENTION PROGRAMS:

Onslow, M., Hayes, B., Hutchins, L., & Newman, D. (1992). Speech naturalness and prolonged-speech treatments for stuttering-further variables and data. *Journal of Speech and Hearing Research*, 35, 274-282. STUTTERING:

Ornstein, Peter A., Larus, Deanna M., & Clubb, Patricia A. (1990). Understanding children's testimony: implications of research on the development of memory. *Annals of Child Development*, 8, LANGUAGE AND MEMORY CHILDREN'S EXPLANATIONS CHILDREN'S SUMMARIES CHILDREN'S DESCRIPTIONS:

Ornstein, Robert E. (1972). The two sides of the brain. In R. E. Ornstein (Ed.), *The psychology of consciousness*. San Francisco, CA: Freeman. LATERALIZATION:

Orsolini, Margherita. (1985). La comprensione di storie: che cosa si sviluppa? (The comprehension of stories: What develops?). *Rassegna di Psicologia*, 3, 31-59. ITALIAN TEXT/STORY GRAMMARS NARRATIVES DISCOURSE COMPREHENSION: ITALIAN

This review discusses the main paradigms of research on the comprehension of stories. The cognitive and linguistic processes which, according to the different paradigms, are involved in story comprehension, are examined. The theoretical ground of different methods and experimental designs is identified. Results of studies on preschool and elementary school children's story comprehension are summarized and compared. Developmental trends are identified.

Orsolini, Margherita. (1985). Lo sviluppo dell'argomento nel gioco simbolico tra bambini in eta prescolare. (Topic development in preschoolers' symbollic play.). *Giornale Italiano di Psicologia*, 2, 235-258. LANGUAGE AND PLAY TOPIC MAINTENANCE TOPIC IDENTIFICATION: ITALIAN

The purpose of this study was to identify the cognitive processes that organize children's pretend activities in play sequences where a topic is shared and developed. Eight subjects, 4-5 years old, were observed in two 30- minute play sessions. The children played in pairs, using miniatures of everyday objects. Both verbal and non verbal productions were analyzed and pretend episodes with topic development were selected and coded. Results show that topic development in pretend activities relies on three major cognitive sources: a) 'scriptal' knowledge, b) knowledge of functional relationships between objects, c) pluri-functionality of objects and actions, as related to the different linguistic ways in which they can be categorized and referred to. These three different sources are discussed in the light of the representational and cognitive abilities involved by them. MO.

Orsolini, Margherita. (1986). 'Ma questa e' una storia.' La costruzione di abilita narrative nell'eta prescolare. ('But this is a story.' The construction of narrative skills in preschool children.). *Bambini*, 10, 22-29. NARRATIVES DISCOURSE COHERENCE EVENTS/SCRIPTS CAUSALITY METALINGUISTICS: ITALIAN

In this review results of a number of studies on children's narratives are examined and compared. The role of schemata, cohesive devices, causal thinking is discussed. Some issues which are not frequently addressed by current trends of research are identified: a) what is the contribution of dialogue to the construction of narrative skills? b) do cultural styles of story-telling affect the children's use of cohesive devices? c) what is the role of metacomunication in narrative discourse? MO.

Orsolini, Margherita. (1988). *Guida al linguaggio orale. (Handbook of spoken language.).* Roma: Editori Riuniti. ITALIAN NARRATIVES METALINGUISTICS DISCOURSE COMPREHENSION CONVERSATIONAL SKILLS LANGUAGE AND EDUCATION: ITALIAN

This book presents theoretical frames and results of research on different areas of preschool children's discourse and language acquisition: conversation, stories' comprehension, story-telling, metalinguistic awareness. Educational implications of these results are discussed.MO

Orsolini, Margherita. (1988). Information exchange in classroom conversation: negotiation and extension of the focus. *European Journal of Psychology of Education*, 3, 341-355. TOPIC INITIATION TOPIC MAINTENANCE LANGUAGE AND EDUCATION SOCIAL SPEECH :

This research is concerned with clarifying whether teacher's communicative strategies affect children's conversational relevance in classroom conversations. 34 conversations between teacher and children in a nursery school in suburban Rome, were collected with a 'quasi-experimental' methodology. 5961 turns at talk were categorized. Categories were aimed at distinguishing different level of relevance in teacher's and children's conversational contributions. The links between the current turn and the topic or the focus of the preceding turn are identified. Frequencies of turn categorizations were computed and transitional probabilities were examined. Results of sequential analysis show that children most often extend or elaborate on the information introduced by the teacher when the teacher has just extended the topic of a previous child speaker. However, in the group observed in this research, peer interaction can take on a function similar to that of teacher-children interaction. high relevance to the preceding child's contribution is significantly followed by a subsequent highly relevant contribution by another child. MO.

Orsolini, Margherita. (1988). Le competenze conversazionali nell'eta prescolare. (Preschoolers' conversational skills.). *Eta Evolutiva*, 31, 69-81. CONVERSATIONAL SKILLS EGOCENTRISM COMMUNICATIVE COMPETENCE PIAGETIAN THEORY DISCOURSE DEVELOPMENT TEXT/STROY GRAMMARS EVENTS/SCRIPTS DISCOURSE STRUCTURE: ITALIAN

This review considers recent research on development and acquisition of conversational abilities in preschool children, focussing on the following issues: 1) empirical evidence provided against the Piagetian hypothesis on egocentrism in child language, 2) relationships between general conversational abilities and specific discourse skills, related to different communicative situations. These issues are discussed analyzing results of studies concerning: a) social and communicative competence involved in conversation, b) relationships between knowledge representation and information-exchange in dialogue, c) children's use of language within specific 'discourse genres,' such as disputes. MO.

Orsolini, Margherita. (1989). Arguing versus co-constructing in children's verbal interaction. *Dossiers de Psychologie*, 37, 53-59. DISCOURSE SUPPORT DISCOURSE FUNCTIONS DISCOURSE STRUCTURE CHILDREN'S EXPLANATIONS CHILDREN'S DISCOURSE:

This study has the exploratory aim of identifying the discourse processes involved in different conversational activities. In particular, oppositive versus consensual verbal exchanges are compared. Twenty-four subjects (of middle-low SE) were observed: 12 kindergarten children (aged 5-6 years) and 12 second-grade children (aged 7-8 years). Each subject took part in two large group discussions (4 participants) on the topic 'balance.' The discussions were led by the children's teacher and occurred after manipulative activities with different types of scales and weights. Results show that in conflictual verbal exchanges children frequently provide support to a preceding claim or opposition move by means of causal explanations, overt appeals to general properties, definitions. These complex discourse processes rarely occurred in consensul verbal exchanges. Results are discussed in the light of the neo-vygostkian and neo-piagetian frameworks. MO.

Orsolini, Margherita. (1990). Episodic structure in children's fantasy narratives: breakthrough to decontextualized discourse. *Language and Cognitive Processes*, 1, 53-79. NARRATIVES DISCOURSE COHERENCE:

In this paper, episodic structure is invoked to explain decontextualized processes of discourse construction and, in particular the use of cohesive devices in children's fantasy narratives. 70 children were tested twice, at 4 and 5 years of age, and their stories were audiotaped and transcribed. The levels of narrative structure, extension of the theme, and use of cohesive devices were identified. A qualitative analysis of three case studies was made, in an attempt to understand on-line discourse processes in episodic and non-episodic stories. The results show that narrative structure, extension of the theme, and cohesion undergo significant development between the first and the second testings, and have strong correlations in both the observations. The qualitative analysis carried out on the case studies suggests that in stories with the least complex narrative structure, the strategies for establishing referential continuity and the processes of maintaining and extending the theme, are 'in competition.' MO.

Orsolini, Margherita, & Devescovi, A. (1988). La comprensione di una storia in bambini di 4 anni. (Story comprehension in 4-year-old children).. In T. DeMauro, & S. Gensini (Ed.), *Dalla parte del ricevente: Percezione, Compresione, Interpretazione*. Roma: Bulzoni. TEXT/STORY GRAMMARS NARRATIVES COMPREHENSION DISCOURSE COMPREHENSION LANGUAGE AND MEMORY: ITALIAN

The 'grammars' of stories predict that items of information which have the functional role of 'Initiating event, Attempts, and Resolution' should be better encoded and retrieved. Research which focuses on the causal structure underlying stories predicts that items of information are better retrieved as a function of the causal links in which they are involved in the text. Both paradigms assume that the processes of encoding of information parallel the processes of information retrieval. These three predictions were tested in this study analyzing the performance of twenty 4-year-old children.

Subjects were requested to recall a story and subsequently, to answer some questions. The story was audiorially presented whereas children were looking at a booklet with 5 pictures depicting some events of the story. Results show that the Focal Events (identified in the way proposed by Omanson, 1982) are more frequently recalled than the non-focal ones, even when there is no picture related to the focal story event. The narrative role of items of information is also significant. 'Reactions' and 'Internal Responses' are the least recalled events, although in the original text they contained a great deal of Focal Events and were also depicted in some of the pictures. Items of information recalled answering the experimenter's questions do no coincide with items of information spontaneously retrieved. This last results suggests that subjects' comprehension is only partially captured in analyses of spontaneous retrieval. MO.

Orsolini, Margherita, & Pontecorvo, Clotilde. (1989). Classroom discussion as a context for learning how to explain. In M. S. Barbieri (Ed.), *La speigazione nell'interazione sociale*. Torino, Italy: Loescher. CHILDREN'S EXPLANATIONS LANGUAGE AND EDUCATION COMMUNICATIVE COMPETENCE: ITALIAN

An analysis of language and interaction in a group of nursery school children while discussing a story. The argumentative value of explanations is pointed out and the contrast of different points of view is seen as a privileged place for the occurence of explanations.MO

Orsolini, Margherita, & Pontecorvo, Clotilde. (1989). Consapevolezza pragmatica e comprensione delle storie. (Pragmatic awareness and comprehension of stories). *Rassegna di Linguistica Applicata*, 1 (2), 179-196. PRAGMATIC DEVELOPMENT NARRATIVES ANAPHORA DISCOURSE COMPREHENSION TEXT/STORY GRAMMARS EVENTS/SCRIPTS: ITALIAN

Pragmatic awareness has been frequently considered correlated to the comprehension processes. For example, judgements of importance have been used by researchers to confirm the prediction that some events have a central role in the subjects's construction of the story's causal chain (Bower, 1982). This study is aimed at clarifying the relationships between pragmatic awareness and story comprehension, and at examining the role played by specific linguistic features of the text. Relationships between pragmatic awareness and story comprehension are inquired into using a correlational design: subjects' recall of an extended story and subjects' judgements of incoherence of four short stories are compared. The role served by the linguistic features of the text is inquired into examining comparing the children's detection of semantic incoherence in two different conditions. In the first one, 'scriptal stories' contain a semantic incoherence created by the violation of the canonical temporal order of actions. In the second one, a canonical relation between actions and characters is violated (for example, a bird goes to the dentist)-however this violation is conveyed by an anaphoric pronoun. 20 four-year old and 20 five-year old children were observed in the recalling and in the 'judgement of incoherence' tasks. Results show that the subjects' scores in the recalling of an extended story are significantly correlated to the scores received in the 'judgement of incoherence' task, when scriptal stories are concerned. The same result does not occur with stories which have a semantic incoherence created by the anaphoric pronoun. Subjects' performance in this last task is very low in both ages and does not correlate with the recalling scores. MO.

Orsolini, Margherita, Pontecorvo, Clotilde, & Amoni, M. (1989). Discutere a scuola: interazione sociale e attivita cognitiva. (School-disputes: social interaction and cognitive ability.). *Giornale Italiano di Psicologia*, 3, 479-510. CHILDREN'S DISCOURSE TURN TAKING DISCOURSE FUNCTIONS: ITALIAN

This study explores the conversational structure of 'classroom discussions.' Fourteen discussions, which were attended by 12 five-year-old children, were analyzed. Discussions were preceded by shared activity and guided by the children's teacher. Discussions were audiotaped and transcribed. Categories of analysis describe the communicative and interactive function of turns at talk. A sequential analysis of frequencies of categories was applied. The most recurrent patterns of teacher-child and child-child discourse were identified. MO.

Oshimatakane, Y. (1992). Analysis of pronominal errors: A case-study. *Journal of Child Language*, 19, 111-131. PRONOUNS ANAPHORA:

Ostigay, Luc, Gagné, Gilles, & Blais, Jean-Guy. (1990). Metalinguistic activities and the development of the use of formal register among elementary school children. In M. A. K. Halliday, J. Gibbons, & H. Nicholas (Eds), *Learning, keeping and using language*. Amsterdam, The Netherlands: John Benjamins. REGISTER METALINGUISTICS:

Otomo, K., & Stoel-Gammon, Carol. (1992). The acquisition of unrounded vowels in English. *Journal of Speech and Hearing Research*, 35, 604-616. VOWELS:

Overes, A. C. M. (1987). Anne, verbal interaction in the first six months of a child (In Dutch). *Reports of the Institute of Phonetic Sciences, University of Amsterdam*, 90, INTERSUBJECTIVITY ADULT-CHILD INTERACTION: DUTCH

Micro-analytic analysis of mother-infant interaction.

Owens, Elmer, & Kessler, Dorcas K. (1989). *Cochlear implants in young deaf children*. San Diego, CA: Singular Publishing Group. DEAF CHILDREN INTEVERVENTION PROGRAMS COCHLEAR IMPLANTS ATYPICAL DEVELOPMENT:

Cochlear implant systems, author contributions, and terminology: an overview. The psychophysics of cochlear implant stimulation. Present status of adults with cochlear implants. Early behavioral assessment. Application of evoked potential audiometry to children with cochlear implants. Hearing aids, cochlear implants, and profoundly deaf children. Tactile aids: developmental issues and current status. Neural prosthetic strategies for young children. Medical and surgical considerations of cochlear implantation in children. Present status of cochlear implants in children. Evaluating speech perception skills: tools for measuring benefits of cochlear implants. Speech production in profoundly hearing-impaired children with reference to cochlear implants. Auditory processing and speech perception: implications for cochlear implants in young children. Issues in language acquisition relevant to cochlear implants in young children. Thoughts on the phychological implications of cochlear implantation in children. Conclusions: current considerations and future directions. Author index. Subject index.

Owens, Maire. (1992). *The acquisition of Irish : a case study.* Philadelphia, PA: Multilingual Matters. IRISH METHODOLOGY-DIARY/CASE STUDY BILINGUALISM:

P

Pačesová, Jaroslava. (1989). Language development: form and function. *Folia Linguistica*, 23, 107-130. OVERVIEW-GENERAL:

Padilla, Jose A. (1990). *On the definition of binding domains in Spanish : evidence from child language.* Dordrecht, The Netherlands: Kluwer Academic. SYNTACTIC STRUCTURES SPANISH ANAPHORA:

Padilla, Raymond V., & Benavides, Alfredo. H. (1992). *Critical perspectives on bilingual education researh.* Tempe, AZ: Bilingual Press/Editoral Bilingue. BILINGUALISM-EDUCATION L2 EDUCATION:

Papers from a series of symposia held April 23-25, 1990, concurrently with the National Association for Bilingual Education annual meeting in Tucson, Arizona.

Palermo, David S. (1978). Semantics and language acquisition: Some theoretical considerations. In R. N. Campbell, & P. T. Smith (Eds), *Recent advances in the psychology of language.* New York, NY: Plenum. ACQUISITION THEORIES-SEMANTICS SEMANTIC DEVELOPMENT LEXICAL DEVELOPMENT:

Palotás, Gábor. (1988). A dyslexia prevencióban részesülö gyermekek differenciál diagnosztikájának nehány kérdéséhez. (Differential diagnostic questions in dyslexia prevention). In M. Gosy (Ed.), *A magyar beszédgyógyítás 100 éve.* Budapest: DYSLEXIA HUNGARIAN: HUNGARIAN

Palotás, Márta. (1988). Összehasonlító szókincsvizsgálat általános iskolás 2-3 osztályos tanulóknal (A comparative examination of the vocabulary of second and third grade elementary school children.). In M. Gosy (Ed.), *A magyar beszédgyógyítás 100 éve.* Budapest: VOCABULARY DEVELOPMENT HUNGARIAN: HUNGARIAN

Pan, Barbara A. (1993). Basic measures of child language. In J. L. Sokolov, & C. E. Snow (Eds), *Handbook of research in language development using CHILDES.* Hillsdale, NJ: Lawrence Erlbaum Associates. METHODOLOGY-ANALYSIS METHODOLOGY-COMPUTERS CHILDES:

Panneton-Cooper, Robin. (1991). The role that prosodic cues play in affecting young infants' perception of speech. In C. Rovee-Collier, & L. P. Lipsitt (Eds), *Advances in infancy research.* Norwood, NJ: Ablex. CUES-PHONOLOGICAL PROSODY SPEECH PERCEPTION:

Pap, Mária, & Pléh, Csaba. (1972). Nyelvhasználat és tarsadalmi helyzet. (Social class and language use). *Szociológia*, 2, 211-234. LANGUAGE AND SOCIAL CLASS HUNGARIAN: HUNGARIAN

Pap, Mária, & Pléh, Csaba. (1972). A szociális helyzet és a beszéd összefüggései az iskoláskor kezdetén. (Relationships between social class and speech at the beginning of school.). *Valoság*, 15, 52-58. EDUCABILITY LANGUAGE AND SOCIAL CLASS LINGUISTIC CODES: HUNGARIAN

A study of Bernstein's hypothesis in Hungarian children. The basic finding is more restricted code usage in 6 year old working class children than in middle class peers.

Pap, Mária, & Pléh, Csaba. (1973). Social class differences in the speech of Hungarian children. *Sociology*, 8, 147-155. LANGUAGE AND SOCIAL CLASS HUNGARIAN:

Papoušek, Mechthild, & Hwang, S. F. C. (1991). Tone and intonation in Mandarin babytalk to presyllabic infants: Comparison with registers of adult conversation and foreign language instruction. *Applied Psycholinguistics*, 12, 481-504. PARENTAL SPEECH-PROSODY MANDARIN L2 EDUCATION:

Papoušek, Mechthild, Papoušek, Hanus, & Symmes, D. (1991). The meanings of melodies in motherese in tone and stress languages. *Infant Behavior and Development*, 14, 415-440. TONE PARENTAL SPEECH-PROSODY CROSSLINGUISTIC STUDY:

Pappas, Christine C. (1990). Acquiring a sense of story genre: An examination of semantic properties. In M. A. K. Halliday, J. Gibbons, & H. Nicholas (Eds), *Learning, keeping and using language* . Amsterdam, The Netherlands: John Benjamins. TEXT/STORY GRAMMARS NARRATIVES SEMANTIC DEVELOPMENT DISCOURSE STRUCTURE:

Pappas, Christine C. (1991). Young children's strategies in learning the book language of information books. *Discourse Processes*, 14, 203-225. LITERACY TEXT/STORY GRAMMARS DISCOURSE STRUCTURE:

Pappas, Dennis G. (1985). *Diagnosis and treatment of hearing impairment in children: a clinical manual.* San Diego, CA: Singular Publishing Group. AUDIOLOGY CLASSIFICATION OF DISORDERS CONGENITAL DISORDERS INTERVENTION PROGRAMS:

> Overview of the hearing mechanism. Pursuing the causes of hearing disorders. Fundamentals of inheritance. Hearing loss associated with perinatal infections. Acquired hearing loss due to other infections and causes. Sensorineural hearing loss associated with trauma. Basic audiological evaluation of congenital hearing loss. Vestibular function in children. Strategies for habilitation. Index.

Parker, Sue T., & Gibson, Kathleen R. (1990). *'Language' and intelligence in monkeys and apes.* New York, NY: Cambridge University Press. LANGUAGE AND OTHER PRIMATES:

> The first collection of articles completely and explicitly devoted to the new field of 'comparative developmental evolutionary psychology' - studies of primate abilities based on frameworks drawn from developmental psychology and evolutionary biology. These frameworks include Piagetian and neo-Piagetian models as well as psycholinguistic ones. These articles represent developmental psychology, cultural and physical anthropology, ethology, and comparative psychology. The book

focuses on such areas as the nature of culture, intelligence, language, and imitation: the differences among species in their mental abilities and their neurological bases. The species studied include the African grey parrot, cebus and macaque monkeys, gorillas, orangutans and both common and pygmy champanzees.

Parodi, Teresa. (1990). The acquisition of word order regularities and case morphology. In M. J. Meisel (Ed.), *Two first languages: Early grammatical development in bilingual children*. Dordrecht: Foris. WORD ORDER CASE BILINGUALISM-SYNTACTIC DEVELOPMENT INFLECTION MORPHOSYNTACTIC DEVELOPMENT BILINGUALISM-MORPHOLOGICAL DEVELOPMENT:

Pask, G. (1975). *Conversation, cognition and learning: A cybernetic theory and methodology*. Amsterdam, The Netherlands: Elsevier-North Holland. ACQUISITION THEORIES METHODOLOGY CONVERSATIONAL SKILLS LANGUAGE AND COGNITIVE DEVELOPMENT:

Pataki, László. (1985). A gyermekkori dysphonia: Kerdések a beszéd- és mentálhigiene szempontjából. (Childhood dysphonia: questions from the viewpoint of speech and mental health.). In I. Hardi, & O. A. Verdes (Eds), *Beszéd es mentálhigiene.*. Budapest: ARTICULATION DISORDERS PHONOLOGICAL DISORDERS HUNGARIAN: HUNGARIAN

Patterson, Francine, & Linden, E. (1981). *The education of Koko*. New York, NY: Holt, Rinehart Winston. LANGUAGE AND OTHER PRIMATES:

A description of the Stanford Gorilla Signing Project. The authors report that in their opinion the gorilla Koko acquired full language capability including linguistic displacement.

Patterson, Karalyn, Seidenberg, Mark S., & McClelland, James L. (1990). Connections and disconnections: Acquired dyslexia in a computational model of reading processes. In R. G. M. Morris (Ed.), *Parallel distributed processing: Implications for psychology and neurobiology*. New York, NY: Oxford University Press. CONNECTIONISM COMPUTER SIMULATIONS DYSLEXIA READING DISORDERS:

Paul, Rhea, & Elwood, T. J. (1991). Maternal linguistic input to toddlers with slow expressive language development. *Journal of Speech and Hearing Research*, 34, 982-988. LANGUAGE DELAY PARENTAL SPEECH-ATYPICAL CHILDREN:

Paul, Rhea, & Jennings, P. (1992). Phonological behavior in toddlers with slow expressive language development. *Journal of Speech and Hearing Research*, 35, 99-107. INDIVIDUAL VARIATION LANGUAGE DELAY PHONOLOGICAL DISORDERS ATYPICAL DEVELOPMENT:

Paul, Rhea, Looney, S. S., & Dahm, P. S. (1991). Communication and socialization skills at ages 2 and 3 in late-talking young children. *Journal of Speech and Hearing Research*, 34, 858-865. RETICENCE-TALKATIVENESS COMMUNICATIVE DEVELOPMENT SOCIAL SPEECH ATYPICAL DEVELOPMENT:

Paul, Rhea, & Shiffer, M. E. (1991). Communicative initiations in normal and late-talking toddlers. *Applied Psycholinguistics*, 12, 419-431. TOPIC INITIATION CONVERSATIONAL SKILLS ATYPICAL DEVELOPMENT RETICENCE-TALKATIVENESS:

Pavchinski, Peter, Evans, Joseph H., & Bostow, Darrel E. (1989). Increasing word recognition and math ability in a severely learning-disabled student with token reinforcers. *Psychology in the Schools*, 26, 397-411. LANGUAGE AND EDUCATION:

> An experiment was conducted in which a learning- disabled youth was treated for a lack of reading and math skills. Token reinforcers were delivered for correct responses to a structured set of math problems and sight words. The subject reached a 90% correct response rate following implementation of a changing criterion experimental design. Part two of the study produced a 100% achievement level for the most difficult multiplication and division items. Results imply that some behaviors identified as learning disabilities may be treatable using motivational strategies. - From Child Development Abstracts.

Pearson, Barbara Zurer. (1990). The comprehension of metaphor by preschool children. *Journal of Child Language*, 17, 185-203. FIGURATIVE LANGUAGE COMPREHENSION:

An elicited repetition task consisting of literal, metaphoric, and anomalous sentences was used to examine 52 preschoolers comprehension of metaphor. Results indicated that there was no significant difference between their literal and metaphoric comprehension, and both were better than their performance on anomalous sentences.

Pellegrini, Anthony D. (1991). *Applied child study: 2. Ed.* Hillsdale, NJ: Lawrence Erlbaum Associates. METHODOLOGY-DESIGN METHODOLOGY-ANALYSIS:

Pellegrini, Anthony D., & Britton, R. (1991). *Narrative thought and narrative language.* Hillsdale, NJ: Lawrence Erlbaum Associates. NARRATIVES COGNITIVE DEVELOPMENT LANGUAGE AND COGNITIVE DEVELOPMENT:

Since before the dawn of history, people have been telling stories to each other and to themselves. Thus stories are at the root of human experience. This volume describes empirical investigations by Jerome Bruner, Wallace Chafe, David Olson, and others on the relationship between stories and cognition. Using philosophical, linguistic, anthropological, and psychological perspectives on narrative, the contributors provide a definitive, highly diversified portrait of human cognition.

Pellegrini, Anthony D., & Galda, Lee. (1991). The joint construction of stories by preschool children and an experimenter. In B. Britton, & A. Pellegrini (Eds), *Narrative thought and narrative language.* Hillsdale, NJ : Lawrence Erlbaum Associates. NARRATIVES:

Penfield, W. (1964). The child's changing brain. *The Atlantic Monthly,* 214(1). LATERALIZATION NEUROLINGUISTICS:

Penning, M. J., & Raphael, T. E. (1991). The impact of language ability and text variables on 6th-grade students' comprehension. *Applied Psycholinguistics*, 12, 397-417. COMPREHENSION LITERACY:

Pennington, Bruce F. (1992). *Reading disabilities: Genetic and neurological influences*. Hingham, MA: Kluwer Academic Press. READING DISORDERS DYSLEXIA AT-RISK CHILDREN:

The result of an international conference held in Boulder, Colorado in 1990, the papers in this book point to the neurological basis of dyslexia.

Pennington, Martha C., & Stevens, Vance. (1991). *Computers in applied linguistics: an international perspective*. London, UK: Multilingual Matters. METHODOLOGY-COMPUTERS C.A.L.L. L2 EDUCATION:

Theoretical and methodological issues of using computers in applied linguistics, second language education, and language teaching.

Pepperberg, I. M. (1993). Cognition and communicaiton in an African Grey parrot. In L. M. Herman, H. L. Roitblat & P. E. Nachtigal, (Eds). *Language and communication: Comparative perspectives*. Hillsdale, NJ: Lawrence Erlbaum Associates. ANIMAL COMMUNICATIONS:

Perdue, Clive. (1990). Complexification of the simple clause in the narrative discourse of adult language learners. *Linguistics*, 28(5), SYNTACTIC STRUCTURES NARRATIVES LANGUAGE AND EDUCATION L2 EDUCATION:

Perdue, Clive. (1991). Crosslinguistic comparisons: Organisational principles in learner languages. In T. Huebner, & C. Ferguson (Eds), *Cross-currents in second language acquisition*. Amsterdam: Benjamins. L2 ACQUISITION STRATEGIES L2 EDUCATION:

Perez-Pereira, Miguel. (1989). The acquisition of morphemes: some evidence from Spanish. *Journal of Psycholinguistic Research*, 18(3), 289-312. SPANISH MORPHOLOGICAL DEVELOPMENT:

Perez-Pereira, Miguel. (1991). The acquisition of gender: What Spanish children tell us. *Journal of Child Language*, 18, 571-590. SPANISH GENDER MORPHOSYNTACTIC DEVELOPMENT:

Perkins, W. H. (1990). What is stuttering. *Journal of Speech and Hearing Disorders*, 55, 370-382. STUTTERING:

Perkins, W. H., Kent, Raymond D., & Curlee, R. F. (1991). A theory of neuropsycholinguistic function in stuttering . *Journal of Speech and Hearing Research*, 34, 734-752. STUTTERING:

Perner, J. (1991). On representing that: The assymetry between belief and desire in children's theory of mind. In D. Frye, & C. Moore (Eds), *Children's theories of mind.* Hillsdale, NJ: Lawrence Erlbaum Associates. THEORY OF MIND REPRESENTATIONS:

Peters, Ann M. (1993). The interdependence of social, cognitive and linguistic development: Evidence from a visually impaired child. In H. Tager-Flusberg (Ed.), *Constraints on language acquisition: Studies of atypical children.* Hillsdale, NJ: Lawrence Erlbaum Associates. ATYPICAL DEVELOPMENT BLIND CHILDREN SOCIAL INTERACTION LANGUAGE AND COGNITIVE DEVELOPMENT:

Peters, S., Shapiro, S. C., & Rapaport, W. J. (1988). Flexible natural language processing and Roschian category theory. In *Proceedings of the Tenth Annual Conference of the Cognitive Science Society.* Hillsdale, NJ: Lawrence Erlbaum. PROTOTYPE THEORY CONCEPT DEVELOPMENT LEXICAL DEVELOPMENT SEMANTIC DEVELOPMENT CATEGORIZATION:

Peterson, Carole. (1990). The who, when and where of child narratives. *Journal of Child Language*, 17, 433-455. NARRATIVES TEXT/STORY GRAMMARS EVENTS/SCRIPTS DISCOURSE STRUCTURE:

> The early development of key orientation (participants, location , and time) was traced with an 18-month longitudinal study of real-experience narratives produced by 10 children aged approximately 2-4 years. There was no developmental improvement. Orientation to when was rare at first and involved formula words indiscriminately applied. When information was more common at all ages, particularly when the narrated events occurred away from home. Overall, very young children can produce narratives in an unscaffolded context to adults unfamiliar with their experiences.

Peterson, Carole, & Dodsworth, Pamela. (1991). A longitudinal analysis of young children's cohesion and noun specification in narratives. *Journal of Child Language*, 18, 397-415. NARRATIVES NOUNS DISCOURSE COHERENCE PRONOUNS CONNECTIVES:

> A study of ten children covering the age range 2:0-3:6 showed that the use of nine cohesive devices increased with age, together with and increased use of pronominal reference and a greater use of conjunctions.

Peterson, Carole, & McCabe, Allyssa. (1990). Linking children's connective use and narrative structure. In A. McCabe, & C. Peterson (Ed.), *Developing narrative structure*. Hillsdale, NJ: Lawrence Erlbaum Associates. NARRATIVES CONNECTIVES:

Peterson, Carole, & McCabe, Allyssa. (1991). On the threshold of the story realm: Semantic versus pragmatic use of connectives in narratives. *Merrill-Palmer Quarterly*, 37, 445-464. CONNECTIVES NARRATIVES:

Peterson, Harold, & Marquardt, Thomas. (1989). *Appraisal and diagnosis of speech and language disorders*. Englewood Cliffs, NJ: Prentice-Hall. ASSESSMENT PROCEDURES CLASSIFICATION OF DISORDERS:

Petitto, Laura A. (1992). Modularity and constraints in early lexical acquisition : evidence from children's early language and gesture. In M. R. Gunnar, & M. Maratsos (Eds), *Modularity and constraints in language and cognition*. Hillsdale, NJ: Lawrence Erlbaum Associates. LEXICAL DEVELOPMENT MODULARITY CONSTRAINTS GESTURE:

Phillips, J. R. (1977). Syntax and vocabulary of mothers' speech to young children. In M. S. Barbieri (Ed.), *Gli inizi del linguaggio: aspetti cognitivi e comunicativi. (The emergence of language: cognitive and communicative aspects.)*. La Nuova, Italy: Firenze. PARENTAL SPEECH-SYNTAX PARENTAL SPEECH-VOCABULARY:

Phillipson, Robert, et al. (1991). *Foreign/second language pedagogy research : a commemorative volume for Claus Farch*. Philadelphia, PA: Multilingual Matters. L2 EDUCATION:

Piaget, Jean, Henriques, Gil, & Ascher, Edgar. (1992). *Morphisms and categories*. Hillsdale, NJ: Lawrence Erlbaum Associates. PIAGETIAN THEORY NEOPIAGETIAN THEORY:

The first English translation of Piaget's later theory which encompasses not only the traditionally expected views concerning transformation and constancy but also introduces new ideas on nontransformatory actions which create morphisms and categories and which are also necessary elements in the acquisition of knowledge.

Pichora-Fuller, M. K., & Benguerel, A. P. (1991). The design of CAST (Computer-aided Speechreading Training). *Journal of Speech and Hearing Research*, 34, 202-212. COMPUTER ASSISTED THERAPY:

Piel, John A. (1990). Unmasking sex and social class differences in childhood aggression: The case for language maturity. *Journal of Educational Research*, 84, 100-106. LANGUAGE AND AGGRESSION SEX DIFFERENCES LANGUAGE AND SOCIAL CLASS LANGUAGE AND AFFECT LANGUAGE AND EDUCATION:

Second- and third-grade students completed the Nancy-Ernie Aggression Test, Apperceptive Aggression Test and a portion of the Paradigmatic-Syntagmatic Language List, to assess language maturity. The results indicated that children who select the physical modal choice on an apperceptive test of aggressive behavior did so regardless of sex or social class. The best predictor for physical aggressive behavior was language immaturity.

Pieraut-Le Bonniec, Gilberte, & Dolitsky, Marlene. (1991). *Language bases-discourse bases: Some aspects of contemporary French psycholinguistics research*. Philadelphia, PA.: John Benjamins. LANGUAGE PRECURSORS FRENCH PRELINGUISTICS DISCOURSE COHERENCE DISCOURSE DEVELOPMENT BIOLOGICAL FOUNDATIONS:

This volume ignores the heavily studied (and usual) mid area of child language acquisition (in and around the two-word stage), to present the recent French focus on prelinguistic speech skills and the development of discourse. From the one side of language acquisition, i.e., prelinguistic speech, the book begins with the physical properties in human development necessary for language to occur. It also offers studies on a child's initial equipment, i.e. intra-uterine skills and skills acquired before first words. At the other side are studies on the development of discourse, the child's acquisition of not only the ability to juxtapose ideas, but to link them into cohesive, coherent texts, and to use argumentation; skills not fully acquired until the child is well into adolescence and nearing adulthood.

Pierce, Amy E. (1992). The acquisition of passives in Spanish and the question of A-chain maturation. *Language Acquisition*, 2, 55-81. PASSIVES SPANISH:

Pierce describes two experiments which investigate 3:0 to 5:0 year old Mexican children's understanding of the passive. She reports a difference in the data which revolves around the position of the subject in morphological passives which she attributes to the development of an A-chain.

Pierce, Amy E. (1992). *Language acquisition and syntactic theory : a comparative analysis of French and English child grammars*. Dordrecht, The Netherlands: Kluwer Academic Publishers. FRENCH SYNTACTIC DEVELOPMENT ACQUISITION AND LINGUISTIC THEORY:

Pimentak, Patricia A., & Kingbury, Nancy A. (1989). *Neuropsychological aspects of right brain injury*. San Diego, CA: Singular Publishing Group. LATERALIZATION TRAUMATIC DISORDERS:

Cerebral dominance and right hemisphere specialization: a neurologist's perspective. The injured right hemisphere: classification of related disorders. Psychological implications of right brain injury: patient and family perspectives. References.

Pine, Julian M. (1992). How referential are referential children: Relationships between maternal-report and observational measures of vocabulary composition and usage. *Journal of Child Language*, 19, 75-86. INDIVIDUAL VARIATION METHODOLOGY-ANALYSIS METHODOLOGY-DESIGN:

Pine, Julian M., & Lieven, Elena V. M. (1990). Referential style at thirteen months: Why age-defined cross-sectional measures are inappropriate for study of strategy differences in early language development. *Journal of Child Language*, 17, 624-631. INDIVIDUAL VARIATION METHODOLOGY-DESIGN:

This study examined the relationship between cross-sectional measures of referential style and measures based on the first 50 words in first-born children. No significant relationship was found.

Pinker, Steven, & Prince, Alan. (1990). Rules and connections in human language. In R. G. M. Morris (Ed.), *Parallel distributed processing: Implications for psychology and neurobiology*. New York, NY: Oxford University Press. CONNECTIONISM RULES REPRESENTATIONS:

The authors examine the differences between rule- driven models of language and connectionist models of language.

Pitkanen-Koli, T., & Kuure, Olli. (1990). *Studier over svenska som andrasprak i skolan (ProSSA). Projektbeskrivning. (Studies on Swedish as a second language in the school. Project presentation.).* Finland: University of Tampere. L2 EDUCATION SWEDISH-FINNISH FINNISH-SWEDISH BILINGUALISM: SWEDISH

Pittam, J., & Ingram, J. (1992). Accuracy of perception and production of compound and phrasal stress by Vietnamese-Australians. *Applied Psycholinguistics*, 13, 1-12. STRESS:

Piven, Joseph, Tsai, Guochuan, Nehme, Eileen, Coyle, Joseph T., Chase, Gary A., & Folstein, Susan E. (1991). Platelet serotonin, a possible marker for familial autism. *Journal of Autism and Developmental Disorders*, 21, 51-59. AUTISM DEVELOPMENTAL DISORDERS:

The 5HT levels of autistic subjects with affected siblings were significantly higher than probands without affected siblings, and autistic subjects without affected siblings had 5HT levels significantly higher than controls.

Pizzuto, E., & Caselli, M. Cristina. (1992). The acquisition of Italian morphology: Implications for models of language development. *Journal of Child Language*, 19, 491-557. ITALIAN MORPHOLOGICAL DEVELOPMENT:

Place, K. S., & Becker, Judith A. (1991). The influence of pragmatic competence on the likeability of grade-school children. *Discourse Processes*, 14, 227-241. PRAGMATIC DEVELOPMENT COMMUNICATIVE COMPETENCE SOCIAL INTERACTION SOCIAL SPEECH:

Plapinger, D., & Kretschmer, R. (1991). The effect of context on the interactions between a normally-hearing mother and her hearing-impaired child. *Volta Review*, 93, 75-87. DEAF CHILDREN PARENTAL SPEECH ADULT-CHILD INTERACTION SOCIAL INTERACTION CONTEXT:

Platt, J., & Coggins, T. E. (1990). Comprehension of social-action games in prelinguistic children-levels of participation and effect of adult structure. *Journal of Speech and Hearing Disorders*, 55, 315-326. SOCIAL INTERACTION ADULT-CHILD INTERACTION PRELINGUISTICS LANGUAGE AND PLAY:

Pléh, Csaba. (1981). Különbözö szórendü mondatok megértése és a dichotikus hallási aszimmetriák 3-6 éves gyermekeknél (The interpretation of sentences with different word orders and dichotic listening asymmetries in children between 3 and 6.). *Pszichológia*, 1, 365-393. WORD ORDER DICHOTIC LISTENING HUNGARIAN LATERALIZATION: HUNGARIAN

Pléh, Csaba. (1981). The role of word order in the sentence interpretation of Hungarian children. *Folia Linguistica*, 15, 331-343. WORD ORDER COMPREHENSION HUNGARIAN:

Pléh, Csaba. (1982). Sentence interpretation strategies and dichotic asymmetries in Hungarian children between 3 and 6 years. In R. Sinz, & M. R. Rosenweig (Eds), *Psychophysiology 1980*. Amsterdam: Jena. COMPREHENSION DICHOTIC LISTENING LANGUAGE AND SOCIAL CLASS HUNGARIAN:

Pléh, Csaba. (1982). Subject or topic in Hungarian: Some psycholinguistic evidence to increase the confusion. In F. Kiefer (Ed.), *Hungarian linguistics*. Amsterdam: Benjamins. CASE TOPIC-COMMENT HUNGARIAN:

Pléh, Csaba. (1983). Some semantic and pragmatic factors of anaphoric interpretation in Hungarian. *Acta Linguistica Academiae Scientiarum Hungaricae*, 33, 201-211. ANAPHORA HUNGARIAN:

Pléh, Csaba. (1986). A gyermeknyelv fejlödésének és kutatásainak modelljeiröl (On models of development and research of child language). In *Pszichológiai Tanulmányok XVI.*. Budapest: OVERVIEW-GENERAL METHODOLOGY HUNGARIAN: HUNGARIAN

Pléh, Csaba. (1988). Sentence understanding in Hungarian. In A. Fusco, & F. M. Battisti, et al. (Eds), *Issues in cognition and social representation*. Milano: Angeli. COMPREHENSION HUNGARIAN COMPLEX SENTENCES:

Pléh, Csaba. (1989). The development of sentence interpretation in Hungarian. In B. MacWhinney, & E. Bates (Eds), *The crosslinguistic study of sentence processing*. New York, NY: Cambridge University Press. COMPREHENSION HUNGARIAN COMPLEX SENTENCES:

Pléh, Csaba. (1989). Formal connexity and pragmatic cohesion in anaphora interpretation. In M. A. Conte, J. S. Petofi, & E. Suzer (Eds), *Text and discourse connectedness*. Amsterdam: Benjamins. ANAPHORA HUNGARIAN DISCOURSE COHERENCE:

Pléh, Csaba, Ackerman, Farrell, & Komlosy, Andreas. (1989). On the psycholinguistics of preverbal modifiers in Hungarian: adult intuition and children's treatment of modifiers. *Folia Linguistica*, 23, 181-213. MODIFIERS HUNGARIAN:

Pléh, Csaba, Jarovinskij, Alexandr, & Balajan, Alexandr. (1984). Szórend és mondatmegértés magyar-orosz kétnyelvü óvodásoknál. (Word order and sentence understanding in Hungarian-Russian bilingual preschoolers.). *Magyar Pszichológiai Szemle*, 41, 282-296. WORD ORDER COMPREHENSION HUNGARIAN-RUSSIAN HUNGARIAN-RUSSIAN BILINGUALISM-SYNTACTIC DEVELOPMENT: HUNGARIAN

In a sentence enactment study a slight tendency to use an agent first interpretation strategy was observed in both languages in bilingual children between 4 and 6 as well as in their monolingual controls. The incidence of this tendency was related to the morphonological difficulties in detecting the accusative in OVS structures. Bilinguals were more sensitive to the correct status of perceptually difficult accusatives. It is concluded that in acquiring simultaneously two unrelated case marking languages, more attention is paid to endings.

Pléh, Csaba, Jarovinskij, Alexandr, & Balajan, Alexandr. (1987). Sentence comprehension in Hungarian-Russian bilingual and monolingual preschool children. *Journal of Child Language*, 14, 587-603. HUNGARIAN-RUSSIAN RUSSIAN-HUNGARIAN RUSSIAN HUNGARIAN BILINGUALISM-SYNTACTIC DEVELOPMENT CASE SEMANTIC RELATIONS ACQUISITION STRATEGIES BILINGUALISM-ACQUISITION STRATEGIES WORD ORDER:

The authors examine the interpretation of transitive sentences with varying word orders /SVO, OVS, SOV, OSV/. The subjects were Hungarian-Russian bilingual preschool children and their Hungarian and Russian monolingual peers. Bever's 'first noun as agent' strategy - as indicated by OVS and OSV errors - appears to be weaker in the bilinguals. An explanation for this is proposed in terms of Slobin's 'attention to the end of the words' factor. The mistaken identification of sentence-initial objects as agents depends on case marking allomorphy. Bilinguals, in general, appear to pay more attention to allomorphy and thus make fewer interpretation errors than their monolingual peers.

Pléh, Csaba, & MacWhinney, Brian. (1985). Formai és szemantikai tényezök egyszerü magyar mondatok megértésében és a megértés fejlödésében. (Formal and semantic factors in understanding simple Hungarian sentences and in the development of understanding.). *Pszichológia*, 5, 321-378. COMPREHENSION HUNGARIAN COMPLEX SENTENCES: HUNGARIAN

Pléh, Csaba, & MacWhinney, Brian. (1988). A visszautaló (anaforikus) elemek és a megértés pragmatikus tényezöi. (Anaphoric elements and the pragmatic factors involved in comprehension.). *Magyar Pszichológiai Szemle*, 44 (45), 21-40. ANAPHORA HUNGARIAN: HUNGARIAN

In children, anaphora interpretation is influenced by the action readiness of the participants in a sequence of sentences.

Pléh, Csaba, & Vargha, András. (1982). Nehány nyelvfejlödési mutató, melyeket nem befolyásol a szociális helyzet. (Some markers of language development that are not influenced by social class position.). *Magyar Pszichológiai Szemle*, 39, 355-371. LANGUAGE AND SOCIAL CLASS HUNGARIAN DICHOTIC LISTENING COMPREHENSION: HUNGARIAN

In a study on over 200 preschoolers using sentence interpretation (enactment) and dichotic asymmetries it was found that neither of these basic data were related to parent's SES.

Pléh, Csaba, & Vargha, András. (1982). Socialnoje polozhenie, ponimanie predlozkenij i dichoticeskie asimmetrii u vengerskih doshkolnikov. (Social class, sentence understanding and dichotic assymetries in Hungarian preschoolers.). *Annales Universitatis Budapestiensis Sectio Paedagogica et Psychologica*, 7, 197-113. HUNGARIAN LANGUAGE AND SOCIAL CLASS DICHOTIC LISTENING COMPREHENSION: RUSSIAN

In a study of over 200 preschoolers using sentence interpretation (enactment) and dichotic asymmetries it was found that neither of these basic data were related to parent's SES.

Pléh, Csaba, & Vargha, András. (1984). Sentence interpretation, dichotic asymmetries, and social status in Hungarian nursery children. In M. Kodyan, & I. Slamenik (Eds), *Psychological development, learning and personality formation*. Prague: Academia. COMPREHENSION DICHOTIC LISTENING LANGUAGE AND SOCIAL CLASS HUNGARIAN:

Pléh, Csaba, & Vargha, András. (1985). A gyermeknyelv fejlödésének és kutatásának modelljeiröl. (On the models of research and development in child language.). *Pszichológiai Tanulmányok*, 16, 105-188. OVERVIEW-THEORY: HUNGARIAN

An extensive review of the international child language literature between 1960 and 1979.

Ploog, D., & Melnechuk, T. (1971). Are apes capable of language? *Neurosciences Research Program Bulletin*, 9(5). LANGUAGE AND OTHER PRIMATES:

Plunkett, Kim, & Marchman, Virginia A. (1991). U-shaped learning and frequency effects in a multi-layer perceptron: Implications for child language acquisition. *Cognition*, 38, 43-102. CONNECTIONISM TENSE UNLEARNING INPUT FACTORS:

A three layer perceptron was used to map associations that are analogous to past tense forms in English. The network showed a U-shaped learning curve in its acquisition of the patterns. Input effects relating to frequency of mappings was examined to see if it was the cause of the U-shaped learning.

Plunkett, Kim, & Sinha, Chris G. (1992). Connectionism and developmental theory. *British Journal of Developmental Psychology*, 10, 209-254. CONNECTIONISM:

Plunkett, Kim, & Stromquist, Sven. (1990). The acquisition of Scandinavian languages. *Gothenburg Papers in Theoretical Linguistics*, 59. SWEDISH DANISH NORWEGIAN MORPHOLOGICAL DEVELOPMENT INFLECTION RELATIVIZATION NEGATION PROSODY DEIXIS ARTICLES BIBLIOGRAPHY:

A more extensive version of the chapter in Slobin's 'Crosslinguistic Study of Language Acquisition' (q.v.) which looks at morphological and syntactic development in the Scandinavian language as as a whole and the individual differences between Danish, Swedish, and Norwegian. The work includes a very full bibliography of Scanidinavian child language research.

Plunkett, Kim, & Stromqvist, Sven. (1992). The acquisition of Scandinavian languages. In D. I. Slobin (Ed.), *The crosslinguistic study of language acquisition (Vol. 3).* Hillsdale, NJ: Lawrence Erlbaum Associates. BIBLIOGRAPHY DANISH SWEDISH NORWEGIAN ICELANDIC MORPHOSYNTACTIC DEVELOPMENT:

This article includes an extensive bibliography of research on the Scandinavian languages. A condensation of Gothenburg Papers in Linguistics # 59 which examinaes morphosyntactic development in the Sacandinavian languages.

Poizner, H., Bellugi, Ursula, & Klima, Edward S. (1990). Brain function for language: Perspectives from another modality. In I. G. Mattingly, & M. Studdert-Kennedy (Eds), *Modularity and the motor theory of speech perception*. Hillsdale, NJ: Lawrence Erlbaum Associates. MODALITY NEUROLINGUISTICS SPEECH PERCEPTION:

Pontecorvo, Clotilde, Orsolini, Margherita, & Zucchermaglio, Cristina. (1989). Metalinguistic skills in children: what develops? *Infancia y Apprendizaje*, 47, 37-54. METALINGUISTICS: ITALIAN

The aim of this study was to identify developmental changes in metalinguistic skills of primary school children, using the notions of 'analyzed knowledge' and 'executive control' (Bialystok, 1986) as two components of metalinguistic awareness. 60 first, second and third grade children were individually interviewed on two tasks. In the first task (guided word substitution) children are asked to substitute an underlined word with five alternatives, thus producing new sentences to be judged on their semantic and/or morphosyntactactic acceptability. In the second task (free word substitution), children have to find out the word that can be cancelled and substituted with a new one. In both tasks children have to express an acceptability judgement, and to give reasons for it. Results from two-way Anova show that the 'control' component does not change much, while the 'analyzed knowledge' changes significantly. However, even third grade children are more aware of the semantic rather than morphosyntactic features of language. MO.

Pontecorvo, Clotilde, & Zucchermaglio, Cristina. (1991). Computer use in learning language. *European Journal of Psychology of Education*, 6, 15-27. METALINGUISTICS LANGUAGE AND EDUCATION L2 EDUCATION:

An observational examination of children's interaction with software and their metalinguistic development. Results indicate that learning language with software has a positive effect on metalinguistic development. From Child Development Abstracts.

Post, K. (1993). Negative evidence. In J. L. Sokolov, & C. E. Snow (Eds), *Handbook of research in language development using CHILDES*. Hillsdale, NJ: Lawrence Erlbaum Associates. NEGATIVE EVIDENCE METHODOLOGY-DESIGN METHODOLOGY-COMPUTERS CHILDES:

Poulos, M. G., & Webster, W. G. (1991). Family history as a basis for subgrouping people who stutter. *Journal of Speech and Hearing Research*, 34, 5-10. STUTTERING:

Poulson, Claire L., Kymissis, Effie, Reeve, Kenneth F., Andreatos, Maria, & Reeve, Lori. (1991). Generalized vocal imitation in infants. *Journal of Experimental Child Psychology*, 51, 267-279. IMITATION:

Effects of modeling and response-contingent social praise on the vocal imitation of three 9- to 13-month-old infants were analyzed. All three infants showed systematic increases in matching during training following the introduction of model-and-praise condition. Probe-trial responding increased systematically with training-trial responding. Non-matching infant vocalizations did not increase systematically with the introduction of the model-and-praise procedure.

Poulson, Claire L., Nunes, L.R., & Warren, Steven F. (1989). Imitation in infancy: A critical review. In H. W. Reese (Ed.), *Advances in child development and behavior*. New York, NY: Academic Press. IMITATION:

Powell, Frank, Finitzo-Hieber, Terese, Friel-Patti, Sandy, & Henderson, Donald. (1985). *Education of the hearing impaired child.* San Diego, CA: Singular Publishing Group. LANGUAGE AND EDUCATION DEAF CHILDREN SIGNING-ASL MORPHOLOGICAL DEVELOPMENT:

Educational programs and services for hearing impaired children: issues and options. The acquisition of three morphological systems in American sign language. Assessment of hearing impaired children: determining typical and optimal levels of performance. Infant deafness and parental grief: psychosocial early intervention. Deafness, mental health, and language. Technology and the education of the hearing impaired. Evaluating changes in communication skills of deaf children using vibrotactile stimulation. Author index. Subject index.

Powell, S. D., & Jordan, R. R. (1992). Remediating the thinking of pupils with autism - principles into practice. *Journal of Autism and Developmental Disorders*, 22, 413-418. AUTISM:

Power, D. J., Wood, David J., & Wood, Heather A. (1990). Conversational strategies of teachers using three methods of communication with deaf children. *American Annals of the Deaf*, 135, 9-13. DEAF CHILDREN LANGUAGE AND EDUCATION SIGNING-CUED SPEECH SIGNING-ENGLISH PARENTAL SPEECH-CONTROL:

Teacher control over conversations with deaf pupils using oral/aural only, signed English or cued speech communication, was related to pupil response, including taking initiative in conversations, misunderstanding the teacher, and length of contributions to the conversation. As teacher control and repair of 'wrong' contributions increased, pupil initiative and length of contribution decreased and misunderstandings of teachers increased.

Power, D. J., Wood, David J., Wood, Heather A., & Macdougall, J. (1990). Maternal control over conversations with hearing and deaf infants and young children. *First Language*, 10, 19-35. DEAF CHILDREN PARENTAL SPEECH-CONTROL:

Mothers talking with their hearing or deaf children aged one to five years were compared on measures of maternal control over conversations and child response to different levels of such control. Maternal input depended upon children's linguistic receptive capacity rather than age or cognitive level, confirming a multi-factor theory of control of maternal input to language learners. - From Child Development Abstracts.

Pozarowska, Elzbieta. (1985). Struktura i proces wspoldzialania oraz jego realizacja jezykowa u dzieci w wieku przedszkolnym. (Structure and process of collaboration and its linguistic realisation in preschool children.). *Studia Psychologiczne*, 22, 114-127.
COLLABORATION TOPIC COLLABORATION PRAGMATIC DEVELOPMENT CONVERSATIONAL COMPETENCE CHILDREN'S DIALOGUES POLISH TOPIC MAINTENANCE TOPIC INITIATION: POLISH

An investigation of topic collaboration in a free play situation with specific reference to the initiation and maintenance of topics of conversation.

Pozarowska, Elzbieta. (1989). Wspoldzialanie w procesie interakcji dzieci w wieku przedszkolnym. (Collaboration in preschoolers as an interactive process). *Kwartalnik Pedagogiczny*, 3, 104-116.
COLLABORATION CHILDREN'S DISCOURSE PRAGMATIC DEVELOPMENT POLISH TOPIC COLLABORATION: POLISH

An investigation of the ontogenesis of collaboration in preschoolers' conversations. Collaboration was shown to vary with age and the structure of the conversational context.

Pozarowska, Elzbieta. (1991). Struktura i strategie dyskursu dzieciecego w sytuacji zadaniowej. (Discourse structure and discourse strategies in task-oriented situation). In B. Bokus, & Z. M. Haman (Eds), *Badan nad kompeteencja komunikacyjna dzieci (Research on children's communicative competence).* CHILDREN'S DISCOURSE DISCOURSE STRUCTURE: POLISH

Precious, A., & Conti-Ramsden, Gina. (1988). Language-impaired children's comprehension of active versus passive sentences. *British Journal of Disorders of Communication*, 23, 229-244.
DISCOURSE COMPREHENSION PASSIVES COMPREHENSION DISORDERS:

Premack, David. (1970). The education of Sarah. *Psychology Today*, 4, 54-58. LANGUAGE AND OTHER PRIMATES:

A description of an experiment to teach language to a chimpanzee, Sarah, using plastic symbols as the medium of communication.

Premack, David. (1971). Language in chimpanzees? *Science* 172, 808-822. LANGUAGE AND OTHER PRIMATES:

A further account of Premack's work with Sarah, a chimpanzee trained to use plastic symbols to communicate.

Premack, David. (1991). The infant's theory of self-propelled objects. In D. Frye, & C. Moore (Eds), *Children's theories of mind*. Hillsdale, NJ: Lawrence Erlbaum Associates. THEORY OF MIND OBJECT PERMANENCE:

Price, Derek W., & Goodman, Gail S. (1990). Visiting the wizard: Children's memory for a recurring event. *Child Development*, 61, 664-680. EVENTS/SCRIPTS SEQUENCING CAUSALITY:

Girls aged 2:6, 4:0, and 5:6 were repeatedly exposed to an episode in a laboratory setting. The number of activities and actions stored in the script increased with age. All ages stored causally related activities but temporal sequencing was age-related. Hierarchical organization of the script emerges gradually over the preschool years.

Prins, D., Hubbard, C. P., & Krause, M. (1991). Syllabic stress and the occurrence of stuttering. *Journal of Speech and Hearing Research*, 34, 1011-1016. STUTTERING STRESS:

Pumfrey, P. D. (1989). Differences in reading strategies among 7 to 8 year old children. *Journal of Research in Reading*, 12, 114-130. LITERACY READING DISORDERS:

The research studied the syntactic, semantic, and graphophonemic miscues made by groups of first year Junior school pupils of high, average, and low reading attainments.

The high reading attainment group made better quality syntactic, semantic and graphophonemic miscues at the lower level of text complexity. As text complexity increased, the miscue quality of high and above average reading attainment groups deteriorated. Higher scores on a word recognition reading test were significantly related to effective use of graphophonemic miscues, but not to the use of syntactic and semantic cues, in reading material from more demanding texts. - From Child Development Abstracts.

Purcell, S. L., & Liles, B. Z. (1992). Cohesion repairs in the narratives of normal-language and language-disordered school-age children. *Journal of Speech and Hearing Research*, 35, 354-362. NARRATIVES DISCOURSE COHERENCE DISCOURSE DISORDERS:

Purushothama, G. (1988). Sequencing and orientation difficulties in reading Kannada script. *Perceptual and Motor Skills*, 65, KANNADA LITERACY READING DISORDERS DYSLEXIA:

In language using phonetic scripts, the frequencies of expected difficulties are fewer. As phonemes are highly abstract, reading difficulties are more frequent in English (an alphabetic system) than in languages using syllabic script. Graphic forms alone may not be responsible for the reading difficulties or fluency but also orthographic system and forms of letters. Ten good readers and ten poor readers from a group of 80 students in Grade 3 were the subjects. Results indicated that both good readers and poor readers showed reversals in reading though the number of reversals made by the poor readers were longer. Orientation reversals were more visual than phonetic unlike those of English. Apart from the script being phonetically regular and syllabic, the ligaturing of consonants with various allographs reduced reversals in reading.GP

Purushothama, G. (1989). Language based concepts and reading acquisition. *FJISHA*, 5 (6), 18-22. LITERACY READING DISORDERS KANNADA DYSLEXIA:

The purpose of the study was to (1) identify the demand of concepts for children to read and (2) finding concepts in which poor readers are deficient. 35 subjects of age 5+ who had been admitted to school and had no earlier experience in learning to read were selected. To list out the demand from concepts, Kannada text book of grade 1 was analyzed and all the words in the book were categorized into various concepts, including morphological constructions. The total score on the test for concepts was correlated with the academic achievement. A significant relationship was found between the certain concepts (time, verb, reference, colour, tense anamotopic words) and school achievement. Whereas no significant correlation was found between number concept and achievement in arithmetic. The study has supported the idea that concepts are important bases for the child on which he/she can build on academic learning.GP

Pustejovsky, J. (1991). Principles versus criteria: on Randall's catapult hypothesis. In J. Weissenborn, H. Goodluck, & T. Roeper (Eds), *Theoretical issues in language acquisition: Continuity and change in development*. Hillsdale, NJ: Lawrence Erlbaum Associates. ACQUISITION THEORIES UNLEARNING:

Pye, Clifton. (1990). The acquisition of ergative languages. *Linguistics*, 28(6), 1291-1330. ERGATIVE LANGUAGES:

Pye, Clifton. (1992). The acquisition of Kiche Maya. In D. I. Slobin (Ed.), *The crosslinguistic study of language acquisition (Vol. 3)*. Hillsdale, NJ: Lawrence Erlbaum Associates. QUICHE MAYAN:

Pynte, J., Girotto, V., & Baccino, T. (1991). Children's communicative abilities revisited: Verbal versus perceptual disambiguating strategies in referential communication. *Journal of Child Language*, 18, 191-213. REFERENTIAL COMMUNICATION OSTENTATION AMBIGUITY:

Q

Quasthoff, Uta M. (1983). Kindliches Erzählen: Zum Zusammenhang von erzählenden Diskursmuster und Zuhöreraktivitaten. (Children's narratives: Cohesion of narrative discourse model and hearer's actions). In D. Boueke, & W. Klein (Eds), *Untersuchungen zur Dialogfahigkeit des Kindes*. Tübingen, Germany: Gunther Narr. NARRATIVES DISCOURSE COHERENCE COMMUNICATIVE COMPETENCE: GERMAN

Quasthoff, Uta M. (1984). On the ontogenesis of doing personal reference: Syntactic, semantic, and interactional aspects. *Folia Linguistica.*, 18, 503-538. PRONOUNS-PERSONAL DEIXIS-PERSONAL SELF-CONCEPT:

Quasthoff, Uta M. (1985). Modèles de discours enfantin la représentation événementielle: savoir social ou procedure interactive? (Models of children's discourse: social knowledge or interactive procedure.). *Bulletin de Psychologie.*, 38, 759-774. DISCOURSE REPRESENTATION CHILDREN'S DISCOURSE: FRENCH

Quasthoff, Uta M. (1986). Narrative discourse pattern as a matter of perspective. In *Pragmatics and Linguistics.* Odense University Press. DISCOURSE STRUCTURE NARRATIVES:

Quasthoff, Uta M. (1987). Kommunikative Muster bei Kindern: Entwicklung oder Interaktion? (Children's communicative models: Development or interaction?). In Narr, et al. (Eds), *Spracherwerb und Mehrsprachigkeit (Language acquistion and multilingualism.).* Tübingen, Germany: Gunther Narr. DISCOURSE STRUCTURE DISCOURSE REPRESENTATION: GERMAN

Quasthoff, Uta M. (1987). Sprächliche Formen des alltaglichen Erzählens: Strukur und Entwicklung. (Grammatical forms of daily reports: Structure and development.). In Erzgaber, et al. (Eds), *Mündliches Erzählen in Alltag, fingiertes mündliches Erzählen in der Literatur*. Tübingen, Germany: Narr. NARRATIVES DISCOURSE STRUCTURE: GERMAN

Quigley, Stephen P., & Paul, Peter V. (1990). *Language and deafness*. San Diego, CA: Singular Publishing Group. ATYPICAL DEVELOPMENT DEAF CHILDREN LITERACY WRITTEN LANGUAGE LANGUAGE AND EDUCATION ASSESSMENT PROCEDURES BILINGUALISM-LANGUAGE DISORDERS L2 EDUCATION BILINGUALISM:

Definitions and historical perspectives. Cognition and language. Primary language development. Reading. Written language. Bilingualism and English as a second language. Assessment and language instruction. Conclusions.

R

Rabain-Jamin, Jacqueline, & Sabeau-Jouannet, Emilie. (1989). Playing with pronouns in French maternal speech to prelingual infants. *Journal of Child Language*, 16(2), 217-238. FRENCH PARENTAL SPEECH-STYLE PRONOUNS:

Rabinowitz, F. Michael, Howe, Mark L., & Lawrence, Joan A. (1989). Class inclusion and working memory. *Journal of Experimental Child Psychology*, 48, 379-409. CLASS INCLUSION PIAGETIAN THEORY:

Three experiments were conducted to investigate the relationship between memory and reasoning used in answering class-inclusion questions. The results reflected the need for a new conceptualization of the class-inclusion task. Performance seems to be dependent upon subjects' abilities to integrate relevant subskills, rather than on deficient reasoning or missing subskills. - From Child Development Abstracts.

Radford, Andrew. (1990). *Syntactic theory and the acquisition of English syntax: The nature of early child grammars of English*. Oxford, UK: Basil Blackwell. EARLY SYNTACTIC DEVELOPMENT LEXICAL DEVELOPMENT:

Radford draws upon an extensive corpus to demonstrate that children's early syntactic development is lexically driven.

Radford, Andrew. (1990). The syntax of nominal arguments in early child English. *Language Acquisition*, 1, 195-223. EARLY SYNTACTIC DEVELOPMENT SEMANTIC RELATIONS BOOTSTRAPPING DETERMINERS SYNTACTIC STRUCTURES NOUNS PRONOUNS PREPOSITIONS:

Radford presents an account of early syntactic development based on the assumption that syntax is bootstrapped by lexical and thematic relations which, he explains, accounts for the absence of nonthematic constituents (e.g. referential and possessive determiners, expletive pronouns, and nonthematic prepositions) in early child language.

Radford, Andrew. (1991). Comments on Roeper and de Villiers. In J. Weissenborn, H. Goodluck, & T. Roeper (Eds), *Theoretical issues in language acquisition: Continuity and change in development*. Hillsdale, NJ: Lawrence Erlbaum Associates. PARAMETER SETTING:

Rado, Maria, & Foster, Lois. (1990). The "bilingual" child as interlanguage hearer: Implications for migrant education. In M. A. K. Halliday, J. Gibbons, & H. Nicholas (Eds), *Learning, keeping and using language* . Amsterdam, The Netherlands: John Benjamins. BILINGUALISM-EDUCATION L2 EDUCATION:

Raghavendra, Parimala, & Fristoe, M. (1990). A spinach with a v on it: What 3-year-olds see in standard and enhanced Blis symbols. *Journal of Speech and Hearing Disorders*, 55, 149-159. BLISS SYMBOLS:

Raghavendra, Parimala, & Leonard, Laurence B. (1989). The acquisition of agglutinating languages: converging evidence from Tamil. *Journal of Child Language*, 16(2), 313-322. TAMIL AFFIXATION LANGUAGE TYPOLOGY:

Raine, Adrian, Hulme, Charles, Chadderton, Helen, & Bailey, Pauline. (1991). Verbal short-term memory span in speech-disordered children: Implications for articulatory coding in short-term memory. *Child Development*, 62, 415-423. LANGUAGE AND MEMORY SPEAKING RATE:

Verbal short-term memory span wass assessed using a task that did not require a verbal response in speech-disordered children and matched controls. The speech-disordered group had a lower short-term memory capacity, a smaller word length effect, and reduced speech-motor activity during rehearsal. These differences were not a function of general intellectual or motor speed differences between groups, and speech rate as a covariate abolished group differences in short-term memory. Speech rate may be a casual determinant of verbal short-term memory capacity.

Randall, Janet H. (1988). Inheritance. In W. Wilkins (Ed.), *Thematic relations*. New York, N.Y.: Academic Press. SEMANTICS AND SYNTAX ACQUISITION AND LINGUISTIC THEORY:

Randall, Janet H. (1990). Catapults and pendulums: The mechanics of language acquisition. *Linguistics*, 28(6), ACQUISITION STRATEGIES ACQUISITION THEORIES UNLEARNING:

Randall, Janet H. (1991). The catapult hypothesis: an approach to unlearning. In J. Weissenborn, H. Goodluck, & T. Roeper (Eds), *Theoretical Issues in Language Acquisition-Continuity and Change in Development*. Hillsdale, NJ: Lawrence Erlbaum Associates. ACQUISITION THEORIES UNLEARNING ACQUISITION STRATEGIES:

Rawson, M. B. (1991). Linguistics and dyslexia in language acquisition. In D. Napoli, & J. Kegl (Eds), *Bridges between psychology and linguistics - A Swarthmore festschrift for Lila Gleitman*. Hillsdale, NJ: Lawrence Erlbaum Associates. DYSLEXIA:

Read, Charles, Buder, E. H., & Kent, Raymond D. (1992). Speech analysis systems - an evaluation. *Journal of Speech and Hearing Research*, 35, 314-332. ASSESSMENT PROCEDURES METHODOLOGY-ANALYSIS:

Reed, C. M., Rabinowitz, W. M., Durlach, N. I., & Delhorne, L. A., et al. (1992). Analytic study of the Tadoma method - improving performance through the use of supplementary tactual displays. *Journal of Speech and Hearing Research*, 35, 450-465. TADOMA METHOD INTERVENTION PROGRAMS:

Réger, Zita. (1979). Bilingual Gypsy children in Hungary: explorations in 'natural' second language acquisition at an early age. *International Journal of the Sociology of Language*, 19, 59-82. BILINGUALISM L2 ACQUISITION HUNGARIAN:

Réger, Zita. (1986). A gyermeknyelvi utánzás kutatása a pszicholingvisztikában. Egy új szempont (The psycholinguistic study of imitation in child language. A new point of view). *Pszichológia*, 6, 93-134. IMITATION HUNGARIAN: HUNGARIAN

Réger, Zita. (1988). Language groups among Gypsies in Hungary and some aspects of their oral culture. In L. M. Mathuna, & N. French, et al. (Ed.), *The less widely taught languages of Europe. Proceedings of the UNESCO/AILA/IRAAL Symposium.*. Dublin: LANGUAGE AND SOCIAL CLASS HUNGARIAN VARIATION:

Rehak, Gizella, & Kovács, Emöke. (1978). Logopedical and orthodontical team work. In B. Ege (Ed.), *IALP Congress Proceedings Copenhagen, 1977, II.*. Copenhagen: Herning. ARTICULATION DISORDERS HUNGARIAN:

Reichart, A. (1986). Speech in relation to surgery in cleft palate infants. In *Report 84, Institute of Phonetic Sciences*. Amsterdam: University of Amsterdam. CLEFT PALATE:

Review of literature on method and age of lip and palate repair.

Reid, Luc. (1990). Young children's difficulty with ambiguous messages: Guessing strategy or comprehension monitoring deficiency? *Journal of Genetic Psychology*, 151, 317-328. AMBIGUITY MONITORING:

Children were assigned to an informed group (showing the inadequacy of guessing) or to a noninformed group. All children listened for 16 trials (8 with informative messages and 8 with ambiguous ones). They were asked to select the referent out of three pictures or to pick a card displaying X if the message did not enable them to distinguish the referent. Informed children were not more adequate in listening behaviors than noninformed children, and all displayed some ability in monitoring their comprehension.

Reilly, Judy Snitzer, McIntire, Marina, & Bellugi, Ursula. (1990). The acquisition of conditionals in American Sign Language: Grammaticized facial expressions. *Applied Psycholinguistics*, 11, 369-392. SIGNING-ASL CONDITIONALS DEAF CHILDREN:

The acquisition of conditional sentences in ASL by deaf children of deaf parents was examined. The results indicate that the children first acquire manual conditional signs before they use the obligatory grammaticized conditional facial expressions. The children acquire the constellation of obligatory non-manual behaviors by component, rather than holistically.

Reilly, Ronan G., & Sharkey, Noel E. (1992). *Connectionist approaches to natural language processing*. Hillsdale, NJ: Lawrence Erlbaum Associates. LANGUAGE PROCESSING CONNECTIONISM REPRESENTATIONS READING DISORDERS COMPUTER SIMULATIONS:

The papers in this comprehensive collection cover both the pros and cons of connectionist models of language processing and range over syntax, semantics, representational adequacy, speech perception and production, and reading deficits.

Reimann, Bernd. (1978). Debilitätsdiagnostik bei schwerhörigen Kindern. (Diagnosis of hard of hearing children.). *Die Sonderschule*, 23 (6), 338-340. CLASSIFICATION OF DISORDERS DEAF CHILDREN ASSESSMENT PROCEDURES: GERMAN

Reimann, Bernd. (1979). Debilität und gleichzeitige Schwerhörigkeit. (Handicap and simultaneous hearing loss.). *Die Sonderschule*, 24 (5), 311-314. DEAF CHILDREN MULTIHANDICAPPED CHILDREN: GERMAN

Reimann, Bernd. (1979). Ein Experiment zur Überprüfung von Aspekten der Begriffsbildung bei schwerhörigen Kindern. (An experiment on the testing of aspects of concept formation by hard of hearing children.). *Wissenschaftliche Zeitschrift der Humboldt-Universität Berlin, Ges.- und Sprachwissenschaftliche Reihe*, 28 (2), 27-32. DEAF CHILDREN LANGUAGE AND COGNITIVE DEVELOPMENT CONCEPT DEVELOPMENT: GERMAN

Reimann, Bernd. (1980). Differentialdiagnostik debiler schwerhöriger Kinder. (Diagnosis of hard of hearing children.). *Die Sonderschule*, 25 (1), 24-28. CLASSIFICATION OF DISORDERS ASSESSMENT PROCEDURES DEAF CHILDREN: GERMAN

Reimann, Bernd. (1981). Zur Psychophänomenologie des debilen schwerhörigen Kindes. (The psychophenomenology of hard of hearing children.). *Die Sonderschule*, 26(2), 83-91. DEAF CHILDREN: GERMAN

Reimann, Bernd. (1982). Probleme des Spracherwerbs schwerhöriger Vorschulkinder. (The problem of language acquisition for hard of hearing preschoolers.). *Die Sonderschule*, 27 (5), 283-288. DEAF CHILDREN: GERMAN

Reimann, Bernd. (1983). Eine empirische Studie zur Figurenwiedererkennung normalhörender und schwerhöriger Kinder. (An empirical study of figure recognition in normal and hard of hearing children.). *Zeitschrift für Psychologie*, 191, 33-49. DEAF CHILDREN LANGUAGE AND COGNITIVE DEVELOPMENT: GERMAN

Reimann, Bernd. (1983). Klassifizierungsleistungen normalhörender und schwerhöriger Kinder. (Categorization in normal and hard of hearing children.). *Zeitschrift für Psychologie*, 191, 182-194. DEAF CHILDREN CATEGORIZATION LANGUAGE AND COGNITIVE DEVELOPMENT: GERMAN

Reimann, Bernd. (1983). Kurzzeitige Speicherung und Strategien der Objekterkennung in Klassifizierungsprozessen bei hörgeschädigten Kindern. (The early development of object recognition strategies and representations by hearing impaired children.). *Zeitschrift für Psychologie*, 191, 410-418. LANGUAGE AND COGNITIVE DEVELOPMENT DEAF CHILDREN: GERMAN

Reimann, Bernd. (1983). Zur Kennzeichnung der Hörschädigung schwerhöriger und gehörlöser Kinder. (On the characteristics of hearing impaired, hard of hearing and deaf children.). *Die Sonderschule*, 28 (6), 333-340. DEAF CHILDREN: GERMAN

Reimann, Bernd. (1984). Kognitive Unterschiede zwischen schwerhörigen und gehörlosen Kindern. (Cognitive differences between hard-of-hearing children and deaf children.). *Die Sonderschule*, 29 (6), 344-347. DEAF CHILDREN LANGUAGE AND COGNITIVE DEVELOPMENT: GERMAN

Reimann, Bernd. (1984). Sprachliche Entwicklung schwerhöriger und gehörlöser Kinder. (Language development by hard of hearing and deaf children.). *Die Sonderschule*, 29 (3), 149-160. DEAF CHILDREN: GERMAN

Reimann, Bernd. (1985). Beziehungen zwischen Hörstatus, sprachlicher und kognitiver Entwicklung hörgeschädigter Kinder. (The relationship between hearing status, and linguistic and cognitive development in deaf children.). *Die Sonderschule*, 30 (3), 157-161. DEAF CHILDREN LANGUAGE AND COGNITIVE DEVELOPMENT: GERMAN

Reimann, Bernd. (1986). Phonetisch orientierte Interpretationen im frühen Spracherwerb des Kleinkindes. (Phonetic information intepretation in early language development by small children.). *Zeitschrift für Psychologie*, 194, 93-103. PHONOLOGICAL DEVELOPMENT PHONEMIC DEVELOPMENT FIS-PHENOMENON PHONETIC INVENTORIES: GERMAN

Reimann, Bernd. (1987). Figurenwiedererkennung und Reproduktion bei hörenden, schwerhörigen und gehörlosen Kindern: eine empirische Analyse. (Figure recognition and reproduction by hearing, hard of hearing, and deaf chidren: An empirical analysis.). *Zeitschrift für Psychologie*, 195, 209-222. DEAF CHILDREN LANGUAGE AND COGNITIVE DEVELOPMENT: GERMAN

Reimann, Bernd. (1987). Kriterien zur Differenzierung hörgeschädigter Kinder. (Criteria for differentiating hearing impaired children.). *Die Sonderschule*, 32 (5), 296-302. DEAF CHILDREN CLASSIFICATION OF DISORDERS: GERMAN

Reimann, Bernd. (1987). *Methodisches Material zur Entwicklung der sprachlichen Tätigkeit bei schwerhörigen Vorschulkindern. (Methodological material on the development of linguistic abilities in hard of hearing children.)*. Berlin: Akademie der Pädagogischen Wissenschaften. DEAF CHILDREN METHODOLOGY: GERMAN

Reimann, Bernd. (1988). Die Entwicklung des Gebrauchs temporaler Mittel in den Vorformen des Erzählens beim Kleinkind. (On the development and use of temporal terms in the "planning(?)" of stories by young children.). *Linguistische Studien/Zentralinstitut für Sprachwissenschaft, Reibe A*, 181, 69-108. TEMPORAL TERMS GERMAN NARRATIVES TEXT/STORY GRAMMARS: GERMAN

Reimann, Bernd. (1988). Die Entwicklung des Objektbegriffes 'auto' und seiner sprachlichen Benennung im Zusammenspiel von Kommunikation und Kognition. (The development of the object concept "Auto" and its use in social play for communication and cognition.). *Zeitschrift für Psychologie*, 196, 189-205. CONCEPT DEVELOPMENT LABELING LEXICAL DEVELOPMENT: GERMAN

Reimann, Bernd. (1988). Zur Bedienung, Pflege und Kontrolle individueller Hörgeräte im Bildungs- und Erziehungsprozess hörgeschädigter Kinder. (On the service, care and control of individual hearing devices in the education and rearing of hearing impaired children.). *Die Sonderschule*, 33 (1), 52-56. DEAF CHILDREN HEARING AIDS: GERMAN

Reimann, Bernd. (1989). Formen und Funktionen elterlicher Korrekturen in der frühen Kind-Eltern-Kommunikation. (Form and function of parental corrections in early child-adult communication.). *Linguistische Studien/Zentralinstitut für Sprachwissenschaft, Reibe A*, 199, 133-142. PARENTAL SPEECH-STYLE PARENTAL INPUT INPUT FACTORS ADULT-CHILD INTERACTION: GERMAN

Reimann, Bernd. (1989). Zum Entwicklungsverlauf hörgeschädigter Kinder. (On the developmental course of hearing impaired children.). *Die Sonderschule*, 34(6), 350-357. DEAF CHILDREN: GERMAN

Reimann, Bernd. (1990). Gesprachsfunktion und sprachliche Struktur reaktiver elterlicher Redebeitrage im frühen Kind-Eltern-Dialog. (Language functions and language stuctures responsive parental speech samples from free play child/parent dialogs.). *Linguistische Studien/Zentralinstitut für Sprachwissenschaft, Reibe A*, 204, 1-38. LANGUAGE FUNCTIONS PARENTAL SPEECH-STYLE ADULT CHILD INTERACTION: GERMAN

Reimann, Bernd. (1990). Pädagogisch-psychologische Diagnostik hörgeschädigter Kinder. (The educational and psychological diagnosis of hearing impaired children.). *Die Sonderschule*, 35, DEAF CHILDREN LANGUAGE AND EDUCATION: GERMAN

Reimann, Bernd, & Eichhorn, Renate. (1984). *Testsystem für hörgeschädigte Kinder. Manual mit Testmaterial. (Test for deaf children-test and manual).* Berlin: Psychodiagnostisches Zentrum. GERMAN DEAF CHILDREN ASSESSMENT PROCEDURE: GERMAN

Reimann, Bernd, & Eichhorn, Renate. (1986). Testsystem für hörgeschädigte Kinder. (Test for deaf children.). *PdZ-Informationen*, 4, 52-55. DEAF CHILDREN ASSESSMENT PROCEDURES: GERMAN

Reitsma, Pieter, & Verhoeven, Ludo Th. (1990). *Acquisition of reading in Dutch.* Dordrecht, Holland: Foris Publications. DUTCH LITERACY:

Rescorla, Leslie A. (1988). Cluster analytic identification of autistic preschoolers. *Journal of Autism and Developmental Disorders*, 18, 475-493. ASSESSMENT PROCEDURES AUTISM:

> The autistic cluster was subdivided according to presence/absence of anxiety and level of functioning. Other clusters included an emotional/behavior disorder group, with some differentiation into externalizing and internalizing clusters, and a group of relatively normal children with few symptoms. - From Child Development Abstracts.

Rescorla, Leslie A., & Schwartz, Ellen. (1990). Outcome of toddlers with specific expressive language delay. *Applied Psycholinguistics*, 11, 393-407. LANGUAGE DELAY ARTICULATION DISORDERS SYNTACTIC DISORDERS MORPHOLOGICAL DISORDERS:

> At follow-up, boys were speaking telegraphic sentences, and many had moderately severe articulation disorders with quite poor intelligibility. All spoke in sentences to some extent, and each displayed some mastery of early morphemes. Few, if any of the children spoke in completely fluent, syntactically complex, and morphologically correct language.

Reynolds, Allan G. (Ed.). (1991). *Bilingualism, multiculturalism, and second language learning. The McGill Conference in honor of Wallace E. Lambert.* Hillsdale, NJ: Lawrence Erlbaum Associates. BILINGUALISM-ATTITUDES BILINGUALISM-COGNITIVE DEVELOPMENT BILINGUALISM-EDUCATION BILINGUALISM-PROBLEMS/EFFECTS BILINGUALISM-CULTURAL FACTORS BILINGUALISM-NEUROLINGUISTICS BILINGUALISM-SEQUENTIAL ACCULTURATION IMMERSION BILINGUALISM-LANGUAGE POLICY L2 AGE INFLUENCES CRITICAL PERIOD:

A festschrift for Wallace E.Lambert which covers the social, psychological, neuropsychological, and cognitive aspects of bilingualism and second language learning, multiculturalism, and language policy and planning.

Reynolds, Allan G. (1991). The cognitive consequences of bilingualism. *ERIC/CLL News Bulletin*, 14(2), pp. 1,4,5,8. BILINGUALISM AND COGNITIVE DEVELOPMENT METHODOLOGY-DESIGN BILINGUALISM-LANGUAGE POLICY BILINGUALISM-PROBLEMS/EFFECTS METHODOLOGY-ANALYSIS:

Most studies since 1962 have shown clear superiority for bilinguals in cognitinve tasks. Unfortunately, this generally uniform pattern of results has lulled us into a state of false complacency, because the designs used have all been the pre-experimental or quasiexperimental designs, with all their attendant weaknesses. The research prior to 1962 has been repeatedly criticized as methodologically inadequate, yet we are not much better off today, even sophisticated statistical techniques like regression analysis, factor analysis, path analysis, etc., do not compensate for inherently trouble-prone designs. Due to the prevelance of design problems, faulty dependant variables, and other logical difficulties, the question we should be asking is whether the thesis that bilinguality positively affects cognitive performance should be so unequivocally embraced. At this juncture, we need a 'third wave' of research, one with sounder designs, better measures, and a more sophisticated theoretical base, before we too readily repeat the mistakes of the first four decades of research in this theoretically, personally, and politically important field.

Reznick, J. Steven. (1990). Visual preference as a test of infant word comprehension. *Applied Psycholinguistics*, 11, 145-166. LEXICAL DEVELOPMENT METHODOLOGY-DESIGN FIRST WORDS COMPREHENSION:

Describes a methodology used to determine whether or not infants had comprehended words. The methodology uses dual screen images and direction of gaze to determine comprehension. Increases in the number of words comprehended increases from 8-14 month old children to 14-20 month old children are reported from. A second experiment confirms the stability of the words comprehended by the older group.

Ribes, E. (1976). Language as behavior: Functional mediation vs. morphological grammatical language in children. In H. Reese, & L. Parrott (Ed.), *Behavioral science: Philosophical, methodological, and empirical advances*. Hillsdale: Erlbaum. ACQUISITION THEORIES LANGUAGE AND BEHAVIORISM:

Ribes, E. (1979). El desarrollo del lenguaje gramatical en niños. (The development of grammatical language in children.). *Revista Mexicana de Analisis de la Conducta*, 5, 83-112. SYNTACTIC DEVELOPMENT SPANISH: SPANISH

Ribes, E. (1985). El concepto de estimulación precoz y su relación con la investigación basica sobre adquisición de lenguaje. (The concept of early stimulation and its relation with basic research on the acquisition of language). *Revista de Logopedia y Fonoaudiología*, 5, 154-156. PRELINGUISTICS LANGUAGE PRECURSORS: SPANISH

Ribes, E. (1985). Que es desde el punto de vista psicológico el lenguaje? (What is language from a psychological point of view?). *Revista de Logopedia y Fonoaudiología*, 5, 139-144. ACQUISITION THEORIES LANGUAGE AND COGNITION: SPANISH

Ribes, E. (1990). Language as contingency-substitution behavior. In L. Hayes, & P. Chase (Eds), *Dialogues in verbal behavior*. Reno: Context Press. LANGUAGE AND COGNITION ACQUISTION THEORIES:

Ribes, E., Botero, M., Cantu, E., & Garcia, V. (1977). El uso generativo del articulo de niños prescolars y su relación con la generalización del estimulo y la respuesta. (The generative use of the article's gender in preschool children and its relation with stimulus and response generalization). In *Analisis de la Conducta: Investugación y Aplicaciónes*. Mexico: Trillas. ARTICLES GENDER LANGUAGE AND BEHAVIORISM SPANISH: SPANISH

Ribes, E., Botero, M., Cantu, E., & Garcia, V. (1977). Un estudio experimental sobre el uso generativo del numero del articulo en niños prescolares. (An experimental study of the generative use of the article's number in preschool children.). In *Analisis de la Conducta: Investigación y Aplicaciónes*. Mexico: Trillas. ARTICLES NUMBER SPANISH: SPANISH

Ribes, E., Brea, L., Solis, R., Dominguez, E., & Surarez, C. (1974). Analisis experimental del uso generativo del genero del articulo en niños prescolares (Experimental analysis of the generative use of the article's gender in preschool children.). In *Aportaciónes al analisis de la conducta: memorias del primer congreso mexicano*. Mexico: Trillas. GENDER ARTICLES SPANISH: SPANISH

Ribes, E., & Cantu, E. (1978). Efectos de la instigación en el 'uso' generativo de partículas gramáticales. (Effects of prompting in the generative 'use' of grammatical particles: Acquisition or maintenance?). *Revista Mexicana de Analisis de la Conducta*, 4, 59-66. GRAMMATICAL CATEGORIES PARTICLES SPANISH: SPANISH

Ribes, E., & Cantu, E. (1978). Efectos del reforzamamiento de respuestas fragmentarias en el 'uso' del articulo en niños prescolares. (Effects of reinforcement of fragmentary responses in the generative 'use' of the article's gender in preschool children.). *Revista Mexicana de Analisis de la Conducta.*, 4, 29-40. ARTICLES GENDER LANGUAGE AND BEHAVIORISM SPANISH: SPANISH

Ribes, E., & Cantu, E. (1986). Efectos de la instigación en el uso generativo del numero del articulo en niños prescolares (Effects of prompting in the generative use of article's number in preschool children). *Revista Mexicana de Analisis de la Conducta*, 12, 33-42. NUMBER ARTICLES SPANISH: SPANISH

Ribes, E., & Cantu, E. (1986). Efectos del reforzamiento de respuestas fragmentarias en el uso del numero articulo en niños prescolares. (Effects of reinforcement of fragmentary responses in the use of article's number in preschool children). *Revista Mexicana de Analisis de la Conducta*, 12, 43-56. NUMBER ARTICLES LANGUAGE AND BEHAVIORISM: SPANISH

Ribes, E., Galesso-Coaracy, S., & Duran, L. (1973). Effects of punishment on the accuracy of reading behavior. *Interamerican Journal of Psychology*, 7, 33-42. LITERACY LANGUAGE AND BEHAVIORISM LANGUAGE AND EDUCATION:

Ribes, E., Garcia, V., Botero, M., & Cantu, E. (1977). Generalización de los efectos del reforzamiento en el comportamiento 'sintactico' de niños prescolares. (Generalization of reinforcement effects in 'syntactic' behavior of school children). *Revista Mexicana de Analisis de la Conducta*, 3, 169-180. LANGUAGE AND BEHAVIORISM: SPANISH

Ribes, E., Gomar, S., & Rivas, L. (1975). Verbal behavior development in preschool children. In T. Thompson, & W. Dokens (Eds), *Applications of behavior modification*. New York, N.Y.: Academic Press. OVERVIEW-THEORY LANGUAGE AND BEHAVIORISM:

Ricciardelli, L. A. (1992). Bilingualism and cognitive development in relation to threshold theory. *Journal of Psycholinguistic Research*, 21, 301-316. BILINGUALISM-COGNITIVE DEVELOPMENT:

Ricciardi, P. W., Voelker, S., Carter, R. A., & Shore, D. L. (1991). K-ABC sequential simultaneous processing and language-impaired preschoolers. *Developmental Neuropsychology*, 7, 523-535. ASSESSMENT PROCEDURES KAUFMAN ASSESSMENT BATTERY FOR CHILDREN:

Ricciuti, Anne E., & Scarr, Sandra. (1990). Interaction of early biological and family risk factors in predicting cognitive development. *Journal of Applied Developmental Psychology*, 11, 1-12. AT-RISK CHILDREN COGNITIVE DEVELOPMENT:

The effects of early biological risks and factors of the home environment on cognitive development was examined. In addition to main effects, the interaction effects of low birth weight and social risks associated with father absence increased the likelihood of cognitive impairment at two.

Ricco, Robert B. (1989). Operational thought and the acquisition of taxonomic relations involving figurative dissimilarity. *Developmental Psychology*, 25, 996-1003. CATEGORIZATION PIAGETIAN THEORY:

Age- and grade-equivalent preoperational and concrete operational groups were given oddity, sort and category membership tasks with pictorial stimuli. Concrete operational subjects showed a greater appreciation for taxonomic relations involving atypical exemplars. Subjects of both levels could appreciate taxonomic relations involving strictly typical or moderately typical exemplars. - From Child Development Abstracts.

Rice, Mabel L. (1991). Children with specific language impairment: toward a model of teachability. In N. A. Krasnegor, et al. (Eds), *Biological and behavioral determinants of language development.* Hillsdale, NJ: Lawrence Erlbaum Associates. TEACHABILITY SPECIFIC LANGUAGE IMPAIRMENT INTERVENTION PROGRAMS:

Rice, Mabel L., Buhr, J. C., & Nemeth, M. (1990). Fast mapping word-learning abilities of language-delayed preschoolers. *Journal of Speech and Hearing Disorders*, 55, 33-42. FAST MAPPING LEXICAL DEVELOPMENT LANGUAGE DELAY:

Rice, Mabel L., Buhr, J. C., & Oetting, J. B. (1992). Specific-language-impaired children's quick incidental learning of words - the effect of a pause. *Journal of Speech and Hearing Research*, 35, 1040-1048. FAST MAPPING SPECIFIC LANGUAGE IMPAIRMENT:

Rice, Mabel L., Sell, M. A., & Hadley, P. A. (1991). Social interactions of speech-impaired and language-impaired children. *Journal of Speech and Hearing Research*, 34, 1299-1307. LANGUAGE DISORDERS SOCIAL SPEECH SOCIAL INTERACTION:

Rice, Mabel L., & Wartella, E. (1981). Television as a medium of communication: Implications for how to regard the child viewer. *Journal of Broadcasting*, 25, 365-372. TELEVISION AND LANGUAGE DEVELOPMENT:

Richard, Richard J., & Snow, Catherine E. (1990). Language use in and out of context. *Journal of Applied Developmental Psychology*, 11, 251-266. CONTEXT COMMUNICATIVE COMPETENCE:

Elementary school children were asked to describe a picture in English under two different instructional conditions assessing judgement to the absence of an interactive interlocutor and to the absence of shared background knowledge with the audience. The native speakers showed greater ability to produce clear and unambiguous messages under more difficult instructional conditions.

Richards, Brian J. (1987). The role of imitation. *Cahiers de l'Institut de Linguistique de Louvain*, 12.3-4, 154-174. IMITATION:

Richards, Brian J. (1988). 'Not wee-wee had he?': Individual differences and the development of tag questions in two and three-year-olds. In G. Collis, A. Lewis, & V. Lewis (Eds), *Proceedings of the 1988 Child Language Seminar.* Warwick, UK: University of Warwick. QUESTIONS-TAGS:

Accounts of children learning tag questions have concentrated on the extension of processing capacity and syntactic knowledge which enable the child to realize previously acquired linguistic functions in a more sophisticated manner. A continuity is frequently assumed from the early stereotypical 'huh?' and 'okay?' to tags containing appropriate verb forms. In the research described here, contrasting styles of development in seven children are identified which are only partially compatible with the outline given above. A consideration of the possible meanings and functions of tags and their relationships with intonation and polarity also leads to a more critical view of the assumption of continuity. Results show that some children develop a repertoire of partially analyzed tags at a remarkably early stage. In some cases specific auxiliary forms are present in tag questions before they have been sampled elsewhere. On the other hand, one child's development is unequivocally analytic and hierarchical. Mastery of the required syntactic transformations is followed by the emergence of tags which gradually increased in complexity. It also becomes evident that mastering the necessary syntax, processing utterances of greater length and complexity than Matrix + Tag, and hearing frequent exemplars is not sufficient for tags to develop. Children have to learn the function of tags in conversation and the circumstances in which they can be uttered felicitously. BJR.

Richards, Brian J. (1990). Access to the agenda: some observations on language development research and its relevance for the practicioner. *Australian Journal of Remedial Education*, 22 (3), 16-20. LANGUAGE AND EDUCATION ADULT-CHILD INTERACTION INPUT FACTORS:

Summary of literature on input and facilatation for teachers.BJR

Richards, Brian J. (1990). Environmental predictors of copula verb development. In M. Forrester, L. Smith, & B. Shire (Eds), *Proceedings of the 1990 Child Language Seminar*. Canterbury: University of Kent. AUXILIARIES COPULA QUESTIONS-YES/NO QUESTIONS-TAGS:

A recurring result from correlational studies which relate the frequency of input variables to rate of language development, is the link between auxiliary verb growth and Yes/No questions (Y/Ns) addressed to children. Explanations for this relationship usually concentrate on the advantages of hearing stressed and non-contracted auxiliary forms in sentence- initial position over heariing unstressed, contracted form in medial position in declaratives. If such accounts are correct, then it can be predicted that Y/Ns which place the copula in initial position will also accelerate the rate of growth of children's copula verb development. This prediction is tested using a sample of 33 children, carefully matched for stages of language development at 1:9 and 2:0 years, whose rate of copula verb growth is measured over the following 9 months. Analyses include an examination of the contribution of sub-categories of Y/Ns, tag questions, and utterances containing sentence-final copulas to the growth of contracted and full copulas. Results confirm that the frequency of inverted copulas in Y/Ns predicts children's copula development, but the overall pattern of correlations obtained is too complex to interpret in terms of a direct causal model.BJR

Richards, Brian J. (1990). *Language development and individual variation: A study of auxiliary verb learning*. New York, NY: Cambridge University Press. INDIVIDUAL VARIATION AUXILIARIES VERBS METHODOLOGY-ANALYSIS:

This study examines the variation between children in their early language development and focusses on their acquisition of the auxiliary verb. Children acquire auxiliaries at different ages and stages of development, and display differences in the rate, style, and sequence of subsequent development. Some developmental differences are related to a tendency to acquire the auxiliary holistically, and others to the quality of interaction with the child's partners in conversation. This book examines some of the syntactic and pragmatic causes of those variations, and addresses methodological issues concerning unanalyzable usage, and real syntactic advance. The book also examines inconsistencies in previous studies of auxiliaries and attempts to resolve them. BJR.

Richards, Brian J. (1991). Investigating relationships between maternal input and rate of children's language development - a reanalysis of Yoder. *Journal of Speech and Hearing Research*, 34, 347-350. PARENTAL INPUT PARENTAL SPEECH INPUT FACTORS DEVELOPMENTAL RATE:

Ricks, D. (1979). Making sense of experience to make sensible sounds. In M. Bullowa (Ed.), *Before speech*. New York, NY: Cambridge University Press. PHONOLOGICAL DEVELOPMENT INFANT PERCEPTION SPEECH PERCEPTION PHONEMIC DEVELOPMENT:

Riddoch, Jane M. (1992). *Neglect and the peripheral dyslexias*. Hillsdale, NJ: Lawrence Erlbaum Associates. DYSLEXIA READING DISORDERS:

A special issue of *Cognitive Neuropsychology* which focuses on peripheral reading disorders caused by functional deficits. Includes neglect dyslexia, letter-by-letter reading and other peripheral reading disorders.

Rieben, Laurence. (1989). Individual differences in word recognition acquisition: A path from an interactive model of reading to an interactive instructional setting. *European Journal of Psychology of Education*, 4, 329-347. LITERACY LANGUAGE AND EDUCATION:

Five first graders were observed four times in an instructional setting where they had to search for words in a reference text. Five different types of searching strategies were inferred: context-oriented, code-oriented, unmediated, copying, passive. Results show a great inter- and intra- individual variability in the use of the different types of strategies. In particular, there are different patterns of occurrence of the code-oriented and context-oriented strategies (simultaneous versus alternate). - From Child Development Abstracts.

Riley, Nancy J. (1989). Piagetian cognitive functioning in students with learning disabilities. *Journal of Learning Disabilities*, 22, 444-451. INVENTORY OF PIAGET'S DEVELOPMENTAL TASKS ASSESSMENT PROCEDURES PIAGETIAN THEORY:

Cognitive abilities as measured by the Inventory of Piaget's Developmental Tasks (IPDT) of male and female fourth and fifth graders with learning disabilities was investigated. A two-way analysis of covariance revealed a significant mean difference in cognitive ability between students with learning disabilities and nondisabled students. - From Child Development Abstracts.

Rintelmann, William F. (1991). *Hearing assessment: 2nd edition*. San Diego, CA: Singular Publishing Group. AUDIOMETRY:

Pure tone audiometry: air and bone conduction. Speech audiometry. Clinical masking. Tumpanometry: basic principles and clinical applications. Acoustic-reflex measurements. Auditory evoked potentials: basic aspects. Auditory evoked responses in site-of-lesion assessment. Auditory evoked potentials in clinical pediatrics. Hearing loss in newborns, infants, and young children. Audiologic assessment of the elderly. Behavioral assessment of the central auditory nervous system. Pseudohypacusis. Classic site-of-lesion tests: foundation of diagnostic audiology. Making clinical decisions. Vestibular system assessment. Instrument calibration.

Ripich, Danielle Newberry, & Spinelli, Francesca M. (1991). *School discourse problems*. San Diego, CA: Singular Group. LANGUAGE AND EDUCATION DISCOURSE DISORDERS RETARDED CHILDREN ASSESSMENT PROCEDURES:

Text covers discourse development and problems in children ranging from pre-schoolers to school-age and older children, and also the problems of special populations in school.

Risholm-Mothander, Pia. (1989). Predictions of developmental patterns during infancy: assessments of children 0-1 years. *Scandinavian Journal of Psychology*, 30(3), 161-167. ASSESSMENT PROCEDURES DEVELOPMENT SCALES:

From Stockholm Bibliographies.

Rispoli, Matthew. (1989). Encounters with Japanese verbs: caregiver sentences and the categorization of transitive and intransitive action verbs. *First Language*, 9(1(25)), 57-80. JAPANESE VERBS-TRANSITIVE VERBS-INTRANSITIVE PARENTAL SPEECH-VERBS:

Rispoli, Matthew. (1991). The mosaic acquisition of grammatical relations. *Journal of Child Language*, 18, 517-551. GRAMMATICAL RELATIONS:

Rispoli, Matthew. (1992). Discourse and the acquisition of 'eat'. *Journal of Child Language*, 19, 581-595. CHILDREN'S DISCOURSE SEMANTIC MAPPING LEXICAL DEVELOPMENT:

Rittenhouse, R. K., & Dancer, J. E. (1992). Educational and legislative issues in students with hearing loss - interdisciplinary considerations. *Volta Review*, 94, 9-17. LANGUAGE AND EDUCATION DEAF CHILDREN:

Rittenhouse, R. K., & Kenyon, P. L. (1991). Conservation and metaphor acquisition in hearing-impaired children-some relationships with communication mode, hearing acuity, schooling, and age. *American Annals of the Deaf*, 136 , 313-320. LANGUAGE AND COGNITIVE DEVELOPMENT FIGURATIVE LANGUAGE DEAF CHILDREN:

Ritter-Brinton, K., & Stewart, D. (1992). Hearing parents and deaf children: Some perspectives on sign communication and service delivery. *American Annals of the Deaf*, 137, 85-91. DEAF CHILDREN SIGNING PARENTAL SPEECH:

Roberts, Jacqueline M. A. (1989). Echolalia and comprehension in autistic children. *Journal of Autism and Developmental Disorders*, 19, 271-281. AUTISM ECHOLALIA COMPREHENSION DISORDERS:

> Those children with poor receptive language skills produced significantly more echolalic utterances than those children whose receptive skills were more age-appropriate. Children who produced fewer echolalic utterances, and had more advanced receptive language ability, evidenced a higher proportion of mitigated echolilia.

Roberts, Joanne E., Burchinal, Margaret R., Davis, B. P., & Collier, A. M., et al. (1991). Otitis media in early childhood and later language. *Journal of Speech and Hearing Research*, 34, 1158-1168. OTITIS MEDIA:

Roberts, Joanne E., Rabinowitch, Shoshanna, Bryant, Donna M., Burchinal, Margaret R., Koch, Matthew A., & Ramey, Craig T. (1989). Language skills of children with different preschool experiences. *Journal of Speech and Hearing Research*, 32(4), 773-786. INPUT FACTORS:

Robin, Donald A., & Eliason, Michele J. (1991). Speech and prosodic problems in children with neurofibromatosis. In C. Moore, K. M. Yorkston, & D. R. Beukelman (Eds), *Dysarthria and apraxia of speech*. Baltimore, MD: Paul H. Brookes. PROSODIC DISORDERS:

Robin, Donald A., Somodi, Lori B., & Luschei, Erich S. (1991). Measurment of tongue strength and endurance in normal and articulation disordered subjects. In C. Moore, K. M. Yorkston, & D. R. Beukelman (Eds), *Dysarthria and apraxia of speech*. Baltimore, MD: Paul H. Brookes. ARTICULATORY DISORDERS ARTICULATION:

Robinson, E. J., & Mitchell, P. (1992). Children's interpretation of messages from a speaker with a false belief. *Child Development*, 63, 639-652. CHILDREN'S DISCOURSE CHILDREN'S JUDGMENTS COMMUNICATIVE COMPETENCE:

Roca, Iggy M. (1990). *Logical issues in language acquisition*. Dordrecht, The Netherlands: Foris Publications. ACQUISITION THEORIES ACQUISITION AND LINGUISTIC THEORY:

Rodda, M., Cumming, C., & Fewer, D. (1992). Memory, learning and language: Implications for deaf education. In M. Marschark, & M. D. Clark (Eds), *Psychological perspectives on deafness*. Hillsdale, NJ: Lawrence Erlbaum Associates. DEAF CHILDREN LANGUAGE AND MEMORY LANGUAGE AND EDUCATION:

Rodrigue, James R., Morgan, Sam B., & Geffken, Gary R. (1991). A comparative evaluation of adaptive behavior in children and adolescents with autism, Down syndrome, and normal development. *Journal of Autism and Developmental Disorders* , 21, 187-196. DOWN SYNDROME AUTISM SOCIAL SPEECH:

Roeper, Thomas, & de Villiers, Jill. G. (1991). Ordered parameters in the acquisition of wh-questions. In J. Weissenborn, H. Goodluck, & T. Roeper (Eds), *Theoretical issues in language acquisition: Continuity and change in development*. Hillsdale, NJ: Lawrence Erlbaum Associates. QUESTIONS-WH PARAMETER SETTING:

Roeper, Thomas, & Weissenborn, Jürgen. (1990). How to make parameters work. In Frazier, & de Villiers, *Language acquisition and processing*. Dordrecht: Kluwer PARAMETER SETTING:

Roitblat, Herbert L., Harley, H. E., & Helweg, D. A. (1993). Cognitive processing in artifical language research. In L. M. Herman, H. L. Roitblat, & P. E. Nachtigall (Eds), *Language and communication: Comparative perspectives*. Hillsdale, NJ: Lawrence Erlbaum Associates. COMPUTER SIMULATIONS LANGUAGE PROCESSING:

Roitblat, Herbert L., Herman, Louis M., & Nachtigall, Paul E. (1993). *Language and communication: Comparative perspectives*. Hillsdale, NJ: Lawrence Erlbaum Associates. LANGUAGE AND OTHER PRIMATES ANIMAL COMMUNICATIONS COMPUTER SIMULATIONS:

Rollins, P., Pan, Barbara A., & Snow, Catherine E. (1991). A brief tutorial. In B. MacWhinney (Ed.), *The CHILDES project: Computational tools for analyzing talk*. Hillsdale, NJ: Lawrence Erlbaum Associates. METHODOLOGY-ANALYSIS CHILDES METHODOLOGY-TRANSCRIPTION METHODOLOGY-COMPUTERS:

Romaine, Suzanne. (1989). The role of children in linguistic change. In L. E. Breivik, & E. H. Jahr (EdS), *Language change: Contributions to the study of its causes*. Berlin, Germany: Mouton-De Gruyter. LANGUAGE CHANGE ACQUISITION AND LINGUISTIC THEORY SOCIOCULTURAL FACTORS:

Romski, Mary Ann, & Sevcik, Rose A. (1991). Patterns of language learning by instruction: evidence from non-speaking persons with mental retardations. In N. A. Krasnegor, et al. (EdS), *Biological and behavioral determinants of language development*. Hillsdale, NJ: Lawrence Erlbaum Associates. RETARDED CHILDREN INTERVENTION PROGRAMS:

Rondal, Jean A. (1973). L'intervention du langage intérieur dans la régulation du comportement moteur et son controle électromyographique. (The intervention of inner speech in the regulation of motor activities and its electromyographic control.). *Revue de Psychologie et des Sciences de l'Éducation*, 8, 491-501. REGULATIVE FUNCTION OF SPEECH LANGUAGE AND COGNITION VYGOTSKYAN THEORY PIAGETIAN THEORY LANGUAGE AND COGNITIVE DEVELOPMENT INNER SPEECH: FRENCH

Rondal, Jean A. (1973). Le rôle régulateur du langage chez l'enfant. (The regulatory role of language for infants.). *Journal de Psychologie Normale et Pathologique*, 3, 307-324. REGULATIVE FUNCTION OF SPEECH LANGUAGE AND COGNITION VYGOTSKYAN THEORY PIAGETIAN THEORY LANGUAGE AND COGNITIVE DEVELOPMENT INNER SPEECH: FRENCH

Rondal, Jean A. (1974). Human intelligence: heritability and malleability. *Psychologica Belgica*, 14, 149-160. HERITABILITY NATIVISM:

Rondal, Jean A. (1974). *The role of speech in the regulation of behavior*. Minneapolis, MN: University of Minnesota, Research and Development Center in Education of Handicapped Children, U.S. Office of Education, Department of Health, Education, and Welfare. REGULATIVE FUNCTION OF SPEECH LANGUAGE AND COGNITION VYGOTSKYAN THEORY PIAGETIAN THEORY LANGUAGE AND COGNITIVE DEVELOPMENT INNER SPEECH:

Rondal, Jean A. (1975). Controle de la latence des réponses dans certaines tâches motrices avec et sans accompagnement verbal. (Control of the response latency in certain motor tasks with and without verbal accompaniment.). *Revue Belge de Psychologie et de Pédagogie*, 37, 29-42. LANGUAGE AND COGNITION VYGOTSKYAN THEORY REGULATIVE FUNCTION OF SPEECH PIAGETIAN THEORY: FRENCH

Rondal, Jean A. (1975). Deaf children: language development and education. *Psychologica Belgica*, 15, 63-74. DEAF CHILDREN LANGUAGE AND EDUCATION:

Rondal, Jean A. (1975). Développement du langage et retard mental. (Language development and mental retardation.). *Liason*, 15, 83-95. RETARDED CHILDREN LANGUAGE AND COGNITIVE DEVELOPMENT LANGUAGE AND COGNITION: FRENCH

Rondal, Jean A. (1975). Développement du langage et retard mental: une revue critique de la littérature en langage anglaise. (Language development and mental retardation: A critical revue of the English language literature.). *L'Année Psychologique*, 75, 513-547. RETARDED CHILDREN LANGUAGE AND COGNITIVE DEVELOPMENT: FRENCH

Rondal, Jean A. (1975). Langage, classe sociale et instruction: une revue sommaire des travaux de B. Bernstein. (Language, social class and education: A review of the work of B. Bernstein). *Revue Française de Pedagogie*, 30, 81-86. LANGUAGE AND SOCIAL CLASS EDUCABILITY: FRENCH

Rondal, Jean A. (1976). *Maternal speech to normal and Down's syndrome children matched for mean length of utterance.* Minneapolis, MN: University of Minnesota, Research and Development Center in Education of Handicapped Children, U.S. Office of Education, Department of Health, Education and Welfare. DOWN SYNDROME PARENTAL INPUT PARENTAL SPEECH:

Rondal, Jean A. (1976). Tests and nontests in psychology in general, and in language assessment in particular: some reflections. *Scientia Paedagogica Experimentalis*, 13, 68-85. ASSESSMENT PROCEDURES METHODOLOGY-ANALYSIS:

Rondal, Jean A. (1977). Aperçu sur le développement du langage envisage sous l'aspect des interactions entre éducateurs et enfants. (Considerations on the development of language gained from interactions between teachers and children.). *Revue Belge de Psychologie et de Pédagogie*, 38, 89-100. LANGUAGE AND EDUCATION INPUT FACTORS: FRENCH

Rondal, Jean A. (1977). *Developmental Sentence Scoring applied to language-learning normal and Down's syndrome children matched for mean length of utterance.* Reston, Virginia: The ERIC Clearinghouse on Handicapped and Gifted Children (The Council for Exceptional Children). ASSESSMENT PROCEDURES DOWN SYNDROME SYNTACTIC STRUCTURES SYNTACTIC DEVELOPMENT:

Rondal, Jean A. (1977). Développement du langage et retard mental: une revue des études ayant utilisé l'Illinois Test of Psycholinguistic Abilities. (The development of language and mental retardation: A revue of studies utilising the ITPA.). *Psychologica Belgica*, 17, 24-34. ILLINOIS TEST OF PSYCHOLINGUISTIC ABILITIES RETARDED CHILDREN: FRENCH

Rondal, Jean A. (1977). Environnement linguistique maternel et retard mental. (Maternal linguistic environment and mental retardation.). *Enfance*, 1, 37-48. PARENTAL SPEECH PARENTAL INPUT RETARDED CHILDREN: FRENCH

Rondal, Jean A. (1977). L'emploi de l'adjectif et de l'article devant le nom des parties du corps dans l'expression de la possession intrinsèque en français: une étude génétique. (Using the adjective and the article before the names of body parts in the expression of intrinsic possesion in French: A developmental study.). *Psychologica Belgica*, 17, 165-181. WORD ORDER FRENCH POSSESSIVES SYNTACTIC STRUCTURES: FRENCH

Rondal, Jean A. (1977). Le développement du langage chez les retards mentaux: retard de développement ou deficit spécifique?. (The development of language by the mentally retarded: delayed development or specific deficit.). In M. Spoelders (Ed.), *Pedagogische Psycholinguistiek*. Gand: Presses de l'Universite de Gand. RETARDED CHILDREN LANGUAGE AND COGNITIVE DEVELOPMENT: FRENCH

Rondal, Jean A. (1977). Maternal speech in normal and Down's syndrome children. In *From research to practice in mental retardation. Proceedings of the 4th Congress of International Association for the Scientific Study of Mental Deficiency.* Baltimore, Maryland: University Park Press. DOWN SYNDROME PARENTAL SPEECH:

Rondal, Jean A. (1978). Developmental Sentence Scoring Procedure and the delay-difference question in language development of Down's syndrome children. *Mental Retardation*, 16, 169-171. ASSESSMENT PROCEDURES DOWN SYNDROME SYNTACTIC STRUCTURES SYNTACTIC DEVELOPMENT:

Rondal, Jean A. (1978). Early language intervention in severely and moderately mentally retarded children. In A. Fink (Ed.), *International perspectives on future special education (First World Congress on Future Special Education, Stirling Scotland, 1978).* Reston, Virginia: The Council for Exceptional Children. RETARDED CHILDREN INTERVENTION PROGRAMS:

Rondal, Jean A. (1978). *Langage et éducation. (Language and education.).* Bruxelles: Dessart et Mardaga. LANGUAGE AND EDUCATION: FRENCH

Rondal, Jean A. (1978). Language delay and language difference in moderately and severely retarded children. In L. Sandals (Ed.), *Proceedings of the Third National Congress*. Winnipeg, Manitoba: The Canadian Council for Exceptional Children. RETARDED CHILDREN:

Rondal, Jean A. (1978). Le développement linguistique des handicapes mentaux est-il simplement retarde ou proprement deficitaire? Une première revue de données avec référence particuliere a la litterature de langue anglaise. (The development of language by the mentally handicapped, is it simply delay or properly a deficit? A first revue of the data with specific reference to the English language literature.). *Journal de Psychologie Normale et Pathologique*, 3, 347-368. RETARDED CHILDREN LANGUAGE AND COGNITIVE DEVELOPMENT: FRENCH

Rondal, Jean A. (1978). Linguistique, psycholinguistique et enseignement de la langue. (Linguistics, psycholinguistics, and the teaching of language.). *L'École Belge*, 5, 257-261. LANGUAGE AND EDUCATION: FRENCH

Rondal, Jean A. (1978). Maternal speech to normal and Down's syndrome children matched for mean length of utterance. In C. Meyers (Ed.), *Quality of Life in Severely and Profoundly Mentally Retarded People: Research Foundations for Improvement.* Washington, DC: American Association on Mental Deficiency. DOWN SYNDROME PARENTAL INPUT ADULT-CHILD INTERACTION INTERSUBJECTIVITY:

Rondal, Jean A. (1978). Maternal speech to normal and Down's syndrome children matched for mean length of utterance. *Down's Syndrome*, 1 (3), 6-7. DOWN SYNDROME PARENTAL SPEECH PARENTAL INPUT:

Rondal, Jean A. (1979). 'Maman est au courant:' une étude des connaissances maternelles quant aux aspects formels du langage du jeune enfant. (Maman are you current: A study of maternal understanding about the formal aspects of young children's language). *Enfance*, 2, 95-105. PARENTAL INPUT FINE TUNING HYPOTHESIS SOCIAL INTERACTION: FRENCH

Rondal, Jean A. (1979). La parole et le langage des mongoliens. (The speech and language of Down syndrome children.). In J. Lambert, & J. Rondal (Eds), *Le mongolisme*. Bruxelles: Mardaga. DOWN SYNDROME: FRENCH

Rondal, Jean A. (1979). Langage paternal et langage maternal dans l'acquisition d'un premier langage. (Paternal and maternal language in first language acquisition). In *Actes du Congres International de Psychologie de l'Enfant*. Paris: PARENTAL SPEECH:

Rondal, Jean A. (1979). Le développement et le fonctionnement cognitif des mongoliens. (Development and the cognitive function of Down sydnrome children.). In J. Lambert, & J. Rondal (Eds), *Le mongolisme*. Bruxelles: Mardaga. DOWN SYNDROME: FRENCH

Rondal, Jean A. (1979). *Votre enfant apprend a parler. (Your child learns to speak.)*. Bruxelles: Mardaga. INTERVENTION PROGRAMS FOR PARENTS OVERVIEW-THEORY: FRENCH

Rondal, Jean A. (1980). Cuestiónes de psicolingüistica y pedagogía de la lenqua. Communicatión presentada en el 'Seminario sobre psicolingüistica'. (Questions about psycholinguistics and language education: Paper presented at the Seminar about Psycholinguistics). *Annuario de Psicológica*, 23, 87-101. LANGUAGE AND EDUCATION: SPANISH

Rondal, Jean A. (1980). The interactive point of view in language development, disorders, and intervention. *Psychologica Belgica*, 20, 185-204. INTERVENTION PROGRAMS SOCIAL INTERACTION HYPOTHESIS SOCIAL INTERACTION:

Rondal, Jean A. (1980). Langage et arrièration mentale: recherches récentes et perspectives. (Language and mental retardation: perspectives and recent research.). *Le Langage et l'Homme*, 42, 3-11. RETARDED CHILDREN LANGUAGE AND COGNITION LANGUAGE AND COGNITIVE DEVELOPMENT: FRENCH

Rondal, Jean A. (1980). Langage paternal et langage maternal dans l'acquisition d'un premier langage. (Paternal and maternal language in first language acquisition). *Enfance*, numero special 4/5, PARENTAL SPEECH PARENTAL INPUT: FRENCH

Rondal, Jean A. (1980). Language development in moderately and severely mentally retarded children: delay, difference, or both? *Special Education in Canada*, 54 (2), 27-32. RETARDED CHILDREN:

Rondal, Jean A. (1980). *Lengaje y educación. (Language and education).* Barcelona: Medica y Technica. LANGUAGE AND EDUCATION: SPANISH

Rondal, Jean A. (1980). Une note sur la théorie cognitive-motivationnelle d'Edward Zigler en matière de retard mental culturel-familial. (A note on the cognitive- motivational theory of Edward Zigler on the matter of cultural-familial mental retardation.). *Psychologica Beligica*, 20, 61-82. RETARDED CHILDREN: FRENCH

Rondal, Jean A. (1981). Comment favoriser le développement de la communication et du langage chez l'enfant exceptionnel par le savoir psycholonguistique et l'application des principes de la psychologie de l'apprentissage? (How to facilitate the development of communication and language by exceptional children through psycholinguistic knowledge and the application of the principles of the psychology of learning?). *Rééducation Orthophonique*, 19, 401-411. LANGUAGE AND EDUCATION INTERVENTION PROGRAMS ATYPICAL CHILDREN: FRENCH

Rondal, Jean A. (1981). La adquisición del lenguaje en sujetos deficientes mentales moderados y heveros. (The acquisition of language in severely and moderately retarded subjects.). *Annuario de Psicológica*, 25, 75-90. RETARDED CHILDREN LANGUAGE AND COGNITIVE DEVELOPMENT: SPANISH

Rondal, Jean A. (1981). Langage et arriération mentale: 'the state of the art.' (Language and mental retardation: 'the state of the art'. In J. A. Rondal, J. Lambert, & H. Chipman (Eds), *Psycholinguistique et handicap mental: Recherches récentes et perspectives*. Bruxelles: Mardaga. RETARDED CHILDREN: FRENCH

Rondal, Jean A. (1981). Langage et handicap socio-culturel: recherches et perspectives. (Language and socio-cultural handicap: researchs and perspectives.). *Le Langage et l'Homme*, 46, 14-25. LANGUAGE AND SOCIAL CLASS: FRENCH

Rondal, Jean A. (1981). Language acquisition in Down's syndrome children: recent studies and problems. In *The Conference on Special Education, Helsinki 1980*. Helsinki: The Finnish Association for Special Education. DOWN SYNDROME LANGUAGE AND COGNITION LANGUAGE AND COGNITIVE DEVELOPMENT:

Rondal, Jean A. (1981). Le point de vue behavioriste en psychologie et en psychologie de l'enfant. (The behaviorist point of view in psychology and in child psychology). In J. Rondal, & M. Hurtig (Eds), *Manual de psychologie de l'enfant* (vol. 1,). Bruxelles: Mardaga. LANGUAGE AND BEHAVIORISM: FRENCH

Rondal, Jean A. (1981). *Psycholinguistique et handicap mental: recherches et perspectives. (Psycholinguistics and mental handicap: research and perspectives.):*. Bruxelles: Mardaga. RETARDED CHILDREN LANGUAGE AND COGNITIVE DEVELOPMENT: FRENCH

Rondal, Jean A. (1981). *Recherches actuelles en psychologie appliquée de langage: les handicapes mentaux modérés et sévères. (Present research in applied psycholinguistics: Moderate and severe mental handicaps.).* Bruxelles: Cercle d'Études, de Diffusion et d'Échanges Rélatifs à l'Enseignement Spécial. RETARDED CHILDREN: FRENCH

Rondal, Jean A. (1981). Spontaneous imitations in Down's syndrome children language development. In P. Mittler (Ed.), *Frontiers of knowledge in mental retardation II: Social, educational and behavioral aspects*. Baltimore, MD: University Park Press. IMITATION DOWN SYNDROME:

Rondal, Jean A. (1982). À propos de l'article 'Difficultes dans la communication mère-enfant et troubles du langage chez les enfants avec retard mental'. (Apropos the article 'Difficulties of mother-child communication and language problems with retarded children' by G. Levi et B. Zollinger. *Enfance*, 3, 211-215. RETARDED CHILDREN PARENTAL SPEECH: FRENCH

Rondal, Jean A. (1982). *El desarollo del lenguaje. (The development of language.).* Barcelona: Medica y Technica. ACQUISITION THEORIES: SPANISH

Rondal, Jean A. (1982). *El mongolísmo.* Barcelona: Herder. DOWN SYNDROME: SPANISH

Rondal, Jean A. (1982). L'acquisition du langage chez les sujets handicapes mentaux modérés et sévères. (The acquisition of language in severely and moderately retarded subjects.). *Revue d'Orientation Scolaire et Professionnelle*, 31, 15-28. RETARDED CHILDREN LANGUAGE AND COGNITIVE DEVELOPMENT: FRENCH

Rondal, Jean A. (1982). Une étude longitudinal des répétitions spontanées dans l'acquisition du langage. (A longitudinal study of spontaneous repetitions in the acquisition of language.). *Le Langage et l'Homme*, 50, 12-24. IMITATION FRENCH: FRENCH

Rondal, Jean A. (1983). El conductísmo social y determinantes interpersonales en el aprendizaje del lenguaje. (Social behaviorism, interpersonal determinants of language acquisition and implications for language intervention.). *Revista de Logopedia y Fonoaudiología*, 3, 13-24. SOCIAL INTERACTION HYPOTHESIS LANGUAGE AND BEHAVIORISM: SPANISH

Rondal, Jean A. (1983). L'acquisizione del linguaggio negli handicappati medi e gravi. (The acquisition of language by severely and moderately mentally retarded subjects.). In *Atti II Congresso Italiano di Logopedia: Communicazione e insufficienza mentale.* Montecatini: Associazione Nazionale Logopedisti. RETARDED CHILDREN LANGUAGE AND COGNITIVE DEVELOPMENT: ITALIAN

Rondal, Jean A. (1983). *L'interaction adulte-enfant et la construction du langage. (Adult-child interaction and the construction of language.)*. Bruxelles: Mardaga. PARENTAL INPUT SOCIAL INTERACTION HYPOTHESIS ADULT-CHILD INTERACTION: FRENCH

Rondal, Jean A. (1983). Langage et déficience mentale: données récentes et perspectives. (Language and mental deficiency: Recent works and perspectives.). *Bulletin d'Audiophonologie*, 16, 603-622. RETARDED CHILDREN LANGUAGE AND COGNITION: FRENCH

Rondal, Jean A. (1983). Language development in Down's syndrome individuals: a systematic and componential approach. In *Proceedings de la Conference on Down's Syndrome.* Madrid: Instituto Internacional Para La Investigacion Y Asesoramiento Sobre La Defiencia Mental. DOWN SYNDROME LANGUAGE AND COGNITIVE DEVELOPMENT:

Rondal, Jean A. (1983). Lenguaje y deficiencia mental: datos recientes y perspectivas. (Language and mental deficiency : recent works and perspectives.). *Revista de Logopedia y Fonoaudiología*, 3, 67-77. RETARDED CHILDREN LANGUAGE AND COGNITIVE DEVELOPMENT: SPANISH

Rondal, Jean A. (1983). Les aspects educatifs langagiers de l'arrieration mentale. (The educational and linguistic aspects of mental retardation.). In *L'Enfant Handicape Mental* . Bruxelles: Presses de L'Universite Libre de Bruxelles. LANGUAGE AND EDUCATION RETARDED CHILDREN LANGUAGE AND COGNITIVE DEVELOPMENT:

Rondal, Jean A. (1983). Quel rôle peut jouer l'imitation verbale dans l'acquisition du langage par l'enfant? (What is the role played by verbal imitation in children's language acquisition?). *Rééducation Orthophonique*, 21, 393-407. IMITATION: FRENCH

Special edition: 'Langage, Fonctionnement Cognitif et Personnalite, I. Psychologie du Langage et Psycholinguistique' (Language, cognitive functions and personality: I. Psychology of language and psycholinguistics).

Rondal, Jean A. (1983). Social behaviorism and the interpersonal determinants of language acquisition. *Social Behaviorism*, 4, 27-31. LANGUAGE AND BEHAVIORISM SOCIAL INTERACTION HYPOTHESIS:

Rondal, Jean A. (1984). Bilingualism and mental handicap: some programmatic views. *Neurolinguistics*, 13, 135-139. RETARDED CHILDREN BILINGUALISM-LANGUAGE DISORDERS LANGUAGE AND COGNITIVE DEVELOPMENT:

Rondal, Jean A. (1984). Commentary on C. Kierman's the development of communication of cognition. In J. Dobbing, A. Clarke, J. Corbett, J. Hogg, & R. Robinson (Eds), *Scientific studies in mental retardation*. Londress: The Royal Society of Medicine and The MacMillan Press. LANGUAGE AND COGNITIVE DEVELOPMENT RETARDED CHILDREN:

Rondal, Jean A. (1984). Développement de la communication et du langage chez l'enfant handicape mental avec référence a l'intérvention précoce. (Development of communication and language by children with mental handicaps with reference to early intervention.). In *Actes du colloque: Aspects de la déficience mentale chez l'enfant* (vol. 42,). RETARDED CHILDREN INTERVENTION PROGRAMS LANGUAGE AND COGNITIVE DEVELOPMENT: FRENCH

Rondal, Jean A. (1984). El papel del entorno en la adquisición del lenguaje en el niño. (The role of the "entorno" in children's language acquisition. *Revista de Logopedia y Fonoaudiología*, 4, ACQUISITION THEORIES: SPANISH

Rondal, Jean A. (1984). Le rôle de l'entourage dans l'acquisition du langage par l'enfant. (The role of the caregivers in the acquisition of language by children.). *Revue Belge de Psychologie et de Pédagogie*, 46, 71-80. SOCIAL INTERACTION HYPOTHESIS PARENTAL INPUT INPUT FACTORS: FRENCH

Rondal, Jean A. (1984). Les déterminants intérpersonnels de l'acquisition du langage chez l'enfant. (The interpersonal determinants of language acquisition by children.). In P. Ferrand (Ed.), *Communiquer demain: données actuelles et perspectives*. Nancy: Unadrio. SOCIAL INTERACTION HYPOTHESIS: FRENCH

Rondal, Jean A. (1984). Linguistic and prelinguistic development in moderate and severe mental retardation. In J. Dobbing, A. Clarke, J. Corbett, J. Hogg, & R. Robinson (Eds), *Scientific studies in mental retardation*. London: The Royal Society of Medicine and The Macmillan Press. RETARDED CHILDREN PRELINGUISTICS LANGUAGE AND COGNITIVE DEVELOPMENT:

Rondal, Jean A. (1984). Vers une théorie environnementaliste-cognitiviste de l'acquisition du langage. (Towards an environmentalist-cognitivist theory of language acquisition.). *Revue de Laryngologie*, 105, 363-368. ACQUISITION THEORIES: FRENCH

Rondal, Jean A. (1985). *Adult-child interaction and the process of language acquisition*. New York, NY: Praeger Press. SOCIAL INTERACTION HYPOTHESIS PARENTAL INPUT ADULT-CHILD INTERACTION:

Rondal, Jean A. (1985). Bilingualism and mental handicap: some perspective views. In Y. Lebrun, & M. Paradis (Eds), *Early bilingualism and child development*. Amsterdam: Swets and Zeitlinger. BILINGUALISM-COGNITIVE DEVELOPMENT RETARDED CHILDREN LANGUAGE AND COGNITIVE DEVELOPMENT:

Rondal, Jean A. (1985). Comme favoire lo sviluppo della communicazione e del linguaggio nel bambino handicappato. (How to facilitate the development of communication and language by handicapped children.). *HD, Giornale Italiano di Psicologia e Pedagogia dell Handicap e della Disabileta di Apprendimento*, 8, 4-8. RETARDED CHILDREN INTERVENTION PROGRAMS LANGUAGE AND COGNITIVE DEVELOPMENT: ITALIAN

Rondal, Jean A. (1985). *Langage et communication chez les handicapes mentaux: théorie, évaluation et intérvention. (Language and communication by the mentally handicapped: theory, evaluation and intervention.)*. Bruxelles: Mardaga. INTERVENTION PROGRAMS ASSESSMENT PROCEDURES RETARDED CHILDREN LANGUAGE AND COGNITIVE DEVELOPMENT: FRENCH

Rondal, Jean A. (1985). Langage et communication chez les jeunes enfants trisomiques 21. État des connaissances, stratégies et perspectives en matière d'intérvention. (Language and communication in young children with trisomia 21. State of the art, strategies and perspectives on intervention matters.). In J. Rondal, & J. Detraux (Ed.), *Recherche et intérvention dans les troubles et difficultés du langage.* TRISOMIA LANGUAGE DISORDERS COMMUNICATIVE DISORDERS RETARDED CHILDREN LANGUAGE AND COGNITIVE DEVELOPMENT: FRENCH

Rondal, Jean A. (1985). Le rôle de l'environnement dans la construction du langage. (The role of the environment in the construction of language.). In *Le développement du langage chez l'enfant. La Médicine Infantile.* Paris: Maloine. SOCIAL INTERACTION ENVIRONMENTAL INFLUENCES LANGUAGE AND BEHAVIORISM: FRENCH

Rondal, Jean A. (1985). Logopédie contemporaine. (Contemporary logopedics.). *Les Dossiers de l'Orthophoniste*, 47, LANGUAGE AND EDUCATION: FRENCH

Rondal, Jean A. (1985). Perspectivas en logopedia. *Revista de Logopedia y Fonoaudiología*, 4, 132-138. LANGUAGE AND EDUCATION: SPANISH

Rondal, Jean A. (1986). Approche de la méthodologie de la recherche en psycholinguistique développementale. (Approaches to research methodology in developmental psycholingistics.). *Glossa*, 3, 4-23. METHODOLOGY: FRENCH

Rondal, Jean A. (1986). Contexte pragmatique et développement du langage. Une note sur les positions théoriques récentes de J. Bruner.. (Pragmatic context and the development of language. A note on the recent theoretical position of J. Bruner.). *Langage et pragmatique*, 24, 151-161. SOCIAL INTERACTION HYPOTHESIS PRAGMATIC DEVELOPMENT: FRENCH

Rondal, Jean A. (1986). Langage et communication chez les jeunes enfants trisomiques 21. État des connaissances, stratégies et perspectives en matière d'intérvention. (Language and communication in young children trisomic 21. State of the knowledge, strategies and perspectives on matters of intervention.). *Questions de Logopedie*, 9 (1), 51-85. LANGUAGE DISORDERS DOWN SYNDROME TRISOMIA INTERVENTION PROGRAMS RETARDED CHILDREN LANGUAGE AND COGNITIVE DEVELOPMENT: FRENCH

Rondal, Jean A. (1986). *Le développement du langage chez l'enfant trisomique 21. (Language development in children with trisomic 21.).* Bruxelles: Mardaga. DOWN SYNDROME TRISOMIA LANGUAGE AND COGNITIVE DEVELOPMENT: FRENCH

Rondal, Jean A. (1986). Le rôle de l'entourage dans l'acquisition du langage chez l'enfant. (The role of the caregivers in the acquisiiton of language by children.). *Glossa*, 2, 18-25. SOCIAL INTERACTION HYPOTHESIS INPUT FACTORS PARENTAL INPUT ENVIRONMENTAL INFLUENCES: FRENCH

Rondal, Jean A. (1986). Lenguaje y communicicación en los niños pequeños trisomicos 21. Situación de los conocimientos, estrategias y perspectivas sobre la intervención (en homenaja a Jorge Perello). (Language and communication in young children "trisomicos 21". State of the knowledge, strategies and perspectives on matters of intervention.). *Revista de Logopedia y Fonoaudiología*, 6 (2), 52-66. LANGUAGE DISORDERS DOWN SYNDROME TRISOMIA INTERVENTION PROGRAMS RETARDED CHILDREN LANGUAGE AND COGNITIVE DEVELOPMENT: SPANISH

Rondal, Jean A. (1986). Psicólingüistica y pratica logopedica. (Psycholinguistics and logopedic practice. In M. Monfort (Ed.), *Investigación y logopedua (III Simposio de Logopedia, Madrid).* Madrid: Ciencías de la Educación Prescolar y Especial. LANGUAGE AND EDUCATION: SPANISH

Rondal, Jean A. (1987). *Aide et intérvention précoce à domicile. La méthode psycho-éducative développée par l'APEM. (Aid and early home intervention: The psycho-educational method developed by APEN.).* Heusy-Verviers: APEM. INTERVENTION PROGRAMS DOWN SYNDROME: FRENCH

Rondal, Jean A. (1987). Bilingüalisma y retraso mental. *Revista de Logopedie, Foniatra y Audiologia*, 4, 224-241. LANGUAGE AND COGNITIVE DEVELOPMENT BILINGUALISM-COGNITIVE DEVELOPMENT RETARDED CHILDREN: SPANISH

Rondal, Jean A. (1987). *L'apprentissage du langage et de la communication. Guide pratique et manuel d'intérvent dans les cas de troubles et de difficultés développementales. (Learning language and communication. A practical guide and an intervention manual for cases of trouble and developmental difficulty.).* Paris: UNESCO. ACQUISITION THEORIES INTERVENTION PROGRAMS REFERENCE MANUAL: FRENCH

Rondal, Jean A. (1987). La surdité profonde dans ses aspects psycholinguistiques et éducatifs: quelques réflexions et suggestions. (The profoundly deaf: psycholinguistic and educational aspects - some reflections and suggestions.). *Questions de Logopédie*, 14, 91-104. DEAF CHILDREN LANGUAGE AND EDUCATION: FRENCH

Rondal, Jean A. (1987). Language development and mental retardation. In W. Yule, & M. Rutter (Eds), *Language development and disorders*. Oxford, Philadelphia: Blackwell, Lippencott. RETARDED CHILDREN LANGUAGE AND COGNITIVE DEVELOPMENT:

Rondal, Jean A. (1987). Les interactions adulte-enfant et la construction du langage. (Adult-child interaction and the construction of language.). *Apprendizagem/Disenvolvimento*, 2(7), 96-100. ADULT-CHILD INTERACTION SOCIAL INTERACTION HYPOTHESIS PARENTAL INPUT: FRENCH

Rondal, Jean A. (1987). Les retards de langage: premiers indices et rééducation. (Language delays: first indications and intervention.). *Glossa*, 4, 28-35. LANGUAGE DELAY INTERVENTION PROGRAMS ASSESSMENT PROCEDURES: FRENCH

Rondal, Jean A. (1987). Los retrasos del lenguaje: primeros indiciós y reeducatión. (Language delay: primary indicators and intervention.). In J. R. Aparicio (Ed.), *Actos del XIV Congreso Naciónal de la A.E.L.F.A.*. Madrid: Cepe. LANGUAGE DISORDERS ASSESSMENT PROCEDURES LANGUAGE DELAY: SPANISH

Rondal, Jean A. (1987). Psycholinguistique et pédagogie du langage: un dialogue encore a construire. (Psycholinguistics and language education: A dialogue under construction.). *Mother-Tongue Teaching*, 2, 14-21. LANGUAGE AND EDUCATION: FRENCH

Rondal, Jean A. (1987). Sections on absence of language, language delays, language deficiencies and deficits. In *Encyclopedia of special education* . Baltimore, MD: University Park Press. LANGUAGE AND EDUCATION LANGUAGE DISORDERS LANGUAGE DELAY:

Rondal, Jean A. (1987). Stratégies d'enseignement parentales et apprentissage du langage par le jeune enfant. (Strategies of parental teaching and the learning of language by young children.). *Les grands courants de recherche sur le langage enfantin*, 13, 103-134. PARENTAL INPUT INPUT FACTORS: FRENCH

Rondal, Jean A. (1988). Accuisizione e strutturazione del linguaggio degli handicappati mentali. Il caso della Trisomia 21. (Acquisition and structure of language by mentally handicapped children ; The case of "trisomia 21".). In C. Cornoldi, & R. Vianello (Eds), *Handicap, comunicazione e linguaggio*. Bergamo: Juvenilia. DOWN SYNDROME TRISOMIA LANGUAGE AND COGNITIVE DEVELOPMENT RETARDED CHILDREN: ITALIAN

Rondal, Jean A. (1988). Come favorise lo sviluppo del linguaggio nel bambino eccezionale. (Faciliatating the development of language in exceptional children.). In R. Cocchi, C. Belacchi, & P. Cercolani (Eds), *Risultati di 8 anni terapia farmacologica nella Sindrome di Down*. Pesaro: Gisstimmai. DOWN SYNDROME INTERVENTION PROGRAMS ATYPICAL DEVELOPMENT: ITALIAN

Rondal, Jean A. (1988). Down's syndrome. In K. Mogford, & D. Bishop (Eds), *Language development in exceptional circumstances*. London, UK: Churchill Livingstone. DOWN SYNDROME:

Rondal, Jean A. (1988). Estrategias de los padres y apprendizaje del lenguaje en los niños. (Paternal strategies and the learning of language by children.). *Revista de Logopedia y Fonoaudiología*, 8, 11-22. PARENTAL SPEECH-SEX DIFFERENCES PARENTAL INPUT INPUT FACTORS: SPANISH

Rondal, Jean A. (1988). Indications positives et negatives dans l'acquisition des aspects grammaticaux de la langue maternelle. (Positive and negative indicators in first language grammatical acquisition.). *European Bulletin of Cognitive Psychology*, 8, 383-398. SYNTACTIC DEVELOPMENT ASSESSMENT PROCEDURES AT-RISK CHILDREN: FRENCH

Rondal, Jean A. (1988). Language development in Down's syndrome: a life-span perspective. *International Journal of Behavioral Development*, 11, 21-36. DOWN SYNDROME LANGUAGE AND COGNITIVE DEVELOPMENT:

Rondal, Jean A. (1988). Parent-child interaction and the process of language acquisition in severe mental retardation: beyond the obvious. In K. Marfo (Ed.), *Parent-Child interaction and developmental disabilities*. New York, NY: Praeger Press. ADULT-CHILD INTERACTION RETARDED CHILDREN PARENTAL INPUT SOCIAL INTERACTION HYPOTHESIS:

Rondal, Jean A. (1988). Psycholinguistique et pédagogie de la langue maternelle: un dialogue encore à construire. (Psycholinguistics and education in the mother tongue: A dialogue still to be built). *Éducation*, 213, 21-28. LANGUAGE AND EDUCATION: FRENCH

Rondal, Jean A. (1988). Tests et non-tests en psychologie en general et dans l'évaluation du langage en particulier: quelques réflexions. (Traduit de l'anglais par J.P. Broonen). (Tests and nontests in psychology in general, and in language assessment in particular: some reflections.). *Questions de Logopédie*, 15, 37-59. ASSESSMENT PROCEDURES METHODOLOGY: FRENCH

Special edition on assessment procedures in language development.

Rondal, Jean A. (1989). *L'interazione adulto-bambino e la costruzione del linguaggio. (Adult-child interaction and the construction of language.)*. Roma: Armando Editore. SOCIAL INTERACTION HYPOTHESIS PARENTAL INPUT ADULT-CHILD INTERACTION: ITALIAN

Rondal, Jean A. (1989). *Language development in the mentally handicapped*. London, UK: Cole & Whurr. RETARDED CHILDREN LANGUAGE AND COGNITIVE DEVELOPMENT:

Rondal, Jean A. (1989). Le langage de l'enfant handicape. (Language and the handicapped child.). *Glossa*. ATYPICAL CHILDREN RETARDED CHILDREN DEAF CHILDREN APHASIAS AUTISM: FRENCH

Special editions of *Glossa*, Part 1 published in 1989, Part 2 published in 1990.

Rondal, Jean A. (1989). *Réflexions sur l'intérvention précoce. Les parents comme partenaires. (Reflections on early intervention: Parents as partners.).* Lille: URAPEI. INTERVENTION PROGRAMS FOR PARENTS: FRENCH

Rondal, Jean A. (1990). Aide et intérvention précoce auprès des enfants et de leur famille avec attention particuliere au problème de la communication et du langage. (Aid and early intervention for children and families with particular attention to problems of communication and language.). In J. Pourtois (Ed.), *Les thématiques de l'éducation familiale*. Bruxelles: Mardaga. INTERVENTION PROGRAMS: FRENCH

Rondal, Jean A. (1990). Conditions, potentialites et limites de l'integration scolaire pour les déficients mentaux. (Conditions, potentials, and limits of the educational integration of the mentally handicapped.). *Le Journal de l'APEM*, 25, 4-20. LANGUAGE AND EDUCATION RETARDED CHILDREN: FRENCH

Rondal, Jean A. (1990). *Guida all' educazione dei bambini Down. (Guide to the education of Down syndrome children.).* Roma: Armando Editore. DOWN SYNDROME LANGUAGE AND EDUCATION LANGUAGE AND COGNITIVE DEVELOPMENT: ITALIAN

Rondal, Jean A. (1990). L'autonomia relativa del linguaggio come systema cognitiva. (The relative autonomy of language within the cognitive system.). *Studi di Psicologia dell' Educazione*, -, LANGUAGE AND COGNITIVE DEVELOPMENT MODULARITY: ITALIAN

Rondal, Jean A. (1990). Language and communication in mental handicap: Semiology of problems and questions of rehabilitation. In O. Schindler (Ed.), *Stato dell'arte in foniatria e logopedia*. Torino: Editrice Omega. INTERVENTION PROGRAMS RETARDED CHILDREN LANGUAGE AND COGNITIVE DEVELOPMENT:

Rondal, Jean A. (1990). Language in Down's syndrome: a life-span and modularity perspective. *Italian Journal of Applied Linguistics.* DOWN SYNDROME LANGUAGE AND COGNITIVE DEVELOPMENT: ITALIAN

Rondal, Jean A. (1990). Le langage de l'enfant trisomique 21 et l'intérvention langagière précoce. (Language and children with trisomia 21 and early language intervention.). In M. Lysens, & J. Rondal (Eds), *Actes du Premier Congrès Européen sur le Syndrome de Down.* Verviers (Heusy): APEM. RETARDED CHILDREN DOWN SYNDROME INTERVENTION PROGRAMS TRISOMIA: FRENCH

Rondal, Jean A. (1990). Lenguaje y comunicación en niños deficientes mentales. (Language and communication in mentally retarded children.). *Revista Galega de Psicópedagoxia.* RETARDED CHILDREN LANGUAGE AND COGNITIVE DEVELOPMENT: SPANISH

Rondal, Jean A. (1990). Perspectives sur le langage dans la trisomie 21. (Perspective on language in trisomia 21.). *European Down Syndrome Association Newsletter*, 1, 5-7. DOWN SYNDROME TRISOMIA LANGUAGE AND COGNITIVE DEVELOPMENT: FRENCH

Rondal, Jean A. (Ed.). (1990). *Principes d'une intérvention psycho-éducative en matière de langage. Actes du Colloque International de Lyon sur la Trisomie 21. (Principles of psycho-educational intervention in matters of language.).* London: MacGraw-Hill. INTERVENTION PROGRAMS DOWN SYNDROME: FRENCH

Rondal, Jean A. (1990). Production en Bliss chez l'infirme moteur cerebral: structuration semantique et syntaxique, et dependance vis-a-vis du dispotif tabulaire. (Productions in Bliss by subjects with cerebral motor problems: Semantic and syntactic structure and dependence...). *Enfance*, 7. LANGUAGE AND MOTOR DEVELOPMENT BLISS SYMBOLS CEREBRAL DISORDERS:

Rondal, Jean A. (1990). Recherches en psycholinguistique développementale (Research on psycholinguistic development.). *Glossa.* OVERVIEW-PSYCHOLINGUISTICS ACQUISITION THEORIES: FRENCH

A special edition.

Rondal, Jean A. (1990). Social behaviorism, interpersonal determinants of language acquisition and implications for language intervention. In G. Eifert, & I. Evans (Eds), *Unifying behavior therapy: Contributions of paradigmatic behaviorism*. New York, NY: Springer. LANGUAGE AND BEHAVIORISM SOCIAL INTERACTION HYPOTHESIS INTERVENTION PROGRAMS:

Rondal, Jean A. (1993). Exceptional cases of language development in mental retardation: The realtive autonomy of language as a cognitive system. In H. Tager-Flusberg (Ed.), *Constraints on language acquisition: Studies of atypical children*. Hillsdale, NJ: Lawrence Erlbaum Associates. ATYPICAL DEVELOPMENT RETARDED CHILDREN MODULARITY LANGUAGE AND COGNITIVE DEVELOPMENT:

Rondal, Jean A., Adrao, M., & Neves, S. (1980). Classe sociale, langage, et instruction: la compréhension du langage de l'école maternelle et élémentaire inférieure. (Social class, language and instruction: The comprehension of language in the "grade school".). *Les Sciences de l'Éducation pour l'Ère Nouvelle*, Oct-Nov-Dec., 245-264. LANGUAGE AND SOCIAL CLASS EDUCABILITY LANGUAGE AND EDUCATION: FRENCH

Rondal, Jean A., Adrao, M., & Neves, S. (1981). Classe sociale, langage, et instruction: la compréhension du langage de l'enseignant par l'enfant au niveau maternel et élémentaire inférieur. (Social class, language, and instruction: The comprehension of the language of education by "kindergarteners and grade schoolers".). In G. Gagné, & M. Page (Eds), *Études sur la langue des jeunes quebecois (1969-1979)*. Montreal: Les Presses de l'Universite de Montreal. FRENCH LANGUAGE AND EDUCATION LANGUAGE AND SOCIAL CLASS EDUCABILITY: FRENCH

Rondal, Jean A., Adrao, M., Neves, S., & Dalle, E. (1982). La compréhension du langage de l'enseignant par l'enfant au niveau de l'école maternelle et élémentaire inférieure dans des milieux scolaires contrastés selon la composition sociale. (The comprehension of the language of education by grade schoolers in the environment of schools contrasted according to social composition.). *Revue Française de Pedagogie*, 58, 29-35. LANGUAGE AND EDUCATION LANGUAGE AND SOCIAL CLASS: FRENCH

Rondal, Jean A., Bachelet, Jean-Francois, Carter, M., Ghiotto, Martine, Haidon, M., & Warland, M. (1988). Parametres de variation lexicale en Langue Belge des Signes (Francophonie). (Lexical variation in Signed Belgian French.). *Psychologica Belgica*, 28, 67-75. SIGNING VARIATION NONSTANDARD DIALECTS: FRENCH

Rondal, Jean A., Bachelet, Jean-Francois, Monteirin, C. Granna, Le Docte, A. M., Perée, F., & Stafilas, E. (1985). Transcripción, segmentación y informatización de un corpus de lenguaje. (Transcription, segmentation, and information from a language corpus). *Revista de Logopedia y Fonoaudiología*, 5, 39-50. METHODOLOGY-TRANSCRIPTION METHODOLOGY-ANALYSIS: SPANISH

Rondal, Jean A., Bachelet, Jean-Francois, & Perée, F. (1985). Analyse du langage et des interactions verbales adulte-enfant. (The analysis of language and verbal interactions between adults and children.). *Bulletin d'Audiophonologie*, 5 (6), 507-535. METHODOLOGY-ANALYSIS ADULT-CHILD INTERACTION SOCIAL INTERACTION HYPOTHESIS: FRENCH

Rondal, Jean A., & Bredart, Serge. (1982). Langage oral: aspects développementaux. (Oral language: developmental aspects.). In J. Rondal, & X. Seron (Eds), *Troubles du langage: Diagnostic et rééducation*. Bruxelles: Mardaga. OVERVIEW-THEORY: FRENCH

Rondal, Jean A., Bredart, Serge, Stafilas, E., Grana, C., Ghiotto, Martine, Perée, F., Giakis, A., André, A., & Antwerpen, S. Van. (1982). Bilinguisme et réussite scolaire chez les enfants d'immigrés espagnols de la région liègeoise. (Bilingualism and educational success in immigrant Spanish children in the Liège region.). *Psychologica Belgica*, 22, 121-142. BILINGUALISM-EDUCATION SPANISH-FRENCH FRENCH-SPANISH L2 EDUCATION LANGUAGE AND EDUCATION: FRENCH

Rondal, Jean A., & Brusset, B. (1981). Problèmes méthodologiques en psychologie de l'enfant.. (Methodological problems in child psychology.). In J. Rondal, & M. Hurtig (Eds), *Manuel de psychologie de l'enfant*, vol. 1. Bruxelles: Mardaga. METHODOLOGY: FRENCH

Rondal, Jean A., & Cession, A. (1988). Intelligence artificielle et psycholinguistique. (Artifical intelligence and psycholinguistics). *Journal de Réflexion sur l'Informatique*, 9, 33-35. COMPUTER SIMULATIONS CONNECTIONISM: FRENCH

Rondal, Jean A., & Cession, A. (1988). Prime manisfestation e sviluppo del linguaggio nella Trisomia 21. (The intial manifestation and development of language in "trisomia 21".). *Risposte*, 11, 19-34. DOWN SYNDROME LANGUAGE AND COGNITIVE DEVELOPMENT TRISOMIA ASSESSMENT PROCEDURES: ITALIAN

Rondal, Jean A., & Defays, D. (1978). Reliability of mean length of utterance as a function of sample size in early language development. *Journal of Genetic Psychology*, 133, 305-306. MEAN LENGTH OF UTTERANCE METHODOLOGY-ANALYSIS:

Rondal, Jean A., & Detraux, J. J. (1986). Recherche et intérvention dans les troubles et difficultés de développement du langage. (Compte rendu du symposium de Liège, 1985). (Research and intervention in troubles and difficulties with language development.). *Questions de Logopédie*, 9, INTERVENTION PROGRAMS LANGUAGE DISORDERS: FRENCH

Rondal, Jean A., Detraux, J. J., & Mercier, M. (1987). Systèmes de communication alternatifs et augumentés: (Compte rendu du symposium international de Liège, 1986) (Augmented and alternative systems of communication.). *Glossa*, 6, INTERVENTION PROGRAMS SIGNING BLISS SYMBOLS: FRENCH

Special editions : Part 1 in *Glossa* (6) and Part 2 in *Glossa* (9).

Rondal, Jean A., & Hamers, J. (1981). Le point de vue de la psychologie sociale. (The point of view of social psychology.). In J. Rondal, & M. Hurtig (Eds), *Manuel de psychologie de l'enfant* (vol. 1,). Bruxelles: Mardega. SOCIAL INTERACTION HYPOTHESIS: FRENCH

Rondal, Jean A., Hamers, J., & Seron, Xavier. (1981). Communication et langage. (Communication and language.). In J. Rondal, & M. Hurtig (Eds), *Manuel de psychologie de l'enfant,* vol. 2. Bruxelles: Mardage. OVERVIEW-THEORY: FRENCH

Rondal, Jean A., Henrot, F., & Charlier, M. (1986). *Le langage des signes: aspects psychologiques, psycholinguistiques et psycho-educatifs. (Sign language: psychological, psycholinguistic, and psycho- educational aspects.)*. Bruxelles: Mardaga. SIGNING: FRENCH

Rondal, Jean A., & Hoffmeister, R. (1975). Pour un apprentissage gestuel par les retardes mentaux: une proposition. (For a gestural apprenticeship for the mentally retarded: a proposition.). *Revue Belge de Psychologie et de Pédagogie*, 37, 51-60. RETARDED CHILDREN SIGNING INTERVENTION PROGRAMS: FRENCH

Rondal, Jean A., & Hoffmeister, R. (1976). Sign language as an alternative language system for the mentally retarded. *Philippine Journal of Mental Health*, 7(2), 57-62. RETARDED CHILDREN SIGNING INTERVENTION PROGRAMS:

Rondal, Jean A., & Lambert, J. L. (1975). A double failure to replicate O'Connor and Hermelin's experimental results in a discriminative learning with reversal in the case of moderately mentally retarded children. *Journal of Genetic Psychology*, 126, 157-158. RETARDED CHILDREN:

Rondal, Jean A., & Lambert, J. L. (1981). L'acquisition du langage chez les déficients mentaux: le problème delai-différence et le développement linguistique avancé. Actes du colloque 'Langage et acquisition du langage'. (Language acquisition by the mentally retarded: The delay-difference problem and advanced linguistic development. Acts of the Colloquium "Language and language acquisition"). *Revue de Phonétique Appliquée*, 57, 93-97. RETARDED CHILDREN LANGUAGE AND COGNITIVE DEVELOPMENT: FRENCH

Rondal, Jean A., & Lambert, J. L. (1982). *Language acquisition by the mentally retarded: the problem of delay - difference and advanced linguistic develompent*. New York, NY: Plenum Press. RETARDED CHILDREN LANGUAGE AND COGNITIVE DEVELOPMENT:

Rondal, Jean A., & Lambert, J. L. (1982). *Questions et réponses sur le mongolisme. (Questions and answers on Down syndrome.)*. Quebec et Paris: Les Éditions La Liberté et Maloine. DOWN SYNDROME: FRENCH

Rondal, Jean A., Lambert, J. L., Chipman, Harold H., & Pastouriaux, F. (1982). Arrièration mentale. (Mental retardation.). In J. Rondal, & X. Seron (Eds), *Troubles du langage: Diagnostic et rééducation*. Bruxelles: Mardaga. RETARDED CHILDREN: FRENCH

Rondal, Jean A., Lambert, J. L., & Sohier, C. (1980). L'imitation verbale et non-verbale chez l'enfant retarde mental mongolien et non-mongolien. (Verbal and non-verbal imitation by Down syndrome children and non-Down syndrome retarded children.). *Enfance*, 3, 107-122. RETARDED CHILDREN DOWN SYNDROME IMITATION: FRENCH

Rondal, Jean A., Leyens, N., Bredart, Serge, & Perée, F. (1983). Factors influencing assignment of anaphoric pronoun coreference in children and adults. In *Proceedings of the Annual Child Language Seminar*. Glasgow: University of Strathclyde. ANAPHORA PRONOUNS:

Rondal, Jean A., Leyens, N., Bredart, Serge, & Perée, F. (1984). Coréférence et stratégie des fonctions parallèles dans le cas des pronoms anaphoriques ambigus. (Coreference and the parallel functions strategy in the case of ambiguous anaphoric pronouns.). *Cahiers de Psychologie Cognitive*, 4 (2), 151-170. ANAPHORA PRONOUNS AMBIGUITY: FRENCH

Rondal, Jean A., Leyens, N., Bredart, Serge, & Perée, F. (1984). Factors influencing assignment of anaphoric pronoun coreference in children and adults. *First Language*, 4, 154. ANAPHORA PRONOUNS:

Rondal, Jean A., & Neves, S. (1979). Quand 'mon papa' est 'ton papa.' Une note sur le développement des adjectifs possessifs. (Why 'my papa' is 'your papa'. A note on the development of possessive adjectives). *Le Langage et l'Homme*, Octobre, 37-46. ADJECTIVES POSSESSIVES WORD CLASS PRONOUNS-POSSESSIVE: FRENCH

Rondal, Jean A., Perée, F., Thorens, J., & Bachelet, Jean-Francois. (1987). *ALGELO: un programme d'analyse lexico-grammaticale d'échantillons de langage par micro-ordinateur (logiciel et manuel d'utilisation). (Algelo, a microcomputer package for the lexico-grammatical analyis of language samples.).* Paris: Unadrio. METHODOLOGY-COMPUTERS METHODOLOGY-ANALYSIS: FRENCH

Rondal, Jean A., & Rodriguez-Sprindall, C. (1985). Hacía una teoría cognitivo-ambientalista de la adquisición del lenguaje. (Towards an environmentalist-cognitivist theory of language acquisition.). *Revista Mexicana de Analisis de la Conducta*, 11 (1 & 2), 55-68. ACQUISITION THEORIES: SPANISH

Rondal, Jean A., & Rondal, R. (1975). *Bibliography on language and speech in relation to mental retardation: 1900-1975.* Reston, Virginia: Resources in Education, The ERIC Clearinghouse on Handicapped and Gifted Children. BIBLIOGRAPHY LANGUAGE AND COGNITION LANGUAGE AND COGNITIVE DEVELOPMENT RETARDED CHILDREN:

Rondal, Jean A., & Rondal, R. (1975). Speech and Language: bibliography on speech and language in mental retardation 1900-1975. (Part I). *Philippine Journal of Mental Health*, 6(2), 39-62. BIBLIOGRAPHY RETARDED CHILDREN LANGUAGE AND COGNITIVE DEVELOPMENT:

Rondal, Jean A., & Rondal, R. (1975). Speech and Language: bibliography on speech and language in mental retardation 1900-1975. (Part II). *Philippine Journal of Mental Health*, 7(1), 51-64. BIBLIOGRAPHY RETARDED CHILDREN LANGUAGE AND COGNITIVE DEVELOPMENT:

Rondal, Jean A., & Seron, Xavier (Ed.). (1982). *Troubles du langage: diagnostic et rééducation. (Language disorders: diagnosis and intervention.), vol..* Bruxelles: Mardaga. ASSESSMENT PROCEDURES INTERVENTION PROGRAMS: FRENCH

Rondal, Jean A., & Seron, Xavier. (1988). *Trastornos del lenguaje. (Language disorders.).* Barcelona: Paidos. LANGUAGE DISORDERS: SPANISH

Rondal, Jean A., Seron, Xavier, & Lambert, J. L. (1982). Problématique du trouble, évaluation du langage et apport de la psycholinguistique. (A troublesome problem, psycholinguistics and the evaluation of language.). In J. Rondal, & X. Seron (Ed.), *Troubles du langage: Diagnostic et rééducation*. Bruxelles: Mardaga. ASSESSMENT PROCEDURES METHODOLOGY: FRENCH

Rondal, Jean A., & Staats, Arthur W. (1985). Paradigm integration versus substitution in psycholinguistics. *International Newsletter of Paradigmatic Psychology*, 1, 23-26. LANGUAGE AND BEHAVIORISM ACQUISITION THEORIES:

Rondal, Jean A., & Thibaut, J. P. (1987). *Problèmes de psycholinguistique. (Psycholinguistic problems.)*. Bruxelles: Mardaga. OVERVIEW-PSYCHOLINGUISTICS METHODOLOGY: FRENCH

Rondal, Jean A., & Thibaut, J. P. (1990). Facteurs de transitivité semantique dans la compréhension des énonces déclaratifs chez l'enfant. (Factors of semantic transitivity in the comprehensoin of declarative utterances by children.). *Glossa*. TRANSITIVITY COMPREHENSION COMPLEX SENTENCES: FRENCH

Rondal, Jean A., Thibaut, J. P., & Cession, A. (1990). Transitivity effects of children's sentence comprehension. *European Bulletin of Cognitive Psychology (Cahiers de Psychologie Cognitive)*, 10 (4), 385-400. TRANSITIVITY COMPREHENSION COMPLEX SENTENCES:

Rondal, Jean A., Thibaut, J. P., Cession, A., Bredart, Serge, & Kaens, A. M. (1988). Semantic and syntactic factors in the comprehension of passives. In F. van Besien (Ed.), *First Language Acquisition*. Gand: Association Belge de Linguistique Appliquee. PASSIVES SEMANTICS AND SYNTAX CUES-SYNTACTIC CUES-SEMANTIC:

Rondal, Jean A., & Turnure, James E. (1976). *Maternal interaction related to linguistic development in normal and Down's syndrome children*. Reston, Virginia: The ERIC Clearinghouse on Handicapped and Gifted Children (The Council for Exceptional Children). DOWN SYNDROME PARENTAL INPUT ADULT-CHILD INTERACTION INTERSUBJECTIVITY:

Rosch, Eleanor H. (1977). Human categorization. In N. Warren (Ed.), *Studies in crosscultural psychology,* vol. 1. New York, NY: Academic Press. PROTOTYPE THEORY CATEGORIZATION:

Rosch, Eleanor H., & Lloyd, B. B. (1978). *Cognition and categorization*. New York, NY: Halstead Press. CATEGORIZATION CONCEPT DEVELOPMENT PROTOTYPE THEORY:

Rose, Clifford F., Whurr, Renata, & Wyke, Maria A. (1990). *Aphasia*. San Diego, CA: Singular Publishing Group. APHASIAS LANGUAGE AND HANDEDNESS CLASSIFICATION OF DISORDERS LATERALIZATION INTERVENTION PROGRAMS:

Classification of aphasia. Linguistic levels in aphasia. Non-verbal communication. The relationship between brainedness and handedness. Phylogical differences between left and right. Observatioons on right hemisphere language function. Language-related functions of the right cerebral hemisphere. Aphasia: new directions in clinical theory. The anatomical and pathological basis of aphasia. The clinical neurology of aphasia. Subcortical aphasia. The relationship between aphasia and motor aphasia. Speech fluency in aphasia. The assessment of non-verbal abilities in aphasic subjects. The assessment of verbal comprehension. The assessment of verbal expression. Addressing disorders of gesture. The speech therapist's assessment of aphasia. Non-vocal approaches to aphasia rehabilitation. The management of the aphasic patient. Assessment of treatment in aphasia.

Rose, J. C., Lincoln, A. J., & Allen, M. H. (1992). Ability profiles of developmental language disordered and learning disabled children-a comparative analysis. *Developmental Neuropsychology*, 8, 413-426 . DEVELOPMENTAL DISORDERS LANGUAGE AND COGNITIVE DEVELOPMENT:

Roseberry, C. A., & Connell, P. J. (1991). The use of an invented language rule in the differentiation of normal and language-impaired Spanish-speaking children. *Journal of Speech and Hearing Research*, 34, 596-603. ASSESSMENT PROCEDURES SPANISH METHODOLOGY RULES:

Rosen, Christine D., & Gerring, Joan P. (1986). *Head trauma: educational reintegration*. San Diego, CA: Singular Publishing Group. TRAUMATIC DISORDERS:

Anatomy of the brain. Early recovery. Long term recovery implications for school planning. Instructional preparation. Applications.

Rosenbek, John C., LaPointe, Leonard L., & Wertz, Robert T. (1989). *Aphasia: a clinical approach*. San Diego, CA: Singular Publishing Group. APHASIAS READING DISORDERS DYSLEXIA AGRAPHIA ANOMIA:

An introduction to clinical aphasiology. Neurological bases of aphasia. Appraisal, diagnosis, prognosis, and treatment. Dyslexia and reading problems associated with aphasias. Treating agraphia and anomia.

Rosenbek, John C., & McNeil, Malcom R. (1991). A discussion of classification in motor speech disorders: Dysarthria and apraxia of speech. In C. Moore, K. M. Yorkston, & D. R. Beukelman (Eds), *Dysarthria and apraxia of speech*. Baltimore, MD: Paul H. Brookes. CLASSIFICATION OF DISORDERS MOTOR DISORDERS DYSARTHRIA APRAXIA:

Rosenbek, John C., McNeil, Malcom R., & Aronson, Arnold E. (1983). *Apraxia of speech: Physiology, acoustics, linguistics, management*. San Diego, CA: Singular Publishing Group. APHASIAS APRAXIA BROCA'S APHASIA PHONOLOGICAL DISORDERS ARTICULATION DISORDERS ACOUSTIC PHONETICS:

Subcortical lesions and verbal apraxia. The elusive lesion-apraxia of speech link in Broca's aphasia. Prediction of site of lesion from speech apraxis error patterns. Articulatory movements in apraxia of speech. Apraxic speakers' vowel duration in consonant-vowel-consonant syllables. An analysis of Voice Onset Time (VOT) in aphasic and normal subjects. Simplification and gesture reduction in phonological disorders of apraxia and aphasia. Response to treatment in patients with apraxia and aphasia. Response to treatment in patients with apraxia of speech. Sequential treatment of split lists.

Rosenblith, Judy F., & Sims-Knight, Judith E. (1989). *In the beginning: Development in the first two years*. Beverley Hills, CA: Sage Publications. INFANT PERCEPTION COGNITIVE DEVELOPMENT LANGUAGE AND COGNITIVE DEVELOPMENT:

Introductory text covering infant development during the first two years.

Rosenhouse, Judith. (1977). A preliminary report: an analysis of some types of a baby's cries. *Journal of Phonetics*, 5, 299-312. CRYING:

Classification and description of cry types stimulated by different internal causes were made here, with the subject being a 1 1/2-month-old baby girl. An important part of the task was to find the main groups of cries that are meaningful in the baby's utterances. Four types were observed in the study: hunger, pain, illness and alarm cries. By spectographic analysis various features being prominent. Normal hunger and illness cry features were found to be comparable in principle with features of certain diseases of babies found in other studies.JR

Rosenhouse, Judith. (1980). Duration in infants' communication by cries. *Journal of Phonetics*, 8, 135-156. CRYING:

This study takes up the aspect of duration of a baby's cries for analysis. From this analysis a distinction was made between three major parts of the cry structure: (1) single cries and pauses: (2) the overall pattern of the whole sequence of cries and pauses: (3) the internal division of the sequence into groups of single cries which form rhythmic cycles of cries. These three parts may be perhaps compared with morphemes, paragraphs (or 'spoken chain') and sentences from the point of view of conventional adult speech communication. The three parts were measured from the recorded graphs of a chart recorder for four types of cries, namely hunger, pain, fatigue and illness cries. The statistical values: average, standard deviation, skewness, kurtosis and the most probable value (for intervals of 100 ms) were then calculated by computer for all the cycles and the whole sequences that served as material of the study, and the results were then compared. These results show interesting and complex differences between the crying types and open the way to future research in this direction so as to enable practical diagnosis of the infants' condition. JR.

Rosenhouse, Judith. (1986). Evaluation of computer-aided instruction to Hebrew-speaking hearing-impaired children. In *Technical Report 88.208*. Haifa, Israel: The IBM Israel Science and Technology and Scientific Center. HEBREW DEAF CHILDREN INTERVENTION PROGRAMS COMPUTER ASSISTED THERAPY:

This report summarizes and evaluates the first stages of computer aided experimental work with hearing impaired children and deaf children at Haifa. The computer's part was the IBM Paris Speech Training Program which by analysis of the voice parameters (frequency, amplitude and time) motivates children to play with voice-eliciting computer games. The various computer games that are included in the program are briefly described, as well as the ways we used them with the children. The experimental teaching included three age groups of children from kindergarten age to the last year of elementary school and with varied hearing-loss rates, linguistic backgrounds, home backings and personalities. The diverse data are here examined in the hope of creating effecient ways of implementing this new device as an aid to teach hearing-impaired and deaf children to talk. The results of the present study are generally positive.JR

Rosenhouse, Judith. (1986). Intonation problems of hearing-impaired Hebrew-speaking children. *Language and Speech*, 29, 62-95. HEBREW PROSODIC DISORDERS DEAF CHILDREN INTONATION:

Intonation of hearing-impaired Hebrew-speaking children in Israel was studied in two speech modes: spontaneous speech and reading aloud a written text. Attention was focused on statements and questions, usually considered basic types of semantic definition and (apparently) of intonation patterns. The subjects were 9-12 year-old hearing-impaired children and a control group of hearing children of the same ages. The utterances were analyzed by an IBM speech training program, which enabled graphical presentation of fundamental frequency and intensity distributions. This report presents preliminary conclusions concerning F ranges and F contours (internal vs. final intonation structure), and duration problems on hearing-impaired children, and considers the possibility and value of defining and studying intonation of the hearing-impaired.JR

Rosenhouse, Judith. (1986). On language problems of Arab children (in Hebrew and Arabic). *Mifgash*, 3 (7), 92-95. LITEARCY ARABIC LANGUAGE DISORDERS READING DISORDERS: HEBREW ARABIC

Rosenhouse, Judith. (1987). Foreign language teaching and Arabic in the country (in Hebrew). *Bulletin of Teachers of Arabic*, 2, 19-22. REGISTER LANGUAGE AND EDUCATION READING DISORDERS ARABIC: HEBREW

This paper describes the different methods in teaching Arabic in Israel, according to the students. Arabic is taught in Israel to both Jewish and Arab school children. But methods, aims and duration vary, and with them also achievements and attitudes. Arab children learn Arabic (i.e., literary Arabic) as their prestige register, while their mother tongue is colloquial. Jewish children learn it as a second or third language (after English) and some learn colloquial dialects, some the literary, and this classification may also run along age groups (the older learn the literary language). Those who learn literary Arabic also learn the Arabic alphabet, unlike those who learn the colloquial dialect. This paper raises the question of difficulties for children with different backgrounds and how the ministry of education should deal with such difficulties.

Rosenhouse, Judith. (1988). Computer-aided teaching of intonation to Hebrew-speaking hearing- impaired children. In *Revised Summaries and 24 Reprinted Abstracts from Posters and Section Papers at the 4th International Congress for the Study of Child Language, Paper No. 2*. Lund, Sweden: Child Language Research Institute. DEAF CHILDREN HEBREW COMPUTER ASSISTED THERAPY INTONATION PHONOLOGICAL DISORDERS:

One of the major problems of deaf speech is intonation, which is often described as 'monotaneous' or 'too jumpy' or 'not in pitch,' etc. As intonation is not easy to teach, it is often left behind other speech aspects. A set of IBM computer programs of voice-activated games, especially designed for the deaf, was donated in 1986 to the local branch of MIHA (the organization which cares for young hearing-impaired children) in Haifa, and this paper describes and sumarizes its use and effectiveness among the kindergarten children (aged 3-4), as well as some older ones (ages 8, 11) and younger ones (aged 2). The games provide various aspects of speech training. It was convenient to start with breath training and pitch modulation games before starting more 'abstract' intonation patterns, by a different program which analyzes the sound wave into its FO and/or intensity components. Relating these aspects to speech was accompanied by work on syllabic rhythm (by e.g. hand claps). Although within the short time of our experiments with the children in 1986 not much could be achieved with the smaller ones, the older ones showed quick grasp of the intonation elements as well as improved performance. Motivation for computer-aided speech-training was overall enhanced.JR

Rosenhouse, Judith. (1989). Bedouin folktales in Arabic lessons (in Hebrew). *Bulletin of Teachers of Arabic*, 5 (6), 53-65. ARABIC LANGUAGE AND EDUCATION: HEBREW

Folk tales are an especially attractive story genre, and in every culture there are story-tellers who pass them on from one generation to another, and often to children. This fact may help in enriching the curricula for Arabic lessons at various levels of age and linguistic knowledge. As Bedouins have (still) the glamour of traditional desert dwellers, their stories form a special group within the genre of Arabic folk stories, and are likely to rouse interest in the children and motivation to learn the linguistic material, as well as the social and cultural background. Two stories in colloquial Arabic and colloquial Bedouin dialects are supplied as examples, with their translation into Hebrew and some notes.JR

Rosenhouse, Judith. (1990). A new frequency-transportation hearing-device for the hearing-impaired. Results of a study with children. *Hearing Journal*, November. DEAF CHILDREN HEARING AIDS INTERVENTION PROGRAMS:

This new device transposes and compresses proportionately and dynamically the frequencies above 2kHz to the lower range. It treats consonants separately from vowels, while yielding joint information at the output. The final output has much lower frequencies than the original signal, but keeps the proportions between the formants. The device is intended to help those hearing impaired subjects, whose audiograms show down-sloping hearing abilities, and who usually have hearing residues only up to about 1KHz. The operation of this device was tested with a small group of children (3 m., 1 f. aged 10). The main purpose was to examine the effect of immediate reactions of the subjects to the device, and long-term training effects on hearing without the device. The subjects were tested by standard hearing tests for the deaf and specially prepared language tests upon their first meeting with the device, and after a period of training with speech-teachers. An additional second stage was appended with only one subject who later had the device for longer-term home use.JR

Rosenhouse, Judith, & Shehadi, C. (1986). Notes of diglossia problems in Arabic: the educational aspect. In I. Idalovichi, & N. Ararat (Eds), *Philosophy, language, arts: Essays in honour of Alexander Barzel*. Haifa, Israel: The Technicon. ARABIC REGISTER SOCIOLINGUISTIC FACTORS LANGUAGE AND EDUCATION LITERACY:

Language problems in the Arabic speaking worlds can best be described by the term 'Diglossia,' which means that a society has a constant state of duality in language usage. Namely, different language systems exist for formal needs on the one hand and for informal needs on the other. Arabic is known for the big chasm between the 'literary language' and the colloquial usage which is not even considered a language by most of its speakers. The problems if this 'schizophrenic' situations begins for native speakers of Arabic at a very young age-as soon as they start school. In this paper some school books used in the two first grades of some elementary schools in Haifa and its vicinity are linguistically and critically examined. The books are non-homogeneous and reveal various types of difference. More literary forms in larger concentration in a book seem to indicate more learning difficulties for the children, whose mother tongue is colloquial Arabic. Emotional reactions to these difficulties have been recorded in the Arabic literature, though the Arabic educational system (also outside Israel) does not support attitudinal changes.JR

Rosenthal-Rollins, P. (1993). Specific language impaired children. In J. L. Sokolov, & C. E. Snow (Eds), *Handbook of research in language development using* . Hillsdale, NJ: Lawrence Erlbaum Associates. SPECIFIC LANGUAGE IMPAIRMENT METHODOLOGY-COMPUTERS CHILDES:

Rost, Detlef H. (1989). Reading comprehension: Skill or skills? *Journal of Research in Reading*, 12, 87-113. LITERACY GERMAN:

To investigate if early reading comprehension is composed of different separate subskills, 38 German reading tests, one spelling test and one speed of information processing test were administered to 220 German second graders (114 girls, 106 boys). A principal component analysis (principal axis extraction) led only to one broad general reading comprehension component, accounting for 61% of the total variance. - From Child Development Abstracts.

Roth, Norbert, Beyresiss, Jutta, Schlenzka, Klaus, & Beyer, Hannelore. (1991). The effects of two levels of linguistic constraint on echolalia and generative language production in children with autism. *Journal of Autism and Developmental Disorders* , 21, 131-157. AUTISM ECHOLALIA:

The effects of specific types of antecedent utterances on the verbal behaviors of three autistic subjects were examined. Adult utterance types were differentiated in terms of the amount of control the adults exhibited in their verbal interactions with the subjects during a free play setting. From Child Development Abstracts.

Rothweiler, Monika. (1991). Spracherwerb und Grammatik: Linguistische Untersuchungen zum Erwerb von Syntax und Morphologie. (Language acquisition and grammar: Lingistic investigations of the acquisition of syntax and morphology.). *Linguistische Berichte*. GERMAN SYNTACTIC DEVELOPMENT MORPHOLOGICAL DEVELOPMENT MORPHOSYNTACTIC DEVELOPMENT: GERMAN

Rotman, B. (1977). *Jean Piaget: Psychologist of the real*. Hassocks, Sussex, England: Harvester Press. PIAGETIAN THEORY LANGUAGE AND COGNITIVE DEVELOPMENT:

Roush, J., Harrison, M., & Palsha, S. (1991). Family-centered early intervention - the perceptions of professionals. *American Annals of the Deaf*, 136, 360-366. INTERVENTION PROGRAMS:

Roussey, Jean-Yves. (1991). Text schemas in a modeling paradigm: Improvements of a narrative and a description by ten-year-olds. *European Journal of Psychology of Education*, 6, 233-242. EVENTS/SCRIPTS TEXT/STORY GRAMMARS WRITTEN LANGUAGE LANGUAGE AND EDUCATION:

Revision of errors in a prewritten text was performed by two experimental groups. One group performed a prereading task in which they were provided with the schema for the text to be revised, and the second group completed the revision without access to the schema information. Access to the schema information had a positive effect on the revision task. From Child Development Abstracts.

Rubin, Donald L., Galda, Lee, & Pellegrini, Anthony D. (1989). Development of informational adequacy in speech and writing. *Applied Psycholinguistics*, 10, 387-399. WRITTEN LANGUAGE COMMUNICATIVE COMPETENCE:

The present study replicates and extends previous research by administering referential and explanatory communication tasks in both speech and writing to children at three grade levels. In addition, an independent measure of social cognitive ability was administered. Results confirmed increasing differentiation with age between speech and writing, with fifth graders displaying greater informational adequacy in writing. Children's performance in written communication, rather than speech, revealed a dependency on social cognitive ability. - From Child Development Abstracts.

Ruff, Holly A., & Lawson, Katharine R. (1990). Development of sustained, focused attention in young children during free play. *Developmental Psychology*, 26, 85-93. ATTENTION LANGUAGE AND PLAY METHODOLOGY-DESIGN:

Children were seen at 1, 2, and 3:6 years in free play. The duration of focused attention increased significantly. In study 2, children at 2:6, 3:6, and 4:6 years were seen in free play. The results replicated the earlier ones. - From Child Development Abstracts.

Ruff, Holly A., Lawson, Katharine R., Parrinello, Roseanne, & Weissberg, Renata. (1990). Long-term stability of individual differences in sustained attention in the early years. *Child Development*, 61, 60-75. ATTENTION METHODOLOGY-DESIGN:

Children were observed at 1, 2, and 3:6 years in free play and in structured situations. Quantitative measures of inattention at 2 years were predictive of comparable measures at 3:6 years. For preterms separately, quantitative measures of inattention at 1 year were predictive of both behavior and the mothers' rating on the Connors Hyperactivity subscale at 3:6 years. Global, qualitative ratings of attentiveness at 1 and 2 years predicted mother's ratings on the Connors at 3:6 years for the group and for full-terms. For full-terms only, the global ratings of attentiveness at 1 and 2 years were predictive.- From Child Development Abstracts.

Rumbaugh, Duane M., Hopkins, W. D., Washburn, D. A., & Savage-Rumbaugh, E. Sue. (1991). Comparative perspectives of brain, cognition, and language. In N. A. Krasnegor, et al. (Eds), *Biological and behavioral determinants of language development*. Hillsdale, NJ: Lawrence Erlbaum Associates. LANGUAGE AND OTHER PRIMATES NEUROLINGUISTICS LANGUAGE AND COGNITION:

Rumbaugh, Duane M., Hopkins, W. D., Washburn, D. A., & Savage-Rumbaugh, E. Sue. (1993). Chimpanzee competence for counting in a video-formatted task situation. In L. M. Herman, H. L. Roitblat, & P. E. Nachtigall (Eds), *Language and communication: Comparative perspectives*. Hillsdale, NJ: Lawrence Erlbaum Associates. LANGUAGE AND OTHER PRIMATES ANIMAL COMMUNICATIONS:

Runyan, C. M., Bell, J. N., & Prosek, R. A. (1990). Speech naturalness ratings of treated stutterers. *Journal of Speech and Hearing Disorders*, 55, 434-438. STUTTERING:

Ruscello, D. M., Louis, K. O. St., & Mason, N. (1991). School-aged children with phonologic disorders: Coexistence with other speech language disorders. *Journal of Speech and Hearing Research*, 34, 236-242. PHONOLOGICAL DISORDERS LANGUAGE DISORDERS:

Rustin, Lena. (1991). *Parents, families, and the stuttering child*. San Diego, CA: Singular Publishing Group. STUTTERING INTERVENTION PROGRAMS FOR PARENTS INTERVENTION PROGRAMS:

The family background of childhood and adolescent stuttering: a long-term study. Young stutterer's speech production: some clinical considerations. Interaction with preschool stutterers: how will this influence therapy? Parents and their preschool stuttering child. Using families to help the school-age stuttering child. Intensive management of the adolescent stutterer. Therapy for adolescents: speech and attitude change. Indexes.

Rustin, Lena, & Kuhr, Armin. (1988). *Social skills and the speech impaired*. San Diego, CA: Singular Publishing Group. SOCIAL SPEECH LANGUAGE DISORDERS INTERVENTION PROGRAMS SIGNING ASSESSMENT PROCEDURES:

Main section headings: fundamental principles. Non-verbal communication behaviors. Cognition and communication. Principles and elements of training. Group therapy. Social skills for training for the speech and language handicapped. Assessment. Ecercises. References. Index.

Rustin, Lena, Purser, Harry, & Rowley, David. (1987). *Progress in the treatment of fluency disorders*. San Diego, CA: Singular Group. DISFLUENCIES STUTTERING INTERVENTION PROGRAMS INTERVENTION PROGRAMS FOR PARENTS:

Neuropsychological models of speech dysfluency. Hemispheric processing and stuttering. An approach to the study of motor speech mechanisms in stuttering. Linguistic profiling of stuttering behavior. Assessment and diagnosis of childhood dysfluency. The treatment of stuttering: recent history and contemporary issues. The Cooper Personalized Fluency Control Therapy Program. Personal construct theory and the treatment of adolescent dysfluency. The treatment of childhood dysfluency through active parental involvement. Paradoxical therapy in the treatment of stuttering. Self-help for stutterers: experience in Britain. Informing stutterers about treatment. The effectiveness of treatment for stuttering. The psychology of treatment evaluation. References. Index.

Rutter, M., & Schopler, Eric. (1992). Classification of pervasive developmental disorders - some concepts and practical considerations. *Journal of Autism and Developmental Disorders*, 22, 459-482. CLASSIFICATION OF DISORDERS DEVELOPMENTAL DISORDERS:

Ryalls, J., & Larouche, A. (1992). Acoustic integrity of speech production in children with moderate and severe hearing impairment. *Journal of Speech and Hearing Research*, 35, 88-95. DEAF CHILDREN ACOUSTIC PHONETICS INTELLIGIBILITY:

Ryan, B. P. (1992). Articulation, language, rate, and fluency characteristics of stuttering and nonstuttering preschool children. *Journal of Speech and Hearing Research*, 35, 333-342. STUTTERING ARTICULATION SPEAKING RATE:

S

Saben, C. B., & Ingham, J. C. (1991). The effects of minimal pairs treatment on the speech-sound production of 2 children with phonologic disorders. *Journal of Speech and Hearing Research*, 34, 1023-1040. PHONOLOGICAL DISORDERS TREATMENT GENERALIZATION:

Sachs, Jacqueline, Donnelly, J., Smith, Cheryl A., & Bookbinder, J. D. (1991). Preschool children's conversation intrusions - behavior and metapragmatic knowledge. *Discourse Processes*, 14, 357-372. PRAGMATIC DEVELOPMENT CONVERSATIONAL SKILLS COMMUNICATIVE COMPETENCE METALINGUISTICS:

Sagart, L., Halle, P., de Boysson-Bardies, Bénédicte, & Arabia-Guidet, C. (1986). Tone production in modern standard Chinese: an electromyographic investigation. *Cahiers de Linguistique Asie Orientale*, 15, 205-220. CHINESE TONE:

Saleemi, Anjum P. (1992). *Universal Grammar and language learnability*. New York, NY: Cambridge University Press. LEARNABILITY PARAMETER SETTING SYNTACTIC DEVELOPMENT ACQUISITION THEORIES-SYNTAX:

The author combines Universal Grammar and Learnability Theory to propose an account of syntactic development. The work is based on the tenet that linguistic theory alone is insufficient to account for language development.

Salmon, Shirley J., & Mount, Kay H. (1991). *Alaryngeal speech rehabilitation: for clinicians by clinicians*. San Diego, CA: Singular Publishing Group. ALARYNGEAL SPEECH INTERVENTION PROGRAMS TRAUMATIC DISORDERS:

Anatomy and physiology of speech. The artificial larynx. Esophageal speech training: the initial phase. Toward advancing esophageal communication. Group therapy. Tracheoesophageal puncture: general considerations. Treatment following tracheoesophageal fistulization. Clinical application of alaryngeal speech judgements. Failure in acquiring esophageal speech. Living with a laryngectomee. Consequences of total laryngectomy in daily living activities. Conducting alaryngeal speech rehabilitation workshops. Indexes.

Samar, Vincent J., & Metz, Dale E. (1991). Scaling and transcription measures of intelligibility for populations with disordered speech: Where's the beef? *Journal of Speech and Hearing Research*, 34, 699-702. ASSESSMENT PROCEDURES INTELLIGIBILITY METHODOLOGY-TRANSCRIPTION:

Samo, Martha T. (Ed.). (1991). *Acquired aphasia, vol.* (2). San Diego, CA: Academic Press. ACQUIRED APHASIA TRAUMATIC DISORDERS CLASSIFICATION OF DISORDERS INTERVENTION PROGRAMS:

A comprehensive account of many aspects of acquired aphasia. The book includes chapters on: childhood aphasia, adult aphasia, traumatic injury, localization, classification, and the psychosocial, intellectual, and linguistic effects of acquired aphasia. In addition recovery and treatment are also covered in the text.

Sanchez-Casas, R. M., Davis, C. W., & Garcia-Albea, J. E. (1993). Bilingual lexical processing: Exploring the cognate-noncognate distinction. In A. M. B. de Groot, & C. Barry (Eds), *The multilingual community*. Hillsdale, NJ: Lawrence Erlbaum Associates. BILINGUALISM-LEXICAL DEVELOPMENT TRANSFER:

Sander, E. (1972). When are speech sounds learned? *Journal of Speech and Hearing Disorders*, 37, 55-63. PHONEMIC DEVELOPMENT PRODUCTION/PERCEPTION:

Sanders, Danielle M. (1988). *Teaching deaf children: techniques and methods*. San Diego, CA: Singular Publishing Group. LANGUAGE AND EDUCATION DEAF CHILDREN INTERVENTION PROGRAMS:

Considerations in the education of hearing impaired children. Deafness, cognition, and language development. Strategies of effective teaching. Planning lessons. Understanding test information. Implementation. Examples of rewritten lessons. References. Subject index.

Sanders, T. J. M., Spooren, W. P. M., & Noordman, L. G. M. (1992). Toward a taxonomy of coherence relations. *Discourse Processes*, 15, 1-35. DISCOURSE COHERENCE:

Sandlin, Robert E. (1988). *Handbook of hearing aid amplification: theoretical and technical considerations*. San Diego, CA: Singular Publishing Group. AUDIOLOGY HEARING AIDS INTERVENTION PROGRAMS:

A historical review. Psychoacoustic and design considerations in hearing aid selection. Principles of high fidelity hearing aid amplification. Principles of signal processing. Compression in hearing aids. Technical considerations for sound field audiometry. Principles of acoustic measurements and ear canal resonances. Hearing aid formulae and their applications. Computer technology and hearing aids. Technical aspects of cochlear implants. Discrimination of acoustic signals. Observations and future considerations.

Sandlin, Robert E. (1990). *Handbook of hearing aid amplification: Clinical considerations and fitting practices*. San Diego, CA: Singular Publishing Group. AUDIOLOGY INTERVENTION PROGRAMS COCHLEAR IMPLANTS HEARING AIDS:

The art of dispensing. Three important considerations in hearing aid selection. Post-fitting and rehabilitative nanagement. Hearing aid amplification and central processing disorders. Pediatric considerations. Considerations for the selecting and the fitting of amplification for geriatric adults. The application of speech stimuli in hearing aid selection and evaluation. Cochlear implants and rehabilitative practices. Hearing aid assessment ant the auditory brainstem response. Clinical application of real-ear probe tube measurement. Clinical application of sound field audiometry.

Sasaki, Y. (1991). English and Japanese interlanguage comprehension strategies-an analysis based on the Competition Model. *Applied Psycholinguistics*, 12, 47-73. INTERLANGUAGE-CONSTRAINTS ENGLISH-JAPANESE JAPANESE-ENGLISH COMPETITION MODEL:

Satake, Nobuo. (1990). A computational model of first acquisition. In *First language acquisition as problem solving*. Singapore: World Scientific. COMPUTER SIMULATIONS:

Saunders, George. (1990). "Artificial" bilingualism: Must it fail? In M. A. K. Halliday, J. Gibbons, & H. Nicholas (Eds), *Learning, keeping and using language* . Amsterdam, The Netherlands: John Benjamins. BILINGUALISM LANGUAGE AND EDUCATION:

Savage-Rumbaugh, E. Sue. (1990). Language acquisition in a nonhuman species: Implications for the innateness debate. *Developmental Psychobiology*, 23(7), NATIVISM LANGUAGE AND OTHER PRIMATES:

Savage-Rumbaugh, E. Sue. (1991). Language learning in the Bonobo: how and why they learn. In N. A. Krasnegor, et al. (Eds), *Biological and behavioral determinants of language development*. Hillsdale, NJ: Lawrence Erlbaum Associates. LANGUAGE AND OTHER PRIMATES:

Savage-Rumbaugh, E. Sue. (1993). Language learnablity in man, ape, and dolphin. In L. M. Herman, H. L. Roitblat, & P. E. Nachtigall (Eds), *Language and communication: Comparative perspectives*. Hillsdale, NJ: Lawrence Erlbaum Associates. LEARNABILITY LANGUAGE AND OTHER PRIMATES ANIMAL COMMUNICATIONS:

Sbisa, -. (1989). Speech acts of explanation. In M. S. Barbieri (Ed.), *La speigazione nell'interazione sociale*. Torino, Italy: Loescher. CHILDREN'S EXPLANATIONS SPEECH ACTS: ITALIAN

From a pragmatic perspective, the author inquires about the nature of explanations: whether they are a type of speech act in their own, or whether, as it is suggested in this chapter, they share some of the features of different types of speech acts.MSB

Scaife, M., & Bruner, Jerome S. (1975). The capacity for joint visual attention in the infant. *Nature*, 253, 265-266. GAZE JOINT REFERENCE PRELINGUISTCIS:

Scales, Barbara, Almy, Millie, Nicolopoulou, Ageliki, & Ervin-Tripp, Susan. (1991). *Play and the social context of development in early care and education*. New York, NY: Teacher's College Press. LANGUAGE AND PLAY:

This volume is a collection of papers from a symposium about play held at the Institute of Human Development, University of California, Berkeley, in May 1988 that considers play as the focus of the child's social world. The contributors offer keen insights into the important role of play in a number of relevant areas including language and literacy, cognitive development, and socialization.

Scarborough, Hollis S. (1990). Very early language deficits in dyslexic children. *Child Development*, 61, 1728-1743. DYSLEXIA AT-RISK CHILDREN READING DISORDERS:

Children who later developed reading disabilities were deficient in the length, syntactic complexity, and pronunciation accuracy of spoken language, but not in lexical or speech discrimination. As 3-year-olds, these children began to show deficits in receptive vocabulary and object-naming abilities, and as 5-year-olds they exhibited weakenesses in object-naming, phonemic awareness, and letter-sound knowledge that have characterized kindergartners who became poor readers.

Scarborough, Hollis S., Leslie, Rescorla., Tager-Flusberg, Helen, Fowler, Anne E., & Sudhalter, Cicki. (1991). The relation of utterance length to grammatical complexity in normal and language-disordered groups. *Applied Psycholinguistics*, 12, 23-45. AUTISM DOWN SYNDROME MEAN LENGTH OF UTTERANCE LANGUAGE DELAY:

Mean length of utterance (MLU) in morphemes was examined as a predictor of the grammatical complexity of natural language corpora of normal preschoolers and of children and adolescents with delayed language, Fragile X syndrome, Down syndrome, and autism. The Index of Productive Syntax (IPSyn) served as the measure of syntactic and morphological proficiency. For all groups, a strong curvilinear association between measures was found across the MLU range from 1.0 to about 4.5.

Scarcella, Robin C., Andersen, Elaine S., & Krashen, Stephen D. (1990). *Developing communicative competence in a second language.* New York, NY: Newbury House. L2 COMMUNICATIVE COMPETENCE L2 EDUCATION:

Scarpa, Ester M. (1985). A emergencia da coesao intonacional. (The emergence of intonational cohesion). *Cadernos de Estudos Linguisticos (IEL, UNICAMP),* 10, 31-41. INTONATION PORTUGUESE: PORTUGUESE

Scarpa, Ester M. (1985). Intonacao e processos dialogicos: fusao ou diferenciacao? (Intonation and dialogue processes: fusion or differentiation?). In *Aquisicao da linguagem. Serie Estudos.* Uberaba. INTONATION CONVERSATIONAL SKILLS PORTUGUESE: PORTUGUESE

Scarpa, Ester M. (1987). Aquisicao da linguagem e aquisicao daescrita: continuidade ou ruptura? (Acquisition of language and acquisition of literacy: continuity or discontinuity? *Estudos Linguisticos (G.E.L., Campinas),* 14, 118-129. CONTINUITY/DISCONTINUITY PORTUGUESE LITERACY: PORTUGUESE

Scarpa, Ester M. (1988). Desenvolvimento da intonacao e a organizacao da fala inicial. (Development of intonation and the organization of early speech). *Cadernos de Estudos Linguisticos (IEL, UNICAMP),* 14, 65-84. INTONATION PORTUGUESE: PORTUGUESE

Scarpa, Ester M. (1990). Forma ediscurso: sobre a organizacao prosodica da fala decriancaspequenas. (Form and discourse: on the prosodic organization of infant speech). In *Anais da XIX Reuniao Anual de Psicologia (Proceedings of the XIX Annual Meeting of Psychology).* Ribeirao Preto: USP. PROSODY INTONATION PORTUGUESE: PORTUGUESE

Scarpa, Ester M. (1991). O jogo, a construcao e o erro. (Play, construction and error). *Ideias* , 8, LANGUAGE AND PLAY SPEECH ERRORS LANGUAGE AND EDUCATION PORTUGUESE: PORTUGUESE

Published by Sao Paulo, Fundacao para o Desenvolvimentoda Educacao.

Scarr, S. (1992). Developmental theories for the 1990s-development and individual differences. *Child Development*, 63, 1-19. INDIVIDUAL VARIATION:

Schaefer, Charles, Gitlin, Karen, & Sandgrund, Alice. (1991). *Play diagnosis and assessment*. New York, NY: John Wiley & Sons. ASSESSMENT PROCEDURES INTERVENTION PROGRAMS LANGUAGE AND PLAY ADULT-CHILD INTERACTION DEVELOPMENTAL SCALES:

A collection of essays dealing with: developmental play scales, diagnostic play scales, parent-child interaction scales, peer interaction scales, projective play techniques, and play therapy scales.

Schaefer, Earl S. (1989). Dimensions of mother-infant interaction: Measurement, stability, and predictive validity. *Infant Behavior and Development*, 12, 379-393. ADULT-CHILD INTERACTION METHODOLOGY-ANALYSIS:

Two dimensions of mother-infant interaction are identified: positive interaction, and gentle/sensitive versus punitive/irritable. Higher reliability was found for positive interaction than the other dimension, and positive interaction correlated with academic competence. No significant correlation was found between the second dimension and infant behavior during kindergarten.

Schaerlaekens, A. M. (1974). Een generatief-transformationeel model voor kindertaalwerving. ((A generative transformational model for child language acquisition.). *Forum der Letteren*, 15 (2), 130-137. ACQUISITION THEORIES-SYNTAX: DUTCH

Schaerlaekens, A. M. (1974). A generative transformational model for child language acquisition: a discussion of L. Bloom, 'Language Development: Form and Function in Emerging Grammars'. *Cognition*, 2 (3), 361-376. ACQUISITION THEORIES-SYNTAX:

Schaerlaekens, A. M. (1976). De periode van de tweewoordzin in de taalontwikkeling van het Nederlandstalig kind. (The period of the two-word sentence in language development of Dutch- speaking children.) . *Tijdschrift voor Logopedie en Audiologie*, 6 (3), TWO-WORD SPEECH EARLY SYNTACTIC DEVELOPMENT DUTCH: DUTCH

Schaerlaekens, A. M. (1976). Kindertaal, generatieve semantiek en markeringstheorie. (Child language, generative semantics and markedness theory.). In M. Spoelders (Ed.), *Psycholinguistisch onderzoek in Belgie*. Gent: Rijksuniversiteit. MARKEDNESS: DUTCH

Schaerlaekens, A. M. (1976). Language development in Dutch-speaking triplets. In G. Drachmanhersg (Ed.), *Akten des I. Salzburger Koloquiums uber Kindersprache*. Tubingen: Gunter Narr. DUTCH MULTIPLE BIRTHS SIBLING EFFECTS:

Schaerlaekens, A. M. (1977). *De taalontwikkeling van het kind: een orientatie in het Nederlandstalig onderzoek. (Child language development: An orinetation based on evidence from Dutch-speaking children.).* Groningen, Holland: Wolters-Noordhoff. DUTCH GENERAL-OVERVIEW: DUTCH

Second edition (derde herziene druk) 1980. Third edition (vierde herziene druk) 1982.

Schaerlaekens, A. M. (1981). Kindertaalontwikkeling. (Child language development.). In R. Dirven (Ed.), *Taalwetenschap: overzicht en inzicht*. ACQUISITION THEORIES-OVERVIEW: DUTCH

Schaerlaekens, A. M. (1985). Taalaanpassing bij guitenlandse adoptiekinderen. (The language adaption of foreign adopted children.). *Kind en Adolescent*, 6 (4), BILINGUALISM-SEQUENTIAL L2 ACQUISITION BILINGUALISM PROBLEMS/EFFECTS CRITICAL PERIOD: DUTCH

Schaerlaekens, A. M. (1986). De rol van het gebruik van kinderboeken in het taalontwikkelingsproces. (The effect of using children's books on the process of language development.). In S. V. D. Meulen (Ed.), *Taalontwikkelingsstoornissen, onderzoek en behandeling*. Lisse, Holland: Swets & Zeitlinger. SOCIAL INTERACTION HYPOTHESIS ADULT-CHILD INTERACTION: DUTCH

Schaerlaekens, A. M. (1986). Taalontwikkeling van het kind. (Children's language development.). In L. Heylen (Ed.), *En kijk op Logopedie*. Leuven: Acco. ACQUISITION THEORIES-OVERVIEW: DUTCH

Schaerlaekens, A. M. (1986). Taalontwikkeling. (Language development.). In P. Paardekoper (Ed.), *De Nederlandse Taalkunde in kaart*. Leuven: ACQUISITION THEORIES-OVERVIEW: DUTCH

Schaerlaekens, A. M. (1987). Aspecten van kindertaalstudie. (Aspects of child language research.). In *Omtrent Logopedie, 2*. Leuven: Acco. ACQUISITION THEORIES-OVERVIEW: DUTCH

Schaerlaekens, A. M. (1989). Spontane taalanalyse als onderzoeksmethode voor taalverwerving. (Analyzing samples of spontaneous speech as a research method for language acquisition.). *Logopedie en Foniatrie*, 61 (5), 156-160. METHODOLOGY-ANALYSIS: DUTCH

> This paper deals with the emergence of linguistic analysis of language samples, as this method resulted in several procedures adapted to the Dutch language. Originally designed for language pathology, this method can also be used in research concerning normal language development, and some research has already been completed in Dutch. A few critical remarks concerning this procedure are formulated and suggestions are made for further use. AS.

Schaerlaekens, A. M. (1989). Taalontwikkeling: van onmondig tot geletterd. (Language development: from speechless childhood to literacy.). In R. Kohnstamm, & G. Cluckers (Ed.), *Problemen en risicosituaties*. Loghum-Slaterus. ACQUISITION THEORIES-OVERVIEW LITERACY: DUTCH

Schaerlaekens, A. M., Forrez, G., & Bael, L. Van. (1989). Mimicry of intonation in 10- to 12-month-old children: a failure to replicate. *Clinical Linguistics and Phonetics*, 4, 139-144. INTONATION BABBLING PROSODY:

It has generally been assumed that children begin to imitate the intonation of adult speakers during the first year of life. Lieberman (1967), on the basis of an experiment with two babies (10 and 13 months of age), argued that babies switch to a lower fundamental frequency while interacting vocally with adults than when they babble alone. This he considered a kind of imitation called mimicry. We duplicated Lieberman's experiment with three babies while increasing the size of the babbling samples, collecting the babbling samples at three different ages for each child (10, 11, and 12 months), and increasing the precision of the voice analysis by using a suitable computer program, thus, in turn, increasing the precision of the measurement of the fundamental frequency. Our conclusions do not confirm Lieberman's results in any way. The fundamental frequency fluctuated for each child, independently of the age and interacting circumstances. The results do not show any coherent pattern. We conclude that further research should focus on the imitation of intonation patterns but not on the pitch as such.

Schaerlaekens, A. M., & Gillis, Steven. (1987). *De taalverwerving van het kind. Een hernieuwde orientatie in het Nederlandstalig onderzoek. (Chldren's language acquisition: A renewed orientation in Dutch research.).* Groningen: Wolters-Noordhoff. DUTCH GENERAL-OVERVIEW: DUTCH

This book is a guide to the acquisition of Dutch as a mother tongue. It reviews most of the existing literature on the acquisition of Dutch and integrates it in a chronological picture.AS

Schaerlaekens, A. M., Huygelier, N., & Dondeyne, A. (1988). Language adjustment in international adoptions. *Journal of Multilingual and Multicultural Development*, 9 (3), 247-266. L2 ACQUISITION CRITICAL PERIOD BILINGUALISM-SEQUENTIAL BILINGUALISM-CULTURAL FACTORS BILINGUALISM PROBLEMS/EFFECTS:

The process of linguistic adaptation of foreign children who are adopted by families with a totally different mother tongue is bound to be a very peculiar one. A survey is given of the existing (scarce) literature addressing this problem. In addition, an investigation was conducted concerning foreign children adopted into Dutch-speaking families. Enquiries concerning this process were made by means of a questionnaire sent to the parents of 118 children born in India and adopted by Dutch-speaking families in Belgium. On the basis of these data, an attempt is made to formulate answers to two questions: (1) How, on average, does linguistic adaptation progress, and what may parents be led to expect? (2) Is this group of children a risk group with regards to lasting language problems that could eventually result in learning problems? On the basis of the accumulated data it is possible to form a picture of the adaptation process, which falls into a short, early period and a further acquisition process. Children who are younger than three years upon their arrival appear to handle both periods differently from children who are older on their arrival. The answer to the second question must be formulated differently for each of these two groups. Striking for the entire group is the increased occurrence of various ear conditions. As is well-known, any hearing problem is a risk factor in language acquisition.AS

Schaerlaekens, A. M., & Timmermans, B. (1986). *Ieder zijn communicatie. (Communication for everybody.).* Leuven, Holland: Acco. COMMUNICATIVE DEVELOPMENT: DUTCH

Schaff, Adam. (1973). *Language and cognition*. New York, NY: McGraw-Hill. SAPIR-WHORF HYPOTHESIS LANGUAGE AND COGNITION CULTURAL FACTORS:

Schaffer, H. R. (1977). Early interactive development. In J. Oates (Ed.), *Early cognitive development.* London, UK: Croom-Helm. INTERSUBJECTIVITY ADULT-CHILD INTERACTION SOCIAL INTERACTION HYPOTHESIS PRELINGUISTICS:

Schaner-Wolles, Chris. (1989). Strategies in acquiring grammatical relations in German: word order or case marking?. *Folia Linguistica*, 23, 131-156. GERMAN CASE WORD ORDER GRAMMATICAL RELATIONS:

Schaner-Wolles, Chris, & Tonelli, L. (1990). The acquisition of affricates in Viennese German. In J. Dosuna, & C. Pensado (Eds), *Naturalists at Krems. Papers from the Workshop on Natural Phonology and Natural Morphology.* Salamanca: Ediciones Universidad de Salamanca. GERMAN AFFRICATES NONSTANDARD DIALECT:

> The paper presents and analyzes the data resulting from a systematic study on the acquisition of affricates by forty monolingual German speaking children, aged between 2:3 and 6:6. Most widespread substitution patterns are compared with data from other languages. A natural process analysis is proposed in order to account for regular substitutions as well as for apparently contridictory ones.CSW

Scherer, Nancy J., & Olswang, Lesley B. (1989). Using structured discourse as a language intervention technique with autistic children. *Journal of Speech and Hearing Disorders*, 54, 383-394. AUTISM INTERVENTION PROGRAMS:

> A structured discourse strategy, employing child echoic imitations and adult expansion, was used to teach 5 autistic children two-term semantic relations. The results showed that an increase in modeling and expansion was related to an increase in the children's initial spontaneous imitations of two-term relations. - From Child Development Abstracts.

Schick, B., & Moeller, M. P. (1992). What is learnable in manually coded English sign systems. . *Applied Psycholinguistics*, 13, 313-340. SIGNING-MANUAL ENGLISH:

Schiefelbusch, Richard L. (1986). *Language competence: assessment and intervention*. San Diego, CA: Singular Publishing Group. CONVERSATIONAL COMPETENCE REQUESTS METHODOLOGY-DESIGN METHODOLOGY-ANALYSIS INTERVENTION PROGRAMS:

The development of conversationsal competence. The development of requests. Observational methods in the study of communicative competence. Sequential analysis of naturalistic communication. Language intervention through sensemaking and fine tuning. Incidental strategies. A review of studies on learning disabled children's communicative competence. Mismatched premises of the communicative competence model and language intervention. Author index. Subject index.

Schiefelbusch, Richard L., & Bricker, D. D. (EdS). (1981). *Early language: Acquisition and intervention.* Baltimore, MD: University Park Press. ACQUISITION THEORIES INTERVENTION PROGRAMS:

Schieffelin, Bambi B. (1990). *The give and take of everyday life.* New York, NY: Cambridge University Press. KALULI LANGUAGE AND SOCIAL TRANSMISSION LANGUAGE SOCIALIZATION:

Schieffelin examines the use of language to transmit social values in Kaluli society.

Schleichkorn, Jay. (1983). *Coping with cerebral palsy: answers to questions parents often ask.* San Diego, CA: Singular Publishing Group. CEREBRAL PALSY:

Cerebral palsy: the condition itself. Causes of cerebral palsy: growth and development. Medical and surgical problems: Professional services. Psychological and social concerns. Educational concerns. Life experiences. Research. References.

Schlesinger, Izchak M. (1977). Al musagim, milim urechishatam (On the Acquisition of Concepts and Words.). *Iyyun: A Hebrew Philosophical Quarterly*, 27, 89-104. CONCEPTUAL DEVELOPMENT LEXICAL DEVELOPMENT SEMANTIC DEVELOPMENT: HEBREW

Schlyter, Suzanne. (1987). Language mixing and linguistic level in three bilingual children. *Scandinavian Working Papers on Bilingualism*, 7, CODE-SWITCHING:

Schlyter, Suzanne. (1990). The acquisition of tense and aspect. In M. J. Meisel (Ed.), *Two first languages: Early grammatical development in bilingual children*. Dordrecht: Foris. ASPECT TENSE:

Schober-Patterson, Debra, & Johnson, Cynthia J. (1989). Conversational topics of 4-year-olds. *Journal of Speech and Hearing Research*, 32(4), 857-870. CHILDREN'S DISCOURSE TOPIC IDENTIFICATION:

Schober-Patterson, Debra, & Johnson, Cynthia J. (1991). Non-dialogue speech during preschool interactions. *Journal of Child Language*, 18, 153-170. PRIVATE SPEECH:

> The portion of preschool verbal interaction which could not be considered successful dialogue was described. Dyads of four-year-olds were videotaped during free play and segments of talk were identified as dialogue or non-dialogue. Thirteen types of non-dialogue were identified. Results revealed that all dyads exhibited non-dialogue, but differences were noted in regard to amount and type.

Scholnick, Ellin K., & Hall, William S. (1991). The language of thinking: metacognition and conditional words. In S. A. Gelman, & J. Byrnes (Ed.), *Perspectives on language and thought*. New York, NY: Cambridge University Press. LANGUAGE AND COGNITION LANGUAGE AND COGNITIVE DEVELOPMENT CONNECTIVES-CONDITIONAL VERBS-CONDITIONAL:

Schrader, Carol T. (1989). Written language and use within the context of young children's symbolic play. *Early Childhood Educational Research Quarterly*, 4, 225-244. SEMIOTIC FUNCTIONS SYSTEMIC THEORY LANGUAGE AND PLAY WRITTEN LANGUAGE:

> The purpose of this study was to answer the following question: In what ways do prekindergarten children use language within the context of their spontaneous symbolic play? The participants, who attended the same preschool, were

seven children ranging in age from 5 to 5:6 years. Oral language, writing and play behaviors were transcribed from videotape. Data were classified using Halliday's seven language functions. Results indicate that children write and read what they write when they are involved in sociodramatic play. Functions of children's writing included instrumental, regulatory, interactional, personal and informational purposes. Children did not write for imaginative or heuristic purposes. - From Child Development Abstracts.

Schrier, A., & Stollnitz, F. (Ed.). (1971). *Behavior of non-human primates: modern research trends.* New York, NY: Academic Press. LANGUAGE AND OTHER PRIMATES:

Schulz, Geralyn M., & Ludlow, Christy L. (1991). Botulinum treatment for orolingual-mandibular dystonia: Speech effects. In C. Moore, K. M. Yorkston, & D. R. Beukelman (Eds), *Dysarthria and apraxia of speech*. Baltimore, MD: Paul H. Brookes. MOTOR DISORDERS ARTICULATORY DISORDERS:

Schusterman, R. J., Gisinger, R., Grimm, B. K., & Hanggi, E. B. (1993). Behavior control by exclusion and attempts at establishing semanticity in marine mammals using match to sample paradigms. In L. M. Herman, H. L. Roitblat, & P. E. Nachtigall (Eds), *Language and communication: Comparative perspectives*. Hillsdale, NJ: Lawrence Erlbaum Associates. ANIMAL COMMUNICATIONS:

Schwanenflugel, P. (Ed.) (1991). *The psychology of word meanings*. Hillsdale, NJ: Lawrence Erlbaum Associates. LEXICAL DEVELOPMENT SEMANTIC DEVELOPMENT REPRESENTATIONS-LEXICAL SEMANTIC MAPPING REPRESENTATIONS-SEMANTIC:

Topics covered include: the nature and structure of word meaning, how new word meanings are acquired in childhood and later on in life, and how research and word processing may tell us something about the way in which word meanings are represented and how they relate to language processor.

Schwartz, Bonnie D. (1992). Testing between UG-based and problem-solving models of L2A: Developmental sequence data. *Language Acquisition*, 2, 1-19. L2 EDUCATION L2 LINGUISTIC THEORY:

Schwartz concludes that the UG-based is a closer fit as it predicts a single developmental sequence whereas the problem-solving model predicts several different sequences.

Schwartz, Richard G. (1982). Lexical styles in early language acquisition. In R. N. St Clair, & W. von Raffler-Engel (Eds), *Language and cognitive styles*. Lisse, The Netherlands: Swets and Zeitlinger. LEXICAL DEVELOPMENT INDIVIDUAL VARIATION:

Scliar-Cabral, Leonor. (1985). Mother tongue education at schools in the third world, problems discussed through an experiment among pre-elementary children in Brazil.. In *Rassegna Italiana di Linguistica Applicata*. Roma: Bulzoni. LANGUAGE AND EDUCATION:

Scliar-Cabral, Leonor. (1985). Un exemplo de psicolinguistica aplicada minorar o insucesson escolar (An example of applied psycholinguistics to help diminish drop-outs.). *Perspectiva.*, 2(4), 73-86. LANGUAGE AND EDUCATION: PORTUGUESE

Scliar-Cabral, Leonor. (1986). Processos psicolinguisticos de leitura e a crianca (Psycholinguistic reading processes in children.). *Letras de Hoje.*, 63, 7-20. LITERACY: PORTUGUESE

Scliar-Cabral, Leonor. (1986). Review of J. M. Meisel's 'Language acquisition'. (Review of adquisicion de lenguaje - Aquisicao da linguagem). *Applied Psycholinguistics*, 10, 237-242. BOOK REVIEW :

Scliar-Cabral, Leoner. (1987). Semelhances e diferencas entre a aquisicao das primeira linguas e a aquisicao sistematica das segundas linguas (Similarities and differences between first language acquisition and systematic second language learning). In H. Bohn, & P. Vandresen (Eds), *Topicos de Linguistica Aplicada: O Ensino de Linguas Estrangeiras.*. Florianopolis: UFSC. L2/L1 ACQUISITION: PORTUGUESE

Scliar-Cabral, Leonor. (1987). Variacoes estilisticas em narrativas de pre-escolares. (Stylistic variations in pre-elementary children's narratives.). In *Anais do V Encontro de Estudos Bilinguis e Variacao Linguistica da Regiao Sul*. Florianopolis: Universidade Federal De Santa Caterina. NARRATIVES INDIVIDUAL VARIATION PORTUGUESE: PORTUGUESE

Scliar-Cabral, Leonor. (1989). Pesquisas sobre aquisicao da linguagem no Brasil nos ultimos quinze anos. (Review of the last 15 years of research on language acquisition in Brazil.). In *Anais do I Encontro Nacional sobre Aquisicao da Linguagem*. Porto Alegre: CEAL-PUCRGS. PORTUGUESE OVERVIEW-GENERAL CROSSLINGUISTIC STUDY: PORTUGUESE

Scliar-Cabral, Leonor. (1990). Disturbios da comunicacao. (Language disorders.). *Cadernos do CED*, 15, PORTUGUESE LANGUAGE DISORDERS: PORTUGUESE

Scliar-Cabral, Leonor. (1990). Polaridades em linguagem. (Language polarities.). *Cadernos do CED*, 15, 9-17. PORTUGUESE LANGUAGE TYPOLOGY VARIATION: PORTUGUESE

Scliar-Cabral, Leonor, & Grimm-Cabral, L. (1987). Research on narrativity in literacy improvement. In G. Gagné (Ed.), *Selected papers in mother tongue education. (Etudes in pedagogie de la langue maternalle.)*. Montreal, Canada: Foris Publications. LITERACY LANGUAGE AND EDUCATION NARRATIVES:

Scliar-Cabras, Leonor. (1990). A narratividade aplicada ao diagnostico e a terapia de disturbios da comunicao. (Narrativity applied to assessment and therapy in language impairment.). In *Anais do lo Encontro Sul Americabo de Fonoaudiologia*. Curitiba: EDUCA. NARRATIVES PORTUGUESE ASSESSMENT PROCEDURES INTERVENTION PROGRAMS: PORTUGUESE

Scopesi, Alda, & Ganci, L. (1988). Strategie comunicative tra maschi e femmine in situazione di piccolo gruppo. (Communicative stratgeies between males and females in small groups.). *Contributi dei Dipartimenti e degli Istituti Italiani di Psicologia*, 1 (2), 79-89. ITALIAN LANGUAGE AND GENDER ROLES: ITALIAN

This paper aims to explore verbal communication between males and females in small groups in order to clarify: 1) whether the presence of an adult in the group influences the verbal behavior of males and females: 2) whether the communication between the children is modified according to the sexual homo/heterogeneity of the group. 26 groups of 3 children from 30 to 36 months are observed: 13 are of the same sex and 13 of mixed sex. The results show substantial similarities between the verbal behavior of males and females, albeit with same differences in the communicative strategies adopted.AS

Scopesi, Alda, & Zanobini, M. (1990). Episodi e contesto nelle interazioni tra bambini ed educatrici in asilo nido. (Conversational episodes and context in the interactions among children and teachers in a day care center.). *Eta Evolutiva*, 37, 19-29. LANGUAGE AND EDUCATION ADULT-CHILD INTERACTION SOCIAL INTERACTION CHILDREN'S DIALOGUES CHILDREN'S DISCOURSE: ITALIAN

Scott, D., Isard, Sarah, & de Boysson-Bardies, Bénédicte. (1985). Perceptual isochrony in English and in French. *Journal of Phonetics*, 13, 155-162. LANGUAGE AND COGNITION LANGUAGE AND PERCEPTION FRENCH PROSODY:

Scott, D., Isard, Sarah, & de Boysson-Bardies, Bénédicte. (1986). On the measurement of rhythmic irregularity: a reply to Benguerel. *Journal of Phonetics*, 14, 327-330. PROSODY DISFLUENCIES:

Seidenberg, Mark S. (1990). Lexical access: Another theoretical soapstone? In D. A. Balota, G. B. Flores d'Arcais, & K. Rayner (Eds), *Comprehension processes in reading*. Hillsdale, NJ: Lawrence Erlbaum Associates. LEXICAL ACCESS LITERACY:

Seidenberg, Mark S., & McClelland, James L. (1989). A distributed, developmental model of word recognition and naming. *Psychological Review*, 96, 523-568. CONNECTIONISM WORD RECOGNITION LEXICAL DEVELOPMENT LITERACY:

The model consists of sets of orthographic and phonological units and an interlevel of hidden units. Weights on connections between units were modified during a training phase using the back-propagation learning algorithm. The model simulates many aspects of human performance, including (a)differences between words in terms of processing difficulty, (b) pronunciation of novel items, (c) differences between readers in terms of word recognition skill, (d)transitions from beginning to skilled reading, and (e) differences in performance on lexical decision and naming tasks. The model's behavior early in the learning phase corresponds to that of children acquiring word recognition skills. - From Child Development Abstracts.

Selinker, Larry. (1992). *Rediscovering interlanguage.* New York, NY: Longmans. INTERLANGUAGE:

Sell, M. A. (1992). The development of children's knowledge structures: Events, slots, and taxonomies. *Journal of Child Language*, 19, 659-676. EVENTS/SCRIPTS SLOT-FILLER CATEGORIES CATEGORIZATION:

Selnes, O. A., & Whitaker, H. (1979). Neurological substrates of language and speech production. In S. Rosenberg (Ed.), *Sentence production; developments in research and theory.* Hillsdale, NJ: Lawrence Erlbaum Associates. NEUROLINGUISTICS NEURAL SUBSTRATES SPEECH PRODUCTION:

Semenza, C., Bisiacchi, P. S., & Romani, L. (1992). Naming disorders and semantic representations. *Journal of Psycholinguistic Research*, 21, 349-364. ANOMIA SEMANTIC MAPPING SEMANTIC DISORDERS REPRESENTATIONS-SEMANTIC:

Sena, Rhonda, & Smith, Linda B. (1990). New evidence on the development of the word 'Big'. *Child Development*, 61, 1034-1052. DIMENSIONAL ADJECTIVES SEMANTIC DEVELOPMENT:

When objects vary extremely, younger and older children take 'big' to mean tall. The object to which big is applied also influences whether height, length or area is attended to. In a production task, adults rarely used the word big to describe the stimuli with which children's understanding of big is typically tested. The meaning and use of big is complex and big may not at any age refer simply to the larger object.

Sereno, M. I. (1991). Language and the primate brain. In K. Hammond, & D. Gentner (Eds), *Proceedings of the Thirteenth Annual Conference of the Cognitive Science Society*. Hillsdale, NJ: Lawrence Erlbaum Associates. LANGUAGE AND OTHER PRIMATES NEUROLINGUISTICS:

Serra, Miquel. (1991). Approximation cognitif a la dysphasie. (Cognitive approximation of dysphasia.). *Glossa*. APHASIAS: FRENCH

Serra, Miquel. (1991). Diferencias Individuales en la adquisición del lenguaje. (Individual differences in language acquisition.). In M. Siguan (Ed.), *Estudios de Psicólingüistica, II*. Madrid: Piramide. INDIVIDUAL VARIATION: SPANISH

Sevin, J. A., Matson, Johnny L., Coe, David A., & Fee, Virginia E., et al. (1991). A comparison and evaluation of 3 commonly used autism scales. *Journal of Autism and Developmental Disorders*, 21, 417-432. AUTISM ASSESSMENT PROCEDURES:

Seyfarth, R. M., & Cheney, D. L. (1993). Meaning, reference, and intentionality in the natural vocalizations of monkeys. In L. M. Herman, H. L. Roitblat, & P. E. Nachtigall (Ed.), *Language and communication: Comparative perspectives*. Hillsdale, NJ: Lawrence Erlbaum Associates. VOCALIZATIONS ANIMAL COMMUNICATIONS LANGUAGE AND OTHER PRIMATES:

Shakhnarovich, Aleksandr M., Iur'eva, Nadezhda M., & Leont'ev, Aleksei A. (1990). *Psikholingvisticheskii analiz semantiki i grammatiki : na materiale ontogeneza rechi. (Psycholinguistic analysis of semantics and grammar.)*. Moscow, Russia: Nauka. LEXICAL DEVELOPMENT MORPHOLOGICAL DEVELOPMENT SEMANTIC DEVELOPMENT RUSSIAN: RUSSIAN

Shaklee, Harriet, & Goldston, David. (1989). Development in causal reasoning: Information sampling and judgement rule. *Cognitive Development*, 4, 269-281. CAUSALITY:

The present study investigated development in the ability to sample and use data about probabilistic relationships in order to test causal hypotheses. Third-grade, seventh-grade, and college students were asked to sample cards representing observations of two potentially related events and then to judge the causal relationship between those events. Overall accuracy of causal judgement was low (67-70%correct), with more errors on the noncontingent than on the two contingent relationships. Causal judgement accuracy improved with age across problem types. - From Child Development Abstracts.

Shank, R. O. (1973). Identification of conceptualizations underlying natural language. In R. O. Shank, & K. M. Colby (EdS), *Computer models of thought and language*. San Francisco, CA: Freeman. COMPUTER SIMULATIONS ACQUISITION AND LINGUISTIC THEORY:

Shank, R. O., & Colby, K. M. (Eds). (1973). *Computer models of language and thought.* San Francisco, CA: Freeman. COMPUTER SIMULATIONS:

Shapiro, Jon, Nix, Gary W., & Foster, Steven F. (1990). Auditory perceptual processing in reading disabled children. *Journal of Research in Reading*, 13, 123-132. READING DISORDERS AUDITORY DISCRIMINATION SPEECH PERCEPTION METALINGUISTICS:

One hundred and three children and matched, average readers were administered a battery of auditory perceptual processing tasks. Discriminant analyses indicated that three of the four factors were able to discriminate between the able and disabled readers. Most notable among these was advanced phonological awareness. Auditory discrimination could not discriminate between the groups.

Sharpe, P. (1990). An assessment of the cognitive abilities of multiply handicapped children-adaptations of the Uzgiris and Hunt Scales and their use with children in Britain and Singapore. *Child Care Health and Development*, 16, 335-353. UZGIRIS-HUNT SCALES MULTIHANDICAPPED CHILDREN CROSSCULTURAL STUDY:

Shatz, Marilyn. (1991). Using cross-cultural research to inform us about the role of language in development: Comparisons of Japanese, Korean, and English, and of German, American English and British English. In M. H. Bornstein (Ed.), *Cultural approaches to parenting*. Lawrence Erlbaum Associates. CROSSLINGUISTIC STUDY-PARENTAL SPEECH:

Shatz, Marilyn, & Ebeling, Karen. (1991). Patterns of language learning-related behaviors: Evidence for self-help in acquiring grammar. *Journal of Child Language*, 18, 295-313. SYNTACTIC DEVELOPMENT MONITORING REPETITION:

Four types of language-related learning behaviors were examined in the home environments of four English speaking children. Analysis revealed that the majority of revisions made by the children were grammatical in nature. From Child Development Abstracts.

Shatz, Marilyn, & Wilcox, Sharon A. (1991). Constraints on the acquisition of English modals. In S. A. Gelman, & J. Byrnes (Eds), *Perspectives on language and thought*. New York, NY: Cambridge University Press. LANGUAGE AND COGNITION LANGUAGE AND COGNITIVE DEVELOPMENT CONSTRAINTS-COGNITIVE MODALS :

Shaw, S., & Coggins, T. E. (1991). Interobserver reliability using the phonetic level evaluation with severely and profoundly hearing-impaired children. *Journal of Speech and Hearing Research*, 34, 989-999. METHODOLOGY-ANALYSIS DEAF CHILDREN ASSESSMENT PROCEDURES:

Sheldon, Amy. (1976). Speakers' intuitions about the complexity of relative clauses in Japanese and English. In S. Mufwene, C. Waska, & S. Steever (Eds), *Papers from the Twelfth Annual Meeting of the Chicago Linguistic Society*. Chicago, IL: Chicago Linguistic Society. RELATIVIZATION CROSSLINGUISTIC STUDY-SYNTAX:

Sheldon, Amy. (1977). Assumptions, methods and goals of language acquisition research. *Indian Journal of Applied Linguistics*, 3(1), 1-18. METHODOLOGY:

Also in F. R. Eckman and A. J. Hastings (eds.) 1979. *Studies in first and second language acquisition.* Rowley, MA: Newbury House.

Sheldon, Amy. (1977). On strategies for processing relative clauses: A comparison of children and adults. *Journal of Psycholinguistic Research*, 6(4), 305-318. RELATIVIZATION:

Sheldon, Amy. (1978). The acquisition of relative clauses in French. *Recherches Linguistiques a Montreal*, 10, 263-278. FRENCH RELATIVIZATION:

Published by the Department of Linguistics, University of Montreal.

Sheldon, Amy. (1978). Language development and literacy. In P. D. Pearson, & R. Beach (Eds), *Minnesota perspectives on literacy*. St. Paul, MN: College of Education, University of Minnesota. LITERACY LANGUAGE AND EDUCATION:

Sheldon, Amy. (1979). The acquisition of relative clauses in French and English: Implications for language learning universals. In F. R. Eckman (Ed.), *Current trends in linguistics: Bilingualism, experimental linguistics, and language typologies*. Hemisphere Publishing Corp. RELATIVIZATION FRENCH LANGUAGE UNIVERSALS CROSSLINGUISTIC STUDY-SYNTAX:

Sheldon, Amy. (1985). The relationship between production and perception of the /r/-/l/ contrast in Korean adults learning English: A reply to Borden, Gerber and Milsark. *Language Learning*, 35(1), 107-113. LIQUIDS L2 PHONOLOGY INTERLANGUAGE-PHONOLOGY KOREAN-ENGLISH ENGLISH-KOREAN:

Sheldon, Amy. (1990). 'Kings are royaler than queens': Language and socialization. *Young Children*, 45, 4-9. LANGUAGE AND SOCIAL TRANSMISSION LANGUAGE SOCIALIZATION LANGUAGE AND GENDER ROLES:

Sheldon, Amy. (1990). Pickle fights: Gendered talk in preschool disputes. *Discourse Processes*, 13, 5-31. CHILDREN'S DISCOURSE LANGUAGE AND GENDER ROLES LANGUAGE AND SOCIAL TRANSMISSION LANGUAGE SOCIALIZATION:

Sheldon, Amy. (1992). Conflict talk: Sociolinguistic challenges to self-assertion and how young girls meet them. *Merrill-Palmer Quarterly*, 38, 95-117. LANGUAGE AND GENDER ROLES CHILDREN'S DISCOURSE LANGUAGE SOCIALIZATION LANGUAGE AND SOCIAL TRANSMISSION:

Sheldon, Amy. (1993). Preschool girls' discourse competence: managing conflict and negotiating power. In *Proceedings of the Berkeley Women and Language Conference*. Berkeley, CA: Berkeley Linguistics Society, University of California-Berkeley. CHILDREN'S DISCOURSE COMMUNICATIVE COMPETENCE LANGUAGE AND GENDER ROLES:

Sheldon, Amy. (1993). Saying it with a smile: Girls' conflict talk as double-voice discourse. In E. Mashira, & G. Iverson (Ed.), *Principles and prediction: The analysis of natural Language. Papers in honor of Jerry Sanders* . Philadelphia, PA: John Benjamins. LANGUAGE AND GENDER ROLES LANGUAGE AND SOCIAL TRANSMISSION DISCOURSE ANALYSIS:

Shemesh, Michael. (1990). Gender-related differences in reasoning skills and learning interests of junior high school students. *Journal of Research in Science Teaching*, 27, 27-34. SEX DIFFERENCES:

Seventh to ninth grade students were assessed for their level of mastery of formal reasoning skills by a test based on videotaped simple experiments. Learning interests were assessed by a written response to an open question. Results showed that adolescent boys develop patterns of formal reasoning before their girl classmates. In addition, boys tend to prefer science and technology subjects, while girls tend to prefer language, social studies and humanities. - From Child Development Abstracts.

Shewan, Cynthia M., & Bandur, Donna L. (1986). *Treatment of aphasia: a language-oriented approach*. San Diego, CA: Singular Publishing Group. APHASIAS INTERVENTION PROGRAMS:

Treatment for auditory processing. Materials for auditory processing. Treatment for visual processing. Materials for visual processing. Treatment for gestural and gestural-verbal communication. Materials for gestural and gestural-verbal communication. Treatment for oral expression. Treatment for graphic expression. Materials for graphic expression. Subjects, procedures, and efficacy data for the LOT study.

Shipley, Elizabeth F., & Shepperson, Barbara F. (1990). Countable entities: Developmental changes. *Cognition*, 34, 109-136. NOUNS-COUNT/MASS CLASS INCLUSION CATEGORIZATION:

When children (3:0-4:0) were asked to count labeled entities such as 'forks,' they counted each detached part of a fork as a separate entity. When asked to count kinds or properties, exemplified by several separate objects, they included each discrete object in their count. Their counts of classes were more accurate in the absence of objects, or in the presence of a single member of each class, than in the presence of several members of each class.

Shriberg, Lawrence D. (1990). *PEPPER-Programs to Examine Phonetic and Phonologic Evaluation Records*. Hillsdale, NJ: Lawrence Erlbaum Associates. METHODOLOGY-COMPUTERS METHODOLOGY-ANALYSIS METHODOLOGY-TRANSCRIPTION PHONOLOGICAL DEVELOPMENT PHONOLOGICAL DISORDERS:

A series of programs for phonological analysis.

Shriberg, Lawrence D., Kwiatkowski, Joan, & Snyder, T. (1990). Tabletop versus microcomputer-assisted speech management - response evocation phase. *Journal of Speech and Hearing Disorders*, 55, 635-655. COMPUTER ASSISTED THERAPY INTERVENTION PROGRAMS:

Shute, Brenda, & Wheldall, Kevin. (1989). Pitch alterations in British motherese: some preliminary acoustic data. *Journal of Child Language*, 16(3), 503-512. PARENTAL SPEECH-PROSODY:

Shyamala, K. C. (1986). *Speech disorders in children - an introduction*. Port Blair: Integrated Education for the Disabled Cell, Directorate of Education, Andaman Nicobar Administration. LANGUAGE DISORDERS INTERVENTION PROGRAMS:

Shyamala, K. C. (1989). Verbal stereotypy in autism - a study of expressive language behaviour. *NIMHANS*, 7 (2), 175-179. AUTISM PHONOLOGICAL DISORDERS SYNTACTIC DISORDERS:

In this study, a few specific, isolated and salient features of phonological and syntactic aspects of expressive language behaviour of a small clinical population are identified and gross similarities and differences across these autistic children are reported. This paper is a small extract of a larger project on the study of speech and language characteristic in a cross linguistic autistic group. The verbal features that have been noted are a few phonological aspects including voice, articulation and prosody. Syntactic aspects including speech output, lexicon, pronominal usage, echolalia, perseveration and idiosyncratic featured in terms of all of these. It was felt that there was certainly a developmental delayed as well as deviance in these children in terms of language use. It is noted that, although certain similarities across these children could be discerned at a gross level, each child presented an idiosyncratic picture as to differentiate himself from others in terms of verbal behaviour.

Shyan, M. R., & Wright, A. A. (1993). The effects of language on information processing and abstract concept learning in dolphins, monkeys, and humans. In L. M. Herman, H. L. Roitblat, & P. E. Nachtigall (Eds), *Language and communication: Comparative perspectives*. Hillsdale, NJ: Lawrence Erlbaum Associates. LANGUAGE AND OTHER PRIMATES ANIMAL COMMUNICATIONS CONCEPT DEVELOPMENT LANGUAGE AND COGNITION:

Sidiropoulou, M. (1992). On the connective 'although'. *Journal of Pragmatics*, 17(3), 201-221. CONNECTIVES CONNECTIVES-CONDITIONAL ADVERBS:

Siegal, Michael. (1991). *Knowing children : experiments in conversation and cognition*. Hillsdale, NJ: Lawrence Erlbaum Associates. LANGUAGE AND COGNITIVE DEVELOPMENT COMMUNICATIVE DEVELOPMENT CONVERSATIONAL SKILLS:

Siegel, Linda S., & Brainerd, C. J. (Eds). (1978). *Alternatives to Piaget: Critical essays on the theory*. New York, NY: Academic Press. PIAGETIAN THEORY NEOPIAGETIAN THEORY:

Siegel, Linda S., & Hodkin, B. (1982). The garden path to the understanding of cognitive development: Has Piaget lead us into poison ivy? In S. Modgil, & C. Modgil (Eds), *Jean Piaget - concensus and controversy*. New York, NY: Praeger. PIAGETIAN THEORY LANGUAGE AND COGNITIVE DEVELOPMENT:

Siegler, Robert S. (Ed.). (1990). *Children's thinking: What develops?* Hillsdale, NJ: Lawrence Erlbaum Associates. COGNITIVE DEVELOPMENT:

Siegler, Robert S. (1992). What do developmental psychologists really want?. In M. R. Gunnar, & M. Maratsos (Eds), *Modularity and constraints in language and cognition*. Hillsdale, NJ: Lawrence Erlbaum Associates. MODULARITY CONSTRAINTS LANGUAGE AND COGNITIVE DEVELOPMENT:

Siegler, Robert S., & Jenkins, Eric A. (1989). *How children discover new strategies*. Hillsdale, NJ: Lawrence Erlbaum Associates. COGNITIVE DEVELOPMENT STRATEGY DEVELOPMENT:

> The authors describe new strategy construction processes as being divided into two parts: discovery and generalization. The authors provide interesting insights into the acquisition and development of strategies as their ideas controvert the popular conceptions of strategy development.

Sigel, I. E., Brodzinsky, D. M., & Golinkoff, Roberta M. (Eds). (1981). *New directions in Piagetian theory and practice*. Hillsdale, NJ: Lawrence Erlbaum Associates. PIAGETIAN THEORY NEOPIAGETIAN THEORY LANGUAGE AND COGNITIVE DEVELOPMENT:

Sigurdson, J. (1993). Frequency modulated whistles as a medium for communication with the bottle-nosed dolphin. In L. M. Herman, H. L. Roitblat, & P. E. Nachtigall (Eds), *Language and communication: Comparative perspectives*. Hillsdale, NJ: Lawrence Erlbaum Associates. ANIMAL COMMUNICATIONS:

Sigurjonsdottir, Sigridur. (1993). Binding in Icelandic: Evidence from language acquisition. *UCLA Working Papers in Psycholinguistics*, 2(1). ICELANDIC PARAMETER SETTING CROSSLINGUISTIC STUDY-SYNTAX:

Silva, M. N. (1991). Simultaneity in children's narratives - the case of when, while and as. *Journal of Child Language*, 18, 641-662. NARRATIVES ADVERBS CONNECTIVES:

Silver, L. S., & Halpern, H. (1992). Word-finding abilities of 3 types of aphasic subjects. *Journal of Psycholinguistic Research*, 21, 317-348. APHASIAS LEXICAL ACCESS WORD RECOGNITION:

Silverman, H. J. (1973). *Consciousness and the acquisition of language*. Evanston, IL: Northwestern University Press. LANGUAGE AND COGNITION LANGUAGE AND COGNITIVE DEVELOPMENT:

Silverman, I. W., & Geiringer, E. (1973). Dyadic intervention and conservation induction: A test of Piaget's equilibration model. *Child Development*, 44, 815-879. CONSERVATION PIAGETIAN THEORY LANGUAGE AND COGNITIVE DEVELOPMENT:

Simonsen, Hanne G. (1983). *En norsk femarings sprakbruk. (Language use of a five-year-old.)*. Oslo: Novus. SYNTACTIC DEVELOPMENT NORWEGIAN: NORWEGIAN

> The book is an investigation of the syntax of a Norwegian five-year- old, based on tape-recorded spontaneous speech samples. Both structural and functional aspects of his use of language are discussed and compared to adult spoken language.HGS

Simonsen, Hanne G. (1983). Om hvordan vi snakker med barn-og hvordan barn snakker med hverandre. (On how we talk to children and how children talk to each other.). In M. Gravir (Ed.), *Barnet og talemalet*. Oslo: Universitetsforlaget. ADULT-CHILD INTERACTION SOCIAL SPEECH PARENTAL SPEECH COMMUNICATIVE COMEPTENCE: NORWEGIAN

Simonsen, Hanne G. (1986). Om toaringers fonologi-system og prosesser. (On the phonology of two-year-olds - systems and processes.). In P. Mjaatvan, & L. Smith (Eds), *Barnesprak*. Trondheim: NAVF's senter for barneforskning. PHONOLOGICAL DEVELOPMENT NORWEGIAN: NORWEGIAN

The phonological system of a Norwegian boy at two stages, 2.0 and 2.3, from two points of view-both independently of the adult system, and as deviation from the adult system.HGS

Simonsen, Hanne G. (1987). Fonologiske hierarkier og barns spraktilegnelse. (Phonological hierarchies and children's language acquisition.). *Norskrift*, 52, 87-101. PHONOLOGICAL PATTERNS PHONOLOGICAL UNIVERSALS PHONOLOGICAL DEVELOPMENT ACQUISTION THEORIES-PHONOLOGY: NORWEGIAN

Different types of phonological hierarchies are described and discussed according to their usefulness as models for children's language acquisition.HGS

Simonsen, Hanne G. (1990). Universal aspects of phonological acquisition. In *Proceedings from the Twelfth Scanidinavian Conference of Lingistics*. Reykjavik, Iceland: PHONOLOGICAL DEVELOPMENT PHONOLOGICAL UNIVERSALS SAMOAN NORWEGIAN LIQUIDS :

A discussion of the "phonetic" (Locke) versus the "phonological" (Ingram) model of phonological acquisition in the light of data from Norwegian and Samoan liquids.HGS

Simonsen, Hanne G., & Christensen, Kirsti K. (1980). Nar man byner a ga sann litt pa skolen a sann: en femarings bruj av "sann". (The use of "sann" by a 5-year-old.). In E. Hovdhaugen (Ed.), *The Nordic languages and modern linguistics*. Oslo: Universitetsforlaget. PLURIFUNCTIONALITY: NORWEGIAN

The article discusses the use of the word 'sann' in the speech of a Norwegian five-year-old. 'Sann' is a multiple-function word with two main types of functions: pro-word functions (where the closest English equivalent is 'such,' 'like'), and pragmatic, hedging functions (equivalent to 'like,''sort of.') We try to show how this word can fill several communicative functions, and how the use differs in children and adults because of their different linguistic abilities and needs.HGS

Sinclair, Anne. (1984). Los procedimientos de traducción en el niño. (The procedures of translation in the child.). In M. Siguan (Ed.), *Adquisición precoz de una segunda lengua*. Barcelona, Spain: Ediciónes de la Universidad. BILINGUALISM: SPANISH

Sinclair, Anne, & Berthoud-Papandropoulou, Ioanna. (1984). Children's thinking about the language and their acquisition of literacy. In J. Downing, & R. Valtin (Eds), *Language awareness and learning to read*. New York, NY: Plenum. LITERACY METALINGUISTICS:

Sinclair, Anne, Siegrist, F., & Sinclair, Hermina. (1983). Young children's ideas about the written number system. In D. Rogers, & J. Sloboda (Eds), *The acquisition of symbolic skills*. New York, NY: Plenum. NUMERALS WRITTEN LANGUAGE:

Sinclair, Anne, & Sinclair, Hermina. (1984). Preschool children's interpretation of written numbers. *Human Learning*, 3, 173-184. NUMERALS WRITTEN LANGUAGE:

Sinclair, Anne, Sinclair, Hermina, & de Marcellus, O. (1971). Young children's comprehension and production of passive sentences. *Archives de Psychologie*, 41, 1-22. PASSIVES COMPREHENSION PRODUCTION/COMPREHENSION:

Sinclair, Hermina. (1967). *Langage et operations: Sous-systemes linguistiques et operations concretes. (Language and operations: Linguistic subsystems and concrete operations.)*. Paris, France: Dunod. PIAGETIAN THEORY LANGUAGE AND COGNITIVE DEVELOPMENT CONCRETE OPERATIONAL STAGE:

Sinclair, Hermina. (1969). Developmental psycholinguistics. In D. Elkind, & J. H. Flavell (Eds), *Studies in cognitive development*. New York, NY: Oxford Unviersity Press. PIAGETIAN THEORY LANGUAGE AND COGNITIVE DEVELOPMENT:

Sinclair, Hermina. (1971). Piaget's theory on language acquisition. In M. F. Rosskopf, L. P. Steffe, & S. Taback (Eds), *Piagetian cognitive-development research and mathematical education*. Reston, VA: National Council of Teachers of Mathematics. PIAGETIAN THEORY LANGUAGE AND COGNITIVE DEVELOPMENT:

Sinclair, Hermina. (1971). Representation and memory. In M. F. Rosskopf, L. P. Steffe, & S. Taback (Eds), *Piagetian cognitive-development research and mathematical education*. Reston, VA: National Council of Teachers of Mathematics. LANGUAGE AND MEMORY REPRESENTATIONS PIAGETIAN THEORY:

Sinclair, Hermina. (1971). Sensorimotor action patterns as a condition for the acquisition of syntax. In R. Huxley, & E. Ingram (Eds), *Language acquisition, models and methods*. New York, N.Y.: Academic Press. LANGUAGE AND COGNITIVE DEVELOPMENT SENSORIMOTOR INTELLIGENCE PIAGETIAN THEORY:

Sinclair, Hermina. (1972). Some comments on Fodor's reflection on L.S. Vygotsky's "Thought and Language". *Cognition*, 1, 317-318. PIAGETIAN THEORY VYGOTSKYAN THEORY LANGUAGE AND COGNITIVE DEVELOPMENT:

Sinclair, Hermina. (1973). L'éxplication en linguistique. (Explanation in linguistics.). In L. Apostel, G. Cellevier, & J. T. Desanti, et al. (Eds), *L'éxplication dans les sciences*. Paris, France: Flammarion. OVERVIEW-LINGUISTICS PIAGETIAN THEORY: FRENCH

Sinclair, Hermina. (1973). Taal en denken. (Language and thought). *Tijdschrift voor Orthopedagogik*, , 255-264. PIAGETIAN THEORY LANGUAGE AND COGNITIVE DEVELOPMENT: DUTCH

Sinclair, Hermina. (1974). Apprentissage verbal portant sur la conservation des quantités continués. (Verbal learning and the convservation of continuous quantity.). In H. Sinclair, M. Bovet, & B. Inhelder (Eds), *Apprentissage des structures de la connaissance*. Paris, France: PUF. CONSERVATION PIAGETIAN THEORY LANGUAGE AND COGNITIVE DEVELOPMENT: FRENCH

Sinclair, Hermina. (1974). Epistemology and the study of language. In *Problemes de Psycholinguistique*. Paris, France: Editions du CNRS. PIAGETIAN THEORY LANGUAGE AND COGNITIVE DEVELOPMENT:

Sinclair, Hermina. (1974). From pre-operational to concrete thinking and parallel development of symbolization. In M. Schwebel, et al. (Eds), *Piaget in the classroom.*. New York, NY: Routledge & Kegan Paul. PIAGETIAN THEORY SYMBOL DEVELOPMENT CONCRETE OPERATIONAL STAGE LANGUAGE AND COGNITIVE DEVELOPMENT:

Sinclair, Hermina. (1974). Jean Piaget y la lingüistica. (Jean Piaget and linguistics.). In *Jean Piaget y las sciencias sociales.*. Salamanca, Spain: Sigueme. PIAGETIAN THEORY LANGUAGE AND COGNITIVE DEVELOPMENT: SPANISH

Sinclair, Hermina. (1974). L'acquisition du langage d'un point de vue Piagetien. (The Piagetian viewpoint on the acquisition of language.). *Folia Phoniatrica*, 26, 1-12. PIAGETIAN THEORY LANGUAGE AND COGNITIVE DEVELOPMENT: FRENCH

Sinclair, Hermina. (1974). Le développement des structures sensori-motrices entant que modèle heuristique pour l'élaboration des premières structures linguistiques. (The development of sensorimotor structures as a heuristic model for the elaboration of primary linguistic structures.). *Bulletin d'Audiophonologie*, 4, 355-366. SENSORIMOTOR INTELLIGENCE PIAGETIAN THEORY LANGUAGE AND COGNITIVE DEVELOPMENT: FRENCH

Sinclair, Hermina. (1975). Language and cognition in subnormals. In N. O'Connor (Ed.), *Language, cognitive deficits and retardation*. London, UK: Butterworth. LANGUAGE AND COGNITION RETARDED CHILDREN LANGUAGE AND COGNITIVE DEVELOPMENT:

Sinclair, Hermina. (1977). Études comparatives. (Comparative studies.). In J. Bronckart, P. Malvieu, M. Siguan, H. Sinclair, & A. Tabouret-Keller (Eds), *La genèse de la parole*. Paris, France: PUF. PIAGETIAN THEORY LANGUAGE AND COGNITIVE DEVELOPMENT: FRENCH

Sinclair, Hermina. (1978). Conflict and progress. In *Psychology and biology of language and thought: Essays in honour of Eric Lenneberg*. New York, NY: Academic Press. PIAGETIAN THEORY ACCOMODATION LANGUAGE AND COGNITIVE DEVELOPMENT:

Sinclair, Hermina. (1978). Developmental psycholinguistics. In B. Inhelder, & H. H. Chipman (Eds), *Piaget and his school*. New York, NY: Springer-Verlag. PIAGETIAN THEORY LANGUAGE AND COGNITIVE DEVELOPMENT:

Sinclair, Hermina. (1978). Epistemology and the study of language. In B. Inhelder, & H. H. Chipman (Eds), *Piaget and his school*. New York, NY: Springer-Verlag. PIAGETIAN THEORY LANGUAGE AND COGNITIVE DEVELOPMENT:

Sinclair, Hermina. (1978). L'apport de la théorie de Piaget a l'étude de l'acquisition du langage. (Applying Piagetian theory to the study of the acquisition of language.). *Cahiers de l'Institut de Linguistique de Louvain*, 51(2), 29-41. PIAGETIAN THEORY LANGUAGE AND COGNITIVE DEVELOPMENT: FRENCH

Sinclair, Hermina. (1978). Note on Piaget and dialectics. *Human Development*, 21, 211-213. PIAGETIAN THEORY LANGUAGE AND COGNITIVE DEVELOPMENT:

Sinclair, Hermina. (1978). The relevance of Piaget's early work for a semantic approach to language acquisition. In B. Presseisen, D. Goldstein, & M. Appel (Eds), *Topics in cognitive development*. New York, NY: Plenum. SEMANTIC DEVELOPMENT PIAGETIAN THEORY ACQUISITION AND LINGUISTIC THEORY SEMANTIC HYPOTHESIS:

Sinclair, Hermina. (1980). Language and mathematics: In acquisition. In R. Karplus (Eds), *Proceedings of the Fourth International Congress on Mathematics Education.*. Berkeley, CA: LANGUAGE AND COGNITIVE DEVELOPMENT PIAGETIAN THEORY:

Sinclair, Hermina. (1982). The development of writing in young children: Problems and perspectives. In E. Ferreiro, & M. Gomez-Palacio (Eds), *Nuevas perspectivas sobre los processos de lectura y escritura*. Mexico: Siglo XXI. WRITTEN LANGUAGE PIAGETIAN THEORY:

Sinclair, Hermina. (1982). L'enfant sourd et l'école: Réalité et perspectives. (The deaf child and the school: Reality and perspectives.). *Cahiers du Service Médico-pédagogique (Geneve)*, 2, 27-30. LANGUAGE AND EDUCATION DEAF CHILDREN PIAGETIAN THEORY: FRENCH

Sinclair, Hermina. (1982). La créativité dans le développement cognitif. (Creativity and the development of language.). In N. Nicolaidis, & E. Schmid-Kitsikis (Eds), *Créativité et/ou symptôme*. Paris, France: Glancier-Guenaud. PIAGETIAN THEORY LANGUAGE AND COGNITIVE DEVELOPMENT: FRENCH

Sinclair, Hermina. (1982). Piaget on language: A perspective. In S. Modgil, & C. Modgil (Eds), *Jean Piaget: Consensus and controversy.*. London, UK: Holt, Rinehart & Winston. PIAGETIAN THEORY LANGUAGE AND COGNITIVE DEVELOPMENT:

Sinclair, Hermina. (1982). Sviluppo cognitivo e linguaggio. (The development of cognition and language.). In L. Camaioni (Ed.), *La teoria di Jean Piaget.*. Florence, Italy: Giunti Barbera. PIAGETIAN THEORY LANGUAGE AND COGNITIVE DEVELOPMENT: ITALIAN

Sinclair, Hermina. (1983). Linguistique déscriptive et psychologie cognitive. (Descriptive linguistics and cognitive psychology.). In *Recherches sur le français parle #5*. Aix en Provence, France: Publications de l'Université de Provence. OVERVIEW-PSYCHOLINGUISTICS: FRENCH

Sinclair, Hermina. (1985). Language and cognitive development in Piaget's view. In L. Camaioni, & C. de Lemos (Eds), *Questions on social explanation: Piagetian themes reconsidered*. Amsterdam, The Netherlands: John Benjamins. PIAGETIAN THEORY LANGUAGE AND COGNITIVE DEVELOPMENT:

Sinclair, Hermina. (1986). The transition from sensory-motor behavior to symbolic activity. *Citation Classic*, 18(13), 16. PIAGETIAN THEORY LANGUAGE AND COGNITIVE DEVELOPMENT:

Sinclair, Hermina. (1987). Activités organisatrices du jeune enfant et début du langage. (Organisational activities of young children at the onset of language.). In G. Pierraut-Le Bonniec (Ed.), *Connaitre et le dire*. Bruxelles, Belgium: Mardaga. PIAGETIAN THEORY LANGUAGE AND COGNITIVE DEVELOPMENT: FRENCH

Sinclair, Hermina. (1987). Comments on Thomas Roeper's paper. In S. Modgil, & C. Modgil (Eds), *Noam Chomsky, consensus and controversy*. Sussex, England: Palmer Press. NATIVISM NATURE/NURTURE ACQUISITION AND LINGUISTIC THEORY:

Sinclair, Hermina. (1987). Conflict and congruence in development and learning. In L. S. Liben, & D. H. Feldman (Eds), *Development and learning*. Hillsdale, N.J.: Lawrence Erlbaum Associates. LANGUAGE AND COGNITIVE DEVELOPMENT ASSIMILATION ACCOMODATION PIAGETIAN THEORY:

Sinclair, Hermina. (1987). Language: A gift of nature or a home-made tool? In S. Modgil, & C. Modgil (Eds), *Noam Chomsky, consensus and controversy*. Sussex, England: Palmer Press. NATIVISM NATURE/NURTURE ACQUISITION AND LINGUISTIC THEORY:

Sinclair, Hermina. (1987). Symbolisme et interaction interpersonnelle. (Symbolism and interpersonal interaction.). *Cahiers de la Fondation Archives Jean Piaget*, 8, 155-168. SYMBOL DEVELOPMENT SOCIAL INTERACTION: FRENCH

Sinclair, Hermina (Ed.). (1988). *La production de notations chez le jeune enfant: Langage, nombre, rythmes et mélodies. (Notational production by young children: Language, number, rhythm, and melody.).* Paris, France: PUF. LANGUAGE AND COGNITIVE DEVELOPMENT NUMERALS LANGUAGE AND EDUCATION: FRENCH

Sinclair, Hermina. (1988). Strutture dell' intelligenza e capacita comunicative. (The structure of intelligence and communicative capacity.). In C. Cornoldi, & R. Vianello (Eds), *Handicap, comunicazione e linguaggio.*. Bergamo, Italy: Juvenilia. LANGUAGE AND COGNITIVE DEVELOPMENT: ITALIAN

Sinclair, Hermina. (1989). Language acquisition: A constructivist view. *Cahiers de la Fondation Archives Jean Piaget*, 10. LANGUAGE AND COGNITIVE DEVELOPMENT ACQUISITION THEORIES PIAGETIAN THEORY:

Sinclair, Hermina. (1992). Changing perspectives in child language acquisition. In H. Beilin, & P. B. Pufall (Eds), *Piaget's theory: Prospects and possibilities*. Hillsdale, NJ: Lawrence Erlbaum Associates. PIAGETIAN THEORY NEOPIAGETIAN THEORY LANGUAGE AND COGNITIVE DEVELOPMENT:

Sinclair, Hermina, & Berthoud-Papandropolou, Ioanna. (1983). Essai d'interprétation de quelques procédés langagièrs chez l'enfant. (Essay on the interpretation of certain language procedures in the child.). *Archives de Psychologie*, 51, 139-144. PIAGETIAN THEORY LANGUAGE AND COGNITIVE DEVELOPMENT: FRENCH

Sinclair, Hermina, Berthoud-Papandropolou, Ioanna, Gerard, J., & Veneziano, Edy. (1985). Constructivisme et psycholinguistique génétique. (Constructivism and genetic psycholinguistics.). *Archives de Psychologie*, 53, 37-60. LANGUAGE AND COGNITIVE DEVELOPMENT PIAGETIAN THEORY: FRENCH

Sinclair, Hermina, Berthoud-Papandropoulou, Ioanna, Bronckart, J. P., Chipman, Harold H., Ferreiro, Emilia, & Rappe du Cher, E. (1976). Recherches en psycholinguistique génétique. (Genetic psycholinguistic research.). *Archives de Psychologie*, 44, 157-175. PIAGETIAN THEORY LANGUAGE AND COGNITIVE DEVELOPMENT: FRENCH

Sinclair, Hermina, & Ferreiro, Emilia. (1970). Étude génétique de la compréhension, production et répétition des phrases au mode passif. (Genetic study of the comprehension, production, and repetition of passives.). *Archives de Psychologie*, 40, 1-42. PASSIVES IMITATION: FRENCH

Sinclair, Hermina, & Sinclair, Anne. (1986). Children's mastery of written numerals and the construction of basic number concepts. In J. Hiebert (Ed.), *Conceptual and procedural knowledge: The Case of mathematics*. Hillsdale, NJ: Lawrence Erlbaum Associates. NUMERALS PIAGETIAN THEORY:

Sinclair, Hermina, Stambak, Mira, Lezine, I., Rayna, S., & Verba, M. (1982). *Les bébés et les choses ou la créativité du développement cognitif. (Babies and things or the creativity of cognitive development.)*. Paris, France: PUF. PIAGETIAN THEORY LANGUAGE AND COGNITIVE DEVELOPMENT COGNITIVE DEVELOPMENT: FRENCH

Singer, Murray. (1990). *Psychology of language: An introduction to sentence and discourse processes*. Hillsdale, NJ: Lawrence Erlbaum Associates. LANGUAGE PROCESSING LITERACY:

An upper level/graduate introduction to language processing with particular reference to reading and discourse comprehension.

Sininger, Yvonne S., Klatzky, Roberta L., & Kirchner, Diane M. (1989). Memory scanning speed in language-disordered children. *Journal of Speech and Hearing Research*, 32, 289-297. LANGUAGE AND MEMORY LANGUAGE DISORDERS:

Children with severe language disorders and age- matched controls were evaluated for short-term memory scanning speed. Average per-item scanning speed for the normal children was 66 ms, which was significantly different from the 253 ms average scanning speed of the language disordered group. Results indicate that children with developmental language disorders may demonstrate reduced processing speed or memory retrieval time, which could contribute to linguistic deficits. - From Child Development Abstracts.

Siren, Kathleen A., & Wilcox, Kim A. (1990). The utility of phonetic versus orthographic transcription methods. *Child Language Teaching and Therapy*, 6, 127-146. METHODOLOGY-TRANSCRIPTION:

This study compared composite orthographic and phonetic transcripts derived from the same language sample collected from a three-year-old hearing child of deaf parents. Discrepancies between the transcripts which involved the use of grammatical morphemes were selected for analysis. The largest group of these discrepancies was subjected to spectographic analysis from which both spectral and temporal measurements were made.

Skarakis-Doyle, Elizabeth, MacLellan, N., & Mullin, K. (1990). Nonverbal indicants of comprehension monitoring in language-disordered children. *Journal of Speech and Hearing Disorders*, 55, 461-467. MONITORING COMPREHENSION DISORDERS:

Skarakis-Doyle, Elizabeth, & Mentis, Michelle. (1991). A discourse approach to language disorders: Investigating complex sentence production. In T. M. Gallagher, & N. Rees (Eds), *Pragmatics of language: Clinical practice issues*. San Diego, CA: Singular Group. DISCOURSE DISORDERS COMPLEX SENTENCES METHODOLOGY-DIARY/CASE STUDY:

A review of the development of complex sentences in children's language use, and a description of a case study of language disordered children.

Skarakis-Doyle, Elizabeth, & Mullin, K. (1990). Comprehension monitoring in language-disordered children-a preliminary investigation of cognitive and linguistic factors. *Journal of Speech and Hearing Disorders*, 55, 700-705. MONITORING LANGUAGE AND COGNITIVE DEVELOPMENT COMPREHENSION DISORDERS:

Slater, Alan, Cooper, Rachel, Rose, David, & Morison, Victoria. (1989). Prediction of cognitive performance from infancy to early childhood. *Human Development*, 32, 137-147. LANGUAGE AND COGNITIVE DEVELOPMENT ASSESSMENT PROCEDURES PRELINGUISTICS:

Two longitudinal studies found that measures of looking behavior in early infancy predicted later problem solving and verbal and general intelligence. - From Child Development Abstracts.

Slator, B. (1991). Using context for sense preference. In U. Zernik (Ed.), *Lexical acquisition: Exploiting on-line resources to build a lexicon*. Hillsdale, NJ : Lawrence Erlbaum Associates. CONTEXT LEXICAL DEVELOPMENT SEMANTIC MAPPING:

Sloan, Christine. (1991). *Treating auditory processing difficulties in children*. San Diego, CA: Singular Group. AUDIOLOGY DEAF CHILDREN INTERVENTION PROGRAMS PROCESSING DISORDERS:

Slobin, Dan I. (1992). Introduction. In D. I. Slobin (Ed.), *The crosslinguistic study of language acquisition* . Hillsdale, NJ: Lawrence Erlbaum Associates, Inc., Publishers. CROSSLINGUISTIC STUDY:

These volumes continue to examine findings on the acquisition of different types of languages. Volumes 3 and 4 include selective critical reviews approaching the languages in question as case studies in potential crosslinguistic typologies of acquisitional problems, considering those data which contribute to issues of general theoretical concern in developmental psycholinguistics and linguistic theory.

Sloper, Patricia, Turner, Stephen, Knussen, Christina, & Cunningham, Cliff. (1990). Social life of school children with Down's syndrome. *Child: Care, Health and Development*, 16, 235-251. DOWN SYNDROME LANGUAGE AND SOCIAL CLASS LANGUAGE AND COGNITIVE DEVELOPMENT SOCIAL INTERACTION:

The social integration of Down syndrome children into groups of other children was related to social class, parental education, marital status, recreational orientation, and achievement. In addition, children at the lower end of the IQ range in the sample had fewer informal play contacts. The importance of the family in stimulating children's social development is highlighted by these results.

Smadja, F. (1991). Macroding the lexicon with co-occurrence knowledge. In U. Zernik (Ed.), *Lexical acquisition: Exploiting on-line resources to build a lexicon*. Hillsdale, NJ : Lawrence Erlbaum Associates. LEXICAL DEVELOPMENT SYNTACTIC DEVELOPMENT CONSTRAINTS-SYNTACTIC:

Smit, Ann B., Hand, L., Freilinger, J. J., & Bernthal, John E., et al. (1990). The Iowa articulation norms project and its Nebraska replication. *Journal of Speech and Hearing Disorders*, 55, 779-798. ARTICULATION PHONOLOGICAL DEVELOPMENT PHONETIC INVENTORIES:

Smith, A. (1990). Toward a comprehensive theory of stuttering-a commentary. *Journal of Speech and Hearing Disorders*, 55, 398-401. STUTTERING:

Smith, A. (1992). A theory of neuropsycholinguistic function in stuttering - commentary. *Journal of Speech and Hearing Research*, 35, 805-809. STUTTERING:

Smith, Bruce L., Brown-Sweeney, Sharon, & Stoel-Gammon, Carol. (1989). A quantitative analysis of reduplicated and variegated babbling. *First Language*, 9, 175-190. BABBLING:

The present study investigated babbling by analyzing the utterances of 10 infants who were followed at approximately 4-month intervals from about 6-18 months of age. Although there was a period during which reduplicated utterances were found to occur somewhat more frequently than variegated productions, followed by a period of more frequent occurrences of variegated productions, both types co-occurred throughout the entire age range studied. - From Child Development Abstracts.

Smith, Bruce L., Macaluso, C., & Brown-Sweeney, Sharon. (1991). Phonological effects shown by normal adult speakers learning new words-implications for phonological development. *Applied Psycholinguistics*, 12, 281-298. PHONOLOGICAL DEVELOPMENT VOCABULARY DEVELOPMENT:

Smith, Cheryl A., & Sachs, Jacqueline. (1990). Cognition and the verb lexicon in early lexical development. *Applied Psycholinguistics*, 11, 409-424. LEXICAL DEVELOPMENT VERBS PRODUCTION/COMPREHENSION:

Twenty-four 12-19-month-old children were studied through observation and maternal report of their acquisition of verbs in comprehension and production of nonverbal behavior reflected in play. There is substantive growth in the comprehension of verbs in this period, with a rapid increase between 14-16 months in the total number of verbs and decontextualized verbs comprehended, but no similar surge in production.

Smith, E. E., & Swinney, D. A. (1992). The role of schemas in reading text - a real-time examination. *Discourse Processes*, 15 , 303-316. LITERACY EVENTS/SCRIPTS COMPREHENSION:

Smith, Suzanne T., Macaruso, Paul, Shankweiler, Donald P., & Crain, Stephen. (1989). Syntactic comprehension in young poor readers. *Applied Psycholinguistics*, 10, 429-454. SYNTACTIC DEFICIT HYPOTHESIS READING DISORDERS COMPREHENSION:

Second-grade good and poor readers were tested on spoken sentences with restrictive relative clauses. A high level of performance by both reader groups, demonstrated knowledge of relative clause structure. The poor readers' performance closely paralleled that of the good readers both in pattern of errors and in awareness of the pragmatic aspects of relative clauses.

Smith, Teresa C., Edmonds, Jane E., & Smith, Billy. (1989). The role of sex differences in the referral process as measured by the Peabody Picture Vocabulary Test-Revised and the Wechsler Intelligence Scale for Children. *Psychology in the Schools*, 26, 354-358. PEABODY PICTURE VOCABULARY TEST WECHSLER SCALES SEX DIFFERENCES:

Sex differences apparent in the Peabody Picture Vocabulary Test-Revised (PPVT-R) and the Wechsler Intelligence Scale for Children-Revised (WISC-R) were examined in a sample of 370 to 432 Arkansas school children who were first-time referrals for a psychological evaluation. A separate 2 x 11 (subjects' sex x subjects' age) analysis of variance was performed for each dependent variable. Results indicated sex differences among WISC-R Full Scale, Verbal, and Performance Iqs and PPVT-R standard scores ($p < .01$). Further significant sex differences were indicated at several age groups on each dependent variable, with males consistently scoring higher than females on 87% of the dependent measure excluding the WISC-R subtest Coding, on which females scored higher. - From Child Development Abstracts.

Snow, Catherine E. (1977). Mothers' speech research: From input to interactions. In C. E. Snow, & C. A. Ferguson (Eds), *Talking to children: Language input and acquisition*. New York, NY: Cambridge University Press. SOCIAL INTERACTION HYPOTHESIS PARENTAL SPEECH INPUT FACTORS:

Snow, Catherine E. (1978). The conversational context of language learning. In R. N. Campbell, & P. T. Smith (Eds), *Recent advances in the psychology of language*. New York, NY: Plenum. SOCIAL INTERACTION HYPOTHESIS ADULT-CHILD INTERACTION PARENTAL SPEECH INPUT FACTORS:

Snowdon, C. T. (1993). Linguistic phenomena in the natural communication of animals. In L. M. Herman, H. L. Roitblat, & P. E. Nachtigall (Ed.), *Language and communication: Comparative perspectives*. Hillsdale, NJ: Lawrence Erlbaum Associates. ANIMAL COMMUNICATIONS:

Snowling, M., Chiat, Shulamuth, & Hulme, C. (1991). Words, nonwords, and phonological processes - some comments on Gathercole, Willis, Emslie, and Baddeley. *Applied Psycholinguistics*, 12, 369-373. METHODOLOGY-DESIGN PHONOLOGICAL PROCESSES VOCABULARY DEVELOPMENT LANGUAGE AND MEMORY:

Snyder, Lynn S., & Downey, D. M. (1991). The language-reading relationship in normal and reading-disabled children. *Journal of Speech and Hearing Research*, 34, 129-140. READING DISORDERS LITERACY:

Soederbergh, Ragnhild. (1974). Barnsprakets grammatik. (The grammar of child language.). In U. Teleman, & T. Hultman (Eds), *Spraket i bruk*. Lund: Liber Laromedel Gleerups. SYNTACTIC DEVELOPMENT SWEDISH: SWEDISH

Soederbergh, Ragnhild. (1975). Barnets sprakutveckling och dess konsekvenser for pedagogiken. (The child's language development: implications for education at school.). In I. Ahlgren (Ed.), *Spraket och skolan*. Lund, Sweden: Liber. LANGUAGE AND EDUCATION: SWEDISH

Soederbergh, Ragnhild. (1975). Language by ear and by eye: review article. *Journal of Child Language*, 2 (1), 153-168. LITERACY:

Soederbergh, Ragnhild. (1975). Reading and stages of language acquisition. In W. McCormack, & S. Wurm (Eds), *Language and man: Anthropological issues*. Dordrecht, The Netherlands: Mouton. LITERACY:

Soederbergh, Ragnhild. (1976). Learning to read between two and five: some observations on normal hearing and deaf children. In R. Lado, & T. Anderson (Eds), *Georgetown University Papers on Language and Linguistics No 13: Early Reading*. Washington, DC: Georgetown University Press. LITERACY DEAF CHILDREN:

Soederbergh, Ragnhild. (1976). Learning to read: breaking the code or attaining functional literacy. In R. Lado, & T. Anderson (Eds), *Georgetown University Papers on Language and Linguistics No 13: Early Reading*. Washington, DC: Georgetown University Press. LITERACY:

Soederbergh, Ragnhild. (1977). *Reading in early childhood: a linguistic study of a preschool child's gradual acquisition of reading ability*. Washington, DC: Georgetown University Press. LITERACY:

Soederbergh, Ragnhild. (1979). Barnets sprakliga kreativitet belyst av exempel fran ordbojning och ordbildning. (Children's linguistic creativity: evidence from word inflection and word formation.). *Sprakform och spaknorm*, 67, SWEDISH INFLECTION LEXICAL DEVELOPMENT MORPHOLOGICAL DEVELOPMENT LINGUISTIC CREATIVITY: SWEDISH

Soederbergh, Ragnhild. (1979). *Barnets tidiga sprakutveckling. (Children's early language development.)* . Lund, Sweden: Liber. SWEDISH PRELINGUISTICS FIRST WORDS EARLY SYNTACTIC DEVELOPMENT ADULT-CHILD INTERACTION LINGUISTIC CREATIVITY CROSSLINGUISTIC STUDY-SYNTAX : SWEDISH

Five chapters: 1) Prespeech, first words. 2) First word combinations, crosslinguistic comparisons with English. 3) Talking to children. 4) Dialogue (from adult supported ritual to conversation) 5) The linguistic creativity of the child (in body language, paralinguistics, inflections, word formation: the child as story teller, actor and poet.) RS.

Soederbergh, Ragnhild. (1979). Ritleken-nagra observationer och kommentarer till sprakligt samspel i lek mellan barn och vuxen. (Playing by making drawings together - some observations on language interaction in adult-child play.). *Nordisk Tidsskrift for Logopedi og Foniatri*. LANGUAGE AND PLAY ADULT-CHILD INTERACTION: SWEDISH

Soederbergh, Ragnhild. (1980). Sprakanvandning vid dockskapslek. (The use of language in playing with a doll's house.). *Nysvenska Studier*. LANGUAGE AND PLAY: SWEDISH

Soederbergh, Ragnhild. (1980). Story-telling, dramatic role play and displaced speech in play with dolls. *First Language*, 1. LANGUAGE AND PLAY NARRATIVES:

Soederbergh, Ragnhild. (1981). Teaching deaf preschool children to read in Sweden. In P. Dale, & D. Ingram (Eds), *Child Language: An International Perspective*. Baltimore, MD: University Park Press. LITERACY DEAF CHILDREN:

Soederbergh, Ragnhild. (1982). Early reading as language acquisition. *System*, 9, 207-213. LITERACY:

Soederbergh, Ragnhild. (1982). Linguistic effects by three years of age of extra contact during the first hour post partum. In C. Johnson, & C. Thew (Eds), *Proceedings of the Second International Congress for the Study of Child Language*. Washington, DC: University Press of America. NEONATES PRELINGUISTICS:

Soederbergh, Ragnhild. (1985). Early reading with deaf children. *Prospects*, 15 (1), LITERACY DEAF CHILDREN:

Soederbergh, Ragnhild. (1986). Acquisition of spoken and written language in early childhood. In I. Kurcz, G. Shugar, & J. Danks (Eds), *Knowledge and Language*. Amsterdam, The Netherlands: North-Holland. LITERACY:

Soederbergh, Ragnhild. (1986). From communication as language to language as communication. In B. Lindblom, & R. Zetterstrom (Eds), *Proceedings of an International Symposium held at The Wenner-Gren Center, Stockholm*. New York, NY: The Macmillan Press-Stockton Press. COMMUNICATIVE DEVELOPMENT:

Soederbergh, Ragnhild. (1988). Children's creative communication. In *The Fourth International Congress for the Study of Child Language*. Lund, Sweden: Lund University Press. LINGUISTIC CREATIVITY INTERSUBJECTIVITY PRELINGUISTICS ACQUISITION THEORIES CHILDREN'S DISCOURSE SOCIAL SPEECH BILINGUALISM LITERACY:

Contributions by Soederbergh (Introduction), Colwyn Trevarthen (Infants trying to talk), Loekie Elbers (How children actively create their own language development),

Grace Wales Shugar (The nature of peer discourse), Els Oksaar (Aspects of creativity: interactional strategies of mono- and multi- lingual children), Margaret M. Clark (Literacy learning in creative contexts), and Jon-Roar Bjorkvold (Our musical mother tongue-world wide).

Soederbergh, Ragnhild. (1989). Towards an integrated model of conversational analysis - verbal and nonverbal. In *Proceedings from The Second Scandinavian Child Language Symposium, Lund, 1-2 (Paper 4).* Lund, Sweden: Lund University: Child Language Research Institute. METHODOLOGY-ANALYSIS:

Soederbergh, Ragnhild. (1990). The parent linguist and her child as metalinguistic collaborators. In *Symposium Balticum.* Hamburg: Buske. METALINGUISTICS:

Soederbergh, Ragnhild, & Bredvad-Jensen, A-Ch. (1987). A dialogue model and its application in a free play situation. In P. Lilius, & M. Saari (Eds), *The Nordic Languages and Modern Linguistics 6.* Helsinki: Helsinki University Press. METHODOLOGY-DESIGN:

Soja, Nancy N., Carey, Susan, & Spelke, Elizabeth S. (1991). Ontological categories guide young children's inductions of word meanings: Object terms and substance terms. *Cognition*, 38, 179-211. NOUNS-COUNT/MASS LEXICAL DEVELOPMENT SEMANTIC DEVELOPMENT:

The ontological distinction between objects and non-solid substances conditions projection of word meanings prior to the child's mastery of count/ mass syntax was examined. Two-year-old subjects' projection of the novel word to new objects respected the shape and number of the original referent. In contrast, their projections of new words for non-solid substances ignored shape and number.

Sokolov, Jeffrey L., & MacWhinney, Brian. (1990). The CHIP framework: Automatic coding and analysis of parent-child conversational interaction. *Behavioral Research Methods, Instruments, and Computers*, 22, 151-161. CHILDES DISCOURSE ANALYSIS METHODOLOGY-ANALYSIS METHODOLOGY-COMPUTERS:

Sokolov, Jeffrey L., & Moreton, J. (1993). Individual differences in linguistic imitativeness. In J. L. Sokolov, & C. E. Snow (Eds), *Handbook of research in language development using CHILDES*. Hillsdale, NJ: Lawrence Erlbaum Associates. IMITATION INDIVIDUAL VARIATION METHODOLOGY-DESIGN METHODOLOGY-COMPUTERS CHILDES:

Sokolov, Jeffrey L., & Snow, Catherine E. (Eds). (1993). *Handbook of research in language using CHILDES*. Hillsdale, NJ: Lawrence Erlbaum Associates. METHODOLOGY-DESIGN METHODOLOGY-ANALYSIS METHODOLOGY-COMPUTERS CHILDES CHILD LANGUAGE CORPORA:

> A guide book for both beginners and seasoned researchers wishing to find out more about computer analysis of child language and the CHILDES package. This work includes research reports as well as tutorials on the use of the CHILDES/CLAN programs.

Sokolov, Jeffrey L., & Snow, Catherine E. (1993). Transcript analysis using CHILDES. In J. L. Sokolov, & C. E. Snow (Eds), *Handbook of research in language development using CHILDES*. Hillsdale, NJ: Lawrence Erlbaum Associates. METHODOLOGY-TRANSCRIPTION CHILDES METHODOLOGY-ANALYSIS METHODOLOGY-COMPUTERS:

Sommers, R. K. (1991). Approaches to the prediction of language abilities in a sample of children who have developmental delays. *Journal of Speech and Hearing Research*, 34, 317-324. DEVELOPMENTAL DISORDERS:

Sonino, Elisabetta Zuanelli. (1989). *Literacy in school and society*. New York, NY: Plenum. LANGUAGE AND EDUCATION LITERACY L2 READING PROFICIENCY:

> A collection of interdisciplinary essays dealing with learning to read in a first and/or second language.

Sorsby, Angela J., & Martlew, Margaret. (1991). Representational demands in mothers' talk to preschool children in two contexts: Picture book reading and a modeling task. *Journal of Child Language*, 18, 373-395. PARENTAL SPEECH-STYLE ADULT-CHILD INTERACTION:

24 mother-child dyads were videotaped in each context and their conversations were analyzed for representational demand, interactive features, and communicative function. The mothers' conversation was at a higher level of abstraction during the reading task than it was in the play-dough modeling task. The accuracy of the children's high level responses was greater during the reading task. There was no significant difference between the task in terms of low-level response. From Child Development Abstracts.

Spector, C. C. (1990). Linguistic humor comprehension of normal and language-impaired adolescents. *Journal of Speech and Hearing Disorders*, 55, 533-541. COMPREHENSION FIGURATIVE LANGUAGE:

Spence-Sutton, R., & Woll, B. (1992). The status and functional role of finger spelling in BSL. In M. Marschark, & M. D. Clark (Eds), *Psychological perspectives on deafness*. Hillsdale, NJ: Lawrence Erlbaum Associates. DEAF CHILDREN SIGNING-FINGER SPELLING:

Spencer, Patricia E., & Gutfrend, Mary. (1990). Characteristics of 'dialogues' between mothers and prelinguistic hearing-impaired and normally-hearing infants. *Volta Review*, 92, 351-360. INTERSUBJECTIVITY DEAF CHILDREN PARENTAL INPUT PARENTAL SPEECH-STYLE PARENTAL SPEECH-ATYPICAL CHILDREN ADULT-CHILD INTERACTION:

'Dialogues' between normally-hearing mothers and their prelinguistic hearing-impaired (HI) or normally-hearing (NH) infants were analyzed to determine relative contributions of mothers and infants. No froup differences were found in responsiveness of mothers or infants, HI infants produced fewer potential topic initiating behaviors and mothers of HI infants contributed a greater percent of dyadic topic initiations.

Square-Storer, Paula A., & Apeldoorn, Suzanne. (1991). An Acoustic study of apraxia of speech in patients with different lesion loci. In C. Moore, K. M. Yorkston, & D. R. Beukelman (Eds), *Dysarthria and apraxia of speech*. Baltimore, MD: Paul H. Brookes. APRAXIA TRAUMATIC DISORDERS:

Sroufe, Alan, & Jacobvitz, Deborah. (1989). Diverging pathways, developmental transformations, multiple etiologies and the problem of continuity in development. *Human Development*, 32, 196-203. CONTINUITY/DISCONTINUITY:

Could homotypic continuity be assumed, determining the degree of continuity in individual development over time would be straight forward. But simple stability is rarely obtained for several reasons, as will be illustrated by research examples. Data from an ongoing longitudinal study following children from birth through age 10-11 illustrate impressive continuity over time. - From Child Development Abstracts.

Stambak, Mira, & Sinclair, Hermina (Eds). (1993). *Pretend play among three-year-olds*. Hillsdale, NJ: Lawrence Erlbaum Associates. LANGUAGE AND PLAY PIAGETIAN THEORY:

An edited collection of papers dealing with the Piagetian premises that social interaction with peers leads to collabarative processing which ultimate leads to objective knowledge via shared meanings of the situation. The authors share the collective opinion that spontaneous free play provides a better insight into the workings of children's minds than experimental and laboratory based designs. This translation into English was carried out by Hermina and Morris Sinclair.

Stark, Rachel E. (1989). Temporal patterning of cry and non-cry sounds in the first eight months of life. *First Language*, 9, 107-136. CRYING VOCALIZATIONS:

Cry and non-cry vocalizations produced by two normal infants in the reflexive, pleasure voicing, and/or expansion periods of vocal development were examined and compared with respect to different aspects of temporal patterning. Overall series duration and number of breath groups per series were significantly greater for cry than later emerging non-cry vocalizations. The subtle differences in temporal patterning that were detected may relate to physiological stress factors present only in cry. - From Child Development Abstracts.

Stark, Rachel E., & Tallal, Paula. (1988). *Language, speech, and reading disorders in children: neuropsychological studies*. San Diego, CA: Singular Publishing Group. READING DISORDERS SPECIFIC LANGUAGE IMPAIRMENT ARTICULATION DISORDERS MOTOR DISORDERS ASSESSMENT PROCEDURES:

Background. Research methods. The children with specific language impairment. The children with articulation impairment. The children with reading impairment. Research implications. Implications for clinical management. Standardized tests. Standard procedures. Neurodevelopmental protocol. Glossary. References. Author index. Subject index.

Starkweather, C. W. (1990). Concomitant speech and language disorders in stuttering children-a critique of the literature - comment. *Journal of Speech and Hearing Disorders*, 55, 802-803. STUTTERING:

Steffenburg, Suzanne, Gillberg, Christopher, Hellgren, Lars, Andersson, Lena, Gillberg, I. Carina, Jakobsson, Gun, & Bohman, Michael. (1989). A twin study of autism in Denmark, Finland, Iceland, Norway and Sweden. *Journal of Child Psychology and Psychiatry*, 30, 405-416. MULTIPLE BIRTHS AUTISM CROSSLINGUISTIC STUDY-DISORDERS CONGENITAL DISORDERS:

The Nordic countries were screened for the occurance of cases of autism with a same-sexed twin under age 25 years. Twenty-one pairs (11 monozygotic and 10 dizygotic) of twins and one set of identical triplets were found and extensively examined. The concordance for autism by pair was 91% in the monozygotic and 0% in the dizygotic pairs. The corresponding concordances for cognitive disorder were 91% and 30%, respectively. In most of the pairs discordant for autism, the autistic twin had more perinatal stress. The results lend support for the notion that autism has a heriditary component and that perinatal stress is involved in some cases.

Steinstrater, Christiane. (1990). *Zur kindlichen Sprechhandlungsfähigkeit : Analyse eines Korpus spontaner Sprechsprache einer Fünfjährigen. (On the language capabilities of children: An analysis of a spontaneous corpus from a five-year-old.).* Frankfurt am Main, Germany: P. Lang. GERMAN METHODOLOGY-DIARY/CASE STUDY: GERMAN

Stemberger, Joseph P. (1989). Speech errors in early child language production. *Journal of Memory and Language*, 28(2), 164-188. SPEECH ERRORS PHONOLOGICAL SUBSTITUTIONS PHONETIC VARIATION:

Stemberger, Joseph P. (1992). A connectionist view of child phonology: Phonological processing without phonological processes. In C. A. Ferguson, L. Menn, & C. Stoel-Gammon (Eds), *Phonological development: Models, research, implications*. Monkton, MD: York Press. CONNECTIONISM PHONOLOGICAL PROCESSES RULES-PHONOLOGICAL:

Stemmer, Nathan. (1971). Some aspects of language acquisition. In Y. Bar-Hillel (EdS), *Pragmatics of Natural Languages.*. Dordrecht: Reidel. ACQUISITION THEORIES-EMPIRICIST:

Stemmer, Nathan. (1973). Language acquisition and classical conditioning. *Language and Speech*, 16, 279-282. LANGUAGE AND BEHAVIORISM ACQUISITION THEORIES-EMPIRICIST:

Stemmer, Nathan. (1975). On semantic approaches to language acquisition. *Language Sciences*, 34, 8-11. ACQUISITION THEORIES-SEMANTICS:

Stemmer, Nathan. (1981). A note on empiricism and structure-dependence. *Journal of Child Language.*, 8, 649-656. ACQUISITION THEORIES-EMPIRICIST:

Stemmer, Nathan. (1982). On cognitive factors in language acquisition: Generalization classes versus concepts. In R. N. St Clair, & W. von R. Engel (Eds), *Language and cognitive styles*. Lisse: Swets and Zeitlinger. ACQUISITION THEORIES-EMPIRICIST CONCEPT DEVELOPMENT LEXICAL DEVELOPMENT:

Stemmer, Nathan. (1983). *The roots of knowledge*. Oxford: Blackwell. ACQUISITION THEORIES-SEMANTICS CONCEPT DEVELOPMENT LEXICAL DEVELOPMENT ACQUISITIOIN THEORIES-EMPIRICIST:

Stemmer, Nathan. (1984). Empiricist versus mentalist theories of language acquisition. *Semiotica*, 49, 139-159. ACQUISITION THEORIES-EMPIRICIST:

Stemmer, Nathan. (1985). The role of generalization classes in language acquisition. *Communication and Cognition*, 18, 263-279. ACQUISITION THEORIES-EMPIRICIST LEXICAL DEVELOPMENT CONCEPT DEVELOPMENT:

Stemmer, Nathan. (1989). The acquisition of the ostensive lexicon: The superiority of empiricist over cognitive theories. *Behaviorism*, 17, 41-61. ACQUISITION THEORIES-EMPIRICIST LEXICAL DEVELOPMENT OSTENTATION:

Stemmer, Nathan. (1989). Empiricist versus prototype theories of language acquisition. *Mind and Language*, 4, 201-221. ACQUISITION THEORIES-EMPIRICIST PROTOTYPE THEORY LEXICAL DEVELOPMENT CATEGORIZATION:

Stemmer, Nathan. (1990). Skinner's 'Verbal Behavior', Chomsky's review, and mentalism. *Journal of the Experimental Analysis of Behavior*, November. LANGUAGE AND BEHAVIORISM ACQUISITION THEORIES-EMPIRICIST:

Stern, Daniel N. (1989). Crib monologues from a psychoanalytic perspective. In K. Nelson (Ed.), *Narratives from the crib*. Cambridge, MA: Harvard University Press. CRIB SPEECH NARRATIVES LANGUAGE AND FREUDIAN THEORY:

Stern, Wilhelm, & Stern, Clara. (1965[1907]). *Die Kindersprache*. Darmastadt, Germany: Wissenschaftliche Buchgesellschaft. GERMAN: GERMAN

This is a 1965 re-issue of the 1928 third edition of the Sterns' classic treatise on child language. The first edition was published in 1907 and the second in 1914.

Sternberg, Robert J., & Berg, Cynthia A. (1992). *Intellectual development*. New York, NY: Cambridge University Press.
LANGUAGE AND COGNITIVE DEVELOPMENT PIAGETIAN THEORY COGNITIVE DEVELOPMENT NEOPIAGETIAN THEORY:

A life-span approach to intellectual development which includes overviews of cognitive development from a variety of perspectives including Piagetian and Neo-Piagetian theory, psychometry, information processing, learning theory, and context. The book attempts to synthesise the various theories into a cohesive model of intellectual development.

Sternberg, Robert J., & Okagaki, Lynn. (1989). Continuity and discontinuity in intellectual development are not a matter of 'either-or'. *Human Development*, 32, 158-166.
CONTINUITY/DISCONTINUITY PIAGETIAN THEORY:

The question of whether intellectual development is continuous or discontinuous is not a meaningful one if these two patterns of development are held to be mutually exclusive. We attempt to demonstrate the validity of our argument successively for psychometric, Piagetian, cognitive and contextual points of view, and then make the same demonstration in somewhat more detail from the standpoint of the triarchic theory of human intelligence. - From Child Development Abstracts.

Stevens, James. (1992). *Applied multivariate statistics for the social sciences*. Hillsdale, NJ: Lawrence Erlbaum Associates.
METHODOLOGY-ANALYSIS:

This volume stresses narrative discussions of the issues, and practical applications of multivariate analysis rather than the complex mathematics that underpin it.

Stevenson, Rosemary J. (1991). Maturation and learning: linguistic knowledge and performance: a commentary on Clahsen and Felix. In J. Weissenborn, H. Goodluck, & T. Roeper (Eds), *Theoretical issues in language acquisition: Continuity and change in development*. Hillsdale, NJ: Lawrence Erlbaum Associates.
ACQUISITION THEORIES NATURE/NURTURE:

Stevenson, Rosemary J. (1993). *Language, thought and representation*. New York, NY: John Wiley & Sons. LANGUAGE AND COGNITION REPRESENTATIONS COMPUTER SIMULATIONS:

An examination of the development of ideas about the relationship between language, thought, and representation from the early days of cognitive psychology to the present. The focus is on psychology, but the book also covers linguistics, philosophy, and artificial intelligence.

Stewart, J., & Sinclair, Hermina. (1975). Comprehension of questions by children between 5 and 9. *International Journal of Psycholinguistics*, 3, 17-26. QUESTIONS COMPREHENSION LATER SYNTACTIC DEVELOPMENT:

Stockman, I. J., & Vaughn-Cooke, F. (1992). Lexical elaboration in children's locative action expressions. *Child Development*, 63, 1104-1125. SPATIAL TERMS LOCATIVES ORIENTATIONAL TERMS:

Stoefen-Fisher, J. M., & Balk, J. (1992). Educational programs for children with hearing loss - least restrictive environment. *Volta Review*, 94, 19-28. DEAF CHILDREN LANGUAGE AND EDUCATION:

Stoel-Gammon, Carol. (1989). Prespeech and early speech development of two late talkers. *First Language*, 9, 207-224. BABBLING FIRST WORDS RETICENCE/TALKATIVENESS LINGUISTIC PRECOCITY:

Speech samples of 34 children were analyzed to determine patterns of babbling and early word productions from 9 to 24 months. The present study focuses on the vocal and verbal development of two 'late talkers.' Analysis of these subjects' prespeech utterances revealed that one of them produced a few canonical babbles from 9 to 21 months. The other displayed an unusual pattern of sound preferences in his babbles. At 24 months, word productions of both late talkers evidenced more phonetic repertoires and simpler syllable shapes than those used by their peers. - From Child Development Abstracts.

Stoel-Gammon, Carol. (1992). Prelinguistic vocal development: measurement and predictions. In C. A. Ferguson, L. Menn, & C. Stoel-Gammon (Eds), *Phonological development: Models, research, implications*. Monkton, MD: York Press. BABBLING VOCALIZATIONS ASSESSMENT PROCEDURES METHODOLOGY-ANALYSIS:

Stoel-Gammon, Carol. (1992). Research on phonological development: recent advances. In C. A. Ferguson, L. Menn, & C. Stoel-Gammon (Eds), *Phonological development: Models, research, implications*. Monkton, MD: York Press. PHONOLOGICAL DEVELOPMENT:

Stoker, R. (1991). Language issues in the education of hearing-impaired children. *Volta Review*, 93, 323-324. LANGUAGE AND EDUCATION DEAF CHLDREN:

Stone, Wendy L., & Caro-Martinez, Lourdes M. (1990). Naturalistic observations of spontaneous communication in autistic children. *Journal of Autism and Developmental Disorders*, 20, 437-453. AUTISM:

> Children with autism were observed during their everyday school activities in order to examine patterns of spontaneous communication. Communication patterns were found to vary as a function of the child's cognitive level and severity of autism.

Strauss, Alfred A., Lehtinen, Laurae, & Kephart, Newell C. (1989). *Psychopathology and education of the brain-injured child*. San Diego, CA: Singular Publishing Group. TRAUMATIC DISORDERS ATYPICAL DEVELOPMENT LANGUAGE AND EDUCATION:

> Historical review. Anatomy of the brain and its function. Perception and perceptual disturbances of brain-injured children. Thinking disorders in brain-injured children. Behavior disorders in brain-injured children. Testing the brain-injured child. Clinic and diagnosis of brain-injury in children. The concept of the exogenous child versus the endogeneous child. General principles in the education of the brain-injured child. Teaching arithmetic to brain- injured children. Teaching writing to brain-injured children. Anatomy and physiology of the central nervous system. Embryology and

brain-injury. Psychopathology of perception. Psychopathology of language. Psychopathology of behavior. Testing the brain-injured child with normal I.Q. References. Index.

Street, Richard L., & Cappella, Joseph N. (1989). Social and linguistic factors influencing adaptation in children's speech. *Journal of Psycholinguistic Research*, 18, 497-519. INDIVIDUAL VARIATION CHILDREN'S RESPONSES COMMUNICATIVE COMPETENCE SOCIOLINGUISTIC FACTORS:

Patterns of adaptation related to specific linguistic and pragmatic abilities, such as verbal responsiveness, involvement in the interaction, and the production of relatively complex syntactic structures were studied. Children generally reciprocated changes in the adult's speech rate and response latency and there were differences in degree and type of adaptation within specific dyads. Chronological age was not useful in accounting for this individual variation, but specific linguistic and social abilities were. - From Child Development Abstracts.

Streri, Arlette, & Spelke, Elizabeth S. (1989). Effects of motion and figural goodness on haptic object perception in infancy. *Child Development*, 60, 1111-1125. OBJECT PERMANENCE:

Four-month-old infants held 2 rings, 1 in each hand, out of view. The rings moved rigidly together and were either the same or different in substance, weight, texture and shape. After haptic habituation to a ring display, patterns of preferential looking to visibly connected vs. separated rings provided evidence that the infants perceived the rings in both experiments as parts of one connected object. - From Child Development Abstracts.

Stromqvist, Sven. (1980). Games of repair and child language development: Some hypotheses and observations. In E. Hovdhaugen (Ed.), *The Nordic languages and modern linguistics*. Oslo, Sweden: Universitersforlaget. CONVERSATIONAL REPAIRS SWEDISH NORWEGIAN DANISH:

Stromqvist, Sven. (1981). The pragmatics of prosody in children's pretend play. In T. Fretheim (Ed.), *Nordic prosody.* Tapir: LANGUAGE AND PLAY PROSODY:

Stromqvist, Sven. (1981). Remarks on referential ambiguity in play. *Gothenburg Papers in Theoretical Linguistics*, 43, LANGUAGE AND PLAY AMBIGUITY REFERENCE:

Stromqvist, Sven. (1983). Utkast till en teori for tillagnandet av personliga pronomen (Towards a theory of the acquisition of personal pronouns.). *Gothenburg Papers in Theoretical Linguistics*, 84, PRONOUNS-PERSONAL SWEDISH: SWEDISH

Stromqvist, Sven. (1984). *Barns sprak: teorier och iakttagelser (Children's language: Theories and observations).* Malmo: Liber. ACQUISITION THEORIES: SWEDISH

Stromqvist, Sven. (1984). Make-believe through words: A linguistic study in children's play with a doll's house. *Gothenburg Monographs in Linguistics*, 4. REFERENCE DEIXIS LANGUAGE AND PLAY SWEDISH:

In this study, aspects of make-believe play are analysed from a linguistic point of view. The data are drawn from video recordings of 26 Swedish three-yearolds and their mothers playing with a doll's house. A set of linguistic devices, mainly deictic, used by the children and mothers to shift between reference to the make-believe world and reference to the real world is analysed. Also, a special type of utterances employed by children during make-believe play as a means to exist actions on the make-believe level is analyzed.

Stromqvist, Sven. (1985). Tre fragor om barns sprakutveckling (Three questions about child language development). In J. H. Ahlsen, & E. Hjelmquist (Eds), *Tal, Ljud, Horsel 2.* Gotenborg, Sweden: University of Gotenborg: Department of Linguistics. OVERVIEW-THEORY: SWEDISH

Stromqvist, Sven. (1988). Svenska i ett ontogenetiskt perspektiv (Swedish in an ontogenetic perspective). In P. Linell (Ed.), *Svenskans beskrivning 16*. Linkoping: University of Linkoping: Department of Communication Studies. SWEDISH: SWEDISH

Stromswold, K. (1993). The acquisition of WH-questions. In J. L. Sokolov, & C. E. Snow (Eds), *Handbook of research in language development using CHILDES*. Hillsdale, NJ: Lawrence Erlbaum Associates. QUESTIONS-WH METHODOLOGY-DESIGN METHODOLOGY-COMPUTERS CHILDES:

Strong, C. J., & Shaver, J. P. (1991). Stability of cohesion in the spoken narratives of language-impaired and normally developing school-aged children. *Journal of Speech and Hearing Research*, 34, 95-111. DISCOURSE COHERENCE NARRATIVES:

Stuckless, E. R. (1991). Reflections on bilingual, bicultural education for deaf children - some concerns about current advocacy and trends . *American Annals of the Deaf*, 136, 270-272. BILINGUALISM-CULTURAL FACTORS BILINGUALISM-EDUCATION BIMODALITY DEAF CHILDREN BIMODALITY:

Studdert-Kennedy, Michael. (1991). Comment: the emergent gesture. In I. G. Mattingly, & M. Studdert-Kennedy (Eds), *Modularity and the motor theory of speech perception*. Hillsdale, NJ : Lawrence Erlbaum Associates. PHONETIC GESTURES SPEECH PERCEPTION:

Studdert-Kennedy, Michael. (1991). Language development from an evolutionary perspective. In N. A. Krasnegor, et al. (Eds), *Biological and behavioral determinants of language development*. Hillsdale, NJ: Lawrence Erlbaum Associates. ACQUISITION THEORIES:

Studdert-Kennedy, Michael. (1992). Leap of faith - a review of language and species. *Applied Psycholinguistics*, 13, 515-527. HUMAN SPECIFICITY LANGUAGE AND OTHER PRIMATES:

Sturmey, P., Matson, Johnny L., & Sevin, J. A. (1992). Analysis of the internal consistency of 3 autism scales. *Journal of Autism and Developmental Disorders*, 22, 321-328. AUTISM ASSESSMENT PROCEDURES:

Subramanyaiah, M. G. (1981). Acquisition of morphological rules for plural allomorphs in Kannada-a pilot study. *Jaiish*, 12, 57-61. KANNADA MORPHOLOGICAL DEVELOPMENT RULES-MORPHOLOGICAL WUG TEST MORPHOSYNTACTIC DEVELOPMENT:

This study was conducted to evaluate the acquisition of morphological rules in children using a test developed in Kannada. This test is based on 'Wug test' developed by Jean Berko in English. The subjects consisted of fourteen children of age range 9-10 years. Three kinds of plural allomorphs were studied (galu, aru and ondiru) which were frequently used by children and adults whose native language was Kannada. Cloze tecniques were used to assess the knowledge about the morphological rules of Kannada language. Results indicated that most of the children did not have any difficulty with usage of /galu/ form. They substituted /galu/ for /aru/. All had difficulty with /andiru/ form. The poor performance may not have been wholly due to the lack of knowledge of these rules but may have been due to other factors also. A general heirarchy in terms of substitution may be suggested. This phenomen suggests the manner by which equilibrium is upset and also the process of how it is slowly gained.

Suffridge, K. H. (1973). Prelinguistics, imagery, cognition: An individual experience. *Volta Review*, 75(2), 82-87. PRELINGUISTICS LANGUAGE AND COGNITIVE DEVELOPMENT INDIVIDUAL VARIATION:

Sugarman, Susan. (1987). *Piaget's construction of the child's reality*. New York, NY: Cambridge University Press. OVERVIEW-PIAGET PIAGETIAN THEORY NEOPIAGETIAN THEORY LANGUAGE AND COGNITIVE DEVELOPMENT:

A close, conceptual critique of select portions of Piaget's theory of mental development in children. The study focuses on six of Piaget's earlier, richer works, and argues that even if his claims were empirically accurate, his theses simply could not describe the way children think, or the way in which their thinking develops. By working through the details of Piaget's arguments, Sugarman suggests alternative lines of inquiry that should result in a clearer understanding of children's mental life, and the origins of adult thought.

Sugárné Kádár, Julia. (1976). *A beszédfejlödés utjai - beszédfejlesztés az óvodában (Modes of speech development - language training in kindergarten)*. Budapest: Tankönyvkiadó. LANGUAGE AND EDUCATION HUNGARIAN: HUNGARIAN

Sugárné Kádár, Julia. (1977). A preverbális kommunikációs készség jellemzöi (Communicative skills in the prelinguistic period). *Magyar Pszichológiai Szemle*, 34, 351-362. PRELINGUISTICS INTENTIONALITY INTERSUBJECTIVITY HUNGARIAN: HUNGARIAN

Sugárné Kádár, Julia. (1982). A beszéd kialakulásának feltételei és megjelenési formai a vokális kommunikációban (Preconditions and forms of the emergence of speech in vocal communication). *Pszichológia*, 2, 259-277. PRELINGUISTICS LANGUAGE PRECURSORS HUNGARIAN: HUNGARIAN

Sugárné Kádár, Julia. (1984). Die Vokalisation des Sauglings und deren Beziehung zur Empathik der Eltern. Psychologie aus Ungarn. Herausgegeben von F. Pataki. (Infants' vocalizations and parental interaction. Psychology from Hungary. The work of F. Pataki). *Zeitschrift für Psychologie*, 6, 67-71. VOCALIZATIONS INTERSUBJECTIVITY HUNGARIAN PARENTAL INPUT INPUT FACTORS SOCIAL INTERACTION HYPOTHESIS: GERMAN

Sugárné Kádár, Julia (Ed.). (1985). *Beszéd és kommunikáció az óvodás és kisiskoláskorban (Speech and communication in preschool and early school years).*, *vol.*. Budapest: Akadémiai Kiadó. LANGUAGE AND EDUCATION HUNGARIAN: HUNGARIAN

Sugárné Kádár, Julia. (1985). A beszéd prozódia szerepének fejlödése (Evolution of the role of prosody in speech). In J. S. Kádár (Ed.), *Beszéd és kommunikáció az óvodás és kisiskoláskorban*. Budapest: Akadémiai Kiadó. PROSODY HUNGARIAN: HUNGARIAN

Sugárné Kádár, Julia. (1985). A szókincs és a szófajok 3-6 éves korü gyermekek beszédében különbözö beszédhelyzetekben. (Vocabulary and parts of speech in 3-6 year old children's speech in various speech situations.). In J. S. Kádár (Ed.), *Beszéd és kommunikáció az óvodás és kisiskoláskorban*. Budapest: Akadémiai Kiadó. WORD CLASS WORD CHOICE VOCABULARY DEVELOPMENT HUNGARIAN: HUNGARIAN

Sugárné Kádár, Julia. (1985). A vizuális és audiovizuális élmény megfogalmazásának fejlödése (The development of the verbalization of visual and audiovisual experiences). In J. S. Kádár (Ed.), *Beszéd és kommunikáció az óvodás és kisiskoláskorban*. Budapest: Akadémiai Kiadó. CHILDREN'S DESCRIPTIONS NARRATIVES HUNGARIAN: HUNGARIAN

Sugárné Kádár, Julia. (1987). Different social ways of kindergartner's speech development. *Studia Psychologica*, 29/3, 185-202. SOCIAL SPEECH LANGUAGE AND SOCIAL CLASS HUNGARIAN:

Sugárné Kádár, Julia. (1988). Early phases of speech development. In A. Fusco, F. M. Battisti, & R. Tomasoni (Eds), *Issues in cognition and social representation.*. Milano: Franco Angeli. PRELINGUISTCIS HUNGARIAN:

Sugárné Kádár, Julia, & Reok, György. (1985). A szociokulturálisan hátrányos és az átlagoszociálishelyzetü 4-6 éves gyermekek beszédkészségénekjellemzöi. (Characteristics of speech readiness in socioculturally disadvantaged and normal socially situated 4-6 year old children.). In J. S. Kádár (Ed.), *Beszéd és kommunikáció az óvodás és kisiskoláskorban*. Budapest: Akadémiai Kiadó. LANGUAGE AND SOCIAL CLASS HUNGARIAN: HUNGARIAN

Sullivan, Ann, Kelso, Jane, & Stewart, Mark. (1990). Mothers' views on the ages of onset for four childhood disorders. *Child Psychiatry & Human Development*, 20, 269-278. AUTISM ATTENTION DEVELOPMENTAL DISORDERS CONGENITAL DISORDERS:

> The mothers of 120 children were asked a series of questions about their views on the ages at which their children became deviant. The symptoms of autism were noted at 15 months and attention-deficit hyperactivity disorder (ADHD), or conduct disorder plus ADHD, did not separate by age of onset. The mean for both groups was the fourth year of life.

Sulzby, E., & Barro, L. (1990). The oral monologue as a form of emergent reading. In A. McCabe, & C. Peterson (Eds), *Developing narrative structure*. Hillsdale, NJ: Lawrence Erlbaum Associates. NARRATIVES LITERACY:

Surian, Luca. (1991). Do children exploit the Maxim of Antecedent in order to interpret ambiguous descriptions. *Journal of Child Language*, 18, 451-457. AMBIGUITY ITALIAN:

20 Italian 6 year olds, and 20 8 year-olds were asked to interpret eight ambiguous and eight unambiguous descriptions. In both conditions there was a clear preference for the use of a comprehension strategy based on the Maxim of Antecedent. From Child Development Abstracts.

Surian, Luca, & Levorato, Maria C. (1988). Comunicazione referenziale e processi di categorizzazione. (Referential communication and categorization processes.). *Rassegna di Psicologia*, 2, 63-82. CATEGORIZATION REFERENTIAL COMMUNICATION PROTOTYPE THEORY: ITALIAN

A typicality effect on the communicative adequacy of messages was observed when typical and atypical basic objects (after Rosche) were used in the classic referential communication task.MCL

Swann, Joan. (1992). *Girls, boys and language*. Oxford, UK: Basil Blackwell. SEX DIFFERENCES LANGUAGE AND EDUCATION:

An overview of gender related language issues and how they relate to educational practice.

Swanson, Lori A., Leonard, Laurence B., & Gandour, Jack. (1992). Vowel duration in mothers' speech to young children. *Journal of Speech and Hearing Research*, 35, 617-625. PARENTAL SPEECH-STYLE PARENTAL SPEECH-PHONOLOGY:

Swigart, Elca T. (1986). *Normal hearing screening*. San Diego, CA: Singular Publishing Group. AUDIOMETRY ASSESSMENT PROCEDURES:

Information to consider in implementing a neonatal hearing screening program. Model programs.

Swisher, M. V. (1992). The role of parents in developing visual turn-taking in their young deaf children. *American Annals of the Deaf*, 137, 92-100. DEAF CHILDREN TURN TAKNG PARENTAL INPUT:

Szatmari, P. (1992). A review of the DSM-III-R criteria for autistic disorder . *Journal of Autism and Developmental Disorders*, 22, 507-523. CLASSIFICATION OF DISRODERS AUTISM:

Szende, Tamás. (1975). Adalék a gyerek beszédhangrendszerének kialakulásához: Az/r/-/j/ hanghelyettesítés. (The evolving sound system: the /r/- /j/ sound substitution). *Nyelvtudományi Közlemények*, 77, 194-199. PHONOLOGICAL SUBSTITUTIONS LIQUIDS GLIDES HUNGARIAN: HUNGARIAN

T

Taeschner, Traute. (1991). *A developmental psycholinguistic approach to second language teaching*. Norwood, NJ: Ablex Pub. L2 EDUCATION BILINGUALISM-EDUCATION LANGUAGE AND EDUCATION:

English translation of "Insegnare la lingua straniera.".

Taft, Marcus. (1992). *Reading and the mental lexicon*. Hillsdale, NJ: Lawrence Erlbaum Associates. LITERACY LEXICAL ACCESS REPRESENTATIONS-LEXICAL CONNECTIONISM:

A review of the research on lexical processing, lexical access, and lexical representation and how they function in reading which leads to the proposal of a connectionist model of the reading process.

Tager-Flusberg, Helen. (1991). Semantic processing in the free recall of autistic children - further evidence for a cognitive deficit. *British Journal of Developmental Psychology*, 9, 417-430. LANGUAGE AND COGNITIVE DEVELOPMENT AUTISM:

Tager-Flusberg, Helen. (1992). Autistic children's talk about psychological states - deficits in the early acquisition of a theory of mind. *Child Development*, 63, 161-172. THEORY OF MIND AUTISM:

Tager-Flusberg, Helen. (1993). *Constraints on language acquisition: Studies of atypical children*. Hillsdale, NJ: Lawrence Erlbaum Associates. ATYPICAL DEVELOPMENT DEAF CHILDREN BLIND CHILDREN CEREBRAL DISORDERS TRAUMATIC DISORDERS DOWN SYNDROME RETARDED CHILDREN AUTISM CONSTRAINTS MODULARITY NEUROLINGUISTICS CORTICAL STRUCTURES LANGUAGE AND PERCEPTION:

Each of the papers in this book throws light on some aspect of the interrelationship of innate language specific mechanisms and cortical structures and social cognition, and their role in the construction of linguistic ability. Information about this interrelationship is drawn from studeis of atypcial language development.

Tager-Flusberg, Helen. (1993). Dissociations of form and function in the acquisition of language by autistic children. In H. Tager-Flusberg (Ed.), *Constraints on language acquisition: Studies of atypical children*. Hillsdale, NJ: Lawrence Erlbaum Associates. ATYPICAL DEVELOPMENT AUTISM:

Tamis-LeMonda, Catherine S., & Bornstein, Marc H. (1989). Habituation and maternal encouragement of attention in infancy as predictor of toddler language, play, and representational competence. *Child Development*, 60(3), 738-751. ATTENTION LANGUAGE PRECURSORS LANGUAGE AND PLAY REPRESENTATIONS:

Tamis-LeMonda, Catherine S., & Bornstein, Marc H. (1990). Language, play, and attention at one year. *Infant Behavior and Development*, 13, 85-98. LANGUAGE AND PLAY LANGUAGE AND COGNITIVE DEVELOPMENT ATTENTION:

Relations among language production, language comprehension, play competence, and attention span were examined in toddlers. Flexible language production and flexible language comprehension covaried, and play competence covaried with flexible language comprehension and with attention span. In contrast, neither language production nor language comprehension related positively to attention span.

Tamis-LeMonda, Catherine S., & Bornstein, Marc H. (1991). Individual variation, correspondence, stability, and change in mother and toddler play. *Infant Behavior and Development*, 14, 143-162. LANGUAGE AND PLAY ADULT-CHILD INTERACTION:

Significant changes were observed in the characteristics of symbolic and nonsymbolic mother-toddler play at 13 and 20 months. The changes were regularly associated at both ages. From Child Development Abstracts.

Taraban, Roman M., McDonald, Janet L., & MacWhinney, Brian. (1989). Category learning in a connectionist model: Learning to decline the German definite article. In R. Corrigan, F. Eckman, & M. Noonan (Eds), *Linguistic categorization*. Philadelphia, PA: John Benjamins. CONNECTIONISM GERMAN ARTICLES MORPHOLOGICAL DEVELOPMENT CUES-MORPHOLOGICAL INFLECTION:

The authors describe three connectionist networks that learned to correctly assign German articles, and propose that language acquisition may be controlled by cues rather than by rules.

Tarplee, C. (1989). Confirmation and repair: an interactional analysis of redoing sequences in child-adult talk. *York Papers in Linguistics*, 14, 279-296. CONVERSATIONAL REPAIRS PARENTAL INPUT ADULT-CHILD INTERACTION:

'Redoing' sequences (subsuming the traditional notions of 'expansion' and 'retreat') in talk involving a child of 1:6 and his caretaker are examined, as one aspect of the 'language-focussed' nature of child-adult talk. Detailed phonetic transcriptions of naturally-occurring sequences are presented and the methods of Conversation Analysis are employed to explore two ways in which redoing sequences are involved in the initiation of repair. Redoings are seen to be a resource which the adult has for simultaneously affirming the child's lexical choice, while repairing phonetic features. Also, the withholding of a confirmatory redoing by the adult may prompt the child to effect self-repair. Redoings pick up an utterance and display it for some kind of corrective, evaluative, or investigative work to be done on it. They are one way in which the talk between adults and children gets worked on as language. As such, they are a significant feature of the talk through and within which language skills develop.

Taylor, J., & Conti-Ramsden, Gina. (1988). Teachers' responses to children with severe learning difficulties: integrated versus segregated settings. *Child Language Teaching and Therapy*, 4, 271-277. LANGUAGE AND EDUCATION:

Taylor, M., Cartwright, B. S., & Bowden, T. (1991). Perspective taking and theory of mind - do children predict interpretive diversity as a function of differences in observer's knowledge. *Child Development*, 62, 1334-1351. PERSPECTIVE TAKING THEORY OF MIND:

Taylor, Marjorie, & Gelman, Susan A. (1989). Incorporating new words into the lexicon: preliminary evidence for language hierarchies in two-year-old children. *Child Development*, 60(3), 625-636. SEMANTIC ORGANIZATION LEXICAL CATEGORIES LEXICAL DEVELOPMENT:

Taylor, Orlando L. (1986). *Nature of communication disorders in culturally and linguistically diverse populations*. San Diego, CA: Singular Publishing Group. LANGUAGE DISORDERS SOCIOLINGUISTIC FACTORS NONSTANDARD DIALECTS BLACK ENGLISH CHICANO ENGLISH NATIVE AMERICAN LANGUAGES:

Historical perspectives and conceptual framework. Cultural and linguistic groups in the United States. Anthropological considerations in the study of communication. Language variation in the United States. Language acquisition in culturally diverse populations: the black child as a case study. Speech and language disorders in blacks. Speech and language disorders in Hispanics. Barriers to the delivery of speech, language, and hearing services to Native Americans. Hearing disorders among the indigenous peoples of North America and the Pacific Basin.

Taylor, Orlando L. (1986). *Treatment of communication disorders in culturally and linguistically diverse populations*. San Diego, CA: Singular Publishing Group. LANGUAGE DISORDERS SOCIOLINGUISTIC FACTORS NONSTANDARD DIALECTS BLACK ENGLISH CHICANO ENGLISH NATIVE AMERICAN LANGUAGES INTERVENTION PROGRAMS:

Issues, historical perspectives, and conceptual framework. The challange of assessing the language of nonmainstream speakers. Nonstandardized approaches to speech and language assessment. Cognitive assessment of nonwhite children. Clinical principles of language intervention for language disorders among nonstandard speakers of English. Clinical intervention for language disorders among nonstandard speakers of English as a second dialect.

Teller, Virginia, & White, Sheila J. (Eds). (1980). *Studies in child language and multilingualism, vol. 345.* New York, NY: New York Academy of Sciences. BILINGUALISM L2/L1 ACQUISITION:

Temple, Christine M., & Vilarroya, Oscar. (1990). Perceptual and cognitive perspective taking in two siblings with callosal agenesis. *British Journal of Developmental Psychology*, 8, 3-8. PERSPECTIVE TAKING COMMISUROTOMY THEORY OF MIND:

Two children with callosal agenesis were tested on the Piagetian and post-Piagetian tasks of perceptual perspective taking and a task of cognitive perspective taking. There is thus no evidence that absence of the corpus callosum causes a failure to establish a 'theory of mind, ' nor do acallosals display duality of mind such that deductions relating to belief states and view points are unavailable to conscious perception and logical verbal analysis. - From Child Development Abstracts.

Thal, Donna, & Bates, Elizabeth. (1990). Continuity and variation in early language development. In J. Columbo, & J. Fagen (Eds), *Individual differences in infancy: Reliablity, stability and prediction.* Hillsdale, NJ: Lawrence Erlbaum Associates. INDIVIDUAL VARIATION CONTINUITY/DISCONTINUITY:

Thal, Donna, Bates, Elizabeth, & Bellugi, Ursula. (1989). Language and cognition in two children with William's syndrome. *Journal of Speech and Hearing Research*, 32(2), 489-500. WILLIAM'S SYNDROME LANGUAGE AND COGNITION:

Thal, Donna, Tobias, S., & Morrison, D. (1991). Language and gesture in late talkers - a 1-year follow-up. *Journal of Speech and Hearing Research*, 34, 604-612. RETICENCE-TALKATIVENESS GESTURE:

Thelen, E. (1991). Motor aspects of emergent speech. In N. A. Krasnegor, et al. (Eds), *Biological and behavioral determinants of language development.* Hillsdale, NJ: Lawrence Erlbaum Associates. LANGUAGE AND MOTOR DEVELOPMENT:

Thirumalai, -., & Shyamala, K. C. (1986). Simultaneous acquisition of two languages: An overview. In *CICL Occasional monograph series 33*. Mysore: CICL. BILINGUALISM-SIMULTANEOUS KODAVA-KANNADA KANNADA-KODAVA:

The authors have presented aspects of the processes of acquiring two languages simultaneously in an Indian context. This monograph is the result of the authors' empirical investigation during 1980-82 and is presented as an introductory text book for Indian students of linguistics and psychology. The book describes bilingualism, methods adopted in language acquisition studies, developmental sequences and processes in simultaneous multiple language acquisition and aspects of simultaneous acquisition of Kodava and Kannada, two Indian languages spoken in India.

Thomas, Margaret. (1989). The acquisition of English articles by first- and second-language learners. *Applied Psycholinguistics*, 10, 335-355. ARTICLES L2/L1 ACQUISITION NOUNS L2 ACQUISITION STRATEGIES:

L2 learners use 'the' in referential indefinite contexts at significantly higher rates than in nonreferential contexts. Thus, both L1 and L2 learners may share an initial hypothesis associating 'the' with referential nouns. - From Child Development Abstracts.

Thomas, M. (1993). Young children's hypotheses about English reflexives. In J. L. Sokolov, & C. E. Snow (Eds), *Handbook of research in language development using CHILDES*. Hillsdlae, NJ: Lawrence Erlbaum Associates. PRONOUNS-REFLEXIVE CHILDES METHODLOGY-DESIGN METHODOLOGY-COMPUTERS:

Thompson, Roger K., & Oden, David L. (1993). "Language training" and its role in the expression of tacit propositional knowledge by chimpanzees. In Roitblat, H. L., Herman, L. M. & Nachtigal, P. E. (Eds). *Language and communication: Comparative perspectives*. Hillsdale, NJ: Lawrence Erlbaum Associates. LANGUAGE AND OTHER PRIMATES:

Thomson, Michael E. (1989). *Developmental dyslexia.* San Diego, CA: Singular Publishing Group. DYSLEXIA DEVELOPMENTAL DISORDERS READING DISORDERS WRITTEN LANGUAGE AGRAPHIA:

Introduction. Case histories. Dyslexia as a phenomenom of written language. Assessment. Remediation: evaluation and assessment. Remediation: principles and techniques.

Thomson, Michael E., & Watkins, Bill. (1990). *Dyslexia: a teaching handbook.* San Diego, CA: Singular Publishing Group. DYSLEXIA INTERVENTION PROGRAMS LANGUAGE AND EDUCATION READING DISORDERS WRITTEN LANGUAGE LITERACY:

Main section headings: introduction. Making a start. From spoken to written language. Reading. Spelling. Writing. The older student. Computers and the dyslexic.

Tieche-Christinat, C. (1990). La segmentation comme conceptualisation de la phrase chez l'enfant. (Segmentation as conceptualization of the phrase by children.). *Bulletin CILA*, 51, 74-82. LANGUAGE AND COGNITIVE DEVELOPMENT SEGMENTATION CATEGORIZATION SYNTACTIC DEVELOPMENT SYNTACTIC STRUCTURES: FRENCH

Tieche-Christinat, C., Rosset, M., Sinclair, Hermina, & Zei, Branky. (1983). Quelques aspects cognitifs dans l'acquisition du langage. (Some cognitive aspects of language acquisition.). In *Actes du Congres International de la Federation Nationale Orthophonistes.* Toulouse, France: LANGUAGE AND COGNITIVE DEVELOPMENT PIAGETIAN THEORY: FRENCH

Tien-min, Wu, & Zheng-yuan, Xu. (1979). A preliminary analysis of children's language development during the first three years. *Acta Psychologica Sinica*, 2, 153-165. CHINESE VOCALIZATIONS BABBLING FIRST WORDS SINGLE-WORD SPEECH TWO-WORD SPEECH COMPLEX SENTENCES INDIVIDUAL VARIATION CONTINUITY/DISCONTINUITY:

Sound records of 5 children taken from birth through first three years of age were analyzed. Three obvious points concerning the development of language in childhood may be shown in the following: the development of language is a continuous, sequential and regular process with transitional changes both quantitatively and qualitatively all through. It is continuous as well as by stages, and may be divided into six stages: 1) the stage of simple vocalizations-from birth to 3 months, 2) the stage of running syllables-4 to 8 months, 3) the germinal stage in learning to talk-9 to 12 months, 4) the stage of one word sentences, formal beginning of speech learning-1 to 1 1/2 years, 5) the stage of simple sentences, grasping elementary language-1 1/2 to 2 years, 6) the stage of beginning to use compound sentences, grasping the most fundamental speech-2 to 3 years. The children's language development proceeds from concrete to abstract, and this may be seen from the process of grasping words and their parts of speech. Individual differences in language developments are quite clear even among infants in such a small group.ZYX

Till, James A., & Alp, Linda A. (1991). Aerodynamic and temporal measures of continuous speech in dysarthric speakers. In C. Moore, K. M. Yorkston, & D. R. Beukelman (Eds), *Dysarthria and apraxia of speech*. Baltimore, MD: Paul H. Brookes. DYSARTHRIA:

Tingey, Carol. (1988). *Down syndrome: a resource handbook*. San Diego, CA: Singular Publishing Group. DOWN SYNDROME INTERVENTION PROGRAMS FOR PARENTS INTERVENTION PROGRAMS LANGUAGE AND EDUCATION:

Physical characteristics, chromosome analysis, and treatment in Down Syndrome immune deciciency in Down Syndrome. Medical considerations. Counseling the family of a child with Down Syndrome. Parents and grandparents of children with Down Syndrome. My brother, Jim. Gross motor development in young children with Down Syndrome. Facilitating speech and language development. Early intervention for infants and preschoolers with Down Syndrome: a review of best practices and effectiveness data. Elementary school experience. Competitive employment training at the high school level. Recreation: a promising vehicle for promoting the community integration of young adults with Down Syndrome.

Tipper, Steven P., Bourque, Tracy A., Anderson, Susan H., & Brehaut, Jamie C. (1989). Mechanisms of attention: A developmental study. *Journal of Experimental Child Psychology*, 48, 353-378. ATTENTION SEMANTIC MAPPING:

A model of selective attention is proposed which contains a number of properties. First, stimuli which are irrelevant to the subjects' task can be analyzed to semantic levels automatically, and such stimuli can produce intrusion/interference effects. Second, two mechanisms by which selection is achieved are habituation to, and inhibition of, these irrelevant stimuli. - From Child Development Abstracts.

Toda, Sueko, Fogel, Alan, & Kawai, Masatoshi. (1990). Maternal speech to three-month-old infants in the United States and Japan. *Journal of Child Language*, 17, 279-294. CROSSLINGUISTIC STUDY-PARENTAL SPEECH JAPANESE PARENTAL SPEECH-STYLE:

American and Japanese mother-infant dyads were videotaped in the laboratory. Maternal speech was analyzed by function and syntactic form. U.S. mothers were more information-oriented than were Japanese mothers and used more question forms, especially yes/no questions. Japanese mothers were affect- oriented, and they used more nonsense, onomatopoeic sounds, baby talk, and babies' names. The differences in maternal speech appear to reflect characteristic culture-specific communicative styles as well as beliefs and values related to child-rearing.

Toivainen, Jorma. (1973). Mita kaksivuotiaat utsjokelaiset puhuvat 1973? (What language do two year olds speak in the northernmost community in Finland in 1973?). *Kaltio*, 77. FINNISH LAPP SOCIOLINGUISTIC FACTORS VARIATION BILINGUALISM-LANGUAGE PREFERENCE: FINNISH

Two thirds of the mothers, who bore a child in 1970 in Utsjoki, were Saami (or Lappish) speaking, but only half of the born children acquired their mother's first language. The fluency of Finnish was roughly estimated.JT

Toivainen, Jorma. (1976). Aikuisten vaikutus lasten kieleen. (The influence of adults on the language of children.). *Kaltio*, , 73-75. STOPS PARENTAL INPUT FINNISH PARENTAL SPEECH: FINNISH

Observations on acquisition of dental stops before labial ones by Finnish child, and on Finnish baby talk words.JT

Toivainen, Jorma. (1976). A hypocristic geminate consonant suffix in Finnish. *Atken des 1. Salzburger Kolloquiums uber Kindersprache. Salzburger Beitrage zur Linguistik*, 2, FINNISH PHONOLOGICAL DEVELOPMENT PARENTAL SPEECH:

Bisyllabic words are the majority of the Finnish baby talk words. In spite of shortness, the words are derivatives having a germinate stop in the middle. Anttila proposed that consonant gradation would have been effective in the formation of those words. The writer disagrees with this view, showing that the derivation is working all the time. JT.

Toivainen, Jorma. (1976). Lapsenkielen tutkimushanke 1970-1976. (Summary of the Oulu Finnic Child Language Project.). In *Research Reports of the Department of Finnish and Lappish*. Oulu: University of Oulu. FINNISH LAPP: FINNISH

During early seventies Finnish (and Saami) child language material was tape-recorded primarily in Oulu town (and Utsjoki Saami villages), e.g. the Oulu sample of 25 randomly selected children born in 1972, a follow-up investigation from the age of 1 year. This booklet includes lists of children with MLU's calculated up to 1976.JT

Toivainen, Jorma. (1977). Menneen ajan muotojen ilmaantuminen suomalaislasten kieleen. (The appearance of past time forms in the language of Finnish children.). *Nakokulmia kieleen (Helsinki)*, 18, 107-112. TENSE FINNISH INFLECTION: FINNISH

Toivainen, Jorma. (1977). The use of past time verb forms by Finnish children in their second and third years as a reflection of their temporal cognitive abilities. *Akten der 3. Salzburger Jahrestagung fur Linguistik (Psycholinguistik), Salzburger Beitrage zur Linguistik* , 4, 143-156. FINNISH TENSE INFLECTION ASPECT VERBS LANGUAGE AND COGNITIVE DEVELOPMENT:

The first to appear is the preterite about 1:4. The perfect does not appear until about 1:8. The pluperfect appears about 2:7.

Toivainen, Jorma. (1980). Inflectional affixes used by Finnish-speaking children aged 1-3 years. In *Suomalaisen Kirjallisuuden Seuran toimituksia 359*. Helsinki: SKS. FINNISH MORPHOSYNTACTIC DEVELOPMENT INFLECTION: FINNISH

The acquisition of Finnish inflectional morphology by 75% of the Oulu sample before age 4 years 4 months. Calculation of the median age of the first users of each suffix and combination, after that, calculation of the affix age for each sample on behalf of existing suffixes. Appearance and early development up to median age of each inflectional suffix (excluded only those which are marginal even adult speech), including basic forms of verbs, modes, personal forms, past time forms, nominal forms of verbs, local cases (demonstratives, eight nominal cases), partitive (meaning non-entirety from partial up to full negation), accusative, genitive as a case of connection, essive and translative as a role case and plural. Altogether 32 morphological categories were studied. All material up to age 2:11 was taken into an appendix, pages 201-302, in each sample the instances were organized and coded by grammatical categories. JT.

Toivainen, Jorma. (1980). Suomalaislasten ensimmaiset on-lauseet. (The first sentences with copular-existential verb 'olla' by Finnish children.);. In *Congressus Quintus Internationalis Fenno-Ugristarum, III. Dissertationes symposiorum linguisticorum*. Turku: Suomen Kielen Seura. FINNISH COPULA EARLY SYNTACTIC DEVELOPMENT INFLECTION WORD ORDER CASE MORPHOSYNTACTIC DEVELOPMENT: FINNISH

The Finnish verb 'ol-la', basic form for the child being on 3rd singular, is used for existential, copular and even auxiliary purposes. It is acquired early: before the age of 2 years on half of Oulu sample use three-word sentences with a demonstrative (sometimes even a noun in Nominative or Habitative adessive) in the Subject place. The second argument is also occupied, as in the adult language, by nouns in Nominative, Genitive (also without the Nominative head), Partitive (meaning non-entirety or even negation) or in local case.JT

Toivainen, Jorma. (1981). Suffiksikielen omaksumisesta aidinkielena. (On the acquisition of a suffix language as a mother tongue.). *Virittaja*, 49-51. MINIATURE LINGUISTIC SYSTEMS INFLECTION LANGUAGE TYPOLOGY: FINNISH

On the explanation of acquisition of Finnish-like suffix language by referring to general learning strategies.JT

Toivainen, Jorma. (1986). Easy for the child, hard for the grammarian: observations on the function of the partitive in Finnish. In I. Kurcz, G. Shugar, & J. Danks (Eds), *Knowledge and language. Advances in Psychology*. Amsterdam: North-Holland. FINNISH CASE MORPHOSYNTACTIC DEVELOPMENT:

The partitive is the most frequent oblique case in Finnish and it is acquired first by children. The main function of the case is proposed to be that of a complement (namely object, predicative or primary local phrase) of the verb in any kind of sentences, meaning non-entirety of the noun. The category of partitive subject is not needed any more, in adult language either. JT.

Toivainen, Jorma. (1987). Kielen aikasuhteet ja lapsi. (Summary: temporal relations in language and their acquisition by Finnish children.). *Journal of Suomen Kielen Seura*, 29, 37-54. FINNISH ASPECT TENSE VERBS INFLECTION MORPHOSYNTACTIC DEVELOPMENT: FINNISH

The acquisition of Finnish temporal system is described by separate categories tense, taxis and aspect. It is proposed that at first (in a sample of 25 children, the age of the first to use it was 1 year 4 months-median 1:11) past tense forms indicate anterior taxis. By the time, however, when the perfect tense is acquired (for the first 1:8-median 2:4) and assumes that function of anterior taxis that it has in adult language, the imperfect begins to refer to a past moment that is separate from the present. When applying Fletcher's (JCL 1981) comparison of the distribution of imperfect and perfect stems, it appears that in Finnish the proportion of shared stems is 64% (as opposed to 20% in English), which together with earlier evidence (see Tovainen 1977 and 1980, above) stands as proof of the existence of inflection, and of the development of the tense and taxis system at an early age.JT

Toivainen, Jorma. (1987). Partivus finski: jego glowne funkcje i ich przyswajanie przez dzieci. (Finnish partitive: its functions and acquisition by children.). In I. Kurcz, G. Shugar, & B. Bokus (Eds), *Wiedza a jezyk. Tom 2: Jezyk dziecka.* Wroclaw: Ossolineum. FINNISH CASE INFLECTION MORPHOSYNTACTIC DEVELOPMENT: POLISH

Toivainen, Jorma. (1988). Eraiden tekijannimien siirtymisesta ea-adjektiivien malliin. (Summary: overlapping of inflectional types: agentive and adjectival derivatives in Finnish dialects.). *Virittaja,* 504-509. LANGUAGE CHANGE CASE FINNISH VARIATION ADJECTIVES NONSTANDARD DIALECTS: FINNISH

The historical change of inflectional category in restricted and separate Finnish and Carelian dialects is explained by reference also to the language acquisition situation.

Tolchinsky-Landsmann, Liliana. (1988). Form and meaning in the development of written representation. *European Journal of Educational Psychology*, 3, 385-398. WRITTEN LANGUAGE LITERACY:

Tolchinsky-Landsmann, Liliana. (1990). Early writing development: evidences from different orthographic systems. In M. Spoelders (Ed.), *Literacy acquisition..* Lier: Communication and Cognition. CROSSLINGUISTIC STUDY-LITERACY WRITTEN LANGUAGE:

Tolchinsky-Landsmann, Liliana. (1990). Genesi delia lingua scritta e ruolo dell'ambiente: tre paradigmi teorici a confronto (Three accounts of literacy development and the role of environment.). In M. Orsolini, & C. Pontecorvo (Eds), *La costruz dei primi testi nei bambino.* Rome, Italy: Nova Italia. LITERACY: ITALIAN

Tolchinsky-Landsmann, Liliana. (1990). Literacy development and pedagogical implications: Evidence from the Hebrew system of writing. In Y. Goodman (Ed.), *How children construct literacy: Piagetian perspectives.* Newark, Deleware: International Reading Association. LANGUAGE AND EDUCATION CROSSLINGUISTIC STUDY-LITERACY HEBREW LITERACY WRITTEN LANGUAGE:

Tolchinsky-Landsmann, Liliana. (1990). Lo practico, lo cientifico y lo literario: tres componentes en la noción de alfabetismo. (The functional, the scientific and the literary: three components in the notion of literacy.). *Comunicación, Lenguaje y Educación*, 6, 53-62. LITERACY WRITTEN LANGUAGE: SPANISH

Tolchinsky-Landsmann, Liliana. (1991). The conceptualization of writing in the confluence of interactive models of development. In L. Tolchinsky-Landsmann (Ed.), *Culture, schooling, and psychological development.* Norwood, NJ: Ablex. LITERACY WRITTEN LANGUAGE:

Tolchinsky-Landsmann, Liliana, & Levin, Iris. (1982). El desarrollo de la escritura en niños israelies prescolares (The development of writing in Israeli preschoolers). In E. Ferreiro, & M. Gomez-Palacio (Eds), *Nuevas perpectivas sobre los procesos de Lectura y Escritura.* Mexico: Siglo XXI. HEBREW CROSSLINGUISTIC STUDY-LITERACY LITERACY: SPANISH

Tolchinsky-Landsmann, Liliana, & Sandbank, A. (1991). Text production and text differentiation: developmental changes and educational influences. In S. Strauss (Ed.), *Learning environments and psychological development.* Norwood, NJ: Ablex. DISCOURSE ANALYSIS NARRATIVES:

Tomasello, Michael. (1992). *First verbs : a case study of early grammatical development*. New York, NY: Cambridge University Press. VERBS SYNTACTIC DEVELOPMENT SOCIAL INTERACTION EVENTS/SCRIPTS:

A diary study of a two year old's early language development which pinpoints the role of verbs in the acquisition of syntax, and the part that social cognition plays inthe development of language.

Tomasello, Michael, Conti-Ramsden, Gina, & Ewart, Barbara. (1990). Young children's conversations with their mothers and fathers: Differences in breakdown and repair. *Journal of Child Language*, 17, 115-130. PARENTAL SPEECH-SEX DIFFERENCES CONVERSATIONAL REPAIRS PARENTAL SPEECH-STYLE BRIDGE HYPOTHESIS:

Examination of the speech addressed by primary and secondary caregivers to 15-21 month olds was examined for breakdown-repair sequences. The speech of between the secondary caregivers (in this instance fathers) and the children experienced more breakdowns than that between primary caregivers and the children. The authors interpret these results as confirmation of the Bridge hypothesis which claims that secondary caregivers present children with communicative challenges which prepare them for interaction with strangers.

Tomasello, Michael, & Kruger, A. C. (1992). Joint attention on actions: acquiring verbs in ostensive and non-ostensive contexts. *Journal of Child Language*, 19, 311-333. VERBS OSTENTATION JOINT REFERENCE LEXICAL DEVELOPMENT:

Tomblin, J. Bruce, Hardy, J. C., & Hein, H. A. (1991). Predicting poor communication status in preschool children using risk factors present at birth. *Journal of Speech and Hearing Research*, 34, 1096-1105. AT-RISK CHILDREN NEONATES ASSESSMENT PROCEDURES:

Tomes, Lucrezia, & Shelton, Ralph L. (1989). Children's categorization of consonants by manner and place characteristics. *Journal of Speech and Hearing Research*, 32(2), 432-438. CONSONANTS PHONETIC FEATURES CATEGORIZATION:

Touretzky, David S., Elvgren, G., III, & Wheeler, D. W. (1990). Phonological rule induction: an architectural solution. In M. Piatelli-Palmarini (Ed.), *Proceedings of the Twelfth Annual Conference of the Cognitive Science Society*. Hillsdale, NJ: Lawrence Erlbaum Associates. RULES-PHONOLOGICAL CONNECTIONISM PHONOLOGICAL PROCESSES:

Toyama, Noriko. (1989). Maternal speech in mother-toddler picture book reading. *Japanese Journal of Educational Psychology*, 37, 151-157. PARENTAL SPEECH ADULT-CHILD INTERACTION JAPANESE: JAPANESE

Five mother-toddler dyads took part in this longitudinal, four-month study. Their interactions including picture book reading were videotaped and five minutes of each observation session were transcribed. The analysis of mothers' strategies of reading labels in the books showed that their strategies did not strictly correspond with children's comprehension level, but that their speech always included labels in some phase of the reading cycle. Mothers gave opportunities to hear again the label of the thing children had misnamed in the preceding cycle. - From Child Development Abstracts.

Trabasso, Tom. (1972). Mental operations in language comprehension. In J. B. Carroll, & R. O. Freedle (EdS), *Language comprehension and the acquisition of knowledge*. Washington, DC: V. H. Winston. COMPREHENSION LANGUAGE AND COGNITION LANGUAGE AND COGNITIVE DEVELOPMENT:

Trabasso, Tom, & Nickels, M. (1992). The development of goal plans of action in the narration of a picture story. *Discourse Processes*, 15, 249-275. NARRATIVES TEXT/STORY GRAMMARS:

Trevarthen, Colwyn. (1974). Conversations with a two-month old. *New Scientist*, 62, 230-235. ADULT-CHILD INTERACTION SOCIAL INTERACTION HYPOTHESIS INTERSUBJECTIVITY PRELINGUISTICS:

Trevarthen, Colwyn. (1974). The psychobiology of speech development. *Neurosciences Research Program Bulletin*, 12, 570-585. INTERSUBJECTIVITY NEUROLINGUISTICS LANGUAGE AND MOTOR DEVELOPMENT:

Trevarthen, colwyn. (1975). Early attempts at speech. In R. Lewin (Ed.), *Child alive: New insights into the development of young children*. New York, NY: Anchor/Doubleday. PRELINGUISTICS BABBLING INTERSUBJECTIVITY NATIVISM:

Trevarthen, Colwyn. (1979). Communication and cooperation in early infancy: A description of primary intersubjectivity. In M. Bullowa (Ed.), *Before speech*. New York, NY: Cambridge University Press. INTERSUBJECTIVITY ADULT-CHILD INTERACTION SOCIAL INTERACTION HYPOTHESIS PRELINGUISTICS:

Trevarthen, Colwyn, Hubley, P., & Sheeran, L. (1976). Psychological actions in early infancy. *La Recherche*. INTERSUBJECTIVITY ADULT-CHILD INTERACTION:

Trevise, Anne, Perdue, Clive, & Deulofeu, J. (1991). Word order and discursive coherence in L2. In *Proceedings of the Conference on Applied Psycholinguistics*. Amsterdam, The Netherlands: John Benjamins. L2 DISCOURSE L2 WORD ORDER:

Truax, R. (1992). Becoming literate - a sketch of a never ending cycle. *Volta Review*, 94, 395-410. LITERACY:

Tuller, B., & Kelso, J. A. S. (1991). The production and perception of syllable structure. *Journal of Speech and Hearing Research*, 34, 501-508. SYLLABLES-STRUCTURE SPEECH PERCEPTION ARTICULATION:

Turnure, C. (1971). Response to voice of mother and stranger by babies in the first year. *Developmental Psychology*, 4, 182-190. INFANT PERCEPTION SPEECH PERCEPTION PARENTAL SPEECH ADULT-CHILD INTERACTION PRELINGUISTICS:

Tversky, Barbara. (1989). Parts, partonomies and taxonomies. *Developmental Psychology*, 25, 983-995. CATEGORIZATION:

This article reports exploratory work on children's partonomic knowledge, and the relation between it and use of taxonomic organization. Shared parts may facilitate the transition from classification based on perception to classification based on function. - From Child Development Abstracts.

Tyack, P. L. (1993). Animal language research needs a broader comparative and evolutionary framework. In L. M. Herman, H. L. Roitblat, & P. E. Nachtigall (EdS), *Language and communication: Comparative perspectives*. Hillsdale, NJ: Lawrence Erlbaum Associates. ANIMAL COMMUNICATIONS:

Tye-Murray, N., Barkmeier, Julie, & Folkins, J. W. (1991). Scaling and transcription measures of intelligibility for populations disordered speech. *Journal of Speech and Hearing Research*, 34, 697-698. ASSESSMENT PROCEDURES INTELLIGIBILITY METHODOLOGY-TRANSCRIPTION:

Tyler, A. A., & Saxman, J. H. (1991). Initial voicing contrast acquisition in normal and phonologically disordered children. *Applied Psycholinguistics*, 12, 453-479. CONTRAST-VOICE PHONOLOGICAL DISORDERS PHONETIC FEATURES PHONEMIC DEVELOPMENT:

Tyler, Lorraine K. (1992). *Spoken language comprehension: An experimental approach to disorderd and normal processing*. Cambridge, MA: Bradford Books. COMPREHENSION COMPREHENSION DISORDERS LANGUAGE PROCESSING DISCOURSE COMPREHENSION APHASIAS:

A description of the "on-line" real time processing of language and how it breaks down in aphasia.

Tzelgov, J., & Eben-Ezra, S. (1993). Components of the between language semantic-priming effect. In A. M. B. de Groot, & C. Barry (EdS), *The multilingual community*. Hillsdale, NJ: Lawrence Erlbaum Associates. BILINGUALISM INTERLANGUAGE L2 ACQUISITION:

U

Uchida, Nobuko. (1989). The development of 'deficit-complement' schema in a semantic integration of narrative sequences in an abstract drawing story. *Japanese Journal of Educational Psychology*, 37, 327-336. NARRATIVES TEXT/STORY GRAMMARS EVENTS/SCRIPTS: JAPANESE

The role of 'deficit-complement' schema played in a semantic integration of narrative sequences and the development of the same schema was examined. 84 four-year-old and five-year-old children were divided into three homogeneous groups, and assigned to one of three conditions: a non-restricted information with an undetermined deficit, a restricted information, or a non- information. The children were shown an abstract drawing story and were asked to describe each picture and perform a free-recall of the story and comprehension tasks. The results showed that deficit information facilitates semantic integration of narrative sequences. - From Child Development Abstracts.

Ulissi, Stephen Mark, Brice, Patrick J., & Gibbins, Spencer. (1989). Use of the Kaufman-Assessment Battery for Children with the hearing impaired. *American Annals of the Deaf*, 134, 283-287. ASSESSMENT PROCEDURES KAUFMAN ASSESSMENT BATTERY FOR CHILDREN DEAF CHILDREN WECHSLER SCALES:

The Kaufman-Assessment Battery for Children was administered to male and female hearing-impaired elementary school students to determine its appropriateness for hearing-impaired children. The Wechsler Intelligence Scale for Children-Revised was also administered. Results showed that both the Simultaneous Processing Scale and the Nonverbal Scale seemed appropriate for hearing-impaired children, whose scores were similar to those of the test's normative sample.

Umbel, V. M., Pearson, Barbara Zurer, Fernandez, M. C., & Oller, D. Kimbrough. (1992). Measuring bilingual children's receptive vocabularies. *Child Development*, 63, 1012-1020. BILINGUALISM-VOCABULARY DEVELOPMENT ASSESSMENT PROCEDURES METHODOLOGY-ANALYSIS:

Umetani, T., Kitao, S., & Katada, S. (1989). Verbalization of appropriate and inappropriate cues in discrimination reversal learning by moderately mentally retarded children. *Journal of Mental Deficiency Research*, 33, 487-492. RETARDED CHILDREN LANGUAGE AND MEMORY LANGUAGE AND COGNITION:

Effects of verbalization on discrimination reversal for moderately mentally retarded children were examined under three training conditions. Predicted results indicated that verbalization of both appropriate and inappropriate cues within relevant dimensions significantly facilitated reversal shift performance, as compared to verbalization of only appropriate cues or non-verbalization.-From Child Development Abstracts.

V

Vaidyanathan, R. (1991). Development of forms and functions of negation in the early stages of language acquisition - a study in Tamil. *Journal of Child Language*, 18, 51-66. NEGATION TAMIL EARLY SYTNACTIC DEVELOPMENT:

Valletutti, Peter J., McKnight-Taylor, Mary, & Hoffnung, Audrey S. (1989). *Facilitating communication in young children with handicapping conditions: a guide for special educators*. San Diego, CA: Singular Publishing Group. ATYPICAL DEVELOPMENT INTERVENTION PROGRAMS ASSESSMENT PROCEDURES LANGUAGE AND EDUCATION:

Faciliting communication: teacher competencies. The nature of language. The development of oral language. The nature and development of nonverbal communication. The role of assessment in the educational evaluation of young children with handicaps. Teacher assessment of speech and language development of infants and other young children. Organizing instructional experience. Stimulating speech and language development of infants and other young children. Speech and language problems and their remediation. The special education teacher as consultant.

van Besien, Fred. (1981) *Kindertaal: de verwerving het nederlands als moedertaal.* Leuven: Acco. DUTCH: DUTCH

van Bourgondien, M. E., Marcus, L. M., & Schopler, Eric. (1992). Comparison of DSM-III-R and Childhood Autism Rating Scale diagnoses of autism. *Journal of Autism and Developmental Disorders*, 22, 493-506. CLASSIFICATION OF DISORDERS AUTISM:

van Dijk, T. (1985). *Handbook of discourse analysis*. San Diego, CA: Academic Press. DISCOURSE ANALYSIS:

van Dyke, Don C., Lang, David J., Heide, Frances, van Duyne, Susan, & Soucek, Joan M. (1990). *Clinical perspectives on the management of Down syndrome*. New York, NY: Springer Verlag. DOWN SYNDROME INTERVENTION PROGRAMS:

A multidisciplinary volume covering many aspects of Down syndrome therapy including speech pathology.

van Evra, Judith. (1990). *Television and child development*. Hillsdale, NJ: Lawrence Erlbaum Associates. TELEVISION AND LANGUAGE DEVELOPMENT:

The book is divided into three sections. Section 1 deals with the cognitive processing of information from the television, the second with television's impact on social and emotional behavior, and the third deals with the theoretical implications of television for psychological and communication research studies.

van Haaren, H. (1988). Imitation in verbal mother-child interaction (in Dutch). In *Report nr 102, Institute of Phonetic Sciences*. Amsterdam: University of Amsterdam. INTERSUBJECTIVITY CLEFT PALATE IMITATION: DUTCH

A comparative study concerning six mother-child pairs with three of the children born with cleft palates.

van Lancker, Diane, Cornelius, Cathleen, & Needleman, Rosa. (1991). Comprehension of verbal terms for emotions in normal, autistic, and schizophrenic children. *Developmental Neuropsychology*, 7, 1-18. PSYCHOPATHOLOGICAL CHILDREN AUTISM LANGUAGE AND AFFECT:

The abilities of autistic and schizophrenic children to recognize the meanings of concrete nouns, nonemotional adjectives, and emotional adjectives were compared to a normal control (NC) group using a picture- matching task. Autistic children performed significantly worse than chronological-age-matched normal and schizophrenic children on emotional adjectives but did not differ in their abilities to recognize the meanings of nouns and neutral adjectives. Schizophrenic children did not differ from normal children in any of the three tasks. When matched on mental age, autistic and normal groups did not differ significantly.

van Lancker, Diane, & Sidtis, J. J. (1992). The identification of affective-prosodic stimuli by left-hemisphere-damaged and right-hemisphere-damaged subjects - all errors are not created equal. *Journal of Speech and Hearing Research*, 35, 963-970. LATERALIZATION TRAUMATIC DISORDERS:

van Langendonck, -, & Schaerlaekens, A. M. (1977). Definiet en indefiniet en de vroege taalontwikkeling. (Definite and indefinite in early language development.). , 49-68. ARTICLES: DUTCH

van Patten, Bill, & Lee, James F. (1990). *Second language acquisition/foreign language learning*. Philadelphia, PA: Multilingual Matters. L2 ACQUISITION L2 EDUCATION:

van Valin, Robert D., Jnr. (1992). An overview of ergative phenomena and their implications for language acquisition. In D. I. Slobin (Ed.), *The crosslinguistic study of language acquisition (Vol. 3)*. Hillsdale, NJ: Lawrence Erlbaum Associates, Inc., Publishers;. CROSSLINGUISTIC STUDY-MORPHOSYNTAX ERGATIVE LANGUAGES:

van den Eynde, K., Dominicy, M., & Verluyten, P. (1985). Een voorloper van linguistische referentie. In *Linguistics in Belgium 6, Antwerp Papers in Linguistics (Special Issue)*. Belgium: University of Antwerp. SINGLE-WORD SPEECH DEIXIS REFERENCE DUTCH: DUTCH

This paper focuses on the use of deictics in a child's one-word stage.

van der Geest, Ton. (1975). *Some aspects of communicative competence and their implications for language acquisition*. Assen, The Netherlands: van Gorcum. COMMUNICATIVE COMPETENCE:

Vanderlely, H. K. J., & Harris, M. (1990). Comprehension of reversible sentences in specifically language-impaired children. *Journal of Speech and Hearing Disorders*, 55, 101-117. REVERSIBILITY COMPREHENSION COMPREHENSION DISORDERS WORD ORDER:

van der Stelt, J. M. (1978). The development of speech in the deaf child (in Dutch). *Ts voor Orthopedagogiek*, 6, 293-298. DEAF CHILDREN BABBLING LANGUAGE AND EDUCATION INTERVENTION PROGRAMS: DUTCH

Oral teaching methods investigated. A more physiological approach could be helpful in teaching deaf children to speak. Relations with normal speech motor milestones.

van der Stelt, J. M. (1978). The influence of Dr. Johan Conrad Amman upon the changes in the education of the deaf (in Dutch). *Ts voor Orthopedagogiek*, 5, 244-249. DEAF CHILDREN LANGUAGE AND EDUCATION DUTCH: DUTCH

Historical study on oral education of the deaf since 1500.JvdS

van der Stelt, J. M. (1979). Early speech development and the deaf child. In *Anniversaries in Phonetics, Studia Gratulatoria dedicated to Hendrik Mol*. The Netherlands: University of Amsterdam, Institute of Phonetic Sciences. DEAF CHILDREN INTERVENTION PROGRAMS ARTICULATION:

Plea for speech motor aspects in deaf articulation lessons based on research.JvdS

van der Stelt, J. M. (1979). Phonetics and speech development (in Dutch). *Logopedie en Foniatrie*, 51, 243-257. ARTICULATION LANGUAGE AND MOTOR DEVELOPMENT PHONOLOGICAL DEVELOPMENT: DUTCH

Speech development as development of movements, mapping of the oral cavity and milestones in sound production.JvdS

van der Stelt, J. M. (1983). Verbal interaction between mother and child. In *Proceedings of Phonetic Sciences*. Amsterdam: University of Amsterdam. ADULT-CHILD INTERACTION PARENTAL SPEECH:

van der Stelt, J. M. (1985). Speech development and the single subject research design. In *Proceedings 9, Institute of Phonetic Sciences*. Amsterdam: University of Amsterdam. METHODOLOGY-DESIGN METHODOLOGY-LONGITUDINAL STUDY:

Methodological issues in relation to longitudinal developmental research.JvdS

van der Stelt, J. M. (1986). Learning to speak, learning to think. In W. van der Grind, & K. van Wouwe (Eds), *Proceedings of the Fourth Workshop of the Forum Humanum*. PARENTAL INPUT ADULT-CHILD INTERACTION INTERSUBJECTIVITY SOCIAL INTERACTION HYPOTHESIS:

Discusses the influence of mother-infant interaction in relation to speech development.JvdS

van der Stelt, J. M. (1987). Facial and gaze behaviour in mother-infant interaction. In *Proceedings of the Institute of Phonetic Sciences*, 11. Amsterdam: University of Amsterdam. GAZE INTERSUBJECTIVITY SOCIAL INTERACTION HYPOTHESIS ADULT-CHILD INTERACTION:

Changes in frequency of mimical movements and shifts in gaze direction in the first 30 weeks of life in two girls.JvdS

van der Stelt, J. M. (1989). Sensitive stages in face-to-face interaction in the first two years of life. In *Proceedings of the Institute of Phonetic Sciences*, 12. Amsterdam: University of Amsterdam. INTERSUBJECTIVITY ADULT-CHILD INTERACTION SOCIAL INTERACTION HYPOTHESIS:

Differences in face-to-face interaction in two mother-infant pairs and the possible influence on visual communication.JvdS

van der Stelt, J. M. (1990). Mother-infant interaction by eyes and ears (in Dutch). *Van Horen Zeggen*, 31 (2), 51-56. INTERSUBJECTIVITY PARENTAL INPUT ADULT-CHILD INTERACTION SOCIAL INTERACTION HYPOTHESIS: DUTCH

Learning to speak, thanks to well-timed maternal lessons.JvdS van der Stelt, J. M., & Jansonius-Schultheiss, Kino. (1990). Book of codes for the communicative analysis of mother-infant interaction 0 to 24 months of age (in Dutch). In *Instituut voor Fonetische Wetenschappen, Report Nr. 12*. Amsterdam: Universiteit van Amsterdam. METHODOLOGY-ANALYSIS METHODOLOGY-TRANSCRIPTION INTERSUBJECTIVITY ADULT-CHILD INTERACTION: DUTCH

Description of a coding system for communicative behaviors in mother-child interaction: mutual proximity, the visual mode (such as gaze direction), mimical behaviors, tactile input, speech-, head-, hand/arm-, body-, and leg movements for the mother as well as the child.JvdS

van der Stelt, J. M., & Koopmans-van Beinum, F. J. (1981). Note on motor analysis of infant sound. In *Proceedings 6, Institute of Phonetic Sciences*. Amsterdam: University of Amsterdam. METHODOLOGY-TRANSCRIPTION:

Outline of narrow transcription for infant sound production taking into account respiratory, phonatory, and articulatory movements.JvdS

Vedeler, Liv. (1981). Spraklig samspill mellom barn med funksjonsvansker og deres lekekamerater (Verbal communication in kindergarten groups with handicapped children and their nonhandicapped peers.). *Norsk Tidsskrift for Logopedi*, 4, 139-156. LANGUAGE AND PLAY SOCIAL SPEECH HANDICAPPED CHILDREN: NORWEGIAN

Observations were taken in 8 different play groups with three children in free play situations. One of the children in each group had a handicap (language and/or social-emotional problems). Transcriptions of the children's utterances were analyzed with use of Vejleskov's model for analyzing utterance functions and group communication. The handicapped children used more egocentric language than their peers. The communication pattern and utterance function changed when the preschool teacher participated in the children's communication.LV

Vedeler, Liv. (1986). The role of play in the education of handicapped infants. *Prospects*, XVI(4), LANGUAGE AND PLAY HANDICAPPED CHILDREN:

Children's play follows a regular course of development closely related to cognitive, communicative and language development. Structural changes in cognitive development manifests itself in play. This gives the grownups 'keys' to how they can promote a child's development by play and communication.LV

Vedeler, Liv. (1987). *Barns kommunikasjon i rollelek. (Children's communication in dramatic play.).* Oslo: Universitetsforlaget. LANGUAGE AND PLAY SOCIAL SPEECH LANGUAGE AND EDUCATION LITERACY: NORWEGIAN

This book describes verbal communication in dramatic play, recorded and analyzed from 14 preschool children playing in small groups of 3-4. It presents a theoretical perspective. A hypotheses is put forth that dramatic play can promote children's literacy development.LV

Vedeler, Liv. (1988). Litt om observasjon av spraklig samspill. (About observation of verbal communication in preschool children's peer groups.) *Nordisk Tidsskrift for Spesialpedagogik,* 2/88, 78-86. SOCIAL SPEECH COMMUNICATIVE COMPETENCE METHODOLOGY-DESIGN HANDICAPPED CHILDREN: NORWEGIAN

Communication partners will have influence on how a child is able to use his language. It is important to be aware of this in working with handicapped children and integration. Methods are being developed and used for observation of verbal communication in children's free play groups.LV

Vedeler, Liv. (1989). *Lek og kommunikasjon i de forste utviklingsar. (Play and communication in the first developmental years: observation and educational use of play for children with and without handicap.).* Namsos: Pedagogisk Psykologisk Forlag. LANGUAGE AND PLAY PRELINGUISTICS HANDICAPPED CHILDREN METHODOLOGY-DESIGN: NORWEGIAN

The book gives a theoretical background for understanding preverbal development in the first two years of life. It shows how to observe the child's development and how to promote development in the handicapped child by using play and communication.LV

Vedeler, Liv, & Vejleskov, Hans. (1987). Language in preschool education in an functional perspective. In K. Sajavaara (Ed.), *Equality in language learning. Proceedings of the 5th Nordic Conference of Applied Linguistics.* SOCIAL SPEECH LANGUAGE AND PLAY LANGUAGE AND EDUCATION LANGUAGE AND COGNITIVE DEVELOPMENT:

This paper gives a brief account of our research on preschool children's speech in small groups. Verbal communication with playmates as well as with teachers influences the thinking, attitudes, and well-being of an individual child.LV

Vejleskov, Hans. (1972). *Om sprog og taekning I: Werner & Kaplans teori (On language and thinking I: The theory of Werner and Kaplan).* Copenhagen: Munksgaard. LANGUAGE AND COGNITION LANGUAGE AND COGNITIVE DEVELOPMENT: DANISH

Vejleskov, Hans. (1973). Psychological views on the development and function of language in preschool children. *Paedagogica Europa*, 9, 33-50. PRELINGUISTICS LANGUAGE PRECURSORS LANGUAGE AND COGNITIVE DEVELOPMENT:

Vejleskov, Hans. (1975). Om egocentrisk tale (On egocentric speech). In H. Vejleskov (Ed.), *Emner og eksperimenter i bornepsykologien.* Copenhagen: Akademisk forlag. EGOCENTRISM PRIVATE SPEECH PIAGETIAN THEORY: DANISH

Vejleskov, Hans. (1975). *Om sprog og taekning II: Mowrer og Berlynes teorier (On language and thinking II: The theories of Mowrer and Berlyne).* Copenhagen: Munksgaard. LANGUAGE AND COGNITION LANGUAGE AND COGNITIVE DEVELOPMENT LANGUAGE AND BEHAVIORISM: DANISH

Vejleskov, Hans. (1975). Sprogprojekt Espelunden I. *Dansk paedagogisk Tidskrift*, 4, LITERACY LANGUAGE AND EDUCATION DANISH WRITTEN LANGUAGE: DANISH

Part one of a research project on language development in school-beginners and an alternative elementary instruction in reading and writing.HV

Vejleskov, Hans. (1975). Sprogprojekt Espelunden II. *Dansk paedagogisk Tidsskrift.*, 5, DANISH LITERACY LANGUAGE AND EDUCATION WRITTEN LANGUAGE: DANISH

Part two of a research project on language development in school-beginners and an alternative elementary instruction in reading and writing.HV

Vejleskov, Hans. (1976). Psycholinguistic descriptions and their relevance to education: Part 1. *Scandinavian Journal of Educational Research*, 123-134. LANGUAGE AND EDUCATION:

Vejleskov, Hans. (1976). Psycholinguistic descriptions and their relevance to education: Part 2. *Scandinavian Journal of Educational Research*, 187-196. LANGUAGE AND EDUCATION:

Vejleskov, Hans. (1977). Psycholinguistic descriptions and their relevance to education: Part 3. *Scandinavian Journal of Educational Research*, 17-32. LANGUAGE AND EDUCATION:

Vejleskov, Hans. (1977). Sprogprojekt Espelunden IV. *Dansk paedagogisk Tidsskrift.*, 4, DANISH LANGUAGE AND EDUCATION LITERACY WRITTEN LANGUAGE: DANISH

Part IV of a research project on language development in school-beginners and an alternative elementary instruction in reading and writing.HV

Vejleskov, Hans. (1978). The educational relevance of a theory of language functions. In *I.A.L.P. Congress Proceedings*. Denmark: Specialpaedagogisk Forlag. LANGUAGE AND EDUCATION LANGUAGE FUNCTIONS:

Vejleskov, Hans. (1978). *Om sprog og taekning III: Udtryk og oplevelse (On language and thinking III: About pragmatics in linguistic, philosophy, and psychology).* Copenhagen: Munksgaard. LANGUAGE AND COGNITION PRAGMATIC DEVELOPMENT: DANISH

Vejleskov, Hans. (1980). *Born, sprog, og undervisning (Children, language, and teaching).* Copenhagen: Gyldendal. DANISH LANGUAGE AND EDUCATION: DANISH

An anthology about psycholinguistic and sociolinguistic issues.HV

Vejleskov, Hans. (1980). Language, acting, and personality. In L. Marckmann (Ed.), *Auditory training of hearing impaired preschool children.* Copenhagen: DEAF CHILDREN LANGUAGE AND EDUCATION INTERVENTION PROGRAMS:

Vejleskov, Hans. (1980). *Mening og udvikling: En kritisk kommentar til Elisabeth Bates' teori i 'Language and Context'.* Copenhagen: Laererforeningernes Materialeugvalg. CONTEXT ACQUISITION THEORIES-PRAGMATICS PRAGMATIC DEVELOPMENT: DANISH

Commentary on Elizabeth Bates' theory of 'Language and Context.HV

Vejleskov, Hans. (1980). *Sprogfunktioner hos born. En model og en undersogelse.* Copenhagen: Laererforeningernes Materialeudvalg. LANGUAGE FUNCTIONS PRAGMATIC DEVELOPMENT: DANISH

A book presenting an investigation into utterance functions in young children.HV

Vejleskov, Hans. (1980). Theory of language function and observations of children's uses of language. In D. Ingram, F. Peng, & P. Dale (Eds), *Proceedings of the First International Congress for the Study of Child Language.* PRAGMATIC DEVELOPMENT LANGUAGE FUNCTIONS:

Vejleskov, Hans. (1982). A functional analysis of natural language in preschool children. In C. Echols-Johnson, & C. Larson-Thew (Eds), *The Second International Congress for the Study of Child Language..* Maryland: University Press of America. LANGUAGE FUNCTIONS:

Vejleskov, Hans. (1982). Ordforrad, ordforklaring eller hvad? En forundersogelse til videreudvikling af 'The WISC Vocabulary Test'. *Skolepsykologi*, 5, 374-388. ASSESSMENT PROCEDURES WECHSLER SCALES: DANISH

Article about the WISC vocabulary test as a word definition test.HV

Vejleskov, Hans. (1985). *Tale, snak og sprog (Speech, talk, and language)*. Copenhagen: Paedagogisk Psykologisk. OVERVIEW-GENERAL: DANISH

Vejleskov, Hans. (1986). *Er der knas med sproget? (Difficulties with language?)*. Copenhagen: Komiteen for Sundhedsoplysning. OVERVIEW-DISORDERS INTERVENTION PROGRAMS FOR PARENTS: DANISH

Vejleskov, Hans. (1988). A Critique of the distinction between 'academic' and 'communicative' language from a pragmatic point of view. In A. Holmen (Ed.), *Bilingualism and the individual*. Copenhagen: Avon. PRAGMATIC DEVELOPMENT ACQUISITION THEORIES-PRAGMATICS BILINGUALISM:

Vejleskov, Hans. (1988). Social and intellectual functions of language: A fruitful distinction? *Journal of Multilingual and Multicultural Development*, 9, 61-66. LANGUAGE FUNCTIONS:

Vejleskov, Hans. (1989). Otto Jespersen's thinking about child language. In A. Juul, & H. F. Nielsen (Eds), *Otto Jespersen: Facets of his life and work.*. Amsterdam: John Benjamin. ACQUISITION THEORIES:

Vejleskov, Hans. (1989). Understanding people's use of language. In I. A. Bjorgen (Ed.), *Basic issues in psychological research*. Soreidgrend, Norway: Sigma Forlag. PRAGMATIC DEVELOPMENT LANGUAGE FUNCTIONS:

Vejleskov, Hans, & Vedeler, Liv. (1988). *Sprogbrug i smabornsgrupper. (Language use in young children's play groups.)*. Denmark: Paedagogisk Psykologisk Forlag. LANGUAGE AND PLAY METHODOLOGY-DESIGN: NORWEGIAN DANISH

The book describes a method for observing and analyzing children's utterances and communication in playgroups. Examples are given.HV/LV

Velardi, P. (1991). Acquiring a semantic lexicon for natural language processing. In U. Zernik (Ed.), *Lexical acquisition: Exploiting on-line resources to build a lexicon*. Hillsdale, NJ : Lawrence Erlbaum Associates. LEXICAL DEVELOPMENT SEMANTIC DEVELOPMENT SEMANTIC MAPPING LANGUAGE PROCESSING:

Veneziano, Edy. (1982). Les échanges conversationnels mère-enfant et les débuts du langage. (Mother-child conversational exchanges and the onset of language.). *Bulletin d'Audiophonologie*, 2(3), 241-262. PARENTAL SPEECH ADULT-CHILD INTERACTION PRELINGUISTICS PARENTAL INPUT INTERSUBJECTIVITY SOCIAL INTERACTION HYPOTHESIS: FRENCH

Veneziano, Edy. (1987). L'adaptation verbale: Mères et enfants. (Verbal adaptation: Mothers and children.). In J. Gerard-Naef (Ed.), *Savoir parler, savoir dire, savoir communiquer*. Neuchatel, France: Delachaux & Niestle. ADULT-CHILD INTERACTION PARENTAL SPEECH-STYLE: FRENCH

Veneziano, Edy. (1987). Les débuts de la communication langagière. (The beginnings of communicative language.). In J. Gerard-Naef (Ed.), *Savoir parler, savoir dire, savoir communiquer.*. Neuchatel, France: Delachaux & Niestle. PRELINGUISTICS INTENTIONALITY LANGUAGE PRECURSORS: FRENCH

Veneziano, Edy. (1987). Mother-child interactional functioning as a compound dyadic unit. *IPRA Bulletin*, 4, ADULT-CHILD INTERACTION SOCIAL INTERACTION HYPOTHESIS:

Veneziano, Edy. (1990). Le rôle de la répétition dans le passage des énonces a un mot aux énonces a deux mots. (The role of repetition in the transiton from the one word to the two word stage.). *Bulletin CILA*, 51, 61-73. SINGLE-WORD SPEECH TWO-WORD SPEECH TRANSITIONAL PHASES IMITATION: FRENCH

Verhoeven, Ludo Th. (1990). Acquisition of reading in a second language. *Reading Research Quarterly*, 25, 90-114. L2 READING PROFICIENCY TURKISH-DUTCH DUTCH-TURKISH:

This study investigated differences in reading acquisition processes between children learning to read in their native language and children learning to read in a second language. The Turkish children were found to be less effecient in various reading processes in Dutch than their monolingual Dutch peers. There was evidence that Turkish and Dutch children rely on highly comparable strategies.

Verhoeven, Ludo Th., & de Jong, John H. A. L. (1992). *The construct of language proficiency: applications of psychological models to language assessment.* Amsterdam, The Netherlands: John Benjamins. ASSESSMENT PROCEDURES COMMUNICATIVE COMPETENCE METHODOLOGY:

Verlinden, A., & Gillis, Steven. (1988). Nouns and verbs in the input: Gentner (1982) reconsidered. In F. van Besien (Ed.), *First Language Acquisition.* DUTCH LEXICAL DEVELOPMENT WORD CLASS NOUNS VERBS INPUT FACTORS PARENTAL INPUT:

This paper evaluates a claim made by Gentner (1982) that structural phenomena like input frequency, word order, morphological transparency and maternal teaching techniques, cannot account for the fact that children initially acquire more 'nouns' than 'verbs.' This claim is replicated using an extensive corpus of child-directed Dutch.SG

Verrips, M., & Weissenborn, Jürgen. (1992). Routes to verb placement in early German and French: The independence of finiteness and agreement. In J. M. Meisel (Ed.), *The acquisition of verb placement: Functional categories and V2 phenomena in language development.* Dordrecht, The Netherlands: Kluwer Academic. VERBS SYNTACTIC DEVELOPMENT CROSSLINGUISTIC STUDY-SYNTAX FRENCH GERMAN AGREEMENT:

Vietze, Peter M., & Vaughan, Herbert G., Jnr (Eds). (1988). *Early identification of infants with developmental disabilities.* Boston, MA: Allyn & Bacon. ASSESSMENT PROCEDURES ATYPICAL DEVELOPMENT INTERVENTION PROGRAMS DEVELOPMENTAL DISORDERS METHODOLOGY:

Vihman, Marilyn May. (1991). Ontogeny of phonetic gestures: speech production. In I. G. Mattingly, & M. Studdert-Kennedy (Eds), *Modularity and the motor theory of speech perception*. Hillsdale, NJ: Lawrence Erlbaum Associates. PHONETIC GESTURES SPEECH PERCEPTION SPEECH PRODUCTION ARTICULATION:

Vihman, Marilyn May. (1992). Early syllables and the construction of phonology. In C. A. Ferguson, L. Menn, & C. Stoel-Gammon (Eds), *Phonological development: Models, research, implications*. Monkton, MD: York Press. SYLLABLES PHONOLOGICAL DEVELOPMENT:

Vihman, Marilyn May, & McLaughlin, Barry. (1982). Bilingualism and second language acquisition in preschool children. In *Verbal processes in children: Progress in cognitive development research*. New York, NY: Springer-Verlag. BILINGUALISM-SIMULTANEOUS BILINGUALISM-SEQUENTIAL L2 ACQUISITION BILINGUALISM-PROBLEMS/EFFECTS:

Vila, Ignasi. (1983). Del gesto a la palabra. Una explicación funciónal. (From gesture to language: A functional approach.). In J. Palacios, & A. Marchesi (Eds), *Psicológia Evolutiva*. Madrid: Alianza Universidad. PRELINGUISTICS GESTURE: SPANISH

Vila, Ignasi. (1984). Yo siempre hablo catalan y castellano. Datos de una investigación en curso sobre la adquisición del lenguaje en niños bilingües. (I always speak Catalan and Spanish. First data about language acquisition in bilingual children.). In M. Siguan (Ed.), *Adquisición precoz de una segunda lengua.*. Barcelona: Publicacións i Edicións de la Universitat de Barcelona. SPANISH-CATALAN CATALAN-SPANISH BILINGUALISM-SIMULTANEOUS: SPANISH

Vila, Ignasi. (1985). La aparición y desarrollo de términos equivalentes en el primer lenguaje del niño bilingüe familiar. (Origin and development of equivalent terms in the first language of children from bilingual families.). In *Actas del II Congreso Naciónal de Lingüistica Aplicada*. Madrid: SGEL-Educación. BILINGUALISM-FAMILY BILINGUALISM-LANGUAGE DIFFERENTIATION SPANISH-CATALAN CATALAN-SPANISH: SPANISH

Vila, Ignasi. (1986). Interacciónes sociales y adquisición del lenguaje: la 'lectura de libros'. (Social interaction and language acquisition: the book-reading context.). In F. Fernandez (Ed.), *Pasado, presente y futuro de la lingüistica aplicada en España*. Valencia: Universidad de Valencia. SOCIAL INTERACTION HYPOTHESIS ADULT-CHILD INTERACTION: SPANISH

Vila, Ignasi. (1987). Notas acerca de un modelo sobre la ontogenesis del lenguaje. (Notes about a model of language ontogenesis.). In M. Siguan (Ed.), *Actualidad de Lev S. Vigotski*. Barcelona, Spain: Anthropos. VYGOTSKYAN THEORY ACQUISITION THEORIES: SPANISH

Vila, Ignasi. (1989). El desarrollo temprano del lenguaje en los bilingües familiares. (Early language development in children from bilingual families.). In *El bilingüismo en la Europa of Year 2000*. Madrid: Ministerio de Educación y Ciencia. BILINGUALISM BILINGUALISM-FAMILY: SPANISH

Vila, Ignasi. (1990). Aspectos lingüisticos y cognitivos en el proceso de adquisición del lenguaje. (Cognitive and linguistic aspects in the process of language acquisition.). In *Ponencias y comunicacciónes del '16 Congreso Naciónal de AELFA'*. Madrid, Spain: Instituto Naciónal de Servicos Sociales. LANGUAGE AND COGNITIVE DEVELOPMENT: SPANISH

Vila, Ignasi. (1990). El desenvolupament del llenguatge. (Language development.). In C. Triado (Ed.), *Psicologia Evolutiva*. Vic: EUMO. OVERVIEW-THEORY OVERVIEW-GENERAL: CATALAN

Vila, Ignasi. (1990). Estructura y función en la ontogenesis del lenguaje. (Structure and function in the ontogenesis of language.). In I. Idiazabel (Ed.), *Adquisición del lenguaje en bilingües y en monolingues*. San Sebastian: Universidad del Pais Vasco. OVERVIEW-THEORY L2/L1 ACQUISITION: SPANISH

Vila, Ignasi. (1990). La adquisición del lenguaje. (Language acquisition). In J. Palacios, et al. (Eds), *Psicólogia Evolutiva*. Madrid: Alianza. OVERVIEW-THEORY OVERVIEW-GENERAL: SPANISH

Vila, Ignasi. (1990). *La adquisición y el desarrollo del lenguaje. (The acquisition and development of language.).* Barcelona: Grao. OVERVIEW-THEORY OVERVIEW-GENERAL: SPANISH

Vila, Ignasi. (1991). El desarrollo tardío del lenguaje. (Language development after 6:0 years.). In M. Siguan (Ed.), *La ensenanza de la lengua.* Barcelona: Horsori. LANGUAGE AND EDUCATION LATER MORPHOLOGICAL DEVELOPMENT LATER SEMANTIC DEVELOPMENT LATER SYNTACTIC DEVELOPMENT: SPANISH

Vila, Ignasi, & Boada, H. (1989). Vigotski et l'ontogenèse du langage. (Vygotsky and the development of language.). *Enfance,* 42 (1-2), 67-74. VYGOTSKYAN THEORY LANGUAGE AND COGNITIVE DEVELOPMENT: FRENCH

Vila, Ignasi, Boada, H., & Siguan, Miguel. (1982). Adquisición del lenguaje en niños bilingües familiares. Primeros de una investigación. (Language acquisition in children from bilingual families.). *Infancía y aprendizaje,* 19 (20), 89-99. BILINGUALISM-FAMILY: SPANISH

Vila, Ignasi, Boada, H., & Siguan, Miguel. (1984). L'adquisicio del llenguatge en nens bilingues familiars. (Language acquisition in children from bilingual families.). In M. Siguan (Ed.), *Estudi Experimental del Bilinguisme.* Barcelona: Fundacio Caixa de Pensions. SPANISH-CATALAN CATALAN-SPANISH BILINGUALISM-FAMILY: CATALAN

Vila, Ignasi, Boada, H., & Triado, C. (1986). El acceso a las primeras palabras. (The acquisition of first words.). *Cahiers de l'Institut de Linguistique de Louvaine,* 13 (1-2), 77-102. FIRST WORDS LEXICAL DEVELOPMENT: SPANISH

Vila, Ignasi, & Cortes, M. (1985). La lenguaje en una niña monolíngue catalano-hablante, de los 2:3 a los 3:2. (Language acquisition in a Catalan monolingual girl age 2:3 to 3:2.). In *Actas del II Congreso Naciónal de Lingüistica Aplicada.* Madrid: SGEL-Educación. CATALAN: SPANISH

Vila, Ignasi, & Cortes, M. (1990). Aspectos relatativos al desarrollo lexical y morfosintactico de los bilingües familiares. (Aspects of lexical and morphosyntactic development in children from bilingual families.). In I. Idiazabal (Ed.), *Adquisición del lenguaje en bilingües y en monolingues..* San Sebastian: Universidad del Pais Vasco. BILINGUALISM-LEXICAL DEVELOPMENT BILINGUALISM-MORPHOLOGICAL DEVELOPMENT BILINGUALISM-SYNTACTIC DEVELOPMENT BILINGUALISM-SIMULTANEOUS: SPANISH

Vila, Ignasi, & Cortes, M. (1990). Uso función de las formas temporales en el habla infantil. (The use and function of time forms in child language.). *Infancía y Aprendizaje*, 50(51). TEMPORAL TERMS TENSE: SPANISH

Vila, Ignasi, Cortes, M., & Zanon, J. (1987). Baby-talk y designaciónes infantiles en el contexto de lectura de libros. (Baby talk and child labels in a book reading context.). *Anuario de Psicólogia*, 36 (37), 89-105. SOCIAL INTERACTION HYPOTHESIS LABELING PARENTAL SPEECH: SPANISH

Vila, Ignasi, & Elgstrom, S. (1987). Imitación y adquisición de lenguaje. (Imitation and language acquisition.). *Infancía y Aprendizaje*, 38, 1-8. IMITATION: SPANISH

Vila, Ignasi, & Luque, A. (1990). El desarrollo del lenguaje. (Language development.). In J. Palacios, et al. (Eds), *Psicólogia Evolutiva.* Madrid: Alianza. OVERVIEW-THEORY OVERVIEW-GENERAL: SPANISH

Vila, Ignasi, Marti, J., & Mas, I. (1985). Aspectos de la comunicación adulto-niño: el lenguaje de la madre. (Aspects of mother-child communication: the mother's language.). In *Actas del Congreso Naciónal de Lingüistica Aplicada.* Madrid: SGEL-Educación. PARENTAL SPEECH SPANISH ADULT-CHILD INTERACTION: SPANISH

Vila, Ignasi, & Munoz, C. (1986). Adquisición y uso los pronombres de primera y segunda persona en castellano. (Acquisition and the use of first and second person pronouns in Castillian Spanish.). In F. Fernandez (Ed.), *Pasado, presente y futuro de la lingüistica aplicada en España.* Valencia: Universidad de Valencia. SPANISH PRONOUNS-PERSONAL DEIXIS-PERSONAL: SPANISH

Vila, Ignasi, Siguan, Miguel, & Colomina, R. (1989). *Metodologia para el estudio del lenguaje infantil. (Methodology for the study of child language.).* Vic: Abril. METHODOLOGY: SPANISH

Vila, Ignasi, & Zanon, J. (1989). Apriendo a regular la acción conjunta: el contexto de 'dar-y-tomar'. (Learning to regulate joint action: the give-and-take context.). *Estudios de Psicólogia*, 38, 41-59. TURN TAKING PRELINGUISTICS LANGUAGE AND PLAY: SPANISH

Vilaseca-Momplet, Rosa M. (1985). Analisis evolutivo de la categoria funcional 'demanda'. (Developmental analysis of the functional category 'request'). *Revista de Logopedia y Fonoaudiología*, 5(2), REQUESTS LANGUAGE FUNCTIONS: SPANISH

Vilaseca-Momplet, Rosa M., & Moerk, Ernst L. (1989). Estrategias reparatorias de discurso en tres comunidades lingüisticas. (Communicational repair sequences in three linguistic communities.). *Revista de Logopedia Foniatria y Audiologia*, 2(9), CONVERSATIONAL REPAIRS CONVERSATIONAL BREAKDOWNS: SPANISH

Vilaseca-Momplet, Rosa M., & Viladrich, Alifonso C. (1985). Analisis de las 'incomprensiónes' desde una perspectiva interactiva. (Analysis of 'miscommunications' from an interactive point of view). *Revista de Logopedia y Fonoaudología*, 3(3), CONVERSATIONAL BREAKDOWNS CONVERSATIONAL REPAIRS: SPANISH

Vilaseca-Momplet, Rosa M., & Viladrich, C. (1988). Estrategias reparatorias de discurso. (Repair strategies in discourse). *Revista de Logopedia y Fonoaudiología*, 8(3), CONVERSATIONAL REPAIRS CONVERSATIONAL BREAKDOWNS: SPANISH

Villaume, Susan K., & Wilson, Lavisa C. (1989). Preschool children's explorations of letters in their own names. *Applied Psycholinguistics*, 10, 283-300. LITERACY WRITTEN LANGUAGE METALINGUISTICS:

Exploration of names was marked by major transitions: a movement from a unidimensional conceptualization of letters to a multidimensional conceptualization, from general principles to an assimilation of specific knowledge regarding the principles, and a movement from independent explorations of the printed and oral scripts to the integration of the two scripts. - From Child Development Abstracts.

Vinter, Shirley. (1987). Control of early vocalizations of the hearing-impaired infant. *Bulletin d'Audiophonologie*, III, 659-670. VOCALIZATIONS DEAF CHILDREN BABBLING:

Contrary to the allegation of numerous authors, the vocal productions of the deaf child would seem to be different from those of the hearing child as early as 6 months old or even earlier. The babbling to be heard in children afflicted with deep hearing loss from birth is debatable. If the fundamental depends on physiological factors, on the other hand the range, the fundamental variations, the duration of items and the phonic repertoire are controlled by ear and require accoustic information.

Vinter, Shirley. (1989). Vocalizations and the hearing aid. *Réédcation Orthophonique*, 27, 17-25. HEARING AIDS BABBLING DEAF CHILDREN VOCALIZATIONS:

Through the analysis of a deaf child aged seven months, spontaneous sound productions with and without hearing aids, we have tried to show the importance of acoustic parameters in early vocalizations and in particular, the role of the hearing aid in the construction of the deaf child's voice.

Vinter, Shirley. (1990). Analyis of verbal interactions between a mother and her deaf child. *Bulletin d'Audiophonologie*, 6, 413-424. DEAF CHILDREN PARENTAL SPEECH-PROSODY PARENTAL SPEECH-ATYPICAL CHILDREN:

We have analyzed the interactions between a profoundly deaf 25 month old child and her mother, and were particularly interested in prosody and content. Taking part in a study on the type of language offered to deaf children, this work attempts to understand the role of verbal stimulation in the acquisition of language by the young deaf child.

Vinter, Shirley. (1990). Évolution des productions vocales enfantines: aspects normaux et pathologiques. (Development of infant vocalization: normal and pathological aspects.). *Glossa*, 21, PHONOLOGICAL DISORDERS VOCALIZATIONS BABBLING: FRENCH

Vinter, Shirley. (1990). Mélodie et rythme dans la parole de l'enfant sourd. (Melody and rhythm in the speech of deaf children.). *Glossa*, 21, 34-37. PROSODY INTONATION DEAF CHILDREN BIBLIOGRAPHY: FRENCH

Vinter, Shirley. (1990). Rôle et modalités du contrôle acoustique dans la construction de la voix d'un bébé sourd profond appareille. (Role and modalities of acoustic control in language acquisition by a profoundly deaf child.). *Glossa*, 21, 24-29. DEAF CHILDREN: FRENCH

Vinter, Shirley, Llorca, R., & Chalmeau, P. (1986). Temporal construction in deaf children speech. *Bulletin d'Audiophonologie*, 2, 479-492. DEAF CHILDREN ACOUSTIC PHONETICS PROSODY:

Temporal construction in deaf children's speech in a normal scholastic milieu is here studied according to a model presented by Llorca in this same volume. For 4 syllable utterances, these deaf children present the same temporal construction as hearing children but at a different tempo.

Violette, J., & Swisher, L. (1992). Echolalic responses by a child with autism to 4 experimental conditions of sociolinguistic input. *Journal of Speech and Hearing Research*, 35, 139-147. AUTISM ECHOLALIA:

Vogel, Deanie, & Cannito, Michael P. (1991). *Treating disordered speech motor control: for clinicians by clinicians*. San Diego, CA: Singular Publishing Group. MOTOR DISORDERS DYSARTHRIA APRAXIA STRUTTERING DISFLUENCIES INTERVENTION PROGRAMS ACQUIRED APHASIA:

Treating disordered speech motor control: an overview. Comanagement of disordered speech motor control: the role of the neuroligist and the speech pathologist. Structural and functional brain imaging in disorders of speech and motor control. A top-down approach to treatment of dysarthric speech. Pharmacologic approaches to speech motor disorders. A breakdown in interpersonal communication. Apraxia of speech versus phonemic paraphasia: theoretical, diagnostic, and treatment considerations. Acquired neurogenic dysfluency. Neurogenic disorders of prosody. Neurobiological interpretations of spadmodic dysphonia. Noninvasive instrumentation in the treatment of stuttering. Developmental apraxia of speech: theory and practice.

Volden, Joanne, & Lord, Catherine. (1991). Neologisms and idiosyncratic language in autistic speakers. *Journal of Autism and Developmental Disorders* , 21, 109-130. AUTISM:

Autistic, retarded, and mormally developing children's language was coded for the presence of neologisms and idiosyncrasies. The use of neologisms was more prevalent in the autistic group than in age and language matched controls. There were similarities across the groups, but autistic children used more inappropriate words, and their usage was often semantically and phonologically deviant. Idiosyncratic usage increased in proportion with language complexity in the autistic groups, whereas it decreased in the retarded group as language skills improved.

Volkmar, F. R., Cicchetti, Dante, Bregman, J., & Cohen, D. J. (1992). 3 Diagnostic systems for autism: DSM-III, DSM-III=R, and ICD-10. *Journal of Autism and Developmental Disorders*, 22, 483-492. CLASSIFICATION OF DISORDERS AUTISM:

Volling, B. L., & Belsky, J. (1992). The contribution of mother-child and father-child relationships to the quality of sibling interaction: a longitudinal study. *Child Development*, 63, 1209-1222. SIBLING EFFECTS PARENTAL INPUT:

Volterra, Virginia, & Ertig, C. J. (Eds). (1990). *From gesture to language in hearing and deaf children.* New York, NY: Springer-Verlag. GESTURE PRELINGUISTICS DEAF CHILDREN:

Compares the gestures and prelinguistic systems of deaf and hearing children.

Vorster, Jan. (1974). Mothers' speech to children: some methodological considerations. *Publikaties van het Instituut voor Algemene Taalwetenschap*, 8. PARENTAL SPEECH METHODOLOGY-DESIGN METHODOLOGY-ANALYSIS:

Vorster, Jan. (1975). Mommy linguist: The case for motherese. *Lingua*, 37(4). PARENTAL SPEECH:

Vorster, Jan. (1979). Towards an empirical model of language acquisition. *South African Journal of Psychology*, 9. ACQUISITION THEORIES-EMPIRICIST:

Vorster, Jan. (1981). 'Motherese' as 'n voorbeeld van taalvariasie in Afrikaans. (Motherese as an example of language variation in Afrikaans). In *Kongresreferate: 17e Nasionale Kongres van die Linguistevereniging van Suider-Afrika*. Bellville: Universiteit van Wes-Kaapland. PARENTAL SPEECH AFRIKAANS: AFRIKAANS

Vorster, Jan. (1982). The last shall be the first: on the acquisition of the Afrikaans double negative. In G. Claassen, & C. V. Rensburg (Eds), *Proceedings of the Second International Congress for the Study of Child Language*. Washington, DC: University Press of America. AFRIKAANS SYNTACTIC DEVELOPMENT NEGATION:

Vorster, Jan. (1983). Die eerste werkwoorde by Afrikaanse taallerende kinders. (The first verbs of children learning Afrikaans.). In A. Sinclair (Ed.), *G S Nienaber-'n huldeblyk*. Bellville, SA: Universiteit van Wes-Kaapland. VERBS AFRIKAANS FIRST WORDS: AFRIKAANS

Vorster, Jan. (1983). Uit die mond van die moeder: eerste proewe van Afrikaanse 'baby talk.' (From the mouth of the mother: first proofs of Afrikaans baby talk.). In G. Claassen, & C. V. Rensburg (Eds), *Taalverskeidenheid: 'n blik op die spektrum van taalvariasie in Afrikaans*. Kaapstad, SA: Human en Rossow Academica. AFRIKAANS PARENTAL SPEECH: AFRIKAANS

Vorster, Jan. (1984). Setselverwerwing: in die begin was die konsep. (The acquisition of adpositions: In the beginning was the concept.). In V. Webb (Ed.), *Kongresreferate. 20ste Nasionale Kongres van die Linguistevereniging van Suider-Afrika*. Pretoria, SA: University of Pretoria. AFRIKAANS CONCEPT DEVELOPMENT MORPHOLOGICAL DEVELOPMENT AFFIXATION LEXICAL DEVELOPMENT: AFRIKAANS

Vorster, Jan. (1985). Die eerste bywoorde by Afrikaanse kinders. (The first adverbs of Afrikaans children.). In I. Hay, & I. Uys (Eds), *Taalverskeidenheid en taalpatologie*. Pretoria, SA: University of Pretoria. AFRIKAANS ADVERBS FIRST WORDS: AFRIKAANS

Vorster, Jan. (1985). Oor die verhouding voornaamwoord/selfstandige naamwoord in kindertaal. (On the pronoun/noun relationship in child language.). In N. Grieshaber, & J. en Venter (Eds), *Kongresreferate. 21ste Jaarlikse Kongres van die Linguistevereniging van Suider-Afrika*. Pietermaritzburg, SA: University of Natal. ANAPHORA PRONOUNS NOUNS: AFRIKAANS

Vorster, Jan. (1988). Paraphrasing: Extending the database for child language research. *Language Sciences*, 10(1), PARAPHRASES METHODOLOGY:

Vorster, Jan. (1989). Language and thought: developmental perspectives on counterfactual conditionals. *South African Journal of Psychology*, 19(1), CONDITIONALS CONNECTIVES:

Vuyk, R. (1981). *Overview and critique of Piaget's genetic epistemology*. New York, NY: Academic Press. PIAGETIAN THEORY LANGUAGE AND COGNITIVE DEVELOPMENT:

Vygotsky, Lev S. (1981). The genesis of higher mental functions. In J. V. Wertsch (Eds), *The concept of activity in Soviet psychology*. New York, NY: Sharpe. VYGOTSKYAN THEORY SOVIET RESEARCH:

Vygotsky, Lev S., & Luria, Alexander R. (1993). *Studies on the history of behavior: Ape, primitive and child*. Hillsdale, NJ: Lawrence Erlbaum Associates. VYGOTSKYAN THEORY LANGUAGE AND COGNITIVE DEVELOPMENT REGULATIVE FUNCTION OF SPEECH:

> This is the first English translation of this classic Russian book. The editors and translators, V. I. Golod and J. E. Knox, have added to the wealth of information in the work with careful footnoting and bibliographic references to the development of the work and Vygotskyan theory after the original publication date.

W

Wadden, N. P. K., Bryson, S. E., & Rodger, R. S. (1991). A closer look at the autism behavior checklist - discriminant validity and factor structure. *Journal of Autism and Developmental Disorders*, 21, 529-541. AUTISM ASSESSMENT PROCEDURES:

Wade, Karen M., & Haynes, William O. (1989). Dynamic assessment of spontaneous language and cue responses in adult-directed and child-directed play: a statistical and descriptive analysis. *Child Language Teaching and Therapy*, 5, 157-173. LANGUAGE AND PLAY ASSESSMENT PROCEDURES:

A examination of normally developing and language-impaired preschoolers' spontaneous language and responses to clinician cues during conditions of child-directed and adult-directed play. No significant differences were found for subject groups or conditions for the spontaneous language variables. Significant differences were found in the responsiveness of the two groups to clinician clues during the adult versus child-directed play conditions.

Waldstein, R. S., & Baum, S. R. (1991). Anticipatory coarticulation in the speech of profoundly hearing-impaired and normally hearing children. *Journal of Speech and Hearing Research*, 34, 1276-1285. COARTICULATION SPEECH PRODUCTION DEAF CHILDREN ARTICULATION:

Walker, J. F., Archibald, L. M. D, Cherniak, S. R., & Fish, V. G. (1992). Articulation rate in 3-year-old and 5-year-old children. *Journal of Speech and Hearing Research*, 35, 4-13. ARTICULATION SPEAKING RATE:

Walker-Andrews, A. S., & Lennon, E. (1991). Infants' discrimination of vocal expressions - contributions of auditory and visual information. *Infant Behavior and Development*, 14, 131-142. INFANT PERCEPTION INTERSUBJECTIVITY ADULT-CHILD INTERACTION:

Wall, M. J. (1990). Concomitant speech and language disorders in stuttering children - a critique of the literature: Comment. *Journal of Speech and Hearing Disorders*, 55, 802-802. STUTTERING:

Wall, Shavaun M., Pickert, Sarah M., & Gibson, Wesley B. (1989). Fantasy play in 5- and 6-year-old children. *The Journal of Psychology*, 123, 245-256. LANGUAGE AND PLAY SEX DIFFERENCES:

The verbal pretend play of 5- and 6-year-old boys and girls were studied to delineate age and sex differences during the later preoperational period. Sixteen children with average language ability were paired by age and sex and were videotaped for three 15-minute intervals. Older children referred to more invented objects than younger ones but primarily in the service of realistic action formats. Girls' conversations were scored as having significantly more verbal pretending than boys' and a higher proportion of it referred to play roles. There were both age and sex differences in the types of themes, toys used, and roles enacted. - From Child Development Abstracts.

Wallace, Catherine. (1990). Learning to read in a second language: A window on the language acquisition process. In M. A. K. Halliday, J. Gibbons, & H. Nicholas (EdS), *Learning, keeping and using language* . Amsterdam, The Netherlands: John Benjamins. L2 READING PROFICIENCY LANGUAGE AND EDUCATION LITERACY L2/L1 ACQUISITION:

Wallach, Geraldine P., & Miller, Lynda. (1988). *Language intervention and academic success*. San Diego, CA: Singular Publishing Group. INTERVENTION PROGRAMS LANGUAGE AND EDUCATION LITERACY FIGURATIVE LANGUAGE DISCOURSE COHERENCE IMPLICATURE VOCABULARY DEVELOPMENT:

An overview. Strategies for organizing information. Teachers, classrooms, and materials. The transition to literacy: narrative and instructional discourse. Inference and cohesion. Analytical strategies: from sentences to words to sounds. Vocabulary and word naming, figurative language, and other meaningful considerations.

Wamman, Sandra R., Shipley, Elizabeth F., & Shepperson, Barbara F. (1991). Establishing new subcategories: The role of category labels and existing knowledge. *Child Development*, 62, 127-138. NOUNS CATEGORIZATION SEMANTIC ORGANIZATION LEXICAL ACCESS:

We provide additional evidence that novel nouns put 3-year-olds at a disadvantage in subordinate classification. Under each of 2 circumstances, novel nouns do not present an obstacle to subordinate classification.

Wang, Qi, Lillo-Martin, Diane C., Best, Catherine T., & Levitt, Andrea G. (1992). Null subject versus null object: Some evidence from the acquisition of Chinese and English. *Language Acquisition*, 2, 221-254. NULL SUBJECTS CROSSLINGUISTIC STUDY-SYNTAX CHINESE:

The authors examine the premise that as adult Chinese allows null subject constructions, the performance of children in the early stages of acquisiton should be the same in both Chinese and English. Their investigation does not support the premise as children learning Chinese also omit objects which the English speaking children never did. The authors, therefore, argue against the notion that, like Chinese, English is a discourse-oriented language.

Ward, Thomas B. (1990). Further comments on the attribute availability hypothesis of children's category learning. *Child Development*, 61, 611-613. CATEGORIZATION PROTOTYPE THEORY:

Ward, Thomas B., Vela, Edward, & Hass, Sally D. (1990). Children and adults learn family-resemblance categories analytically. *Child Development*, 61, 593-605. CATEGORIZATION OVERGENERALIZATION UNDERGENERALIZATION PROTOTYPE THEORY:

Authors argue that categorization by both children and adults involves primarily analytical modes of learning.

Warren, Steven F., & Reichle, Joe E. (1991). *Causes and effects in communication and language intervention*. Baltimore, MD: Paul H. Brookes. INTERVENTION PROGRAMS ASSESSMENT PROCEDURES RETARDED CHILDREN TURN TAKING COMMUNICATIVE COMPETENCE INTERVENTION PROGRAMS FOR PARENTS:

Topics covered include: stages of development and intervention, communicative competence, turn-taking and conversational skills, parent focussed intervention, effects of mental retardation.

Wartella, E. (Ed.). (1979). *Children communicating: Media and the development of thought, speech, understanding, vol.*. Beverley Hills, CA: Sage Publications. TELEVISION AND LANGUAGE DEVELOPMENT CHILDREN'S DISCOURSE:

Wasserman, Gail A., & Allen, Rhianon. (1990). Aspects of communicative development in physically handicapped toddlers. In E. H. Bendix (Ed.), *The uses of linguistics*. New York, NY: New York Academy of Sciences. ATYPICAL DEVELOPMENT HANDICAPPED CHILDREN COMMUNICATIVE DEVELOPMENT:

Waterson, Natalie. (1976). Perception and production in the acquisition of phonology. In W. von Raffler-Engel, & Y. Lebrun (Eds), *Baby talk and infant speech*. Lisse, The Netherlands: Swets and Zeitlinger. PRODUCTION/PERCEPTION PROSODY PHONOLOGICAL DEVELOPMENT PHONEMIC DEVELOPMENT:

Watkins, R. V., & Rice, Mabel L. (1991). Verb particle and preposition acquisition in language-impaired preschoolers. *Journal of Speech and Hearing Research*, 34, 1130-1141. PREPOSITIONS PARTICLES LANGUAGE DISORDERS:

Watson, B. U. (1991). Some relationships between intelligence and auditory discrimination. *Journal of Speech and Hearing Research*, 34 , 621-627. AUDITORY DISCRIMINATION LANGUAGE AND COGNITIVE DEVELOPMENT:

Watson, Marie M. (1989). Comparison of three methods for eliciting phonological processes. *Perceptual and Motor Skills*, 69, 771-778. METHODOLOGY-DESIGN PHONOLOGICAL PROCESSES ARTICULATION DISORDERS RULES-PHONOLOGICAL:

Eight articulatory disordered children were studied to compare the occurrence of phonological processes using three elicitation methods, including single-word productions, imitated sentences, and continuous speech sampling. A total of 11 phonological processes were shown by the subjects, with only the process of gliding indicative of significantly different rates of occurrence among the three procedures. - From Child Development Abstracts.

Watson, Rita. (1989). Monologue, dialogue, and regulation. In K. Nelson (Ed.), *Narratives from the crib*. Cambridge, MA: Harvard University Press. REGULATIVE FUNCTION OF SPEECH CRIB SPEECH NARRATIVES:

Author describes how the child uses monologues to regulate her environment and herself.

Waxman, Sandra R. (1991). Convergences between semantic and conceptual organization in the preschool years. In S. A. Gelman, & J. Byrnes (Eds), *Perspectives on language and thought*. New York, NY: Cambridge University Press. LANGUAGE AND COGNITION LANGUAGE AND COGNITIVE DEVELOPMENT SEMANTIC MAPPING CONCEPT DEVELOPMENT SEMANTIC ORGANIZATION CATEGORIZATION:

Waxman, Sandra R., & Hatch, T. (1992). Beyond the basics - preschool children label objects flexibly at multiple hierarchical levels. *Journal of Child Language*, 19, 153-166. SEMANTIC MAPPING LEXICAL DEVELOPMENT CATEGORIZATION MUTUAL EXCLUSIVITY LABELING SEMANTIC ORGANIZATION:

Waxman, Sandra R., & Kosowski, Toby D. (1990). Nouns mark category relations: Todlers' and preschoolers' word-learning biases. *Child Development*, 61, 1461-1473. WORD CLASS LEXICAL DEVELOPMENT NOUNS SEMANTIC MAPPING SEMANTIC ORGANIZATION CATEGORIZATION:

Preschool children approach word learning equipped with implicit biases. The noun-category bias proposes that children favor category relations when interpreting the meaning of novel nouns. Children participated in a 5-item match-to-sample task. A target item (e.g., a cow) is given with 4 choices, 2 of which belong to the same superordinate category as the target and 2 of which were thematically related to the target. Novel nouns prompt preschoolers to attend to superordinate-level category relations, even in the presence of multiple thematic alternatives. The bias is specific to nouns, and this noun-category bias exists in 2-year-olds.

Webster, Alec, & McConnell, Christine. (1987). *Children with speech and language difficulties*. Baltimore, MD: Paul H. Brookes Publishing Co. LANGUAGE AND EDUCATION INTERVENTION PROGRAMS ASSESSMENT PROCEDURES:

Written primarily for teachers in ordinary schools, this book covers language and special needs, language tests, intervention, and more. It gives teachers a framework for thinking about language and developing their own insights.

Weeks, L. A. (1989). The lexicon and language acquistion: Crosslinguistic and word-class considerations. *Toegepaste Taalwetenschap in Artikelen.*, 34, 107-114. LEXICAL DEVELOPMENT CROSSLINGUISTIC STUDY WORD CLASS:

Weeks, L. A. (1992). Preschoolers production of tag questions and adherence to the polarity-contrast principle. *Journal of Psycholinguistic Research*, 21, 31-40. QUESTIONS-TAG:

Wei-yao, Gong, Zheng-yuan, Xu, Keats, J. A., & Keats, D. M. (1983). The cooperative research group in studying concept acquisition in bilingual children. *Acta Psychologica Sinica*, 15 (2), 162-168. LANGUAGE AND COGNITION LANGUAGE AND EDUCATION BILINGUALISM-COGNITIVE DEVELOPMENT TRANSFER CONCEPT DEVELOPMENT CHINESE BIDIALECTISM HAN UYGUR:

The aim was to determine whether logical concepts acquired in one language could be transferred to another language. Following Keats & Keats, the Australian psychologists' earlier studies with bilingual children in Australia and Malaysia, a group of 4 to 7 year old children bilingual in Chinese (the language of the Han nationality) and the language of the Uygur nationality and a group of 5 year-old children bilingual in Shanghai dialect and Beijing dialect were presented in both languages and dialects respectively. They were then trained in one language or dialect on the conservation of weight, post-tested in their other language or dialect, and again one month later in both languages or dialects. Results showed that the concept acquired in one of their languages or dialects was immediately available in the other, thus confirming Keats' previous findings that language played a minor part in the acquisition of cognitive concepts in children of this age group, except it seemed that these children would do slightly better on these tasks if trained in their native language.ZYX

Weinberg, Amy. (1990). Markedness versus maturation: The case of subject-auxiliary inversion. *Language Acquisition*, 1, 165-194. MARKEDNESS LEARNABILITY SYNTACTIC STRUCTURES AUXILIARIES INDIVIDUAL VARIATION:

Weinberg provides an elegant explanation of the development of subject-auxiliary inversion that is grounded in government-binding theory and learnability, and attempts to deal with individual variations observed in the development of this construction.

Weinert, Sabine. (1988). Entwicklung schlüssfolgernden Denkens: Eine Untersuchung zur Verarbeitung von Sätzen und Texten im Kindesalter. (Developmental conclusions of thought: An investigation of the processing of sentences and texts by children.). *Zeitschrift für Entwicklungspsychologie und Pädagogische Psychologie*, 20, 15-37. CAUSALITY NARRATIVES IMPLICATURE DISCOURSE COHERENCE: GERMAN

The study is concerned with developing ability of 5-to-8-year-old children to produce causal inferences to connect given events. Using a cued recall procedure. Experiment 1 shows that highly predictable events are not inferred spontaneously when they are not required to integrate explicitly stated text. Inferences contributing to coherence are drawn by the 7/8 year-old -children but not to the same extent by the younger ones. Experiment 2 investigated whether the 'production deficit' of the two younger age groups results in corresponding problems in the reproduction of coherent text. For all age groups, the results showed that causally related events in narratives are remembered better than purely referentially related ones. This holds even if an implicit event has to be inferred to establish a causal connection. Only the 5-year old children show some deficits in drawing causal inferences.

Weinert, Sabine, Grimm, Hannelore, Delille, G., & Scholten-Zitzewitz, R. (1989). Was macht sprachgestorten Kinder das Textverstehen so schwer? (What makes text comprehension so difficult for dysphasic children?). *Heilpädagogische Forschung*, 15, 25-37. APHASIAS SYNTACTIC STRUCTURES SYNTACTIC DISORDERS NARRATIVES TEXT/STORY GRAMMARS: GERMAN

The present study investigates whether the dysphasic children's language deficits are restricted to the acquisition of grammatical 'sentence structures,' or whether these children have additional problems in dealing with 'text structures' that cannot be reduced to their problems in processing complex sentences. Sixteen dysphasic children (age range: 6:6-8:6) and 16 normally developing children (age range: 6:10-7:7) were investigated. All children showed a nonverbal IQ within normal range: the children showed no signs of hearing disorders or severe neurological damage. The language ability was tested by the Heidelberger Sprachentwicklungstest (Heidelberg Language Development Test: Grim & Scholer 1978). We interpret the findings as demonstrating that dysphasic children have problems in recalling relatively independent story events especially if these events are not semantically well integrated. When the individual events are semantically well integrated (e.g., a cow gives milk, likes to eat hay, etc.) the dysphasics are not able to take further advantage of a hierarchical story structure connecting these events. Such an overall structure can only help them to compensate for a low semantic integration of individual events. Thus, the data are in support of the hypothesis that dysphasic children have specific difficulties in using text structure to enhance their understanding and/or recall of comprehensible stories. (Also available as an English translation in the *German Journal of Psychology*, 14, pages 135-137.).

Weismer, Gary, & Liss, Julie M. (1991). Acoustic/perceptual taxonomies of speech production deficits in motor speech disorders. In C. Moore, K. M. Yorkston, & D. R. Beukelman (Eds), *Dysarthria and apraxia of speech*. Baltimore, MD: Paul H. Brookes. MOTOR DISORDERS ACOUSTIC PHONETICS ARTICULATION DISORDERS:

Weiss, D. M., & Sachs, Jacqueline. (1991). Persuasive strategies used by preschool children. *Discourse Processes*, 14, 55-72. CHILDREN'S DISCOURSE:

Weiss, Michael J., Papageorgiou, Apostolos N., & Laplante, David P. (1989). Recovery and dishabituation of sound localization among normal-, moderate-, and high-risk newborns: Discriminant validity. *Infant Behavior and Development* , 12, 321-340. NEONATES INFANT PERCEPTION AT-RISK CHILDREN ASSESSMENT PROCEDURES:

The discriminant validity of new born localized head-turning to speech sounds was assessed using a "familiarization recovery dishabituation" paradigm. Neonates (72 hours corrected age) born at normal, moderate, or high-risk for delayed mental development were identified. Percentage of trial blocks with head-turns toward the sound source and the difference in number of turns toward and away served as principal dependant measures. Comparable percentage of head-turning and rates of orientation and habituation occurred during initial familiarization trials. However, degree of recovery to the novel word and return of the original word and habituation to the novel word discriminated among groups, particularly between normal neonates and those at high risk for subsequent mental delays. - From Child Development Abstracts.

Weissenborn, Jürgen. (1988). Von der 'demonstratio ad oculos' zur 'Deixis am Phantasma'. Die Entwicklung der lokalen Referenz bei

Kindern. (From 'demonstratio ad oculos' to 'Deixis amPhantasma'. The development of local reference by children.). In A. Eschbach (Ed.), *Karl Bühler's theory of language*. Amsterdam: Benjamins. REFERENCE DEIXIS SPATIAL TERMS ORIENTATIONAL TERMS: GERMAN

Weissenborn, Jürgen. (1990). Subjectlose Sätze in der frühen Kindersprache. Ein theoretisches und empirisches Problem der Spracherwerbsforschung. (Subjectless sentences in early child language. A theoretical and empirical problem from language acquisition research.). *Der Deutschunterricht*, 42, 35-47. EARLY SYNTACTIC DEVELOPMENT PARAMETER SETTING NULL SUBJECTS: GERMAN

Weissenborn, Jürgen. (1991). Functional categories and verb movement in early German: The acquisition of German syntax reconsidered. In M. Rothweiler (Ed.), *Spracherwerb und Grammatik: Linguistische Untersuchungen zum Erwerb von Syntax und Morphologie*. GERMAN SYNTACTIC DEVELOPMENT SYNTACTIC STRUCTURES VERBS:

A special issue of *Linguistiche Berichte*.

Weissenborn, Jürgen. (1992). Null subjects in early grammars: implications for parameter setting theories. In J. Weissenborn, H. Goodluck, & T. Roeper (Eds), *Theoretical issues in language Acquisition: Continuity and change in development*. Hillsdale, NJ: Lawrence Erlbaum Associates. NULL SUBJECTS PARAMETER SETTING:

Weissenborn, Jürgen, Goodluck, Helen, & Roeper, Thomas. (1992). Introduction: old and new problems in the study of language acquisition. In J. Weissenborn, H. Goodluck, & T. Roeper (Eds), *Theoretical issues in language acquisition: Continuity and change in development*. Hillsdale, NJ: Lawrence Erlbaum Associates. ACQUISITION THEORIES METHODOLOGY ACQUISITION AND LINGUISTIC THEORY:

Weissenborn, Jürgen, Goodluck, Helen, & Roeper, Thomas. (1992). *Theoretical issues in language acquisition: Continuity and change in development*. Hillsdale, NJ: Lawrence ERlbaum Associates. VARIATION QUESTIONS NULL SUBJECTS PASSIVES PRONOUNS ACQUISITION THEORIES PARAMETER SETTING:

In recent linguistic theory, there has been an explosion of detailed studies of language variation. This volume applies such recent analyses to the study of child language, developing new approaches to change and variation in child grammars and revealing both early knowledge in several areas of grammar and a period of extended development in others. Topics dealt with include question formation, 'subjectless' sentences, object gaps, rules for missing subject interpretation, passive sentences, rules for pronoun interpretation and argument structure. Leading developmental linguists and psycholinguists show how linguistic theory can help define and inform a theory of the dynamics of language development and its biological basis, meeting the growing need for such studies in programs in linguistics, psychology, and cognitive science.

Weissenborn, Jürgen, Kail, Michéle, & Friederici, Angela D. (1990). Language-particular or language-independent factors in acquisition? Children's comprehension of object pronouns in Dutch, French and German. *First Language*, 10, 141-166. DUTCH PRONOUNS FRENCH GERMAN CROSSLINGUISTIC STUDY-SYNTAX:

The comprehension of object pronouns in three languages was studied to determine the role of language-particular factors in acquisition. The results indicate that language-particular factors do not play the role assumed in some theories of language development. More abstract, language independent factors of the pronouns are relevant for acquisition.

Weissenborn, Jürgen, Roeper, Thomas, & de Villiers, Jill. G. (1991). The acquisitiion of Wh-movement in German and French. In T. L. Maxfield, & B. Plunkett (Eds), *Papers on the acquisition of Wh: Proceedings of the University of Massachusetts Roundtable*. Amherst, MA: University of Massachusetts. CROSSLINGUISTIC STUDY-SYNTAX FRENCH GERMAN QUESTIONS-WH:

A special edition of *University of Massachusetts Occasional Papers*.

Weist, Richard M. (1990). Neutralization and the concept of subject in child Polish. *Linguistics*, 28(6), 1331-1349. POLISH GRAMMATICAL RELATIONS CASE SYNTACTIC DEVELOPMENT:

Weist, Richard M. (1991). Spatial and temporal location in child language. *First Language*, 11, 253-267. SPATIAL TERMS TEMPORAL TERMS LANGUAGE AND COGNITIVE DEVELOPMENT:

A sentence-picture matching task was used to determine the relationship between the development of spatial and temporal location. Changes in the spatio-temporal lingistic systems were related to both cognitive and linguistic development. From Child Development Abstracts.

Weist, Richard M., Wysocka, Janna, & Lyytinen, Paula. (1991). A cross-linguistic perspective on the development of temporal systems. *Journal of Child Language*, 18, 67-92. CROSSLINGUISTIC STUDY DEIXIS-TEMPORAL TEMPORAL RELATIONS TEMPORAL TERMS POLISH FINNISH:

The development of temporal location within a cross-linguistic experimental design was evaluated. A comprehension test was constructed with problems which were diagnostic of two salient distinctions within each of three temporal systems. Children from Poland, the USA, and Finland participated. The Polish and American children solved problems requiring absolute temporal location at 2:6, and the older children eventually solved most of the problems requiring relative location. The Finnish children followed a different pattern taking longer to comprehend both types of problems.

Welkowitz, J., Bond, R. N., Feldman, L., & Tota, M. E. (1990). Conversational time patterns and mutual influence in parent child interactions - a time series approach. *Journal of Psycholinguistic Research*, 19, 221-243. INTERSUBJECTIVITY ADULT-CHILD INTERACTION:

Wellman, Henry M. (1990). *The child's theory of mind*. Cambridge, MA: MIT/Batsford. COGNITIVE DEVELOPMENT SELF-CONCEPT THEORY OF MIND LANGUAGE AND MEMORY:

Wellman presents evidence that children as young as three possess a theory of mind. They differentiate between mental and physical acts and understand the relationship between mental states and actions.

Wells, Gordon. (1981). *Learning through interaction: The study of language development*. New York, NY: Cambridge University Press. SOCIAL INTERACTION HYPOTHESIS ADULT-CHILD INTERACTION SOCIAL SPEECH INTERSUBJECTIVITY:

Wells, R. (1970). Comprehension and expression. In J. L. Cowan (Ed.), *Studies in thought and language*. Tucson, AZ: Arizona University Press. PRODUCTION/COMPREHENSION:

Wenk, B. (1989). *Enseigner aux enfants. (Teaching children.)*. Paris: CLE-International/ Larousse. LANGUAGE AND EDUCATION: FRENCH

Werker, Janet F. (1991). The ontogeny of speech performance. In I. G. Mattingly, & M. Studdert-Kennedy (Eds), *Modularity and the motor theory of speech perception*. Hillsdale, NJ : Lawrence Erlbaum Associates. PHONETIC GESTURES SPEECH PRODUCTION SPEECH PERCEPTION:

Werker, Janet F., & Pegg, Judith E. (1992). Infant speech perception and phonological acquisition. In C. A. Ferguson, L. Menn, & C. Stoel-Gammon (Eds), *Phonological development: Models, research, implications*. Monkton, MD: York Press. SPEECH PERCEPTION INFANT PERCEPTION PHONOLOGICAL DEVELOPMENT:

Werner, Lynne, & Bargones, Jill Y. (1991). Auditory psychophysical development in human infants. In *Advances in infancy research*. Norwood, NJ: Ablex. AUDITORY DEVELOPMENT NEUROLINGUISTICS AUDIOLOGY:

Wertsch, James V. (1985). *Culture, communication, and cognition*. New York, NY: Cambridge University Press. VYGOTSKYAN THEORY:

The ideas of the Soviet semiotician and psychologist L.S. Vygotsky are only now beginning to have a major impact in the West. In this volume, distinguished scholars influenced by his approach consider the foundations of Vygotsky's psychology, explain the current significance of his work, and discuss its implications for problems in child development, education, and the study of language and thought. An extended introductory chapter relates the most comprehensive view of Vygotsky's contributions and potential contributions thus far, and will be important reading for cognitive and developmental psychologists, educational researchers, linguists, and semioticians.

West, M. J., King, A. P., & Duff, Michelle A. (1990). Communicating about communication: When innate is not enough. *Developmental Psychobiology*, 23(7), NATIVISM:

Wetherby, Amy M. (1991). Profiling pragmatic abilities in the emerging language of young children. In T. M. Gallagher, & N. Rees (Eds), *Pragmatics of language: Clinical practice issues*. San Diego, CA: Singular Group. ASSESSMENT PROCEDURES PRAGMATIC DEVELOPMENT SYMBOL DEVELOPMENT:

The cognitive, social and communicative bases of symbol use in young children, and the application of research on symbol development to the assessment of normal and disordered progress in children.

Wetherby, Amy M., & Rodriguez, G. P. (1992). Measurement of communicative intentions in normally developing children during structured and unstructured contexts. *Journal of Speech and Hearing Research*, 35, 130-138. INTENTIONALITY COMMUNICATIVE DEVELOPMENT:

Wexler, Kenneth. (1990). Innateness and maturation in linguistics development. *Developmental Psychobiology*, 23(7), NATIVISM NATURE/NURTURE:

Wexler, R. (1978). Empirical questions about developmental psycholinguistics raised by a theory of language acquisition. In R. N. Campbell, & P. T. Smith (Eds), *Recent advances in the psychology of language*. New York, NY: Plenum. ACQUISITION AND LINGUISTIC THEORY:

Whalen, D. H., Levitt, Andrea G., & Wang, Qi. (1991). Intonational differences between the reduplicative babbling of French-learning and English-learning infants. *Journal of Child Language*, 18, 501-516. REDUPLICATION BABBLING CROSSLINGUISTIC STUDY-PHONOLOGY FRENCH PROSODY INTONATION:

White, Burton L. (1975). Critical influences in the origins of competence. *Merrill-Palmer Quarterly*, 21(4), 243-266. INPUT FACTORS ENVIRONMENTAL FACTORS SOCIOLINGUISTIC FACTORS AT-RISK CHILDREN PRELINGUISTICS:

White, Burton L. (1975). *The first three years of life*. Englewood Cliffs, NJ: Prentice-Hall. LANGUAGE AND COGNITIVE DEVELOPMENT INFANT PERCEPTION NEONATES:

White, Lydia. (1990). Implications of learnability theories for second language learning and teaching. In M. A. K. Halliday, J. Gibbons, & H. Nicholas (EdS), *Learning, keeping and using language* . Amsterdam, The Netherlands: John Benjamins. L2 EDUCATION L2 ACQUISITION LEARNABILITY:

White, Lydia. (1991). The verb-movement parameter in second language acquisition. *Language Acquisition*, 1, 337-360. L2 LINGUISTIC THEORY PARAMETER SETTING VERBS ENGLISH-FRENCH FRENCH-ENGLISH ADVERBS:

An examination of the educational implications of teaching parameter resetting for verb-movement in francophone learners of English as a second language. (French allows verb-movement in questions whereas English does not.) Only those learners who received specific instruction on adverb placement came to an understanding of adverbial placement restrictions in English.

Whitehurst, G. J., Smith, M., Fischel, J. E., & Arnold, D. S., et al. (1991). The continuity of babble and speech in children with specific expressive language delay. *Journal of Speech and Hearing Research*, 34, 1121-1129. BABBLING LANGUAGE DELAY:

Whorton, James E., & Morgan, Robert L. (1990). Comparison of the Test of Nonverbal Intelligence and Wechsler Intelligence Scale for Children-Revised in rural Native American and white children. *Perceptual and Motor Skills*, 70, 12-14. WECHSLER SCALES

CROSSCULTURAL STUDY METHODOLOGY ASSESSMENT PROCEDURES TEST OF NONVERBAL INTELLIGENCE:

The Test of Nonverbal Intelligence (TONI) and Wechsler Intelligence Scale for Children-Revised (WISC-R) were administered to 46 Native American and white students who were suspected by their classroom teachers of having learning handicaps. Pearson correlations between these sets of IQs ranged from 0.42 (TONI and WISC-R performance) to 0.89 (WISC-R Verbal and Full Scale).-From Child Development Abstracts.

Wiener, Morton, Rubano, Maureen, & Shilkret, Robert. (1990). A measure of semantic complexity among predictions. *Journal of Psycholinguistic Research*, 19, 103-123. SEMANTIC RELATIONS METHODOLOGY-ANALYSIS:

A scale for assessing the complexity or density of utterances was developed using 10 categories of semantic relations. The categories are inferable from the particular 'meanings' of the words used in an utterance and was applied to three samples of subjects to assess its interjudge reliability and to compare the utterances of fourth-, sixth-, and eighth-grade children from middle and working-class neighborhoods. Interjudge reliabilities were acceptable and significant differences in semantic density were found across grade, between children from working-class and middle-class neighborhoods, and for the stimuli used to elicit the utterances.

Wier, Ruth. (1966). Some questions on the child's learning of phonology. In F. Smith, & G. A. Miller (EdS), *The genesis of language*. Cambridge, MA: MIT Press. PHONOLOGICAL DEVELOPMENT:

Wigglesworth, Gillian. (1990). Children's narrative acquisition: A study of some aspects of reference and anaphora. *First Language*, 10, 105-125. REFERENCE ANAPHORA NARRATIVES:

The author reports an experiment which required children to insert a new character into a story and to maintain reference to the new and existing characters. The results indicate that children's anaphoric and referential skills do not match adult levels.

Wilbur, Ronnie B. (1987). *American sign language: linguistic and applied dimensions: 2nd edition*. San Diego, CA: Singular Publishing Group. SIGNING-ASL LANGUAGE AND EDUCATION DEAF CHILDREN SOCIOLINGUISTIC FACTORS:

Introduction. Sign phonology: traditional approaches. Sign phonology: current approaches. Sign morphology: word formation. Sign morphology: inflection. ASL syntax. Psycholinguistics and neurolinguistics of sign usage. Sign language acquisition. Sociolinguistic aspects of sign language and deaf culture. Sign systems used in educational settings. Sign language and the education of deaf children. Signs and communicatively handicapped people who are not deaf.

Wilcox, M. J., Kouri, T. A., & Caswell, S. (1990). Partner sensitivity to communication behavior of young children with developmental disabilities. *Journal of Speech and Hearing Disorders*, 55, 679-693. DEVELOPMENTAL DISORDERS:

Williams, A. L. (1991). Generalization patterns associated with training least phonological knowledge. *Journal of Speech and Hearing Research*, 34, 722-733. PHONOLOGICAL DISORDERS TREATMENT GENERLAIZATION:

Wilson, R. Graham, & Lynn, Richard. (1990). Personality, intelligence components and foreign language attainment. *Educational Psychology*, 10, 57-71. L2 EDUCATION BILINGUALISM-SEX DIFFERENCES L2 PERSONALITY EFFECTS IRISH:

Twelve-hundred children from the Irish Republic were tested for intelligence abilities, attainment in Irish, psychoticism, neuroticism, and extroversion and attitude to learning foreign languages. Females had a higher N score and had a significantly more positive attitude towards learning a second language and males had a significantly higher P score.

Wimmer, H., & Hummer, P. (1990). How German-speaking 1st graders read and spell - doubts on the importance of the logographic stage.

Applied Psycholinguistics, 11, 349-368. GERMAN LITERACY WRITTEN LANGUAGE:

Winner, Ellen, & Leekman, Susan. (1991). Distinguishing irony from deception: Understanding the speaker's second-order intention. *British Journal of Developmental Psychology*, 9, 257-270. FIGURATIVE LANGUAGE PRAGMATIC DEVELOPMENT COMMUNICATIVE COMPETENCE:

Children listened to stories which contained irony and 'white lies', and were asked to distinguish between them. They appeared to use two strategies to determine the differnces: was the speaker being mean/nice, and did the speaker wish the hearer to believe him/her to be mean/nice. Almost all of the subjects failed to distinguish correctly between when the speaker was being mean and when they were being nice. The speaker's intonaton did not appear to have any impact on the children's ability to distinguish between the two. From Child Development Abstracts.

Wise, Barbara W., & Olson, Richard K. (1990). Subsyllabic units in computerized reading instruction: Onset-rime vs. postvowel segmentation. *Journal of Experimental Child Psychology*, 49, 1-19. SYLLABLES SEGMENTATION LITERACY COMPUTER ASSISTED THERAPY C.A.L.L. LANGUAGE AND EDUCATION:

This study investigated whether children can learn more words segmented at the onset-rime boundary (e.g. CL-AP, D-ISH) than words segmented after the vowel (CLA-P, DI-SH). In all three experiments, onset-rime segmentation proved more helpful than postvowel segmentation in short-term learning of the words. - From Child Development Abstracts.

Wodala, K. A. (1985). *The development of reading skills in an English-Hungarian bilingual child*. Szeged. BILINGUALISM-LITERACY ENGLISH-HUNGARIAN HUNGARIAN-ENGLISH L2 READING PROFICIENCY HUNGARIAN:

Wode, Henning. (1992). Categorical perception and segmental coding in the ontogeny of sound systems: A universal approach. In C. A. Ferguson, L. Menn, & C. Stoel-Gammon (Eds), *Phonological development: Models, research, implications*. Monkton, MD: York Press. PHONEMIC DEVELOPMENT PHONETIC INVENTORIES SPEECH PERCEPTION INFANT PERCEPTION:

Wolf, D. P., Moreton, J., & Camp, L. (1993). Narrative analyses. In J. L. Sokolov, & C. E. Snow (Eds), *Handbook of research in language development using CHILDES*. Hillsdale, NJ: Lawrence Erlbaum Associates. NARRATIVES METHODOLOGY-ANALYSIS METHODOLOGY-COMPUTERS CHILDES:

Wolf, M., & McQuillian, M. K. (Eds). (1980). *Thought and language: Language and reading*. Cambridge, MA: Harvard Educational Review. LANGUAGE AND COGNITIVE DEVELOPMENT LITERACY:

Wolfe, V. I., & Blocker, S. D. (1990). Consonant-vowel interaction in an unusual phonological system. *Journal of Speech and Hearing Disorders*, 55, 561-566. PHONOLOGICAL DISORDERS PHONOLOGICAL DEVELOPMENT VOWELS CONSONANTS:

Wolff, Anthony B., & Thatcher, Robert W. (1990). Cortical reorganization in deaf children. *Journal of Clinical and Experimental Neuropsychology*, 12, 209-221. DEAF CHILDREN LATERALIZATION NEUROLINGUISTICS CORTICAL STRUCTURES:

Topographic mapping of the cerebral cortex of 79 deaf children and a group of matched hearing children was performed, using measures of electroencephalographic coherence, phase, and power. Deaf children had higher total power in bilateral frontal cortex than did hearing children.

Wolff, S., Narayan, S., & Moyes, B. (1991). Family characteristics of autistic children-response. *Journal of Autism and Developmental Disorders*, 21, 558-559. AUTISM PARENTAL INPUT INPUT FACTORS AT-RISK CHILDREN ADULT-CHILD INTERACTION SOCIAL INTERACTION:

Wood, David J., & Wood, Heather A. (1991). Signed English in the classroom: Teaching style and child participation. *First Language*, 11, 189-217. DEAF CHILDREN LANGUAGE AND EDUCATION SIGNING-ENGLISH:

The relationships between teaching style and child participation closely reflect those previously reported for the mainstream classroom. The extent to whic children participate in the discourse is controlled by the teaching style. From Child Development Abstracts.

Woodyatt, G., & Ozanne, A. (1992). Communication abilities and Rett syndrome. *Journal of Autism and Developmental Disorders*, 22, 155-173. DEVELOPMENTAL DISORDERS COMMUNICATIVE DEVELOPMENT COMMUNICATUIVE DISORDERS:

Word, B. S. (1976). *Children and communication: Verbal and nonverbal language*. Englewood Cliffs, NJ: Prentice-Hall. NONLINGUISTIC STRATEGIES SIGNING COMMUNICATIVE DEVELOPMENT:

Workinger, Marilyn S., & Kent, Raymond D. (1991). Perceptual analysis of the dysarthrias in children with athetoid and spastic cerebral palsy. In C. Moore, K. M. Yorkston, & D. R. Beukelman (EdS), *Dysarthria and apraxia of speech*. Baltimore, MD: Paul H. Brookes. CEREBRAL PALSY DYSARTHRIA:

Wray, Alison. (1991). *The focusing hypothesis - The theory of left hemisphere lateralised language re-examined*. Amsterdam, The Netherlands: John Benjamins. LATERALIZATION NEUROLINGUISTICS METHODOLOGY-DESIGN:

This book explores the nature of the control of language processing by the hemispheres of the neocortex. The author expounds a novel hypothesis 'The Focusing Hypothesis' which holds that language processing in the brain is achieved through analytic and holistic systems, the former through left and the latter through right hemisphere processing. This hypothesis differs from current thinking in so far as it proposes that the involvement of the two systems (and two hemispheres) depends on the strategy selected by the speaker and that the engagement by one hemisphere over another will depend upon the communicative intent of the speaker and the propositionality of the utterance under production. The authors proposes that the methodology of current psycholinguistics research predisposes the subject to use the analytic hemisphere. The Focusing Hypothesis is tested by comprehensive review of the existing experimental psycholinguistic, neuropsychological and neurophysiological literature and a range of predictions which follow from the hypothesis are detailed.

Wynn, Karen. (1990). Children's understanding of counting. *Cognition*, 36, 155-193. NUMERALS:

Two- and 3-year-olds counted objects, actions, and sounds. Children counted objects best, but most showed some ability to generalize their counting to actions and sounds. However, when asked 'how many' following counting, only older children gave the last number word used in the count a majority of the time. The same children were asked to give a puppet one, two, three, five, and six items from a pile. The older children counted the items, showed a clear understanding of the cardinal word principle. The younger children succeeded only at giving one and sometimes two items, and never used counting to solve the task.

Y

Yaacov, Katz, et al. (1990). Reading and cognitive abilities: Research note on a longitudinal study in Israel. *Perceptual and Motor Skills*, 70, 47-50. LITERACY HEBREW LANGUAGE AND EDUCATION:

This article reports a 9-year longitudinal study of cognitive factors associated with reading comprehension in an achievement-oriented upper-middle socioeconomic status Israeli population. Reading comprehension was assessed at age 6 and at age 13. The cognitive factors measured were verbal intelligence (age 5), general intelligence (age 13), and academic achievement as assessed by the mean score achieved in language, arithmetic, history and bible (age 13). Verbal intelligence in kindergarten significantly correlated with and predicted reading comprehension in grade 1 but did not correlate with the cognitive measures assessed in grade 8. Reading comprehension in grade 1 significantly correlated with and predicted reading comprehension as well as general intelligence in grade 8. Eighth-grade academic achievement, however, was not predicted by first-grade reading achievement. From Child Development Abstracts.

Yairi, E., & Ambrose, N. (1992). A longitudinal study of stuttering in children - a preliminary report. *Journal of Speech and Hearing Research*, 35, 755-760. STUTTERING METHODOLOGY-LONGITUDINAL STUDY:

Yairi, E., & Ambrose, N. (1992). Onset of stuttering in preschool children-selected factors. *Journal of Speech and Hearing Research*, 35, 782-788. STUTTERING:

Yamada, Jeni E. (1990). *Laura: A case for the modularity of language*. Cambridge, MA: MIT/Batsford. RETARDED CHILDREN LANGUAGE AND COGNITION LANGUAGE AND COGNITIVE DEVELOPMENT MODULARITY LANGUAGE ACQUISITION DEVICE:

Laura, a subject with a testable IQ of 40, provides evidence to support the notion that language is an independent cognitive ability. This case shows that language can develop in spite of extreme cognitive deficit, and counters the claims that cognitive, social/interactive, and perceptual factors can wholly account for language development.

Yamane, Ritsuko. (1989). Integrating process of communicative mode in demanding situation during preverbal period. *Japanese Journal of Educational Psychology*, 37, 345-352. GESTURE INTENTIONALITY ADULT-CHILD INTERACTION JAPANESE: JAPANESE

Three infants were observed for seven months during their preverbal period, and developmental changes in communicative expression were analyzed. The results of the observation suggested that acquisition of 'pointing' in a preverbal period coincided with the establishment of a developmental basis in intentional operation of multiple sensory modalities. - From Child Development Abstracts.

Yavas, Mehmet S. (Ed.) (1991). *Phonological disorders in children*. New York, NY: Routledge. PHONOLOGICAL DISORDERS INTERVENTION PROGRAMS CLINICAL LINGUISTICS:

Yavas, Mehmet S., Hernandorena, C. L. M., & Lamprecht, Regina R. (1991). *Avaliacao fonologica da crianca. (Phonological assessment of the child.)*. Porto Alegre: Artes Medicas. PORTUGUESE ASSESSMENT PROCEDURES INTERVENTION PROGRAMS METHODOLOGY-DESIGN METHODOLOGY-ANALYSIS: PORTUGUESE

Aimed at speech pathologists, AFC introduces the notion of phonological analysis of disordered speech, shows how to elicit spontaneous speech data by way of a new instrument-five thematic drawings based on 125 words containing at least 3 tokens of every sound of Brazilian Portuguese in each of the 4 permitted positions in the syllable and in the word. Three different approaches to phonological analysis, distinctive feature analysis and natural phonological process analysis. Implications for therapy are discussed.RRL

Yavas, Mehmet S., & Lamprecht, Regina R. (1985). Aquisicao da linguagem e o professor alfabetizador. (Language acquisition and the first-grade teacher.). *Letras de Hoje*, 18 (4), 7-31. PORTUGUESE LANGUAGE AND EDUCATION: PORTUGUESE

Trying to ascertain what first-grade teachers know about language acquisition and about the language of children entering school (ages 6 to 7), 102 teachers-with classroom experience ranging from a few months to 40 years-were asked questions syntactic, semantic and pragmatic aspects, language acquisition theories, textbook language, etc. Results show that classroom experience does not compensate for the lack of formal language acquisition studies, which are strongly recommended in teacher-training courses.RRL

Yavas, Mehmet S., & Lamprecht, Regina R. (1988). Processes and intelligibility in disordered phonology. *Clinical Linguistics and Phonetics*, 2 (4), 329-345. PORTUGUESE PHONOLOGICAL DISORDERS INTELLIGIBILITY PHONOLOGICAL PROCESSES RULES-PHONOLOGICAL:

This study investigated the phonological processes in four Brazilian children with phonological disorders. The purpose of the study was to identify the phonological processes, their prevalence, strength and their relative contribution to the intelligibility of the subjects' speech. Results reveal differential effects of sequential and substitution processes and of the consistency/variability of the application of those processes.RRL

Yde, Philip, & Spoelders, Marc. (1990). Cohesive ties in written narratives: A developmental study with beginning writers. In M. A. K. Halliday, J. Gibbons, & H. Nicholas (Eds), *Learning, keeping and using language* . Amsterdam, The Netherlands: John Benjamins. WRITTEN LANGUAGE NARRATIVES DISCOURSE COHERENCE:

Yirmiya, Nirut, Sigman, Marian D., Kasari, Connie, & Mundy, Peter. (1992). Empathy and cognition in high-functioning children with autism. *Child Development*, 63, 150-160. AUTISM LANGUAGE AND AFFECT LANGUAGE AND COGNITIVE DEVELOPMENT:

Ylvisaker, Mark. (1985). *Head injury rehabilitation: children and adolescents*. San Diego, CA: Singular Publishing Group. TRAUMATIC DISORDERS CEREBRAL DISORDERS INTERVENTION PROGRAMS:

Pathophysiology and outcome. The family. Comprehensive medical management. Physical rehabilitation. Cognitive rehabilitation. Behavioral and psychosocial intervention. Educational and vocational rehabilitation. Program management.

Yoder, P. J., & Davies, B. (1992). Greater intelligibility in verbal routines with young children with developmental delays. *Applied Psycholinguistics*, 13, 77-91. INTELLIGIBILITY:

Yoder, P. J., Kaiser, A. P., & Alpert, C. L. (1991). An exploratory study of the interaction between language teaching methods and child characteristics. *Journal of Speech and Hearing Research*, 34, 155-167. LANGUAGE AND EDUCATION L2 EDUCATION:

Yorkston, Kathyrn M., Hammen, Vicky L., & Dowden, Patricia. (1991). Index of contextual intelligibility: A perceptual analysis of intelligible versus unintelligible productions in severe dysathria. In C. Moore, K. M. Yorkston, & D. R. Beukelman (Eds), *Dysarthria and apraxia of speech*. Baltimore, MD: Paul H. Brookes Publishing Co. CONTEXT DYSARTHRIA INTELLIGIBILITY ARTICULATION DISORDERS:

Yoshina-Gaitano, C., & Downey, D. M. (1992). When a story is not a story - a process analysis of the written language of hearing-impaired children. *Volta Review*, 94, 131-158. DEAF CHILDREN NARRATIVES WRITTEN LANGUAGE:

Yoshina-Gaitano, C., & Stredler-Brown, A. (1992). Learning to communicate - babies with hearing impairments make their needs known. *Volta Review*, 94, 107-129. DEAF CHILDREN COMMUNICATIVE DEVELOPMENT INTERSUBJECTIVITY:

Yoshina-Gaitano, C., Stredler-Brown, A., & Jancosek, E. (1992). From phone to phoneme - what can we understand from babble. *Volta Review*, 94, 283-314. BABBLING PHONEMIC DEVELOPMENT:

Young, Copeland H., Savola, Kristen L., & Phelps, Erin. (1991). *Inventory of longitudinal studies in the social sciences*. Newbury Park, CA: Sage Publications, Inc. METHODOLOGY-LONGITUDINAL STUDY METHODOLOGY-DESIGN:

A synopsis of the major longitudinal studies conducted over the last 60 years in North America. Offering clear descriptions of the key attributes of each study. Each study is described in detail, including information on the purpose of the study, the names and addresses of the principle investigators, how the study was conducted (sample size, racial and gender mix, the research instrument used and what they were designed to measure), the current status of the study, and a list of related references. The studies were selected on the following criteria: information must have been collected during a minimum of two time points across a span of at least one year, the original sample must have had a low attrition rate to maintain the quality of the study, and finally, each study must have used multiple measures across more than one domain.

Young, G., & Gagnon, M. (1990). Neonatal laterality, birth stress, familial sinistrality, and left-brain inhibition. *Developmental Neuropsychology*, 6, 127-150. NEONATES LATERLAIZATION LANGUAGE AND HANDEDNESS HERITABILITY:

Young, Richard. (1991). *Variation in interlanguage morphology*. New York, NY: P. Lang. INTERLANGUAGE-MORPHOLOGY:

Younger, Barbara. (1990). Infant categorization: Memory for category-level and specific item information. *Journal of Experimental Child Psychology*, 50, 131-155. CATEGORIZATION LANGUAGE AND MEMORY:

Three experiments assessed retention of category-level information specific to category members. Ten- and 13-month-old infants were familiarized with category instances containing both shared dimensional information and idiosyncratic features. Results of within-category test comparisons indicated that 10-month-old infants regarded information common to all members of the category as more familiar than information specific to individual exemplars.

Youssef, V. (1991). Can I put - I want a slippers to put on: Young children's development of request forms in a code-switching environment. *Journal of Child Language*, 18, 609-624. REQUESTS CODE-SWITCHING:

Yuill, Nicola., & Oakhill, Jane. (1991). *Children's problems in text comprehension : an experimental investigation.* New York, NY: Cambridge University Press. LITERACY READING DISORDERS COMPREHENSION DISORDERS DISCOURSE DISORDERS LANGUAGE AND EDUCATION INTERVENTION PROGRAMS:

A specific look at children's problems with the comprehension of continuous discourse which identifies several problem areas and suggests some methods of dealing with them.

Yussen, Steven R., Rembold, Karen L., & Mazor, Aviva. (1989). Identifying main ideas in picture stories and written narratives. *Journal of Applied Developmental Psychology*, 10, 313-335. LITERACY NARRATIVES WRITTEN LANGUAGE TEXT/STORY GRAMMARS DISCOURSE ANALYSIS:

Two sets of equivalent stories and main idea alternatives were developed with undergraduates. One set was verbal, the other was pictorial. Second, fifth, and eighth graders, ranked the alternative main idea statements for each of the stories in one of the modalities. There was improvement with age in ability to select the best main idea alternatives and increased differentiation in judging quality. There was little difference in responses to main idea alternatives, based on verbal vs. pictorial format. - From Child Development Abstracts.

Z

Zammuner, V. L., & Levorato, Maria C. (1985). La comprensione ed il ricordo delle discontinuita semantiche nelle storie nei bambini. (Comprehension of semantic discontinuities and recall of stories by children. *Giornale Italiano di Psicologia*, 12, 495-515. CONNECTIVES-CONDITIONAL NARRATIVES CONGRUENCY-SEMANTIC: ITALIAN

A study of 'but' and its effect upon children's recall of stories with the adversative 'but' embedded in them.MCL

Zani, B., Carelli, M. G., Benelli, Beatrice, & Cicognani, E. (1991). Communicative skills in childhood - the case of twins. *Discourse Processes*, 14, 339-356. MULTIPLE BIRTHS:

Zebrowski, P. M. (1991). Duration of the speech disfluencies of beginning stutterers. *Journal of Speech and Hearing Research*, 34, 483-491. STUTTERING:

Zeidner, M., & Feitelson, D. (1989). Probing the validity of intelligence tests for preschool children: A smallest space analysis. *Journal of Psychoeducational Assessment*, 7, 175-193. ASSESSMENT PROCEDURES METHODOLOGY-ANALYSIS METHODOLOGY-DESIGN:

An investigation of intra- and intertest associations between subtest scores on two preschool intelligence measures using Guttman's smallest space analysis. A sample of 168 Israeli preschoolers were tested on two intelligence test batteries. Projections of subtests in the two batteries on to the smallest space resulted in highly similar spacial configurations, an indication that there are indeed some underlying intrinsic relationships among the abilities tested.Zelazo, Philip R.,

Zentella, Ana C. (1990). Integrating qualitative and quantitative methods in the study of bilingual code switching. In E. H. Bendix. (Eds), *The uses of linguistics*. New York, NY: New York Academy of Sciences. CODE-SWITCHING METHODOLOGY-DESIGN METHODOLOGY-ANALYSIS:

Zernik, Uri (Ed.). (1991). *Lexical acquisition: Exploiting on-line resources to build a lexicon*. Hillsdale, NJ: Lawrence Erlbaum Associates. LEXICAL DEVELOPMENT:

> On-line information-and free text in particular-has emerged as a major, yet unexploited, resource available in raw form. Available, but not accessible. The lexicon provides the major key for enabling accessibility to on-line text. The expert contributors to this book explore the range of possibilities for the generation of extensive lexicons. In so doing, they investigate the use of existing on-line distionaries and thesauri, and explain how lexicons can be acquired from the corpus-the text under investigation-itself. Leading researchers in four related fields offer the latest investigations: computational linguists cover the natural language processing aspect. Statisticians point out the issues involved in the use of massive data: experts discuss the limitations of current technology, and lexicographers share their experience in the design of the traditional dictionaries.

Zernik, Uri. (1991). Tagging word sense in corpus. In U. Zernik (Ed.), *Lexical acquisition: Exploiting on-line resources to build a lexicon*. Hillsdale, NJ: Lawrence Erlbaum Associates. LEXICAL DEVELOPMENT SEMANTIC DEVELOPMENT SEMANTIC MAPPING:

Zettersten, A. (1986). *New technologies in language learning*. New York, NY: Pergamon. C.A.L.L. LANGUAGE AND EDUCATION L2 TEACHING:

> An examination of the effects of technological advance on language teaching and learning. The text covers: microcomputers, videotex, teletext, videotape and disk, artificial intelligence, speech synthesizers, robotics, satellite communication, film, television, and teleconferencing.

Zukow, Patricia G. (1990). Socio-perceptual bases for the emergence of language: An alternative to innatist approaches. *Developmental Psychobiology*, 23(7), NATIVISM SOCIAL INTERACTION HYPOTHESIS ACQUISITION THEORIES:

Zurif, Edgar B., & Caramazza, Alfonso. (1976). Psycholinguistic structures in aphasia: Studies in syntax and semantics. In Whitaker, H. A. & whitaker, H. (Eds). *Studies in neurolinguistics*, vol. 1. New York, NY: Academic Press. APHASIAS SEMANTICS AND SYNTAX:

Zwicky, Arnold M., et al. (Eds). (1980). *Language development, grammar and semantics: The contribution of linguistics to bilingual education.* Arlington, VA: Center for Applied Linguistics. LANGUAGE AND EDUCATION BILINGUALISM-EDUCATION L2 EDUCATION:

AUTHOR INDEX

SUBJECT INDEX